Advances in Experimental Medicine and Biology

Volume 929

More information about this series at http://www.springer.com/series/5584

Subash Chandra Gupta · Sahdeo Prasad
Bharat B. Aggarwal
Editors

Drug Discovery from Mother Nature

Springer

Editors
Subash Chandra Gupta
Banaras Hindu University
Varanasi, Uttar Pradesh
India

Bharat B. Aggarwal
Inflammation Research Institute
San Diego, CA
USA

Sahdeo Prasad
MD Anderson Cancer Center
University of Texas
Houston, TX
USA

ISSN 0065-2598 ISSN 2214-8019 (electronic)
Advances in Experimental Medicine and Biology
ISBN 978-3-319-41341-9 ISBN 978-3-319-41342-6 (eBook)
DOI 10.1007/978-3-319-41342-6

Library of Congress Control Number: 2016947753

Printed on acid-free paper

This Springer imprint is published by Springer Nature
The registered company is Springer International Publishing AG Switzerland
The registered company address is: Gewerbestrasse 11, 6330 Cham, Switzerland

Contents

About the Editors

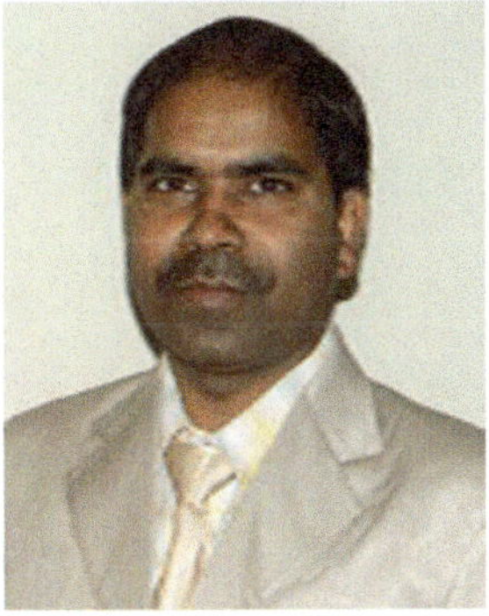

Dr. Subash Chandra Gupta is currently an assistant professor at Department of Biochemistry, Institute of Science, Banaras Hindu University, India.

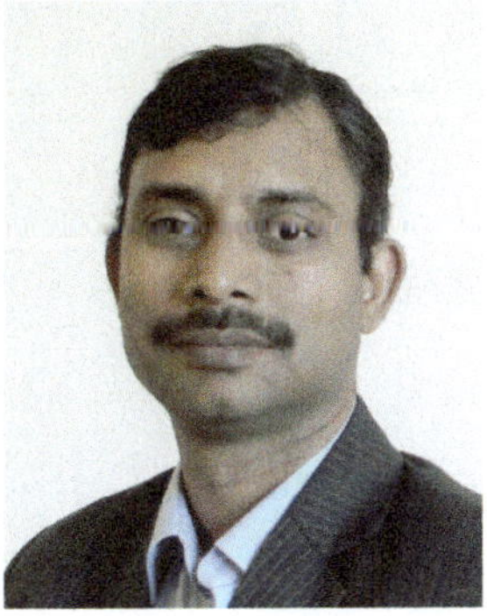

Dr. Sahdeo Prasad is currently at the Department of Experimental Therapeutics, The University of Texas MD Anderson Cancer Center, USA.

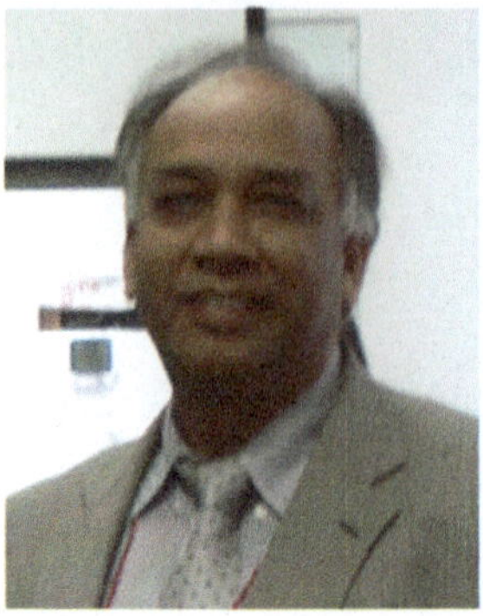

Dr. Bharat B. Aggarwal is currently a founding director of Inflammation Research Institute, San Diego, CA, USA. He was a Ransom Horne, Jr., distinguished professor of Experimental Therapeutics, Cancer Medicine and Immunology, The University of Texas MD Anderson Cancer Center, USA.

Cinnamon and Chronic Diseases

Mitra Hariri and Reza Ghiasvand

Abstract Cinnamon (*Cinnamomum zeylanicum* and Cinnamon cassia), the eternal tree of tropical medicine, belongs to the Lauraceae family and is one of the most important spices used daily by people all over the world. It contains a lot of manganese, iron, dietary fiber, and calcium. Cinnamon contains derivatives, such as cinnamaldehyde, cinnamic acid, cinnamate, and numerous other components such as polyphenols and antioxidant, anti-inflammatory, antidiabetic, antimicrobial, anticancer effects. Several reports have dealt with the numerous properties of cinnamon in the forms of bark, essential oils, bark powder, and phenolic compounds, and each of these properties can play a key role in human health. Recently, many trials have explored the beneficial effects of cinnamon in Alzheimer's disease, diabetes, arthritis, and arteriosclerosis, but still we need further investigations to provide additional clinical evidence for this spice against cancer and inflammatory, cardioprotective, and neurological disorders.

Keywords Cinnamon · Cinnamaldehyde · Cinnamate · Cinnamic acid · Chronic disease

1 Introduction

According to Malaysian researchers and researchers from the United States (US) Department of Agriculture, cinnamon is one of the most important spices used daily by people all over the world. It contains about 38 % of your daily requirement

M. Hariri
Department of Basic Medical Sciences, Neyshabur University of Medical Sciences, Neyshabur, Iran
e-mail: Hariri.mitra@yahoo.com

R. Ghiasvand (✉)
Department of Community Nutrition, School of Nutrition and Food Sciences, Isfahan University of Medical Sciences, Isfahan, Iran
e-mail: ghiasvand@hlth.mui.ac.ir

S.C. Gupta et al. (eds.), *Drug Discovery from Mother Nature*,
Advances in Experimental Medicine and Biology 929,
DOI 10.1007/978-3-319-41342-6_1

of manganese and contains 10 % of your daily requirement for iron and dietary fiber [1]. It also is high in calcium. Beyond this, there are several other reasons why cinnamon is a must-have spice. Cinnamon primarily contains vital oils and other derivatives, such as cinnamaldehyde, cinnamic acid, cinnamate, and numerous other components such as polyphenols [2]. In addition to being an antioxidant, anti-inflammatory, antidiabetic [3], antimicrobial [4], anticancer [5], lipid-lowering [6], and cardiovascular disease-lowering compound [7], cinnamon has also been reported as useful for metabolic syndrome, insulin sensitivity, polycystic ovary syndrome, increasing lean body mass, and gastric emptying [8, 9]. It is useful against neurological disorders, such as Parkinson's and Alzheimer's diseases [10].

Cinnamon is a common ingredient used in tea for nausea during pregnancy. It is also used following delivery to decrease hemorrhage. The health benefits of cinnamon can be attributed to its antibacterial, antifungal, antimicrobial, astringent, and anticlotting properties [11].

Researchers in Europe, the Middle East, India, China, and the United States are not necessarily using the same type of cinnamon when they do their research. This sometimes leads to confusion and to contradictory research findings. There is overwhelming evidence that cinnamon has numerous therapeutic benefits; however, these benefits are not universally reported by researchers in all countries. Also, cinnamon powder rapidly loses its freshness, which means that its active components may volatilize into the air. Thus, research that was done with different types of cinnamon, with an old inventory of cinnamon, with irradiated cinnamon, or cinnamon that was given with certain pharmaceutical drugs may not produce the same results when compared to other cinnamon studies.

In the United States, the word cinnamon can refer to spices that come from various parts of the world and from quite different varieties of plants. Thus, not all cinnamon or all cinnamon essential oil is the same.

This is important, because the different plant varieties do not have the same composition of active components. Ground cinnamon and cinnamon sticks are made from the bark of several related tropical evergreen trees in the Lauraceae (laurel) family. Cinnamon essential oil is distilled from the bark, stems, and leaves of these trees [12].

Most cinnamon spice sold is actually not true cinnamon. It is a closely related spice called cassia. Cassia (*Cinnamomum cassia*): also known as "Chinese Cinnamon," is what is usually sold as cinnamon.

True cinnamon is Ceylon Cinnamon (*Cinnamomum zeylanicum* or sometimes *Cinnamomum verum*). This "true cinnamon" is the preferred variety in Europe and Mexico. It is milder than cassia, but has a more subtle and complex flavor than cassia.

Most of the scientific studies that we will review in this chapter have used ground cinnamon or specific components of cinnamon that have been derived from cinnamon by use of a water process. Some studies have used essential oil of cinnamon, which is produced from distillation.

Conflict between studies about useful effect of cinnamon may be related to various methodological factors such as the use of different varieties of cinnamon, to the use of an old stock of ground cinnamon, to using an inappropriately high or low dose of cinnamon, to using irradiated cinnamon, to the simultaneous use of pharmaceutical medications, or to other problems in research methodology.

2 Physiochemical Properties of Cinnamon

Cinnamon consists of a variety of resinous compounds, including cinnamaldehyde, cinnamate, cinnamic acid, and numerous essential oils [13] (Table 1). Singh et al. [14] reported that the spicy taste and fragrance are due to the presence of cinnamaldehyde and occur due to the absorption of oxygen. As cinnamon ages, it darkens in color, improving the resinous compounds [14]. Sangal reported various physiochemical properties of cinnamon (Table 2). The presence of a wide range of essential oils, such as trans-cinnamaldehyde, cinnamyl acetate, eugenol, L-borneol, caryophyllene oxide, b-caryophyllene, L-bornyl acetate, E-nerolidol, -cubebene, -

Table 1 Chemical constituents of different parts of cinnamon

Part of the plant	Compound
Leaves	Cinnamaldehyde: 1.00–5.00 % Eugenol: 70.00–95.00 %
Bark	Cinnamaldehyde: 65.00–80.00 % Eugenol: 5.00–10.00 %
Root bark	Camphor: 60.00 %
Fruit	Trans-Cinnamyl acetate (42.00–54.00 % and caryophyllene (9.00–14.00 %)
C. zeylanicum buds	Terpene hydrocarbons: 78.00 % alpha-Bergamotene: 27.38 % alpha-Copaene: 23.05 % Oxygenated terpenoids: 9.00 %
C. zeylanicum flowers	(E)-Cinnamyl acetate: 41.98 % Trans-alpha-Bergamotene: 7.97 % Caryophyllene oxide: 7.20 %

Table 2 Physicochemical properties of cinnamon

Parameter	Leaf oil	Bark oil
Specific gravity (20 °C)	1.030–1.050	1.010–1.030
Optical rotation (°) (20 °C)	1·96′–0.40′	Slightly laevorotatory
Refractive index (20 °C)	1.529–1.537	1.573–1.591
Aldehyde content	4 %	65–76 %
Eugenol content	77.3–90.5 %	4–10 %
Solubility characteristics	Soluble in 1.5 volumes of 70 % alcohol	Soluble in 2.0–3.0 volumes of 70 % alcohol

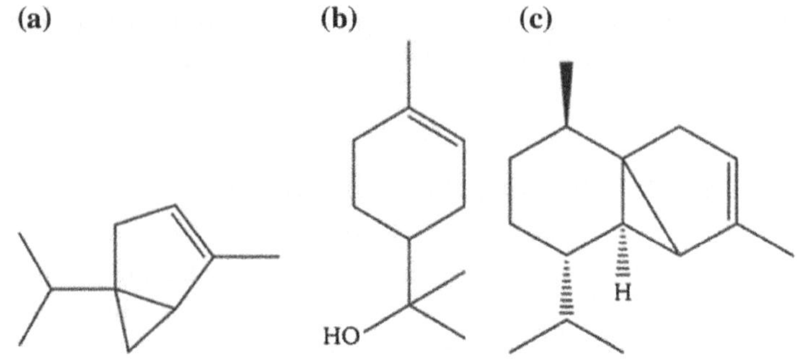

Fig. 1 Endocyclic double bond-containing compounds

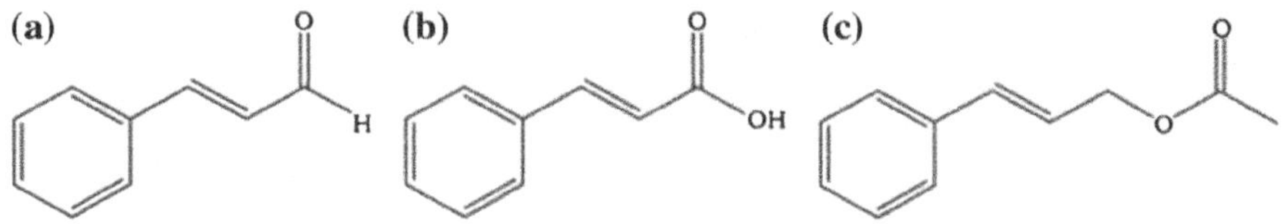

Fig. 2 Cinnamyl group-containing compounds

terpineol, terpinolene, and -thujene, has been reported. The chemical structures of some important constituents of cinnamon are shown in Figs. 1 and 2.

3 Modulation of Cell Signaling Pathways by Cinnamon

New evidence recently demonstrated that a mixture of polyphenols from an aqueous extract of cinnamon possessed anticancer properties by blocking cell cycle progression of leukemic cell lines at the G2/M phase [15]. They indicated treatment of asynchronously growing cells with cinnamon caused an enhancement of cell percentage in G2/M that is because of an increase in activated p38 MAPK by phosphorylation of p38 MAPK in cinnamon-treated cells compared with the non-treated control cells.

Cinnamon has been said to have an insulin-mimetic and insulin-sensitizing action [16]. *Cinnamon cassia* plays a significant role in phosphorylation of signaling proteins and enhancement of expression of insulin-sensitive glucose transporters, which results in mitigation of the insulin resistance [16, 17]. Eugenol component in cinnamon oil can inhibit peroxynitrite-induced nitration and lipid peroxidation in in vitro models [18].

A recent study reported that 2′-hydroxycinnamaldehyde isolated from *C. cassia* bark exhibited an inhibitory effect on the production of nitric oxide by inhibiting the activation of the nuclear factor kappa-light-chain enhancer of activated B cells (NF-κB), indicating that this substance can potentially be used as an anti-inflammatory agent [19]. The ethanolic extract of *C. cassia* showed significant anti-inflammatory effects by reducing the activation of Src/spleen tyrosine-kinase (Src/Syk)-mediated NF-κB [20, 21]. Various compounds contained in *Cinnamomum ramulus* showed anti-inflammatory effects by suppressing the expression of inducible nitric oxide synthesis (iNOS), cyclooxygenase-2 (COX-2), and nitric oxide (NO) production in the central nervous system (CNS). Cinnamophilin is a novel thromboxane A2 receptor antagonist isolated from *Capillaria philippinensis* [22]. A study reported that cinnamophilin confers protection against ischemic damage in rat brains when administered at 80 mg/kg at different time intervals (2, 4, and 6 h) after insult. The effects were found to have a considerable effect (by 34–43 %) on abridged brain infarction [23] and further enhance neurobehavioral outcomes. Cinnamophilin also dramatically condenses the oxygen glucose deprivation-induced neuronal damage in organotypic hippocampal slices in experimental rats. A substance called procyanidin type A trimer (trimer 1) isolated from cinnamon's water-soluble extract showed that trimer 1 may reduce cell swelling by controlling the movement of intracellular calcium [Ca^{2+}] [24]. Trimer 1 also considerably alleviates the oxygen glucose deprivation-induced diminishing effects on glutamate uptake. The protective effects of trimer 1 in attenuating the diminution in glutamate uptake are possibly arbitrated via their effects on the mitochondria.

4 Role of Cinnamon in Chronic Diseases

4.1 Cinnamon Used to Reduce Blood Sugar in Diabetics

C. zeylanicum [true cinnamon] is a popular kitchen spice widely investigated for insulin potentiating effects. Researchers in India investigated water-soluble polyphenols (oligomeric procyanidins) to evaluate their effect on insulin and blood sugar [25]. The polyphenol-enhanced extracts were shown to be safe, while offering good antioxidant potential. The diabetic rats that were treated with the polyphenol-enhanced extracts experienced reduced blood sugar during the 30-day experiment [3]. The same benefit was obtained by a group of 15 human volunteers with chronically elevated fasting blood sugar levels who were not using medication to control blood sugar [26].

A review of studies conducted by California researchers examined cinnamon's effect on blood sugar and lipid (blood fat) levels in diabetic patients. Ten random control trials with a total of 543 patients were examined. Cinnamon doses of 120 mg per day to 6 g per day were given for a period of 4–18 weeks. (6 g is slightly more than 2 teaspoons.) Among the findings was an average reduction in fasting blood sugar levels of 24.59 mg/dL. The reductions ranged from 40.52 to 8.67 mg/dL depending on the study. The studies did not affect hemoglobin A1c levels [27].

A group of researchers from England investigated the blood glucose lowering effect of cinnamon on HbA1c, blood pressure, and lipid profiles in poorly controlled type 2 diabetic patients. Fifty-eight type 2 diabetic patients aged 45–65 years of age, who were being treated only with hypoglycemic agents and who had HbA1c test results of more than 7 % were randomly assigned to receive either 2 g of cinnamon or placebo per day for 12 weeks. At the end of the study, the cinnamon group had an 8.22 % average reduction in HbA1c. Average blood pressures were also significantly reduced [28]. Systolic blood pressure fell from 132.6 to 129.2 mmHg, and the diastolic pressure fell from 85.2 to 80.2 mmHg.

A significant reduction in fasting plasma glucose, waist circumference, and body mass index was observed at week 12 compared with the values at the beginning of the study for the cinnamon group. However, these changes were not significant when compared to the placebo group. The researchers concluded that intake of 2 g (slightly less than a teaspoon) of cinnamon for 12 weeks significantly reduces the HbA1c and blood pressure for poorly controlled type 2 diabetes patients. Cinnamon supplementation could be considered as an additional dietary supplement option to regulate blood glucose and blood pressure levels along with conventional medications to treat type 2 diabetes mellitus [29].

In a study conducted by Chinese researchers, the effects of giving cinnamon polyphenols to diabetic mice were investigated. The mice were fed a high-sugar, high-fat diet. Their results were similar with other studies, which produced reductions in blood sugar, blood insulin levels, and markers of oxidative stress. What was even more interesting was that damage to the pancreatic beta cells in the islets of the pancreas was ameliorated. These benefits may have actually resulted from the repair of pancreatic beta cells and from improvements in their antioxidative capacity, which came from the use of cinnamon polyphenols [30].

Studies which employed the largest doses of cinnamon relative to carbohydrate in the test meal (carbohydrate/cinnamon ratio of 15 or lower [31, 32]) appear to have had the most potent effects on reducing postprandial glycemia [33]. Recent data indicate that the addition of 3 g cinnamon to a low-fat rice pudding test meal had no significant effect on postprandial glycemia in healthy individuals [34]. However, cinnamon did significantly lower serum insulin levels and increase glucagon-like peptide-1 (GLP-1) concentrations, a gastric inhibitory (GI) peptide, which has been shown to increase glucose-dependent secretion of insulin, delay gastric emptying (GE) and reduce glucose absorption and postprandial glycemia [35, 36].

Scientists from Spain also conducted research on polyphenols. They noted that polyphenols have been reported to prevent chronic diseases such as cardiovascular disease, cancer, diabetes, and neurodegenerative diseases [37]. In one study, rats were fed a high-fat and high-sugar diet and were given various polyphenolic plant extracts. They tested extracts from almond, apple, cinnamon, orange blossom, hamamelis, lime blossom, grape vine, and birch. Rats were treated for 56–64 days. Their results showed that only apple and cinnamon extracts were finally considered as potentially important anti-obesity extracts due to their ability to reduce body fat.

They also noted that apple polyphenols reduced metabolic complications associated with obesity [38].

Chinese researchers were interested in studying the ability of Chinese cinnamon (*C. cassia*) to prevent diabetic nephropathy (kidney disease). This disease is very difficult to treat, and prevention is a much better option.

Chinese cassia is one of the most popular natural spices and flavoring agents in many parts of the world. Since previous reports indicated that Chinese cinnamon extract could be used for the treatment of diabetes, the researchers studied its ability to prevent diabetic kidney disease. They isolated several compounds from cinnamon extract. Their results showed that some of the isolates did prevent certain actions which would lead to kidney disease. Thus, they suggested that Chinese cinnamon could be used as a functional food against diabetic nephropathy [39]. Cinnamon can be a natural herb used to lower the high creatinine level and high blood urea nitrogen (BUN) level as a home remedy. Cinnamon can be regarded as a diuretic, which can help increase the urine output. If patients still have urine, they can take cinnamon to lower their high creatinine and high BUN level, because with the increase in the urine output, the wastes in blood can also be filtered out into urine, which contain the creatinine and BUN [40].

Canadian researchers reviewed and evaluated the effects of short-term administration of cinnamon on blood pressure regulation in patients with prediabetes and type 2 diabetes by looking at randomized, placebo-controlled clinical trials. They found that cinnamon significantly decreased systolic blood pressure by an average of 5.39 mm Hg (reductions ranged from 6.89 to 3.89). Diastolic blood pressure was reduced by an average of 2.6 mm Hg (ranging from 4.53 to 0.66) [41]. Cinnamon can decrease weight in diabetic patients too. Researchers prepared a water-based extract from cinnamon bark and gave it to obese rats for 5 weeks. They observed two important changes. First, the rats voluntarily reduced their intake of food, and there was an increase in a neurotransmitter called 5-HT serotonin (5-hydroxy tryptamine). Elevated levels of this neurotransmitter are seen in persons with anorexia. Thus, cinnamon seems to increase this level in overweight rats, which reduces their desire to overeat [42]. The antidiabetic effect of cinnamon has generated broad interest during the past decade. Researchers from Taiwan investigated the ability of essential oil of cinnamon to reduce blood sugar and to protect the pancreas from damage [43]. The essential oil was made from indigenous cinnamon leaves. Several groups of diabetic rats were tested with different doses of cinnamon oil.

All the doses of cinnamon oil significantly lowered fasting blood sugar and fructosamine. A very interesting finding involved the levels of insulin levels in the blood. They found that the lowest dose of cinnamon oil reduced plasma insulin levels better than higher doses. The low dose was 12.5 mg per kg of body weight for the rats; 25 and 50 mg per kg of body weight was not effective for ameliorating the accumulation of insulin.

In addition, the low dose of cinnamon oil significantly reduced pancreatic values of thiobarbituric acid-reactive substances and activities of superoxide dismutase and glutathione reductase in diabetics to an extent greater than that of higher cinnamon doses. In conclusion, appropriate doses of cinnamon of the linalool chemotype exhibited therapeutic potential in blood sugar control that partially resulted from improved insulin secretion. The reduction in oxidative stress and inflammation in the pancreas by cinnamon oil may provide a protective effect on pancreatic cells [43].

4.2 Cinnamon for Arthritis and Pain Relief

Rheumatoid arthritis is a disease of inflammation, so adding anti-inflammatory herbs and spices to your diet might sound like a good idea. Arthritis is a general term that refers to pain, swelling, and stiffness in your joints [44]. There are a variety types of arthritis. Osteoarthritis is known as the wear-and-tear arthritis and occurs as you age or due to an injury. Other forms of arthritis are autoimmune in nature and include rheumatoid arthritis and juvenile rheumatoid arthritis [45]. These conditions are caused when your body's immune system attacks the joints in your body. According to the National Institutes of Health, there are more than 100 types of arthritis. "U.S. News" reports that 46 million Americans suffer with some form of arthritis and that by 2030, 40 % of all American adults are expected to suffer from arthritis [46]. While pain medications are used to treat arthritis, many are turning to natural alternatives like honey and cinnamon. Cinnamon bark from *C. zeylanicum* (verum) is one of the oldest traditional medicines used in India for inflammatory and pain-related disorders. Researchers in India evaluated the efficacy of the polyphenol fraction from *C. zeylanicum* bark in animal models of inflammation and rheumatoid arthritis. They worked with several groups of rats that were induced with various health conditions. These included rat paw inflammation, localized immune system distress (granuloma), or adjuvant-induced polyarthritis. Many scientific pharmacological investigations have also reported on the anti-inflammatory potential cinnamon [47]. The anti-inflammatory action of the Japanese species *Cinnamomum seiboldii* and Cinnamomi cortex [48] has been attributed to a series of tannins. An herbal ophthalmic medicament called Ophthacare, which contains 0.5 % cinnamon, was tested for its anti-inflammatory activity on ocular inflammation in rabbits and found to be effective [49]. The antinociceptive activity (analgesic) [50] and antipyretic (fever-reducing) activity of cinnamon (*C. verum*) bark were also reported.

Another important activity is the immunomodulatory effects exerted by cinnamon. An interesting fact about cinnamon is that it can act both as an immune stimulant and an immune suppressant depending on the species and dose [51]. In vitro inhibitory activity against the complement formation has been documented for cinnamon cortex and cinnamon oil [51]. The extract of cinnamon bark is reported to have anticomplementary activity [52] and immunosuppressive activity [53]. Cinnamon bark's potential for relieving inflammation and pain, and enhancing the immune system, makes it a good candidate as an antiarthritic agent.

Furthermore, cinnamon polyphenol extract (CPE) from the cinnamon bark of various varieties has shown potential for the management of certain human health conditions.

Procyanidins or condensed tannins are flavonoid oligomers whose building blocks are catechin and epicatechin. They are oligomeric end products of the flavonoid biosynthetic pathway and are now identified and recognized for their favorable effects in human beings.

Recently, the immunomodulatory effect of the water extract of cinnamon on anti-CD3-induced cytokine responses and p38, JNK, ERK1/2, and STAT4 activation [53] has been shown. CPE is known to affect immune responses by regulating anti- and pro-inflammatory and glucose transporter type 4 (GLUT4) gene expression as seen in an in vitro study on mouse RAW264.7 macrophages [54]. However, a functional outcome of these effects in an animal model of rheumatoid arthritis has not been investigated.

Researchers observed dose-dependent decreases in inflammation, edema, pain reactions, and cytokine activity. In conclusion, they determined that cinnamon polyphenols have prominent action in animal inflammation and arthritis and therefore can be considered a potential antirheumatic agent, which can be used to treat these diseases [55].

4.3 Cinnamon and Heart Disease

Cinnamon inhibits the release of inflammatory fatty acids such as arachidonic acid, from the blood's platelet membranes. It also works to reduce the formation of thromboxane A2, which is an inflammatory molecule found in the blood stream. This is helpful as an anti-inflammatory, but in addition, it helps to keep the blood the proper thickness. Platelets help the blood to clot together whenever there is an emergency, such as a cut. In many people, the platelets work too hard and can thicken the blood significantly [32]. This can cause a rise in blood pressure, which in turn can damage the arteries and other organs of the body. Cinnamon stops the platelets from thickening the blood too much. The result of study by McGowan et al. [57] demonstrated that cinnamon water extract (CWE) was able to interfere with monocyte differentiation and macrophage scavenger activity, indicating its potential in preventing the development of atherosclerotic lesions [56]. According to study by Jin S at 2011, cinnamon has anti-atherosclerotic activity in hypercholesterolemic zebrafish. In this study, cinnamon had the strongest inhibition of activity against copper-mediated low-density lipoprotein (LDL) oxidation and LDL phagocytosis by macrophages [7]. In addition to the benefits already listed, another way that cinnamon is helpful in preventing heart disease is by simply providing nutrients to the body. The high level of calcium and fiber in cinnamon aids the body in flushing toxins from the body [57]. In addition, many believe cinnamon to be helpful in reducing high cholesterol levels in some people. This can help preventing atherosclerosis and the development of heart disease. Several studies have demonstrated that abnormal blood lipids and lipoproteins are the major risk factors for cardiovascular diseases including ischemic heart disease and atherosclerosis [58, 59]. Dyslipidemia is one of the symptoms of metabolic syndrome that associates with obesity, diabetes, and other comorbidities. Dyslipidemia and hypercholesterolemia result in endothelial dysfunctions, decreased nitric oxide production, and increased reactive oxygen species (ROS) generation [60]. On the other hand, it is suggested that supplementation with antioxidant nutrients and other medicinal plants in humans and animals can attenuate ROS-mediated damage to the heart after an ischemic insult. Cinnamon usually has excellent antioxidant activities.

New evidence shows methanol extract has maximum antioxidant property as compared to the ethanolic and water extract [61]. The antioxidant property is due to the eugenol component, which inhibited peroxynitrite-induced nitration and lipid peroxidation in in vitro models [18]. The oil is said to form a phosphomolybdenum complex, which is responsible for its antioxidant activity [62]. Antioxidant activity of leaf and fruit extracts and essential oils has been reported in several in vitro and in vivo studies [63].

4.4 Cinnamon and Alzheimer's Disease

Alzheimer's disease (AD) is a progressive, irreversible brain disorder with an unclear etiology and no cure. Symptoms include memory loss, confusion, impaired judgment, disorientation, and loss of language skills [64]. In the past two decades, a large number of experimental studies have established a pathological role for amyloid beta (Aß) in AD [65]. However, recent debates have focused on whether Aß amyloid fibrils or Aß-soluble oligomers are the main neurotoxic species, which contribute to neurodegeneration and dementia. Recent studies have shown inhibition of Aß plaque formation in vitro and in vivo by compounds from natural sources [66–68]. Still, evidence for the capability of common edible elements to inhibit Aß oligomerization in vivo remains a challenge.

Researchers from California [69] found that cinnamon contains cinnamaldehyde and epicatechin, which inhibit the aggregation of a particular protein called tau. Tau is needed for the normal structure and function of neurons in the brain. However, if this protein begins to accumulate, it can form neurofibrillary tangles, which is a characteristic of Alzheimer's disease. Cinnamaldehyde and epicatechin were found to protect tau from oxidative damage that can lead to dysfunction [69]. A study found that cinnamon extract (CE) inhibits the formation of toxic Aβ oligomers and prevents the toxicity of Aβ on neuronal PC12 cells. In another study, the oral administration of CE to an aggressive AD transgenic mice model led to the reduction in plaques and improvement in cognitive behavior. The results showed that the use of natural compounds such as cinnamon can inhibit toxic oligomeric Aβ species formation in AD [70].

Uncontrolled activation of microglia results into neuroinflammation, which is strongly involved in the progression of neurodegenerative diseases such as Alzheimer disease, Parkinson's disease, and multiple sclerosis [71]. Activation of microglia occurs in response to some stimuli such as β-amyloid, glutamate, arachidonate, and lipopolysaccharides. Regarding the lower rate of neurodegenerative diseases in Asians, especially those who regularly consume spices, Ho and colleagues at 2013 decided to conduct a series of studies to evaluate the effect of cinnamon on progression of neuroinflammation. They showed that cinnamon has strong antioxidant activity and can scavenge NO, superoxide anion, and peroxynitrite [72], and also cinnamon can effectively suppress synthesis of NO and iNOS in LPS-activated macrophage [73]. Also they showed that cinnamon can suppress TLR4 oligomerization and attenuate the LPS-elicited intracellular signaling process, and hence, it can restore redox capacity and alleviate NFκB activation of LPS-activated microglia [72]. Additionally, other investigations show that cinnamon has some other neuroprotective effects and proanthocyanidin trimer and cinnamaldehyde of cinnamon can suppress the formation of intracellular tau neurofibrillary tangles, in Alzheimer's disease [74]. Also Frydman-Marom et al. [70] at 2011 showed that cinnamon decreased transformation of amyloid monomers into the toxic oligomer in Alzheimer's disease animal models. In conclusion, aforementioned studies suggest cinnamon as a nutraceutical agent with antineuroinflammatory effects that can be used as a dietary adjuvant against neurodegenerative diseases.

5 Anti-inflammatory Effects of Cinnamon in Allergies

During the last decades, prevalence of allergic diseases has increased dramatically. Regarding the major side effects of pharmaceutical treatment, it is actually a matter of great concern to find new therapies for allergic diseases. Therefore, using foods as a nutraceutical agent with less side effects and more acceptance should be considered. According to recent studies, it has been reported that cinnamon may have anti-inflammatory effects in allergies due to its role in inhibition of histamine production from lipid precursors during allergic diseases. Corren and colleagues during a double-blind randomized clinical trial stated that [75] a botanical product containing cinnamon may be helpful to reduce nasal allergy symptoms and PG D2 release in patients with seasonal allergic rhinitis. They demonstrated that a treatment with a botanical product containing cinnamon has both statistically and clinically significant meaningful effect on allergic symptoms in comparison with placebo group. This result was also consistent with their previous in vitro study which reported the same effect. Although they were unable to determine which of the ingredients of the product contributed most to these effect—which is very common in botanical products!—they stated that cinnamon that was found in the product inhibited complement-dependent allergic reaction by reducing immunological hemolysis, chemotactic migration of neutrophils, and the generation of chemotactic factors by mast cells in response to complement-activated serum [75, 76]. Another in vivo study, which studied the anti-inflammatory and immunoregulatory effects of cinnamon and concluded that cinnamon can be suggested as a new nutraceutical treatment candidate for anti-allergic therapy, was conducted by Hagenlocher et al. [77] in 2013. They orally administrated cinnamon to mice and then analyzed the release of mediators and phosphorylation of signaling molecules. They stated that oral administration of cinnamon resulted in statistically significant lower expression of the mast cell MCP6 and MC-CPA also lowers expression of tryptase in human mast cells isolated from intestinal tissue. In this study, cinnamon treatment also almost completely blocked the de novo synthesis of cysteinyl leukotrienes and cytokines. In addition, 80 % of the release of β-hexosaminidase was reduced by cinnamon in human mast cells isolated from intestinal tissue. As commonly known, mast cells are key effector cells of mediated-type allergic reactions and other inflammatory pathways [77]. Mast cells apply their pro-inflammatory effects by producing a wide variety of inflammatory compounds such as stored histamine and proteases, as well as de novo synthesized cytokines such as TNFα, CXCL8, CCL2, CCL3, CCL4, and eicosanoids upon activation. By downregulation of such cytokines and by blocking of degranulation, cinnamon can act as a prophylactic agent for treatment of allergic diseases. According to the results of the aforementioned study, oral administration of cinnamon leads to a strong inhibition of release of mast cell mediators, and it also reduces the expression of mast cell mediators and proteases in mice duodenal tissue, and human mast cells isolated from intestinal tissue. Thus, they suggested that cinnamon can be used as a new nutraceutical agent capable of attenuating allergic reactions, according to its beneficial effects on inhibition of mast cell activation. A recent animal study also demonstrated that a cinnamon-based herbal product showed significant anti-allergic effects on animal model with allergic rhinitis when administered intranasal [78], and according to their results, cinnamon may be helpful to attenuate symptoms of allergic rhinitis due to downregulation of IgE and histamine release.

6 Anti-inflammatory Effect of Cinnamon on Colitis

Inflammatory bowel disease is a group of inflammatory condition of the colon and small intestine, which falls into class of autoimmune diseases. Antigen-presenting cells are a heterogeneous population constituting different types of cells including dendritic cells, B cells, and macrophages that produce and present a wide range of antigens on major histocompatibility complex molecules and play critical roles in various immune responses. Antigen-presenting cells can activate the immune system against pathogens or cause an immunotolerance to self-antigens. So antigen-presenting cells play pivotal roles in maintenance of immunological homeostasis and regulation of these cells has a possible therapeutic effect to block diverse types of inflammatory and autoimmune disorders [79]. Kwon and colleagues at 2011 evaluated the effect of cinnamon on regulation of antigen-presenting cells' activity. They administered cinnamon extract containing 2.9 and 7.9 mg/g trans-cinnamic acid to 6- to 8-week-old male mice for 20 days. Then, experimental colitis was induced by intrarectal injection of 2,4,6-trinitrobenzenesulfonic acid (TNBS). Clinical symptoms such as weight loss were detectable in both treatment and control groups after 2 days of injection. Cinnamon-treated group began to regain weight after day 3 and day 5, while the control group continued to lose weight. In addition, the survival rate in cinnamon-treated mice was about 90 %, while control group had a 50 % rate of survival. In line with weight loss and survival rate, symptoms of colonic inflammation were significantly reduced in cinnamon-treated group compared with control group. They demonstrated that treatment with cinnamon extract resulted in more tolerogenic characteristics of antigen-presenting cells, which inhibited T-cell proliferation, T-cell polarization into Th1 type, while leading to IL-10 produced by CD4 T cells. In addition, oral cinnamon treatment significantly inhibited the progression of experimental colitis by increasing IL-10 production while decreasing the levels of pro-inflammatory cytokines. In addition, treatment with cinnamon significantly downregulated expression levels of MHCII and costimulatory molecules (B7.1 and B7.2) in macrophage cell lines, primarily MCHII + APCs and CD11c + DCs. Administration of cinnamon in a dose-dependent manner also significantly increased expression of B7-DC (PD-L2) as a result of primary MCHII + APCs, which has strong anti-inflammatory properties to suppress T-cell activation [80]. Hence, an increment in B7-DC expression levels by cinnamon possibly will mediate its anti-inflammatory properties [81]. Taking together, Kwon and colleagues stated that cinnamon strongly inhibits maturation of APCs and provides them with abilities to produce high levels of anti-inflammatory cytokines. In addition, cinnamon strongly betters TNBS-induced experimental inflammatory bowel disease due to increasing IL-10 levels while downregulating pro-inflammatory cytokines. Also in another study, Lima and colleagues showed that methyl cinnamate, which is the methyl ester of cinnamic acid and is widely used as a flavoring agent, is able to inhibit the gastrointestinal spasms according to involvement of tyrosine kinase pathways. It also has some anti-inflammatory effects to ameliorate experimental model of acute colitis [82]. On the other hand, some evidence from a cross-sectional study suggest that consumption of spicy foods including cinnamon may be associated with lower gastrointestinal disorders that are related to mast cells and inflammatory pathways. Hence, it seems that the use of cinnamon to treat inflammatory GI disorders may still need more investigations [83].

7 Anti-inflammatory Effects of Cinnamon on *Helicobacter pylori*-induced Gastritis

From old times, cinnamon is used to treat a wide range of GI disorders such as gastritis, dyspepsia, bloating, vomiting, and diarrhea [84, 85].

Helicobacter pylori (formerly *Campylobacter pylori*) is a helical shape, gram-negative, noninvasive bacteria, which usually found in the stomach. More than 50 % of the world population harbor it in their stomach. This infection is more prevalent in less developed countries and is tending to decrease in developed countries. Although *H. pylori* infection is a noninvasive infection and more than 80 % of infected individuals are asymptomatic, it is associated with gastritis, GI ulcers, and even stomach cancer [86]. It also stimulates inflammatory and immune responses and results in increased levels of inflammatory cytokines such as IL-1, IL-6, IL-8, and TNF-α. In addition, *H. pylori* has an indirect effect on IL-8 (which is a major chemotactic agent and activates neutrophils and recruits acute inflammatory cell into the mucosa [87] through activation of NF-κB which in turn stimulates IL-8 production). Zaidi and his colleagues in their study examined the effects of cinnamon on inflammatory pathways causing *H. pylori*-induced gastritis. They showed that cinnamon has some anti-inflammatory effects in *H. pylori*-induced gastritis, and unlike several other medicinal plants, cinnamon did not show any anti-adhesive characteristics against *H. pylori*. Hence, its effect is not due to interference with binding of *H. pylori* to the stomach cells. They stated that cinnamon has a strong IL-8 inhibitory effect on *H. pylori*-infected and TNF-α-stimulated cells [88] and this effect was dose dependent. Moreover, cinnamon resulted in inhibition of phosphorylation of p56 and degradation of IκBα, which caused inactivation and downregulation of NF-κB, and hence reduction in IL-8. In this study, they also showed that cinnamon is an activator of Nrf2-orchestrated antioxidant response in epithelial cells of human's colon and it enhances cellular inflammation response by NF-κB. In conclusion, they demonstrated that cinnamon may play a role at suppressing the gastritis by IL-8 expression via deactivation of NF-κB. So cinnamon can be considered as potential nutraceutical agent to treat *H. pylori*-induced gastritis [88].

Regarding the usefulness of cinnamon to alleviate the *H. pylori* inflammation and despite its well-known antibacterial effects [89], there is no strong evidence to support such an effect in vivo. The only article on the antibacterial effect of cinnamon on *H. pylori* is a clinical trial conducted by Nir et al. [90], which evaluates the effect of 40 mg of an alcoholic extract of cinnamon twice daily for 4 weeks. They concluded that cinnamon extract at aforementioned dose as a single treatment is not effective to eradicate *H. pylori*. However, combination of cinnamon with other antimicrobial herbals or higher doses may be useful [90]. There are other researchers who conducted evaluation on antimicrobial effects of cinnamon. Quale and Rosti at 1996 reported beneficial effects of cinnamon to treat candidiasis in HIV patients and chronic salmonellosis, respectively [74, 91], but clinical trials are necessary to prove these claimed antimicrobial effects of cinnamon.

8 Biological Activity of Cinnamon in Human

A wide range of cinnamon compounds may actively participate in biological processes and have the ability to affect a biological pathway. In vivo effects of various species of cinnamon include the following: lowering HbA1c and fasting blood glucose, reduction in LDL-C, triglycerides, circulating insulin level, and increasing HDL-C. Cinnamon also inhibits excess weight loss during acute phase of diabetes [92].

The biological effect of CZ on glycemic control may be due to its ability to reduce intestinal absorption of glucose by blocking the activity of pancreatic α-amylase and α-glucosidase the enzymes which actively control the metabolism of carbohydrates in intestine. CZ also increases the number of GLUT-4 receptors in cell membrane and increases the tyrosine phosphorylation activity of insulin receptors. In addition, results of studies on CZ suggest that cinnamon zeylanicum consumption leads to stimulation of glycogen synthesis and insulin secretion and blocking of gluconeogenesis. Hydroxychalcone derived from CZ can also act as a mimetic for insulin in adipocytes [93]. Hence, it would actively improve glycemic control in diabetic subject and reduce the risk factors related to diabetes [94]. Some researchers have suggested that at least some these biological activities of cinnamon are related to its polyphenols.

A several of the many few in vivo studies in human to investigate the effect of cinnamon on lipid profile showed that it could not significantly affect lipid concentration [95–98]. While the mechanism for the lipid-lowering effects is not clearly described in literature, there is evidence that supports the hypothesis that cinnamon may reduce serum TG, LDL-C, and total cholesterol due to its effect on increased insulin sensitivity [99] and the high dietary fiber content of CZ.

Cinnamon zeylanicum is found to be a strong antioxidant and to be effective in free radical scavenging activity particularly against DPPH radicals (2,2-diphenyl-1-picrylhydrazyl), ABTS radicals (2,2′-azino-bis (3-ethylbenzothiazoline-6-sulfonic acid)), hydroxyl and superoxide radicals. The majority of antioxidant activity of cinnamon is due to phenolic constituents of it. Results from human studies show that cinnamon can cause a significant reduction in lipid peroxidation level and can improve total antioxidant power and total thiol molecules, in human subjects [100].

Other studies also support from the anti-inflammatory and antimicrobial activities of cinnamon, which are, respectively, considered to arise mainly from the potential of tristetraprolin to destabilizing of pro-inflammatory mRNA and hydrophobic aromatic oils to disrupt the bacterial membrane, which results in ion leakage, but these studies have used a small sample size and the exact mechanism for these effects is not established yet [54, 101].

9 Biological Activity of Cinnamon in Animals

Like human studies on cinnamon, animal researches on the effect of cinnamon have also focused on its antidiabetic and lipid-lowering biological activities. Reviewing the literature shows that the effect of cinnamon on insulin sensitivity [102], insulin secretion [103], and its insulin-like activity improves glycemic control in animal models [104]. Qin et al. [105] also suggested that early administration of cinnamon extract to rats prohibited the development of insulin resistance through improving insulin signaling. Couturier also showed that cinnamon extract would alter the body composition by enhancing insulin sensitivity [106].

Several animal experiments were conducted to investigate effects of cinnamon on lipid profile. They showed that cinnamon may be able to improve lipid profile in animal models [105, 107, 108]. These effects are considered to be related to the effect of cinnamon to regulation of the expression of genes involved in insulin sensitivity and metabolism of lipids. In addition, it has been stated that cinnamon may ameliorate postprandial production of apo B-48 by improving intestinal insulin sensitivity and regulation of TNF-α production in rats [107].

Cinnamon (cinnamomum aromaticum) is claimed to have anti-inflammatory and anticancer effects. Cinnamomum aromaticum can effectively inhibit production of Cox-2 and NO and transcriptional activity of NF-κB [19, 109].

Another biological activity of cinnamomum aromaticum is its antimicrobial characteristics. Results from animal studies show that antimicrobial activity of cinnamon is mainly due to the destabilizing effect of its essential oils on membranes of microorganisms [110]. It has been stated that cinnamomum aromaticum extract is a potent inhibitor of HIV-1 and HIV-2 replication in MT-4 cells infected with HIV [111].

Several studies also have investigated the antioxidant properties of cinnamon zeylanicum and cinnamomum aromaticum and stated that the polyphenolic compounds in cinnamon show potent antioxidant activities in animals [61, 62, 112], which can reduce the complications of diabetes and metabolic syndrome in animal models [106]. The structure of these polyphenolic compounds is very stable and their antioxidant properties are dose dependent [113].

10 How Much Cinnamon Can Be Consumed Per Day

Recommended ranges for cinnamon include 1–4 g per day or 1–6 g per day [11, 114, 115]. According to the European Food Safety Authority, a teaspoon of cassia cinnamon powder contains 5.8–12.1 mg of coumarin. The tolerable daily intake for humans is 0.1 mg/kg body weight, meaning a daily teaspoon might exceed the limit for smaller individuals [116]. People with irritable bowel disease might experience diarrhea. Some people might experience overall warming and even sweating. Taking too much cinnamon can cause nausea and vomiting. In small amounts, cinnamon can calm a queasy stomach.

11 Conclusion

According to scientific evidence, cinnamon has numerous health benefits, but there is some confusion about which type of cinnamon is best, and how much ground cinnamon or cinnamon essential oil is needed for a certain condition. People will need to start slowly and evaluate how the treatment is helping their ailments.

References

1. Tulunay M, Aypak C, Yikilkan H, Gorpelioglu S (2015) Herbal medicine use among patients with chronic diseases. J Intercult Ethnopharmacol 4(3):217–220. PubMed PMID: 26401410. Pubmed Central PMCID: PMC4579486. Epub 2015/09/25. eng
2. Chan KW, Khong NM, Iqbal S, Ch'ng SE, Younas U, Babji AS (2014) Cinnamon bark deodorised aqueous extract as potential natural antioxidant in meat emulsion system: a comparative study with synthetic and natural food antioxidants. J Food Sci Technol 51 (11):3269–3276. PubMed PMID: 26396320. Pubmed Central PMCID: PMC4571215. Epub 2015/09/24. eng
3. Shalaby MA, Saifan HY (2014) Some pharmacological effects of cinnamon and ginger herbs in obese diabetic rats. J Intercult Ethnopharmacol 3(4):144–149. PubMed PMID: 26401364. Pubmed Central PMCID: PMC4576807. Epub 2015/09/25. eng
4. Shan B, Cai YZ, Brooks JD, Corke H (2007) Antibacterial properties and major bioactive components of cinnamon stick (*Cinnamomum burmannii*): activity against foodborne pathogenic bacteria. J Agric Food Chem 55(14):5484–5490. PubMed PMID: 17567030. Epub 2007/06/15. eng
5. Shahwar D, Ullah S, Khan MA, Ahmad N, Saeed A, Ullah S (2015) Anticancer activity of Cinnamon tamala leaf constituents towards human ovarian cancer cells. Pak J Pharm Sci. 28 (3):969–972. PubMed PMID: 26004731. Epub 2015/05/26. eng
6. Javed I, Faisal I, Rahman Z, Khan MZ, Muhammad F, Aslam B et al (2012) Lipid lowering effect of *Cinnamomum zeylanicum* in hyperlipidaemic albino rabbits. Pak J Pharm Sci 25 (1):141–147. PubMed PMID: 22186322. Epub 2011/12/22. eng
7. Jin S, Cho KH (2011) Water extracts of cinnamon and clove exhibits potent inhibition of protein glycation and anti-atherosclerotic activity in vitro and in vivo hypolipidemic activity in zebrafish. Food Chem Toxicol Int J Published Br Ind Biol Res Assoc 49(7):1521–1529. PubMed PMID: 21443916. Epub 2011/03/30. eng
8. Medagama AB, Bandara R (2014) The use of complementary and alternative medicines (CAMs) in the treatment of diabetes mellitus: is continued use safe and effective? Nutr J 13:102. PubMed PMID: 25331834. Pubmed Central PMCID: PMC4210501. Epub 2014/10/22. eng
9. Chen J, Jiang QD, Wu YM, Liu P, Yao JH, Lu Q et al (2015) Potential of essential oils as penetration enhancers for transdermal administration of ibuprofen to treat dysmenorrhoea. Molecules 20(10):18219–18236. PubMed PMID: 26457698. Epub 2015/10/13. eng
10. Anderson RA, Qin B, Canini F, Poulet L, Roussel AM (2013) Cinnamon counteracts the negative effects of a high fat/high fructose diet on behavior, brain insulin signaling and Alzheimer-associated changes. PLoS One 8(12):e83243. PubMed PMID: 24349472. Pubmed Central PMCID: PMC3862724. Epub 2013/12/19. eng
11. Kawatra P, Rajagopalan R (2015) Cinnamon: mystic powers of a minute ingredient. Pharmacognosy Res 7(Suppl 1):S1–S6. PubMed PMID: 26109781. Pubmed Central PMCID: PMC4466762. Epub 2015/06/26. eng
12. Jayaprakasha GK, Rao LJ (2011) Chemistry, biogenesis, and biological activities of *Cinnamomum zeylanicum*. Crit Rev Food Sci Nutr 51(6):547–562. PubMed PMID: 21929331. Epub 2011/09/21. eng
13. Rao PV, Gan SH (2014) Cinnamon: a multifaceted medicinal plant. Evid Based Complement Altern Med eCAM 2014:642942. PubMed PMID: 24817901. Pubmed Central PMCID: PMC4003790. Epub 2014/05/13. eng
14. Singh G, Maurya S, DeLampasona MP, Catalan CA (2007) A comparison of chemical, antioxidant and antimicrobial studies of cinnamon leaf and bark volatile oils, oleoresins and their constituents. Food Chem Toxicol Int J Published Br Ind Biol Res Assoc 45(9):1650–1661. PubMed PMID: 17408833. Epub 2007/04/06. eng

15. Schoene NW, Kelly MA, Polansky MM, Anderson RA (2009) A polyphenol mixture from cinnamon targets p38 MAP kinase-regulated signaling pathways to produce G2/M arrest. J Nutr Biochem 20(8):614–620. PubMed PMID: 18835704. Epub 2008/10/07. eng
16. Cao H, Graves DJ, Anderson RA (2010) Cinnamon extract regulates glucose transporter and insulin-signaling gene expression in mouse adipocytes. Phytomedicine Int J Phytotherapy Phytopharmacol 17(13):1027–1032. PubMed PMID: 20554184. Epub 2010/06/18. eng
17. Jitomir J, Willoughby DS (2009) Cassia cinnamon for the attenuation of glucose intolerance and insulin resistance resulting from sleep loss. J Med Food 12(3):467–472. PubMed PMID: 19627193. Epub 2009/07/25. eng
18. Chericoni S, Prieto JM, Iacopini P, Cioni P, Morelli I (2005) In vitro activity of the essential oil of *Cinnamomum zeylanicum* and eugenol in peroxynitrite-induced oxidative processes. J Agric Food Chem 53(12):4762–4765. PubMed PMID: 15941312. Epub 2005/06/09. eng
19. Lee SH, Lee SY, Son DJ, Lee H, Yoo HS, Song S et al (2005) Inhibitory effect of 2′-hydroxycinnamaldehyde on nitric oxide production through inhibition of NF-kappa B activation in RAW 264.7 cells. Biochem Pharmacol 69(5):791–799. PubMed PMID: 15710356. Epub 2005/02/16. eng
20. Yu T, Lee S, Yang WS, Jang HJ, Lee YJ, Kim TW et al (2012) The ability of an ethanol extract of *Cinnamomum cassia* to inhibit Src and spleen tyrosine kinase activity contributes to its anti-inflammatory action. J Ethnopharmacol 139(2):566–573. PubMed PMID: 22155395. Epub 2011/12/14. eng
21. Youn HS, Lee JK, Choi YJ, Saitoh SI, Miyake K, Hwang DH et al (2008) Cinnamaldehyde suppresses toll-like receptor 4 activation mediated through the inhibition of receptor oligomerization. Biochem Pharmacol 75(2):494–502. PubMed PMID: 17920563. Epub 2007/10/09. eng
22. Yu SM, Ko FN, Wu TS, Lee JY, Teng CM (1994) Cinnamophilin, a novel thromboxane A2 receptor antagonist, isolated from *Cinnamomum philippinense*. Eur J Pharmacol 256(1):85–91. PubMed PMID: 8026563. Epub 1994/04/11. eng
23. Lee EJ, Chen HY, Hung YC, Chen TY, Lee MY, Yu SC et al (2009) Therapeutic window for cinnamophilin following oxygen-glucose deprivation and transient focal cerebral ischemia. Exp Neurol 217(1):74–83. PubMed PMID: 19416670. Epub 2009/05/07. eng
24. Panickar KS, Polansky MM, Graves DJ, Urban JF Jr, Anderson RA (2012) A procyanidin type A trimer from cinnamon extract attenuates glial cell swelling and the reduction in glutamate uptake following ischemia-like injury in vitro. Neuroscience 202:87–98. PubMed PMID: 22166344. Epub 2011/12/15. eng
25. Dagli N, Dagli R, Mahmoud RS, Baroudi K (2015) Essential oils, their therapeutic properties, and implication in dentistry: a review. J Int Soc Prev Commun Dent 5(5):335–340. PubMed PMID: 26539382. Pubmed Central PMCID: PMC4606594. Epub 2015/11/06. eng
26. Im K, Issac A, Nm J, Ninan E, Maliakel B, Kuttan R (2014) Effects of the polyphenol content on the anti-diabetic activity of *Cinnamomum zeylanicum* extracts. Food Funct 5(9):2208–2220. PubMed PMID: 25051315. Epub 2014/07/23. eng
27. Allen RW, Schwartzman E, Baker WL, Coleman CI, Phung OJ (2013) Cinnamon use in type 2 diabetes: an updated systematic review and meta-analysis. Ann Fam Med 11(5):452–459. PubMed PMID: 24019277. Pubmed Central PMCID: PMC3767714. Epub 2013/09/11. eng
28. Bernardo MA, Silva ML, Santos E, Moncada MM, Brito J, Proenca L et al (2015) Effect of cinnamon tea on postprandial glucose concentration. J Diabetes Res 2015:913651. PubMed PMID: 26258147. Pubmed Central PMCID: PMC4516848. Epub 2015/08/11. eng
29. Akilen R, Tsiami A, Devendra D, Robinson N (2010) Glycated haemoglobin and blood pressure-lowering effect of cinnamon in multi-ethnic Type 2 diabetic patients in the UK: a randomized, placebo-controlled, double-blind clinical trial. Diabet Med J Br Diabet Assoc 27 (10):1159–67. PubMed PMID: 20854384. Epub 2010/09/22. eng
30. Li R, Liang T, Xu L, Li Y, Zhang S, Duan X (2013) Protective effect of cinnamon polyphenols against STZ-diabetic mice fed high-sugar, high-fat diet and its underlying

mechanism. Food Chem Toxicol Int J Published Br Ind Biol Res Assoc 51:419–425. PubMed PMID: 23127600. Epub 2012/11/07. eng
31. Solomon TP, Blannin AK (2007) Effects of short-term cinnamon ingestion on in vivo glucose tolerance. Diabetes Obes Metab 9(6):895–901. PubMed PMID: 17924872. Epub 2007/10/11. eng
32. Hlebowicz J, Darwiche G, Bjorgell O, Almer LO (2007) Effect of cinnamon on postprandial blood glucose, gastric emptying, and satiety in healthy subjects. Am J Clin Nutr 85(6):1552–1556. PubMed PMID: 17556692. Epub 2007/06/09. eng
33. Mettler S, Schwarz I, Colombani PC (2009) Additive postprandial blood glucose-attenuating and satiety-enhancing effect of cinnamon and acetic acid. Nutr Res 29(10):723–727. PubMed PMID: 19917452. Epub 2009/11/18. eng
34. Hlebowicz J, Hlebowicz A, Lindstedt S, Bjorgell O, Hoglund P, Holst JJ et al (2009) Effects of 1 and 3 g cinnamon on gastric emptying, satiety, and postprandial blood glucose, insulin, glucose-dependent insulinotropic polypeptide, glucagon-like peptide 1, and ghrelin concentrations in healthy subjects. Am J Clin Nutr 89(3):815–821. PubMed PMID: 19158209. Epub 2009/01/23. eng
35. Deane AM, Nguyen NQ, Stevens JE, Fraser RJ, Holloway RH, Besanko LK et al (2010) Endogenous glucagon-like peptide-1 slows gastric emptying in healthy subjects, attenuating postprandial glycemia. J Clin Endocrinol Metab 95(1):215–221. PubMed PMID: 19892837. Epub 2009/11/07. eng
36. Naslund E, Bogefors J, Skogar S, Gryback P, Jacobsson H, Holst JJ et al (1999) GLP-1 slows solid gastric emptying and inhibits insulin, glucagon, and PYY release in humans. Am J Physiol 277(3 Pt 2):R910–R916. PubMed PMID: 10484511. Epub 1999/09/14. eng
37. Palma A, Ruiz Montoya M, Arteaga JF, Rodriguez Mellado JM (2014) Determination of antioxidant activity of spices and their active principles by differential pulse voltammetry. J Agric Food Chem 62(3):582–589. PubMed PMID: 25264569. Epub 2014/09/30. eng
38. Boque N, Campion J, de la Iglesia R, de la Garza AL, Milagro FI, San Roman B et al (2013) Screening of polyphenolic plant extracts for anti-obesity properties in Wistar rats. J Sci Food Agric 93(5):1226–1232. PubMed PMID: 23080265. Epub 2012/10/20. eng
39. Luo Q, Wang SM, Lu Q, Luo J, Cheng YX (2013) Identification of compounds from the water soluble extract of *Cinnamomum cassia* barks and their inhibitory effects against high-glucose-induced mesangial cells. Molecules 18(9):10930–10943. PubMed PMID: 24013407. Epub 2013/09/10. eng
40. Muthenna P, Raghu G, Kumar PA, Surekha MV, Reddy GB (2014) Effect of cinnamon and its procyanidin-B2 enriched fraction on diabetic nephropathy in rats. Chem Biol Interact 222C:68–76. PubMed PMID: 25199697. Epub 2014/09/10. Eng
41. Akilen R, Pimlott Z, Tsiami A, Robinson N (2013) Effect of short-term administration of cinnamon on blood pressure in patients with prediabetes and type 2 diabetes. Nutrition 29 (10):1192–1196. PubMed PMID: 23867208. Epub 2013/07/23. eng
42. Bano F, Ikram H, Akhtar N (2014) Neurochemical and behavioral effects of *Cinnamomi cassiae* (Lauraceae) bark aqueous extract in obese rats. Pak J Pharm Sci 27(3):559–563. PubMed PMID: 24811817. Epub 2014/05/09. eng
43. Lee SC, Xu WX, Lin LY, Yang JJ, Liu CT (2013) Chemical composition and hypoglycemic and pancreas-protective effect of leaf essential oil from indigenous cinnamon (*Cinnamomum osmophloeum* Kanehira). J Agric Food Chem 22;61(20):4905–4913. PubMed PMID: 23627599. Epub 2013/05/01. eng
44. Aletaha D (2015) Management of rheumatoid arthritis: what happens and what does not happen in real life. Rheumatol Int. PubMed PMID: 26687684. Epub 2015/12/22. eng
45. Catrina AI, Joshua V, Klareskog L, Malmstrom V (2016) Mechanisms involved in triggering rheumatoid arthritis. Immunol Rev 269(1):162–174. PubMed PMID: 26683152. Epub 2015/12/20. eng
46. Arthritis AFWir (2015) www.arthritis.org/about-arthritis/types/rheumatoid-arthritis/what-is-rheumatoid-arthritis.php

47. Kirtikar KR, Basu BEB (1975) Indian medicinal plants. In: Dun D (ed) Bishen Singh Mahendra Pal Singh
48. Kubo M, Ma S, Wu J, Matsuda H (1996) Anti-inflammatory activities of 70 % methanolic extract from Cinnamomi Cortex. Biol Pharm Bull 19(8):1041–1045. PubMed PMID: 8874812. Epub 1996/08/01. eng
49. Mitra SK, Sundaram R, Venkataranganna MV, Gopumadhavan S, Prakash NS, Jayaram HD et al (2000) Anti-inflammatory, antioxidant and antimicrobial activity of Ophthacare brand, an herbal eye drops. Phytomed Int J Phytotherapy Phytopharmacol 7(2):123–127. PubMed PMID: 10839215. Epub 2000/06/06. eng
50. Atta AH, Alkofahi A (1998) Anti-nociceptive and anti-inflammatory effects of some Jordanian medicinal plant extracts. J Ethnopharmacol 60(2):117–124. PubMed PMID: 9582001. Epub 1998/05/15. eng
51. Ravindran PN, Nirmal-Babu K, Shylaja M (2003) Cinnamon and cassia: the genus Cinnamomum. CRS Press
52. Chang H-M, But P-H (1886) Pharmacology and applications of Chinese materia medica. Singapore: World Scientific
53. Lee BJ, Kim YJ, Cho DH, Sohn NW, Kang H (2011) Immunomodulatory effect of water extract of cinnamon on anti-CD3-induced cytokine responses and p38, JNK, ERK1/2, and STAT4 activation. Immunopharmacol Immunotoxicol 33(4):714–722. PubMed PMID: 22053946. Epub 2011/11/08. eng
54. Cao H, Urban JF Jr, Anderson RA (2008) Cinnamon polyphenol extract affects immune responses by regulating anti- and proinflammatory and glucose transporter gene expression in mouse macrophages. J Nutr 138(5):833–840. PubMed PMID: 18424588. Epub 2008/04/22. eng
55. Garella S, Matarese RA (1984) Renal effects of prostaglandins and clinical adverse effects of nonsteroidal anti-inflammatory agents. Medicine (Baltimore) 63(3):165–181. PubMed PMID: 6371441. Epub 1984/05/01. eng
56. Kang H, Park SH, Yun JM, Nam TG, Kim YE, Kim DO et al (2014) Effect of cinnamon water extract on monocyte-to-macrophage differentiation and scavenger receptor activity. BMC Complement Altern Med 14:90. PubMed PMID: 24602512. Pubmed Central PMCID: PMC3973967. Epub 2014/03/08. eng
57. McGowan MP, Proulx S (2009) Nutritional supplements and serum lipids: does anything work? Curr Atherosclerosis Rep 11(6):470–476. PubMed PMID: 19852889. Epub 2009/10/27. eng
58. Brites F, Zago V, Verona J, Muzzio ML, Wikinski R, Schreier L (2006) HDL capacity to inhibit LDL oxidation in well-trained triathletes. Life Sci 78(26):3074–3081. PubMed PMID: 16488445. Epub 2006/02/21. eng
59. Kloner RA, Simkhovich BZ (2005) Benefit of an exercise program before myocardial infarction. J Am Coll Cardiol 45(6):939–940. PubMed PMID: 15766832. Epub 2005/03/16. eng
60. Chenni A, Yahia DA, Boukortt FO, Prost J, Lacaille-Dubois MA, Bouchenak M (2007) Effect of aqueous extract of *Ajuga iva* supplementation on plasma lipid profile and tissue antioxidant status in rats fed a high-cholesterol diet. J Ethnopharmacol 109(2):207–213. PubMed PMID: 16949233. Epub 2006/09/05. eng
61. Mancini-Filho J, Van-Koiij A, Mancini DA, Cozzolino FF, Torres RP (1998) Antioxidant activity of cinnamon (*Cinnamomum Zeylanicum*, Breyne) extracts. Boll Chim Farm 137 (11):443–447. PubMed PMID: 10077878. Epub 1999/03/17. eng
62. Jayaprakasha GK, Jagan Mohan Rao L, Sakariah KK (2003) Volatile constituents from *Cinnamomum zeylanicum* fruit stalks and their antioxidant activities. J Agric Food Chem 51 (15):4344–4348. PubMed PMID: 12848508. Epub 2003/07/10. eng
63. Lee JS, Jeon SM, Park EM, Huh TL, Kwon OS, Lee MK et al (2003) Cinnamate supplementation enhances hepatic lipid metabolism and antioxidant defense systems in high cholesterol-fed rats. J Med Food 6(3):183–191. PubMed PMID: 14585184. Epub 2003/10/31. eng

64. Querfurth HW, LaFerla FM (2010) Alzheimer's disease. N Engl J Med 362(4):329–344. PubMed PMID: 20107219. Epub 2010/01/29. eng
65. van Leuven F (2000) Single and multiple transgenic mice as models for Alzheimer's disease. Prog Neurobiol 61(3):305–312. PubMed PMID: 10727777. Epub 2000/03/23. eng
66. Chauhan NB, Sandoval J (2007) Amelioration of early cognitive deficits by aged garlic extract in Alzheimer's transgenic mice. Phytotherapy Res 21(7):629–640. PubMed PMID: 17380553. Epub 2007/03/24. eng
67. Ono K, Condron MM, Ho L, Wang J, Zhao W, Pasinetti GM et al (2008) Effects of grape seed-derived polyphenols on amyloid beta-protein self-assembly and cytotoxicity. J Biol Chem 283(47):32176–32187. PubMed PMID: 18815129. Pubmed Central PMCID: PMC2583320. Epub 2008/09/26. eng
68. Kim DS, Kim JY, Han YS (2007) Alzheimer's disease drug discovery from herbs: neuroprotectivity from beta-amyloid (1–42) insult. J Altern Complement Med 13 (3):333-340. PubMed PMID: 17480132. Epub 2007/05/08. eng
69. George RC, Lew J, Graves DJ (2013) Interaction of cinnamaldehyde and epicatechin with tau: implications of beneficial effects in modulating Alzheimer's disease pathogenesis. J Alzheimers Dis 36(1):21–40. PubMed PMID: 23531502. Epub 2013/03/28. eng
70. Frydman-Marom A, Levin A, Farfara D, Benromano T, Scherzer-Attali R, Peled S et al (2011) Orally administrated cinnamon extract reduces beta-amyloid oligomerization and corrects cognitive impairment in Alzheimer's disease animal models. PLoS ONE 6(1): e16564. PubMed PMID: 21305046. Pubmed Central PMCID: PMC3030596. Epub 2011/02/10. eng
71. Glass CK, Saijo K, Winner B, Marchetto MC, Gage FH (2010) Mechanisms underlying inflammation in neurodegeneration. Cell 140(6):918–934. PubMed PMID: 20303880. Pubmed Central PMCID: PMC2873093. Epub 2010/03/23. eng
72. Ho SC, Chang KS, Chang PW (2013) Inhibition of neuroinflammation by cinnamon and its main components. Food Chem 138(4):2275–2282. PubMed PMID: 23497886. Epub 2013/03/19. eng
73. Tsai PJ, Tsai TH, Yu CH, Ho SC (2007) Evaluation of NO-suppressing activity of several Mediterranean culinary spices. Food Chem Toxicol Int J Published Br Ind Biol Res Assoc 45 (3):440–447. PubMed PMID: 17074427. Epub 2006/11/01. eng
74. Quale JM, Landman D, Zaman MM, Burney S, Sathe SS (1996) In vitro activity of *Cinnamomum zeylanicum* against azole resistant and sensitive Candida species and a pilot study of cinnamon for oral candidiasis. Am J Chin Med 24(2):103–109. PubMed PMID: 8874667. Epub 1996/01/01. eng
75. Corren J, Lemay M, Lin Y, Rozga L, Randolph RK (2008) Clinical and biochemical effects of a combination botanical product (ClearGuard) for allergy: a pilot randomized double-blind placebo-controlled trial. Nutr J 7:20. PubMed PMID: 18625073. Pubmed Central PMCID: PMC2491648. Epub 2008/07/16. eng
76. Nagai H, Shimazawa T, Matsuura N, Koda A (1982) Immunopharmacological studies of the aqueous extract of *Cinnamomum cassia* (CCAq). I. Anti allergic action. Jpn J Pharmacol 32 (5):813–822. PubMed PMID: 6184511. Epub 1982/10/01. eng
77. Hagenlocher Y, Bergheim I, Zacheja S, Schaffer M, Bischoff SC, Lorentz A (2013) Cinnamon extract inhibits degranulation and de novo synthesis of inflammatory mediators in mast cells. Allergy 68(4):490–497. PubMed PMID: 23409834. Epub 2013/02/16. eng
78. Aswar UM, Kandhare AD, Mohan V, Thakurdesai PA (2015) Anti-allergic effect of intranasal administration of type-A procyanidin polyphenols based standardized extract of cinnamon bark in ovalbumin sensitized BALB/c mice. Phytotherapy Res 29(3):423–433. PubMed PMID: 25504814. Epub 2014/12/17. eng
79. Fillatreau S, Gray D, Anderton SM (2008) Not always the bad guys: B cells as regulators of autoimmune pathology. Nat Rev Immunol 8(5):391–397. PubMed PMID: 18437156. Epub 2008/04/26. eng
80. Greenwald RJ, Freeman GJ, Sharpe AH. The B7 family revisited. Annu Rev Immunol. 2005;23:515–48. PubMed PMID: 15771580. Epub 2005/03/18. eng

81. Kwon HK, Hwang JS, Lee CG, So JS, Sahoo A, Im CR et al (2011) Cinnamon extract suppresses experimental colitis through modulation of antigen-presenting cells. World J Gastroenterol 17(8):976–986. PubMed PMID: 21451725. Pubmed Central PMCID: PMC3057159. Epub 2011/04/01. eng
82. Lima FJ, Cosker F, Brito TS, Ribeiro-Filho HV, Silva CM, Aragao KS et al (2014) Antispasmodic and myorelaxant effects of the flavoring agent methyl cinnamate in gut: potential inhibition of tyrosine kinase. Eur J Pharmacol 740:192–199. PubMed PMID: 25046838. Epub 2014/07/22. eng
83. Esmaillzadeh A, Keshteli AH, Hajishafiee M, Feizi A, Feinle-Bisset C, Adibi P (2013) Consumption of spicy foods and the prevalence of irritable bowel syndrome. World J Gastroenterol 19(38):6465–6471. PubMed PMID: 24151366. Pubmed Central PMCID: PMC3801318. Epub 2013/10/24. eng
84. Kaefer CM, Milner JA (2008) The role of herbs and spices in cancer prevention. J Nutr Biochem 19(6):347–361. PubMed PMID: 18499033. Pubmed Central PMCID: PMC2771684. Epub 2008/05/24. eng
85. Gruenwald J, Freder J, Armbruester N (2010) Cinnamon and health. Crit Rev Food Sci Nutr 50(9):822–834. PubMed PMID: 20924865. Epub 2010/10/07. eng
86. Parkin DM, Bray F, Ferlay J, Pisani P (2001) Estimating the world cancer burden: Globocan 2000. Int J Cancer 94(2):153–156. PubMed PMID: 11668491. Epub 2001/10/23. eng
87. Crabtree JE, Covacci A, Farmery SM, Xiang Z, Tompkins DS, Perry S et al (1995) Helicobacter pylori induced interleukin-8 expression in gastric epithelial cells is associated with CagA positive phenotype. J Clin Pathol 48(1):41–45. PubMed PMID: 7706517. Pubmed Central PMCID: PMC502260. Epub 1995/01/01. eng
88. Zaidi SF, Muhammad JS, Shahryar S, Usmanghani K, Gilani AH, Jafri W et al (2012) Anti-inflammatory and cytoprotective effects of selected Pakistani medicinal plants in *Helicobacter pylori*-infected gastric epithelial cells. J Ethnopharmacol 141(1):403–410. PubMed PMID: 22433535. Epub 2012/03/22. eng
89. Tabak M, Armon R, Neeman I (1999) Cinnamon extracts' inhibitory effect on *Helicobacter pylori*. J Ethnopharmacol 67(3):269–277. PubMed PMID: 10617061. Epub 2000/01/05. eng
90. Nir Y, Potasman I, Stermer E, Tabak M, Neeman I. Controlled trial of the effect of cinnamon extract on *Helicobacter pylori*. Helicobacter 5(2):94–97. PubMed PMID: 10849058. Epub 2000/06/10. eng
91. Rosti L, Gastaldi G (2005) Chronic salmonellosis and cinnamon. Pediatrics 116(4):1057. PubMed PMID: 16199729. Epub 2005/10/04. eng
92. Ranasinghe P, Jayawardana R, Galappaththy P, Constantine GR, de Vas Gunawardana N, Katulanda P (2012) Efficacy and safety of 'true' cinnamon (*Cinnamomum zeylanicum*) as a pharmaceutical agent in diabetes: a systematic review and meta-analysis. Diabet Med J Br Diabet Assoc 29(12):1480–1492. PubMed PMID: 22671971. Epub 2012/06/08. eng
93. Jarvill-Taylor KJ, Anderson RA, Graves DJ (2001) A hydroxychalcone derived from cinnamon functions as a mimetic for insulin in 3T3-L1 adipocytes. J Am Coll Nutr 20 (4):327–336. PubMed PMID: 11506060. Epub 2001/08/17. eng
94. Bandara T, Uluwaduge I, Jansz ER (2012) Bioactivity of cinnamon with special emphasis on diabetes mellitus: a review. Int J Food Sci Nutr 63(3):380–386. PubMed PMID: 22007625. Epub 2011/10/20. eng
95. Mang B, Wolters M, Schmitt B, Kelb K, Lichtinghagen R, Stichtenoth DO et al (2006) Effects of a cinnamon extract on plasma glucose, HbA, and serum lipids in diabetes mellitus type 2. Eur J Clin Invest 36(5):340–344. PubMed PMID: 16634838. Epub 2006/04/26. eng
96. Suppapitiporn S, Kanpaksi N, Suppapitiporn S (2006) The effect of cinnamon cassia powder in type 2 diabetes mellitus. J Med Assoc Thailand = Chotmaihet Thangphaet 89(Suppl 3): S200–S205. PubMed PMID: 17718288. Epub 2007/08/28. eng
97. Vanschoonbeek K, Thomassen BJ, Senden JM, Wodzig WK, van Loon LJ (2006) Cinnamon supplementation does not improve glycemic control in postmenopausal type 2 diabetes patients. J Nutr 136(4):977–980. PubMed PMID: 16549460. Epub 2006/03/22. eng

98. Markey O, McClean CM, Medlow P, Davison GW, Trinick TR, Duly E et al (2011) Effect of cinnamon on gastric emptying, arterial stiffness, postprandial lipemia, glycemia, and appetite responses to high-fat breakfast. Cardiovasc Diabetol 10:78. PubMed PMID: 21899741. Pubmed Central PMCID: PMC3180260. Epub 2011/09/09. eng
99. Khan A, Safdar M, Ali Khan MM, Khattak KN, Anderson RA (2003) Cinnamon improves glucose and lipids of people with type 2 diabetes. Diabet Care 26(12):3215–3218. PubMed PMID: 14633804. Epub 2003/11/25. eng
100. Roussel AM, Hininger I, Benaraba R, Ziegenfuss TN, Anderson RA (2009) Antioxidant effects of a cinnamon extract in people with impaired fasting glucose that are overweight or obese. J Am Coll Nutr 28(1):16–21. PubMed PMID: 19571155. Epub 2009/07/03. eng
101. Meades G Jr, Henken RL, Waldrop GL, Rahman MM, Gilman SD, Kamatou GP et al (2010) Constituents of cinnamon inhibit bacterial acetyl CoA carboxylase. Planta Med 76(14):1570–1575. PubMed PMID: 20379951. Epub 2010/04/10. eng
102. Khan A, Bryden NA, Polansky MM, Anderson RA (1990) Insulin potentiating factor and chromium content of selected foods and spices. Biol Trace Elem Res 24(3):183–188. PubMed PMID: 1702671. Epub 1990/03/01. eng
103. Berrio LF, Polansky MM, Anderson RA (1992) Insulin activity: stimulatory effects of cinnamon and brewer's yeast as influenced by albumin. Horm Res 37(6):225–229. PubMed PMID: 1292975. Epub 1992/01/01. eng
104. Ping H, Zhang G, Ren G (2010) Antidiabetic effects of cinnamon oil in diabetic KK-Ay mice. Food Chem Toxicol Int J Published Br Ind Biol Res Assoc 48(8–9):2344–2349. PubMed PMID: 20561948. Epub 2010/06/22. eng
105. Qin B, Nagasaki M, Ren M, Bajotto G, Oshida Y, Sato Y (2003) Cinnamon extract (traditional herb) potentiates in vivo insulin-regulated glucose utilization via enhancing insulin signaling in rats. Diabet Res Clin Pract 62(3):139–148. PubMed PMID: 14625128. Epub 2003/11/20. eng
106. Couturier K, Batandier C, Awada M, Hininger-Favier I, Canini F, Anderson RA et al (2010) Cinnamon improves insulin sensitivity and alters the body composition in an animal model of the metabolic syndrome. Arch Biochem Biophys 501(1):158–161. PubMed PMID: 20515642. Epub 2010/06/03. eng
107. Qin B, Dawson H, Polansky MM, Anderson RA (2009) Cinnamon extract attenuates TNF-alpha-induced intestinal lipoprotein ApoB48 overproduction by regulating inflammatory, insulin, and lipoprotein pathways in enterocytes. Horm Metab Res = Hormon und Stoffwechselforschung = Hormones et metabolisme 41(7):516–522. PubMed PMID: 19593846. Epub 2009/07/14. eng
108. Qin B, Polansky MM, Sato Y, Adeli K, Anderson RA (2006) Cinnamon extract inhibits the postprandial overproduction of apolipoprotein B48-containing lipoproteins in fructose-fed animals. J Nutr Biochem 20(11):901–908. PubMed PMID: 18993048. Epub 2008/11/11. eng
109. Hong CH, Hur SK, Oh OJ, Kim SS, Nam KA, Lee SK (2002) Evaluation of natural products on inhibition of inducible cyclooxygenase (COX-2) and nitric oxide synthase (iNOS) in cultured mouse macrophage cells. J Ethnopharmacol 83(1–2):133–139. PubMed PMID: 12413723. Epub 2002/11/05. eng
110. Oussalah M, Caillet S, Lacroix M (2006) Mechanism of action of Spanish oregano, Chinese cinnamon, and savory essential oils against cell membranes and walls of *Escherichia coli* O157:H7 and Listeria monocytogenes. J Food Prot 69(5):1046–1055. PubMed PMID: 16715803. Epub 2006/05/24. eng
111. Premanathan M, Rajendran S, Ramanathan T, Kathiresan K, Nakashima H, Yamamoto N (2000) A survey of some Indian medicinal plants for anti-human immunodeficiency virus (HIV) activity. Indian J Med Res 112:73–77. PubMed PMID: 11094851. Epub 2000/11/30. eng
112. Dudonne S, Vitrac X, Coutiere P, Woillez M, Merillon JM (2009) Comparative study of antioxidant properties and total phenolic content of 30 plant extracts of industrial interest using DPPH, ABTS, FRAP, SOD, and ORAC assays. J Agric Food Chem 57(5):1768–1674. PubMed PMID: 19199445. Epub 2009/02/10. eng

113. Kitazuru ER, Moreirac AVA, Mancini-Filhoc J, Delincee H, Villavicencioa ALCH (2004) Effects of irradiation on natural antioxidants of cinnamon (*Cinnamomum zeylanicum* N.). Radiat Phys Chem 71(1–2):37–49. Epub 2004/04/14.eng
114. Sharma V, Rao LJ (2014) An overview on chemical composition, bioactivity and processing of leaves of *Cinnamomum tamala*. Crit Rev Food Sci Nutr 54(4):433–448. PubMed PMID: 24236996. Epub 2013/11/19. eng
115. Ranasinghe P, Pigera S, Premakumara GA, Galappaththy P, Constantine GR, Katulanda P (2013) Medicinal properties of 'true' cinnamon (*Cinnamomum zeylanicum*): a systematic review. BMC Complement Altern Med 13:275. PubMed PMID: 24148965. Pubmed Central PMCID: PMC3854496. Epub 2013/10/24. eng
116. Lin LT, Wu SJ, Lin CC (2013) The anticancer properties and apoptosis-inducing mechanisms of cinnamaldehyde and the herbal prescription Huang-Lian-Jie-Du-Tang (Huang Lian Jie Du Tang) in human hepatoma cells. J Tradit Complement Med 3(4):227–233. PubMed PMID: 24716182. Pubmed Central PMCID: PMC3924998. Epub 2014/04/10. eng

Silymarin and Its Role in Chronic Diseases

Neha, Amteshwar S. Jaggi and Nirmal Singh

Abstract Silymarin is the active constituent of *Silybum marianum* (milk thistle) which is a C-25 containing flavonolignan. Milk thistle has a lot of traditional values, being used as a vegetable, as salad, as bitter tonic, and as galactogogue in nursing mothers and in various ailments such as liver complications, depression, dyspepsia, spleenic congestions, varicose veins, diabetes, amenorrhea, uterine hemorrhage, and menstrual problems. In this present chapter, a comprehensive attempt has been made to discuss the potential of silymarin in chronic disorders. An insight into modulation of cellular signaling by silymarin and its implication in various disorders such as liver disorders, inflammatory disorders, cancer, neurological disorders, skin diseases, and hypercholesterolemia is being provided.

Keywords *Silybum marianum* · Silymarin · Silybin · Isosilybin · Hepatitis · Cancer · Oxidative stress · Immunomodulation

1 Introduction

The commonly known plant milk thistle (*Silybum marianum* L. Gaertn., *Cardus marianus* L., Compositae/Asteraceae) is an ancient plant which is used over 2000 years for the treatment of various disorders [1]. Milk thistle is a tall, biennial herb up to 5–10 ft. with large prickly leaves, large purple flowering heads, and strongly spinescent stems (Fig. 1). The plant derives its name due to the presence of milky veins on the leaves [2]. The plant grows in Kashmir, southern and Western Europe, Southern America, and North America [3]. Traditionally, milk thistle was used as a vegetable in Europe. Leaves were used as salad, and seeds were used as galactogogue in nursing mothers, bitter tonic, and antidepressant, in liver complications (including gallstones), dyspepsia, spleenic congestions, varicose veins,

Neha · A.S. Jaggi · N. Singh (✉)
Pharmacology Division, Department of Pharmaceutical Sciences and Drug Research, Faculty of Medicine, Punjabi University, Patiala 147002, Punjab, India
e-mail: nirmal_puru@rediffmail.com

S.C. Gupta et al. (eds.), *Drug Discovery from Mother Nature*,
Advances in Experimental Medicine and Biology 929,
DOI 10.1007/978-3-319-41342-6_2

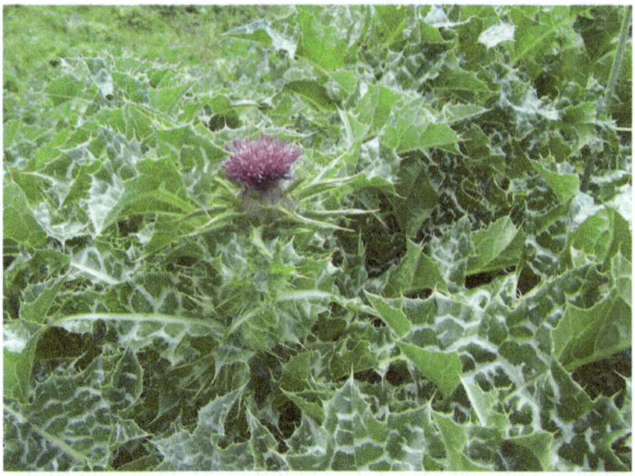

Fig. 1 Milk thistle (*Silybum marianum*) plant with large prickly leaves, purple flowering heads, and spine scent stems

diabetes, amenorrhea, uterine hemorrhage, and menstrual problems [4]. Presently, milk thistle seed, its purified extracts, and its active constituents are mainly used in liver diseases. The active constituent of *S. marianum* (milk thistle) is silymarin, which is a C-25 containing flavonolignan. It is a mixture of 65–80 % of flavonolignans, i.e. silybin A and silybin B, isosilybin A, isosilybin B, silychristin and silydianin, small amounts of flavonoids, and 20–30 % of fatty acids, betaine, apigenin, silybonol, proteins, fixed oil, and polyphenolic compounds (Figs. 2, 3 and 4) [5]. Among these chemical constituents, silybin is the biological active component. Silybin is a mixture of two diastereomers A and B in approximately 1:1 proportion. Silymarin is insoluble in water so usually given in capsule form. It is excreted in bile and its half-life is 6–8 h [6].

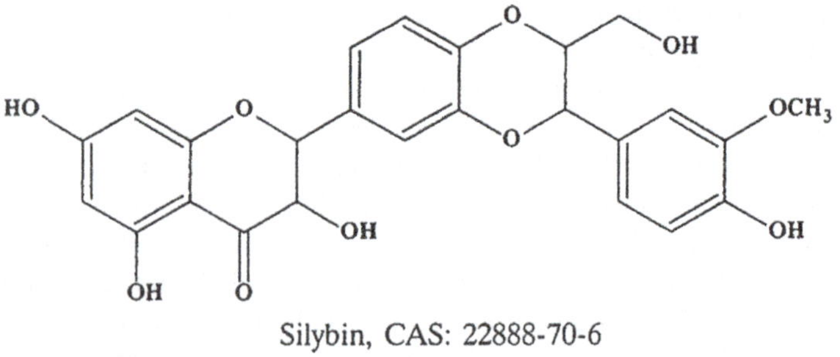

Fig. 2 Chemical structure of silybin

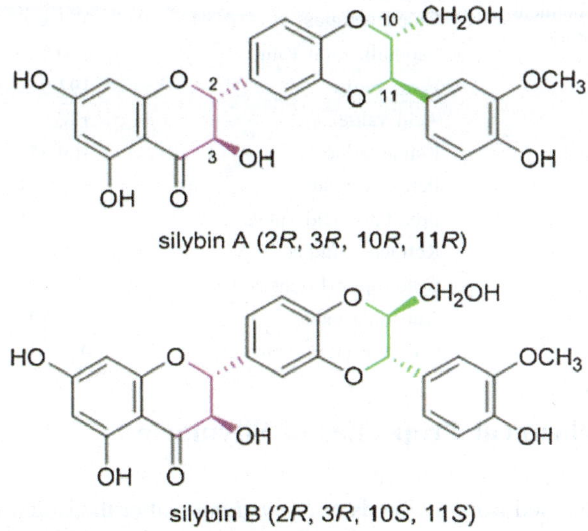

Fig. 3 Chemical structures of silybin A and silybin B

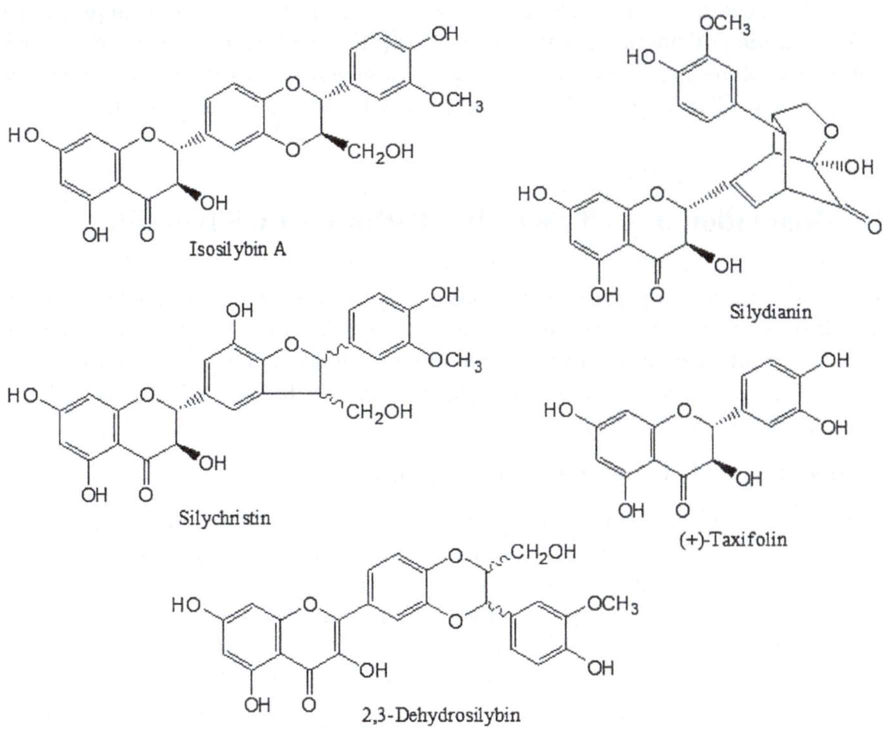

Fig. 4 Chemical structures of isosilybin A, silychristin, silydianin, taxifolin, and 2,3-dehydrosilybin

Table 1 Physiochemical properties of *Silybum marianum*

Characteristics	Value (%)
Saponification value	180.9
Ester value	193.9–195
Acid value	1.82
Iodine value	109.57
Peroxide value	14.97–17.37
Free fatty acid value	16.62–19.22
Refractive index	1.452
Color/optical density	0.3413
Anisidine value	1.8979
Chlorophyll content	0.55

2 Physicochemical Properties of Silymarin

Silymarin is extracted from the seeds of *S. marianum* after the isolation of fatty oils. Seeds are rich in fatty acid composition. The concentration of fatty oils is about 17–31 % and has similar fatty acid composition, i.e. linoleic acid > oleic acid > palmitic acid > stearic acid [7]. It has been reported that seeds of milk thistle have very low moisture content in the range of 4.24–4.72. The physiochemical properties of *S. marianum* oil are described in Table 1 [8]. From Table 1, it has been reported that *S. marianum* is rich in oil and fatty acids which is important from medicinal point of view. The seeds could be utilized as edible oil and proteins [9].

3 Modulation of Cell Signaling Pathways by Silymarin

Apart from its hepatoprotective and antioxidant effects, the use of silymarin has been broadened to other actions such as cardioprotection, skin protection, neuroprotection, and chemoprotection. This mounting attention in use of silymarin is due to its effect on cellular and molecular levels. The modulation of various cell signaling pathways is described as follows:

1. **Modulation of steroid hormone receptors**

Many compounds have been reported to inhibit or activate the expression of nuclear receptors. Polyphenolic compounds inhibit the steroid receptors due to their anti-androgenic and anti-estrogenic activities. Reports suggest that silymarin partially activates estrogen receptors (ER) whereas silybin has weak ER-mediated activity and diastereomer silybin A was found to be inactive [10]. It has been reported that both silymarin and silybin showed an anti-androgenic activity in prostate cancer cells [11].

2. **Modulation of drug transporters**

Multidrug resistance (MDR) occurs as a result of prolonged exposure of cells to a single drug. This causes a problem in the treatment of various bacterial infections and cancers. This resistance may occur via a number of mechanisms. Among these, the drug depletion in cells by membrane efflux proteins such as P-glycoprotein (Pgp) is an important mechanism. Pgp is a phosphorylated glycoprotein of size 170 kDa encoded by human MDR1 gene. This Pgp is important for the systemic disposition of various lipophilic, amphipathic drugs, toxins, carcinogens, etc. [12]. Reports suggest that silymarin is inhibitor of Pgp. Silymarin augments the doxorubicin cytotoxicity in Pgp-positive cells [13]. Silymarin has been reported to inhibit the Pgp-mediated efflux of digoxin and vinblastine resulting in their accumulation in intestinal Caco-2 cells [14]. Reports indicate that silymarin increases the accumulation of daunomycin and vinblastine by inhibiting the other drug transporter such as MRP1 (multidrug resistance-associated protein 1) [15]. Silybin was reported to be a potent, non-competitive inhibitor of trypanosomal purine transporter TbAT1. Silybin also inhibited melarsen-induced lysis of bloodstream form trypanosomes. This makes silybin a good contender for anti-parasital and/or adjuvant anti-parasite treatment [16].

3. **Modulation of inflammation and apoptosis**

Silymarin modulates inflammation by the inhibition of transcription factor NF-κB that is involved in the production of interleukins (IL-1, IL-6), tumor necrosis factor (TNF-α), lymphotoxin, interferon (IFN-γ), and granulocyte-macrophage colony-stimulating factor (GM-CSF) [17]. Silymarin inhibits TNF-α-induced activation of NF-κB which is mediated through the inhibition of phosphorylation and degradation of inhibitory protein IκBa [18]. Silymarin also inhibits TNF-α-induced activation of mitogen-activated protein kinase and c-Jun N-terminal kinase. Silybin has been reported to depress the growth and induce the apoptosis of ECV 304 cells. This occurs as a result of DNA fragmentation, cleaved and condensed nuclear chromatin, and DNA hypoploidy. Silymarin decreases the nuclear level of p65 subunit of NF-κB and change in the ratio of Bax/Bcl-2 that favors apoptosis. It also induces the release of cytochrome c and activation of caspase-3, caspase-9, cleavage of poly (ADP-ribose) polymerase (PARP), and inhibition of cell growth [19]. These results propose that silybin may exert its anti-cancer effect by inhibiting angiogenesis through induction of endothelial apoptosis via modulation of NF-κB, Bcl-2 family of proteins, and caspases.

4. **Modulation of β-catenin signaling**

It has been reported that nuclear β-catenin accumulation results in tumor progression and metastasis. Non-phosphorylated β-catenin interacts with T-cell factor transcription factor and controls the target genes such as cyclins, c-myc, and matrix metalloproteinases that are involved in cellular proliferation and migration [20]. Presence of mutated β-catenin is related to the tumor progression [21]. It has been reported that silymarin increases the expression of GSK-3β and CK-1α that leads to phosphorylation of β-catenin. This results in degradation of β-catenin and decline in nuclear accumulation [22]. Many reports also indicate that silymarin increases the binding of β-TrCP to phosphorylated β-catenin which results in degradation or inactivation of β-catenin [23].

5. **Modulation of EGFR-MAPK/ERK1/2/AKT/mTOR/PP2A signaling**

It has been evidenced that silymarin treatment inhibits transforming growth factor α-mediated activation of erbB1 in human prostate carcinoma cells. Along with this, it also inhibits the tyrosine phosphorylation of an adaptor protein Shc which is the immediate downstream target erbB1 [24]. It is reported that silymarin treatment inhibits activation of ERK1/2 that further impairs the activation of erbB1 [25]. Silymarin is suggested to be involved in suppressing the PP2Ac/AKT Ser473/mTOR pathway in colorectal cancer [26].

6. **Modulation of IGF receptor Signaling**

Silymarin is documented to increase accumulation of insulin-like growth factor binding protein-3 (IGFBP-3) in androgen-independent prostate cancer PC-3 cells. In addition to this, silybin is suggested to decrease insulin receptor substrate 1 (IRS-1) tyrosine phosphorylation that indicates the inhibitory effect on the IGF-R1 receptor-mediated signaling pathway [27].

7. **Modulation of PPAR-Gamma Pathway**

One of the components of silymarin extract such as isosilybin is reported to act as a PPAR-gamma agonist [28]. Therefore, it is suggested as a good candidate for the treatment of diabetes. Isosilybin causes transactivation of PPAR-gamma-dependent luciferase reporter in a concentration-dependent manner. This effect is reversed by PPAR-gamma antagonist T0070907 that indicates agonistic activity of isosilybin [28].

8. **Modulation of LXR pathway**

Administration of silymarin has been reported to increase the expression of peroxisome proliferator-activated receptor gamma coactivator (PGC)-1α/β, peroxisome proliferator-activated receptor (PPAR)-α, forkhead box protein O1 (FOXO1), sterol regulatory element-binding protein (SREBP)-1c, liver X receptor (LXR)-β, and fatty acid synthase (FAS) [29].

9. **Modulation of nitric oxide pathway**

Silymarin is reported to have restorative potential in endothelial damage and vascular tone which is dependent on nitric oxide [30]. Silymarin is reported to inhibit the iNOS gene expression and NO production that is responsible for its anti-inflammatory action.

4 Role of Silymarin in Chronic Diseases

Silymarin is being explored for a wide variety of disorders such as oxidative stress, inflammatory disorders, cancer, liver disorders, gastrointestinal disorders, dyspepsia, spleenic congestions, varicose veins, diabetes, amenorrhea, uterine hemorrhage, and menstrual problems. The exhaustive role of silymarin in various disorders is described below (Fig. 5):

1. **Silymarin and oxidative stress**

Many evidences report that silymarin is powerful antioxidant. It acts as a free radical scavenger and inhibits lipid peroxidation. It protects from oxidative stress by decreasing the levels of reduced glutathione [31]. It has been reported that silibinin is a powerful iron chelator, thereby inhibiting the oxidation of linoleic acid catalyzed by Fe^{2+} salts [32]. Silymarin maintains the normal membrane fluidity by directly interacting with cell membrane components, thereby preventing alteration in the content of lipid fraction [33].

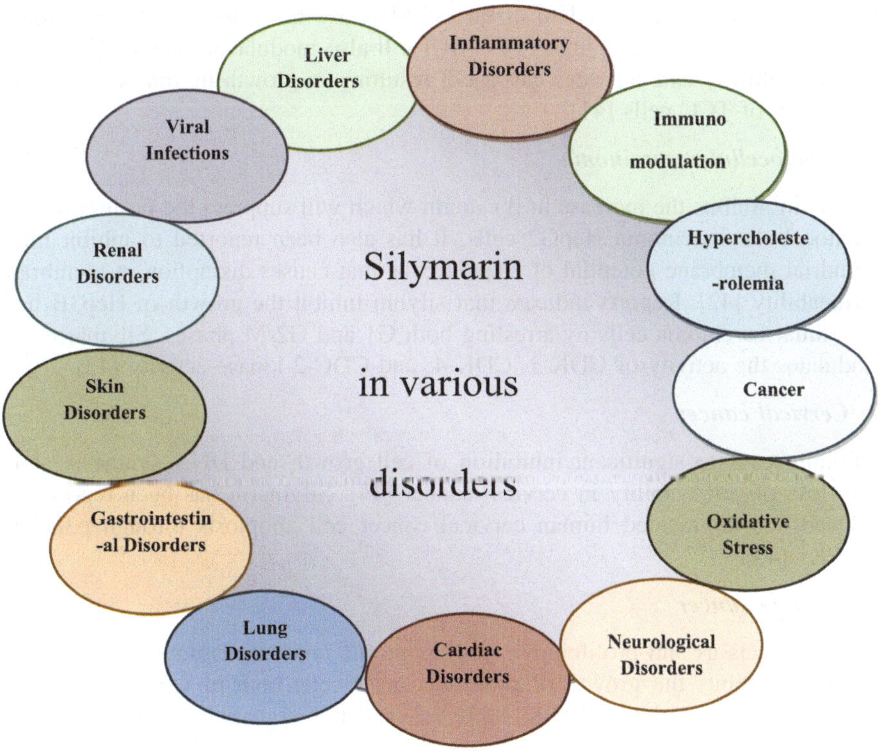

Fig. 5 Therapeutic profile of silymarin in various disorders

2. Silymarin and inflammatory disorders

Silymarin acts as an anti-inflammatory agent in the treatment of arthritis. It acts as an anti-inflammatory agent as it inhibits the migration of neutrophils to the site of inflammation [34]. It inhibits the Kupffer cells, prostaglandins, leukotrienes, and transcription factor NF-κB which regulates various genes involved in the inflammatory process [35–37]. Silymarin has been reported to inhibit the tumor necrosis factor-alpha (TNF-α), interferon-γ, IL-2, and inducible nitric oxide synthase (iNOS) [38, 39].

3. Silymarin and cancer

Silymarin has been used in variety of cancers. Silymarin has been to inhibit the growth of tumors and regression of established tumors. The chemoprotective effect of silymarin is due to its antioxidant and free radical scavenger activity. It has also been reported to modulate the multiple signaling pathways such as NF-κB, EGFR-MAPK/ERK 1/2 signaling, and IGF signaling [40]. The use of silymarin in various types of cancers is explained as follows:

- ***Bladder carcinoma***

Silymarin has been reported to arrest G2/M phase in transition cell carcinoma-human bladder cancer cell lines (TCC-SUP). It also modulates CDK1-CDK cyclin cascade pathway and activates caspase-3 resulting in growth inhibition and apoptotic death of TCC cells [41].

- ***Hepatocellular carcinoma***

Silymarin inhibits the increase in β-catenin which will suppress the proliferation of hepatocellular carcinoma HepG2 cells. It has also been reported to inhibit mitochondrial membrane potential of HepG2 cells that causes disruption in membrane permeability [42]. Reports indicate that silybin inhibit the growth of Hep3B hepatocellular carcinoma cells by arresting both G1 and G2-M phases. Silymarin also modulates the activity of CDK-2, CDK-4, and CDC-2 kinase activity [43].

- ***Cervical cancer***

Silibinin leads to significant inhibition of cell growth and DNA synthesis along with loss of cell viability in cervical cancer [44]. Silymarin has been reported to induced and augmented human cervical cancer cell apoptosis through p38/JNK MAPKs [45].

- ***Prostate cancer***

Silymarin acts as anti-proliferative, pro-apoptotic, and anti-angiogenic in prostate tumor. It inhibits the growth of prostate cancer cells both in vitro and in vivo. Silymarin also modulates MAPK, ERK 1/2, and IGF signaling pathways [46].

- ***Skin cancer***

Skin cancers occur due to ultraviolet light-induced immunosuppression and oxidative stress. It has been noticed that topical and dietary administration of silymarin to mouse prevents photocarcinogenesis. This can occur by inducing apoptosis, increase in catalase activity, and induction in cyclo-oxygenase and ornithine decarboxylase activity [47].

- ***Lung cancer***

Silibinin significantly induces growth inhibition, a moderate cell cycle arrest, and a strong apoptotic cell death in small-cell and non-small-cell human lung carcinoma cells [48]. Treatment of human lung cancer A549 cells with silymarin inhibits phosphorylation of ERK 1/2 and reduces the level of MMP-2 and u-PA [49].

4. Silymarin and Liver disorders

Liver plays a major role in detoxification of drugs and homeostasis. Exposure to toxins and pharmaceutical drugs may lead to liver damage. Silymarin has been reported to be effective in a variety of liver disorders. This effect is attributed due to its antioxidant, anti-inflammatory, anti-fibrotic activity, and many others. The role of silymarin in various liver disorders is as follows:

- ***Anti-hepatotoxic potential***

Silymarin is one of the common plant extracts used for the treatment of liver diseases. Silymarin has shown its efficacy in toxin-induced liver damage such as acetaminophen [50], arsenic [51], and carbon tetrachloride [52]. Silymarin has been reported to protect from hepatic injury induced by *Amanita phalloides*, phenothiazines, and butyrophenones [53]. These toxins disrupt liver membrane and block hepatic protein synthesis. Silymarin blocks the binding sites of these toxins.

- ***Alcoholic liver disease/cirrhosis***

Much evidence suggests that metabolism of ethanol results in the production of free radicals leading to oxidative stress in liver. Silymarin restores the normal liver function due to its antioxidant and hepatoprotective activities [54]. In addition to this, it has also been noticed that silymarin lowers the level of bilirubin, aspartate aminotransferase (AST), alanine aminotransferase (ALT) levels in alcoholic cirrhosis while the level of gamma glutamyl transferase and procollagen III peptide level decreased [55].

- ***Hepatitis***

Silymarin is reported to be effective in both acute and chronic hepatitis. Silymarin decreases the serum bilirubin, AST, and ALT levels. Liver function tests and histological improvement are noted after the administration of silymarin in chronic hepatitis [56].

- ***Liver Fibrosis***

In liver fibrosis, the hepatic stellate cells start converting into myofibroblasts leading to remodeling in the liver structure. Silymarin has been reported to inhibit the conversion of stellate cells into myofibroblasts, indicating the downregulation gene expression involved in fibrosis [57].

- ***Liver tissue regeneration***

Silymarin acts not only on the cell membrane, but also on the nucleus where it increases the formation of ribosomes and DNA synthesis resulting in protein synthesis by stimulating RNA polymerase I and the transcription of rRNA. This is an important step in the repair of cellular injury and is essential for restoring structural proteins and enzymes damaged by toxins [58].

5. **Silymarin and Immunomodulation**

Silymarin exhibits immunomodulatory effect by inhibiting the activation of human T-lymphocytes, human polymorphonuclear leukocyte, inflammatory mediators (IFN-γ, IL-2, 4, TNF-α, and nitric oxide), expression of histocompatibility complex, and nerve cell damage [59]. Silymarin has also been reported to suppress ultraviolet radiation-induced immune suppression [60].

6. **Silymarin and Hypercholesterolemia**

Reports suggest that silymarin affects the metabolism of cholesterol in different ways. Silybin has been reported to inhibit the key enzyme HMG-CoA reductase involved in the synthesis of cholesterol [61]. Silymarin inhibits the synthesis of phospholipids and triacylglycerols which is the major mechanism behind its anti-atherosclerotic and anti-hypocholesterolemic activities. Silymarin also inhibits lipids peroxidation and thereby inhibits the synthesis of triglycerides. It has been reported to reduce the level of biliary cholesterol and phospholipids in both rats and humans [62]. Silymarin decreases the plasma level of cholesterol and low-density lipoproteins (LDL) in hyperlipidemic rats. In type II hyperlipidemic patients, silymarin reduces the total cholesterol and high-density lipoproteins [63, 64].

7. **Silymarin and Neurological disorders**

Silymarin has been used in a number of neurological disorders due to its antioxidant activity and various other mechanisms. Silymarin inhibits the activation of microglia, TNF-α, NF-κB, and nitric oxide, thereby protecting the dopaminergic neurons from lipopolysaccharide-induced neurotoxicity [65]. A comparative 8-week pilot double-blind study on 35 patients suffering from obsessive compulsive disorder was conducted to evaluate the efficacy of silymarin. Results indicated that silymarin has positive effects on obsession and compulsion starting from the fifth week [66].

8. Silymarin and Cardiac Disorders

During chemotherapy some drugs such as doxorubicin results in cardio-toxicity mediated by oxidative stress and apoptosis. Silymarin has been reported to protect from cardio-toxicity due to its antioxidant activity [67]. Silymarin has been reported to be involved in cardiac preconditioning and hence protects the cardiac tissue from ischemia [68]. Amiodarone is an anti-arrhythmic drug, but due to some serious side effects, its use has been limited. Amiodarone leads to toxicity due to free radical generation, direct cytotoxicity, development of lysosomal phospholipids, indirect immunologically mediated toxic effects, and membrane destabilization. Silymarin administration along with amiodarone decreases the development of lysosomal phospholipids [69].

9. Silymarin and Lung Disorders

Silymarin has shown activity against bronchial anaphylaxis, post anaphylactic, or platelet-activating factor-induced hyper-reactivity in guinea pigs. Silymarin has been reported to be effective in asthmatic disorders by decreasing responsiveness to histamine [70]. In addition to this, silymarin has been used in lung cancer which is discussed above.

10. Silymarin and Gastrointestinal Disorders

Silymarin has been reported to exhibit anti-ulcer activity in rats. Reports suggest that silymarin undergoes excessive entero-hepatic circulation which forms a loop between intestine and liver. This prevents the disturbance in the secretion of bile resulting in the increased secretion of bile, cholate, and bilirubin excretion. It has been observed that alloxan induces diabetes mellitus. Alloxan results in the production of hydrogen peroxide and free radicals. Administration of silymarin along with alloxan prevented high plasma glucose levels and damage in pancreatic cells [71]. Silymarin has shown its efficacy in colitis and colon cancer.

11. Silymarin and Skin Disorders

Exposure to UV radiation results in a number of skin disorders such as erythema, edema, sunburn, cell formation, hyperplasia, immune suppression, DNA damage, photoaging, melanogenesis, and skin cancers. This may be due to the generation of free radicals, which causes oxidative stress in skin cells. It has been noticed that topical and dietary administration of silymarin to mouse prevents photocarcinogenesis. This can occur by inducing apoptosis, increase in catalase activity, and induction in cyclo-oxygenase and ornithine decarboxylase activity [59]. Silymarin has been reported to shown efficacy in psoriasis because it inhibits cAMP phosphodiesterase and leukotriene synthesis [72]. Silymarin decreases intracellular production of hydrogen peroxide, nitric oxide, and catalase activity in UVB-irradiated mouse skin. It also inhibits COX-2, PGE2, PGF2, PGD2 expression which plays a major role in tumor production [73]. Silymarin has been reported to inhibit the skin edema, formation of sunburn and apoptotic cells, and infiltration of inflammatory mediators [74]. Many experiments suggest that silymarin is effective against sunburn response, DNA damage, and immunosuppression. Moreover, further studies need to be investigated to determine the effect of silymarin on skin.

12. **Silymarin and Renal Disorders**

Silymarin helps to maintain normal renal function. Alloxan-induced diabetes mellitus in rats produces free radicals which damage renal tissues. Administration of silymarin along with alloxan protects the renal tissues from oxidative damage via increase gene expression of antioxidant enzymes. Therefore, silymarin is useful in the treatment of diabetic nephropathy [75]. Silymarin inhibits the expression of NF-κB, which is involved in the activation of oncogenic process. Therefore, silymarin is useful in the treatment of renal carcinoma [76]. It has been noticed that silymarin (210 mg/day for 8 weeks) in peritoneal dialysis patients inhibits the effect of pro-inflammatory cytokines such as TNF-α [77].

13. **Silymarin and Viral Infections**

Silymarin does not affect viral replication, but it has beneficial role in viral hepatitis due to its inhibitory action on inflammatory and cytotoxic processes induced by viral infection. It has also been reported to inhibit mitochondrial membrane potential of HepG2 cells that causes disruption in membrane permeability [54]. Reports indicate that silybin inhibit the growth of Hep3B hepatocellular carcinoma cells by arresting both G1 and G2-M phases. Silymarin also modulates the activity of CDK-2, CDK-4, and CDC-2 kinase activity [55]. Silymarin exerts anti-viral effect by inhibited expression of TNF-α and NF-κB in human hepatocellular carcinoma cells [78].

5 Biological Activities of Silymarin in Animal Models

(a) **Cardiovascular effects**

It has been reported that silymarin is effective in carbon tetrachloride-induced cardiac damage [79]. It has been found that silymarin ameliorates the inflammatory response-induced cardiac infarction as well as oxidative DNA damage and apoptosis caused by the toxic effects of CCl_4.

(b) **Renal effects**

Silymarin has been reported to prevent cisplatin-induced glomerular and tubular nephrotoxicity in rats [80]. Silymarin has been reported to protect the kidney tissues of rat from ischemic reperfusion injury [81]. Silymarin is shown to prevent tubular dilatation and vacuolization, pelvic inflammation, interstitial inflammation, perirenal adipose infiltration, and tubular and glomerular necrosis in Sprague Dawley rats. Along with this, Silymarin prevented I/R-induced renal damage on the basis of various kidney markers such as serum creatinine, urea, and cystatin C concentrations, serum enzymatic activity of glutathione peroxidase and serum and tissue MDA and NO levels [81].

(c) **Hepatoprotection and hepatitis**

Many reports indicate that administration of silymarin to rats, mice, rabbits, and dogs showed a significant protection against *Amanita* mushroom poisoning [82]. Before exposure to chemical hepatotoxins, pretreatment of rats and mice with silymarin attenuates lipid peroxidation and hepatotoxicity [83]. It has also been evidenced that silymarin protects the liver from alcohol toxicity. In rats with bile duct obstruction, silymarin protects due to its anti-fibrotic effect [84].

(d) **Anti-lipemic effects**

Treatment of silymarin to rats fed with cholesterol-enriched diet increases hepatic LDL clearance, which indicates silymarin has protective role in diet-induced hypercholesterolemia [85]. Silymarin has been reported to be useful in high-fat diet-induced dementia in mouse [86].

(e) **Anti-diabetic and pancreatic protectant**

Silymarin has been reported to protect the pancreas from damage in experimentally induced diabetes mellitus [87]. Silymarin and Silibinin stimulate insulin secretion from β-pancreatic cells of rats which is attributed to its anti-diabetic potential. It has been found that silymarin induces insulin resistance in Wistar rats through an increase of PTEN (Phosphatase and Tensin Homolog) [88].

(f) **Anticancer**

Silymarin has been used in different mouse models of cancer. Reports suggest that silymarin treatment protects the mice from chemical and UVB tumors [89]. The chemoprotective effect of silymarin is due to its antioxidant and free radical scavenger activity. It has also been reported to modulate the multiple signaling pathways such as NF-κB, EGFR-MAPK/ERK 1/2 signaling, and IGF signaling [40]. Silymarin inhibits the increase in β-catenin which suppresses the proliferation of hepatocellular carcinoma HepG2 cells.

(g) **Antioxidant**

Pretreatment of rats with silymarin has efficacy against ischemia-induced gastric ulcers [90]. Silymarin has been reported to act as antioxidant in three ways, i.e., by direct free radical scavenging activity, by preventing the free radical formation by inhibiting specific enzymes responsible for free radical production, and by maintenance of optimal redox status of the cell by activating a range of antioxidant enzymes and non-enzymatic antioxidants, mainly via transcription factors, including Nrf2 and NF-κB [90].

6 Biological Activities of Silymarin in Humans

As we know the use of herbal drugs is increasing throughout the world and among these herbal preparations many formulations are derived from milk thistle. Mainly this drug is used in the treatment of liver diseases from Greco-Roman era, but till now no convincing clue is obtained on its clinical efficacy. A number of clinical trials have been carried out, but these trials fail due to the number of shortcomings such as small sample size, lack of etiology, and severity of disease. Some of the biological activities of silymarin in humans are described as follows:

(a) **Hepatoprotection**

Silymarin is the most commonly used drug when liver damage and alcohol are the major factors for the liver cirrhosis. It has been observed that Europeans use silymarin in larger extent to cure liver damage due to different factors. It has been noticed that administration of milk thistle extract (Legalon) in an open label study of 2367 patients in different liver disorders for eight weeks showed a significant decline in increased liver enzymes [91]. Administration of silybin to *Amanita* mushroom poisoning protects from severe liver damage [92]. It has been evidenced that administration of silymarin in alcohol-induced liver disease in 300 patients showed a significant improvement in liver enzymes within 4 weeks [93].

(b) **Hepatitis**

Reports showed that administration of silymarin to patients with chronic hepatitis twice daily for two months results in a significant decrease in AST and ALT levels [94]. In other study, 57 patients with viral hepatitis receiving silymarin at the dose of 140 mg thrice a day for three weeks indicates lowering of bilirubin, AST, and ALT levels in 3–4 weeks as compared to the placebo-treated humans [95].

(c) **Anti-lipemic**

Reports indicate that silymarin inhibits the hepatic synthesis of cholesterol. On the basis of this, the efficacy of silymarin has been investigated in hypercholesterolemia. Studies showed that patients receiving silymarin (420 mg daily for 1 month) had significant decrease in biliary cholesterol when compared to placebo indicating inhibition of hepatic cholesterol synthesis [96].

(d) **Anti-diabetic**

In a study comprising 60 patients with hepatic cirrhosis and insulin-resistant/insulin-dependent diabetes, administration of silymarin (200 mg thrice a day daily) is observed to result in a decrease in fasting glycemia, blood glucose, glycosuria, and insulin levels within 6 months of treatment [97].

(e) **Anti-inflammatory**

Silymarin has shown anti-inflammatory potential in some clinical studies. In a double-blind placebo-controlled trial involving 40 patients with alcoholic cirrhosis, treatment of silymarin is reported to elevate lectin-induced lymphoblast transformation, and attenuate percentage of $OKT8^+$ cells [98]. Silymarin has also been reported to enhance leukocyte motility.

(f) **Anticancer**

It has been indicated that self-medication with 450 mg silymarin daily to 52-year-old man with hepatocellular carcinoma is resolved spontaneously [99]. Silymarin and silybin demonstrated chemopreventive effects in human epidermal, prostrate, and breast and cancer cell lines.

(g) **Antioxidant**

Silymarin showed an antioxidant effect by increasing the levels of superoxide dismutase in erythrocyte and lymphocytes in patients with alcoholic cirrhosis [100]. In human mesangial cell cultures incubated with glucose, silybin acts as an antioxidant by inhibiting the formation of malondialdehyde. In human leukocytes, silymarin protected against hydrogen peroxide-induced DNA damage. Silymarin has also shown antioxidant effects in human platelets.

7 Conclusion

Since herbal drugs are used for a number of approaches as they are safer and better than the standard medical drugs. Extensive research has been carried to use herbal drugs for the treatment of number of disorders. Silymarin is a well-researched drug and nowadays being explored in a variety of disorders due to its number of properties such as antioxidant, anti-inflammatory, and anti-carcinogenic. It is shown to be quite safe, has less serious side effects, and well tolerated in humans. Sufficient data are now available that document silymarin as an important therapeutic agent with lot of potential in the treatment of liver disorders, cancer, inflammatory disorders, renal disorders, skin disorders, lung disorders, and many more. Nonetheless, more effective clinical trials are required to fully explore the benefits of silymarin in these chronic disorders.

References

1. Pradhan SC, Girish C (2006) Hepatoprotective herbal drug, silymarin from experimental pharmacology to clinical medicine. Ind J Med Res 124:491–504
2. Luper S (1998) A review of plants used in the treatment of liver diseases: Part 1. Altern Med Rev 3:410–421
3. Pepping J (1999) Milk thistle: *Silybum marianum*. Am J Health Syst Pharm 56:1195–1197
4. Barceloux DG (2008) Medical toxicology of natural substances. Wiley, New Jersey
5. Hackett ES, Twedt DC, Gustafson DL (2013) Milk thistle and its derivative compounds: a review of opportunities for treatment of liver disease. J Vet Intern Med 27:10–16

6. Morazzoni P, Montalbetti A, Malandrino S et al (1993) Comparative pharmacokinetics of silipide and silymarin in rats. Eur J Drug Metab Pharmacokinet 18:289–297
7. Ruzickowa G, Fojlova J, Souckova M (2011) *Silybum marianum* (L.) Gaertn. Seed oil from the perspective of environment and genotype- a pilot study. Acta Fytotechnica Zootechnica 14:9–12
8. Goli SAH, Kadivar M, Bahrami B, Sabzalian MR (2008) Physical and chemical characteristics of *Silybum marianum* seed oil. Iran J Food Sci Technol 4:27–32
9. Khan I, Khattak HU, Ullah I, Bangash FK (2007) Study of physicochemical properties of *Silybum marianum* seed oil. J Chem Soc Pak 29:545–548
10. Pliskova M, Vondracek J, Kren V et al (2005) Effects of silymarin flavonolignans and synthetic silybin derivatives on estrogen and aryl hydrocarbon receptor activation. Toxicology 215:80–89
11. Zhu W, Zhang JS, Young YF (2001) Silymarin inhibits function of the androgen receptor by reducing nuclear localization of the receptor in the human prostate cancer cell line LNCaP. Carcinogenesis 22:1399–1403
12. Krena V, Walterov D (2005) Silybin and silymarin—new effects and applications. Biomed Papers 149:29–41
13. Zhang SH, Morris ME (2003) Effects of the flavonoids biochanin A, morin, phloretin, and silymarin on P-glycoprotein-mediated transport. J Pharmacol Exp Ther 304:1258–1267
14. Zhang SZ, Morris ME (2003) Effect of the flavonoids biochanin A and silymarin on the P-glycoprotein-mediated transport of digoxin and vinblastine in human intestinal Caco-2 cells. Pharm Res 20:1184–1191
15. Nguyen H, Zhang SZ, Morris ME (2002) Effect of flavonoids on MRP1-mediated transport in Panc-1 cells. J Pharm Sci 92:250–257
16. Maser P, Vogel D, Schmid C et al (2001) Identification and characterization of trypanocides by functional expression of an adenosine transporter from *Trypanosoma brucei* in yeast. J Mol Med 79:121–127
17. Saliou C, Valacchi G, Rimbach G (2001) Assessing bioflavonoids as regulators of NF-κB activity and inflammatory gene expression in mammalian cells. Meth Enzymol 335:380–386
18. Morishima C, Polyak SJ, Lohmann V et al (2010) Identification of hepatoprotective flavonolignans from silymarin. Proc Natl Acad Sci U S A 107:5995–5999
19. Yoo HG, Jung SN, Hwang YS et al (2004) Involvement of NF-κB and caspases in silibinin-induced apoptosis of endothelial cells. Int J Mol Med 13:81–86
20. Sinnberg T, Menzel M, Kaesler S et al (2010) Suppression of casein kinase 1alpha in melanoma cells induces a switch in betacatenin signaling to promote metastasis. Cancer Res 70:6999–7009
21. Klaus A, Birchmeier W (2008) Wnt signalling and its impact on development and cancer. Nat Rev Cancer 8:387–398
22. Liu C, Li Y, Semenov M et al (2002) Control of beta-catenin phosphorylation/degradation by a dual-kinase mechanism. Cell 108:837–847
23. Hart M, Concordet JP, Lassot I et al (1999) The F-box protein beta-TrCP associates with phosphorylated beta-catenin and regulates its activity in the cell. Curr Biol 9:207–210
24. Tyagi A, Agarwal C, Agarwal R (2002) Inhibition of retinoblastoma protein (Rb) phosphorylation at serine sites and an increase in Rb-E2F complex formation by silibinin in androgen-dependent human prostate carcinoma LNCaP cells: role in prostate cancer prevention. Mol Cancer Ther 1:525–532
25. Agarwal R (2000) Cell signaling and regulators of cell cycle as molecular targets for prostate cancer prevention by dietary agents. Biochem Pharmacol 60:1051–1059
26. Wang JY, Chang CC, Chiang CC et al (2012) Silibinin suppresses the maintenance of colorectal cancer stem-like cells by inhibiting PP2A/AKT/mTOR pathways. J Cell Biochem 113:1733–1743
27. Singh RP, Agarwal R (2004) Prostate cancer prevention by silibinin. Curr Cancer Drug Targets 4:1–11

28. Pferschy-Wenzig EM, Atanasov AG, Malainer C et al (2014) Identification of Isosilybin A from milk thistle seeds as an agonist of peroxisome proliferator-activated receptor gamma. J Nat Prod 77:842–847
29. Prakash P, Singh V, Jain M et al (2014) Silymarin ameliorates fructose induced insulin resistance syndrome by reducing de novo hepatic lipogenesis in the rat. Eur J Pharmacol 727:15–28
30. Demirci B, Demir O, Dost T et al (2013) Treated effect of silymarin on vascular function of aged rats: dependant on nitric oxide pathway. Pharm Biol [Epub ahead of print]
31. Zhao F, Shi D, Li T et al (2015) Silymarin attenuates paraquat-induced lung injury via Nrf2-mediated pathway in vivo and in vitro. Clin Exp Pharmacol Physiol. doi:10.1111/1440-1681.12448. [Epub ahead of print]
32. Ferenci P, Dragosics B, Dittrich H et al (1989) Randomized controlled trial of silymarin treatment in patients with cirrhosis of the liver. J Hepatol 9:105–113
33. Muriel P, Mourelle M (1990) Prevention by silymarin of membrane alterations in acute CCl_4 liver damage. J Appl Toxicol 10:275–279
34. Mayer KE, Myers RP, Lee SS (2005) Silymarin treatment of viral hepatitis: a systematic review. J Viral Hepatitis 12:559–567
35. Vargas-Mendoza N, Madrigal-Santillan E, Morales-Gonzalez A et al (2014) Hepatoprotective effect of silymarin. World J Hepatol 6:144–149
36. Loguercio C, Festi D (2011) Silybin and the liver: from basic research to clinical practice. World J Gastroenterol 17:2288–2301
37. Dixit N, Baboota S, Kohli K et al (2009) Silymarin: a review of pharmacological aspects and bioavailability enhancement approaches. Ind J Pharmacol 39:172–179
38. Dehmlow C, Erhard J, De Groot H (1996) Inhibition of kupffer cell functions as an explanation for the hepatoprotective properties of silibinin. Hepatology 23:749–754
39. Dehmlow C, Murawski N, De Groot H (1996) Scavenging of reactive oxygen species and inhibition of arachidonic acid metabolism by silibinin in human cells. Life Sci 58:1591–1600
40. Manna SK, Mukhopadhyay A, Van NT et al (1999) Silymarin suppresses TNF-induced activation of NF-kB, c-Jun N-terminal kinase and apoptosis. J Immunol 163:6800–6809
41. Haddad Y, Vallerand D, Brault A et al (2011) Antioxidant and hepatoprotective effects of silibinin in a rat model of nonalcoholic steatohepatitis. Evid Based Complement Altern Med 1–10
42. Colturato CP, Constantin RP, Maeda AS Jr et al (2012) Chem Biol Interact 195:119–132
43. DerMarderosian A (2001) The reviews of natural products, 1st edn. Facts and Comparisons, St. Louis
44. Meeran SM, Katiyar S, Elmets CA et al (2006) Silymarin inhibits UV radiation induced immunosuppression through augmentation of interleukin-12 in mice. Mol Cancer Ther 7:1660–1668
45. Strazzabosco M (1999) Effects of silybinin on biliary lipid composition. J Hepatol 12: 290–292
46. Bhattacharya S (2011) Milk thistle (*Silybum marianum* L. Gaert.) seeds in health. In: Preedy VR, Watson RR, Patel V (eds) Nuts and seeds in health and disease prevention, 1st edn. Academic Press (an imprint of Elsevier), London, Burlington, San Diego
47. Kshirsagar A, Ingawale D, Ashok P et al (2009) Silymarin: a comprehensive review. Pharmacognosy Rev 3:116–124
48. Kreeman V, Skottova N, Walterova D (1998) Silymarin inhibits the development of diet-induced hypercholesterolemia in rats. Planta Med 64:138–142
49. Gazak R, Walterova D, Kren V (2007) Silybin and silymarin—new and emerging applications in medicine. Curr Med Chem 14:315–338
50. Tyagi A, Agarwal C, Harrison G et al (2004) Silibinin causes cell cycle arrest and apoptosis in human bladder transitional cell carcinoma cells by regulating CDKI-CDK-cyclin cascade, and caspase 3 and PARP cleavages. Carcinogenesis 25:1711–1720
51. Das S, Roy P, Auddy RG et al (2011) Silymarin nanoparticle prevents paracetamol-induced hepatotoxicity. Int J Nanomed 6:1291–1301

52. Jain A, Yadav A, Bozhkov AI et al (2011) Therapeutic efficacy of sylimarin and naringenin in reducing arsenic-induced hepatic damage in young rats. Ecotoxicol Environ Saf 74: 607–614
53. Mohamed O, Salam EA, Saleem AA et al (2010) Hepatoprotective effects of the nitric oxide donor isosorbide-5-mononitrate alone and in combination with the natural hepatoprotectant, silymarin on carbon tetrachloride-induced hepatic injury in rats. Inflammopharmacology 18:87–94
54. Shaker E, Mahmoud H, Mnaa S (2010) Silymarin, the antioxidant component and *Silybum marianum* extracts prevent liver damage. Food Chem Toxicol 48:803–806
55. Das SK, Vasudevan DM. Protective effects of silymarin, a milk thistle (*Silybum marianum*) derivative on ethanol induced oxidative stress in liver. Indian J Biochem Biophys 43: 306–311
56. Zhang W, Hong R, Tian T (2013) Silymarin's protective effects and possible mechanisms on alcoholic fatty liver for rats. Biomol Ther (Seoul) 30:264–269
57. Ramakrishnan G, Lo Muzio L, Elinos-Baez CM et al (2009) Silymarin inhibited proliferation and induced apoptosis in hepatic cancer cells. Cell Prolif 42:229–240
58. Varghese L, Agarwal C, Tyagi A et al (2005) Silibinin efficacy against human hepatocellular carcinoma. Clin Cancer Res 11:8441–8448
59. Bhatia N, Zhao J, Wolf DM et al (1999) Inhibition of human carcinoma cell growth and DNA synthesis by silibinin, an active constituent of milk thistle: comparison with silymarin. Cancer Lett 147:77–84
60. Huang Q, Wu LJ, Tashiro S et al (2005) Silymarin augments human cervical cancer HeLa cell apoptosis via P38/JNK MAPK pathways in serum-free medium. J Asian Nat Prod Res 7:701–709
61. Sharma Y, Agarwal C, Singh AK et al (2001) Inhibitory effect of silibinin on ligand binding to erbB1 and associated mitogenic signaling, growth, and DNA synthesis in advanced human prostate carcinoma cells. Mol Carcinog 30:224–236
62. Katiyar SK, Korman NJ, Mukhtar H et al (1997) Protective effects of silymarin against photocarcinogenesis in a mouse skin model. J Natl Cancer Inst 89:556–566
63. Das SK, Mukherjee S, Vasudevan DM (2008) Medicinal properties of milk thistle with special reference to silymarin: an overview. Nat Prod Radiance 7:182–192
64. Chen PN, Hsieh YS, Chiou HL et al. Silibinin inhibits cell invasion through inactivation of both PI3K-Akt and MAPK signaling pathways. Chem Biol Interact 156:141–150
65. Wang MJ, Lin WW, Chen HL et al (2002) Silymarin protects dopaminergic neurons against lipopolysaccharide-induced neurotoxicity by inhibiting microglia activation. Eur J Neurosci 16:2103–2112
66. Sayyah M, Boostani H, Pakseresht S et al (2010) Comparison of *Silybum marianum* (L.) Gaertn. with fluoxetine in the treatment of obsessive-compulsive disorder. PNBP 34:362–365
67. Chlopeikova A, Psotova J, Miketova P et al (2004) Chemopreventive effect of plant phenolics against anthracycline-induced toxicity on rat cardiomyocytes. Part I. Silymarin and its flavonolignans. Phytotherapy Res 18:107–110
68. Zholobenko A, Modriansky M (2014) Silymarin and its constituents in cardiac preconditioning. Fitoterapia 97:122–132
69. Vereckei AS, Blazovics A, Gyorgy I et al (1993) The role of free radicals in the pathogenesis of amiodarone toxicity. J Cardiovasc Electrophysiol 4:161–177
70. Breschi MC, Martinotti E, Apostoliti F et al (2002) Protective effect of silymarin in antigen challenge- and histamin-induced bronchoconstriction in vivo guinea-pigs. Eur J Pharmacol 437:91–95
71. Soto C, Mena R, Luna J et al (2004) Silymarin induces recovery of pancreatic function after alloxan damage in rats. Life Sci 75:2167–2180
72. Kock HP, Bachner J, Loffler E (1985) Silymarin: potent inhibitor of cyclic AMP phosphodiesterase. Meth Find Exp Clin Pharmacol 7:409–413

73. Khan AQ, Khan R, Tahir M et al (2014) Silibinin inhibits tumor promotional triggers and tumorigenesis against chemically induced two-stage skin carcinogenesis in Swiss albino mice: possible role of oxidative stress and inflammation. Nutr Cancer 66:249–258
74. Katiyar SK (2002) Treatment of silymarin, a plant flavonoid, prevents ultraviolet light-induced immune suppression and oxidative stress in mouse skin. Int J Oncol 21: 1213–1222
75. Soto C, Perez J, Garcia V et al (2010) Effect of silymarin on kidneys of rats suffering from alloxan-induced diabetes mellitus. Phytomedicine 17:1090–1094
76. Kaur G, Athar M, Alam MS (2010) Dietary supplementation of silymarin protects against chemically induced nephrotoxicity, inflammation and renal tumor promotion response. Invest New Drugs 28:703–713
77. Nazemian F, Karimi GH, Moatamedi M et al (2010) Effect of Silymarin administration on TNF-α serum concentration in peritoneal dialysis patients. Phytotherapy Res 24:1654–1657
78. Polyak SJ, Morishima C, Shuhart MC et al (2007) Inhibition of T-cell inflammatory cytokines, hepatocyte NF-Kappa B signaling and HCV infection by standardised silymarin. Gastroenterology 132:1925–1936
79. Al-Rasheed NM, Al-Rasheed NM, Faddah LM et al (2014) Potential impact of silymarin in combination with chlorogenic acid and/or melatonin in combating cardiomyopathy induced by carbon tetrachloride. Saudi J Biol Sci 21:265–274
80. Nabila EA, Hania NC, Noura SAZ et al (2010) Protective effect of silymarin on cisplatin-induced nephrotoxicity in rats. Pak J Nutr 9:624–636
81. Shahbazi F, Dashti-Khavidaki S, Khalili H et al (2012) Potential renoprotective effects of silymarin against nephrotoxic drugs: a review of literature. J Pharm Pharm Sci 15:112–123
82. Laekeman G, De Coster S, De Meyer K (2003) St. Mary's thistle: an overview. J Pharm Belg 58:28–31
83. Muriel P, Garciapina T, Perez-Alvarez V et al (1992) Silymarin protects against paracetamol-induced lipid peroxidation and liver damage. J Appl Toxicol 12:439–442
84. Boigk G, Stroedter L, Herbst H et al (1997) Silymarin retards collagen accumulation in early and advanced biliary fibrosis secondary to complete bile duct obliteration in rats. Hepatology 26:643–649
85. Skottova N, Krecman V (1998) Dietary silymarin improves removal of low density lipoproteins by the perfused rat liver. Acta Univ Palackianae Olomucensis Facultatitis Med 141:39–40
86. Neha, Kumar A, Jaggi AS et al (2014) Silymarin ameliorates memory deficits and neuropathological changes in mouse model of high-fat-diet-induced experimental dementia. Naunyn Schmiedebergs Arch Pharmacol 387:777–787
87. Soto CP, Perez BL, Favari LP et al (1998) Prevention of alloxan-induced diabetes mellitus in the rat by silymarin. Comp Pharmacol Toxicol 119:125–129
88. Cheng KC, Asakawa A, Li YX et al (2014) Silymarin induces insulin resistance through an increase of phosphatase and tensin homolog in wistar rats. PLOS ONE
89. Zi X, Mukhtar H, Agarwal R (1997) Novel cancer chemopreventive effects of a flavonoid antioxidant silymarin: inhibition of mRNA expression of an endogenous tumor promoter TNF alpha. Biochem Biophys Res Commun 239:334–339
90. De La Lastra CA, Martin MJ, Motilva V et al (1995) Gastroprotection induced by silymarin, the hepatoprotective principle of *Silybum marianum* in ischemia-reperfusion mucosal injury: role of neutrophils. Planta Med 61:116–119
91. Albrecht M (1992) Therapy of toxic liver pathologies with Legalon. Z Klin Med 47:87–92
92. Salhanick SD, Wax PM, Schneider SM, Tong TC et al (2008) Comparative treatment of alpha-amanitin poisoning with N-acetylcysteine, benzylpenicillin, cimetidine, thioctic acid, and silybin in a murine model. Ann Emerg Med 52:184–185
93. Feher J, Deak G, Muzes G et al (1989) Liver-protective action of silymarin therapy in chronic alcoholic liver diseases. Orv Hetil 130:2723–2727
94. Moscarella S, Giusit A, Marra F et al (1993) Therapeutic and antilipoperoxidant effects of silybin-phosphatidylcholine complex in chronic liver disease. Curr Ther Res 53:98–102

95. Magliulo E, Gagliardi B, Fiori GP (1978) Results of a double blind study on the effect of silymarin in the treatment of acute viral hepatitis, carried out at two medical centres. Med Klin 73:1060–1065
96. Nassuato G, Iemmolo RM, Strazzabosco M et al (1991) Effect of Silibinin on biliary lipid composition experimental and clinical study. J Hepatol 12:290–295
97. Velussi M, Cernigoi AM, De Monte A et al (1997) Long-term (12 months) treatment with an anti-oxidant drug (silymarin) is effective on hyperinsulinemia, exogenous insulin need and malondialdehyde levels in cirrhotic diabetic patients. J Hepatol 26:871–879
98. Lang I, Nekam K, Gonzalez-Cabello R et al (1990) Hepatoprotective and immunological effects of antioxidant drugs. Tokai J Exp Clin Med 15:123–127
99. Grossmann M, Hoermann R, Weiss M et al (1995) Spontaneous regression of hepatocellular carcinoma. Am J Gastroenterol 90:1500–1503
100. Feher J, Lang I, Nekam K et al (1990) In vivo effect of free radical scavenger hepatoprotective agents on superoxide dismutase (SOD) activity in patients. Tokai J Exp Clin Med 15:129–134

Eugenol and Its Role in Chronic Diseases

S. Fujisawa and Y. Murakami

Abstract The active components in cloves are eugenol and isoeugenol. Eugenol has recently become a focus of interest because of its potential role in alleviating and preventing chronic diseases such as cancer, inflammatory reactions, and other conditions. The radical-scavenging and anti-inflammatory activities of eugenol have been shown to modulate chronic diseases in vitro and in vivo, but in humans, the therapeutic use of eugenol still remains to be explored. Based on a review of the recent literature, the antioxidant, anti-proliferative, and anti-inflammatory activities of eugenol and its related compounds are discussed in relation to experimentally determined antioxidant activity (stoichiometric factor *n* and inhibition rate constant) and theoretical parameters [phenolic O–H bond dissociation enthalpy (BDE), ionization potential (IP according to Koopman's theorem), and electrophilicity (ω)], calculated using a density functional theory method. Dimers of eugenol and its related compounds showed large antioxidant activities and high ω values and also exerted efficient anti-inflammatory activities. Eugenol appears to possess multiple antioxidant activities (dimerization, recycling, and chelating effect) in one molecule, thus having the potential to alleviate and prevent chronic diseases.

Keywords Eugenol · Antioxidant activity · Theoretical parameter · Anti-inflammatory activity · Preventing chronic diseases

1 Introduction

Cloves are an important spice with a wide range of traditional uses in non-Western countries, mainly as a medicinal antiseptic, analgesic, and antimicrobial agent [1, 2]. The main component of cloves is eugenol, and its isomer—isoeugenol—is produced

S. Fujisawa (✉) · Y. Murakami
School of Dentistry, Meikai University, 1-1 Keyakidai Sakado, Saitama 350-0283, Japan
e-mail: fujisawa33@nifty.com

S.C. Gupta et al. (eds.), *Drug Discovery from Mother Nature*,
Advances in Experimental Medicine and Biology 929,
DOI 10.1007/978-3-319-41342-6_3

from eugenol via a reaction that occurs naturally in cloves. These compounds are incorporated into a variety of dental materials and household and personal hygiene products including perfumes, cream lotions, soaps, and detergents and are used as flavoring agents in non-alcoholic drinks, baked foods, and chewing gum [1]. Eugenol and its related compounds are effective antioxidants that can prevent free radical-mediated diseases such as cancers, inflammatory conditions, type-2 diabetes mellitus (DM), cardiovascular disease, neurodegenerative disorders, and periodontal disease [2–4]. They can act as free radical scavengers or generators, depending on their nature and concentration, and this dual effect may influence cell viability and anti-inflammatory activity to various degrees [5]. Investigations in our laboratory have focused on the antioxidant, anti-proliferative, and anti-inflammatory activities of eugenol and its related compounds, particularly dimers of eugenol and isoeugenol. Various dimers have been previously synthesized from 4-allyl-2-methoxyphenol (eugenol), 4-hydroxy-3-methoxy-1-propenylbenzene (isoeugenol), 2-*t*-butyl-4-methoxyphenol (BHA), 2-methoxy-4-methylphenol (MMP), and 4-hydroxy-3-methoxycinnamic acid (ferulic acid) monomers; and eugenol-dimer, dehydrodi-isoeugenol (DHDI), α-diisoeugenol (R-1-ethyl-5-hydroxy-*t*-3-(4-hydroxy-3-methoxy phenyl)-6-methoxy-c-2-methylindane), MMP-dimer, BHA-dimer, and ferulic acid-dimer (*bis*-ferulic acid) (Fig. 1) [3, 6–9]. The antioxidant, anti-proliferative, and anti-inflammatory activities of these compounds together with curcumin, tetrahydrocurcumin (THC), magnolol, honokiol, 2,2′-biphenol, 4,4′-biphenol, etc., have also been investigated [10–24]. Their antioxidant activity was determined using the induction period method developed in our laboratory [6–9] and also the well-known 1,1-diphenyl-2-picrylhydrazyl (DPPH) assay. The anti-proliferative activity was determined by the [3-(4,5-di-methylthazol-2-yl)-2,5-diphenyltetrazolium bromide, yellow tetrazole (MTT)] assay, and the anti-inflammatory activity by the assessment of the inhibitory effects of cyclooxygenase (Cox)-2 and/or nuclear factor kappa B (NF-κB) on lipopolysaccharide (LPS)- or *Porphylomonas gingivalis* (Pg)-fimbria-stimulated RAW264.7 cells (a murine macrophage-like cell line) using northern blotting, Western blotting, and other techniques [10–24]. Here, we present our results and discuss the antioxidant, anti-proliferative, and anti-inflammatory activities of eugenol and its related compounds, which are of significance for selecting and designing novel nonsteroidal anti-inflammatory drug (NSAID)-like phenolic compounds for the treatment of chronic diseases. Also, the role of eugenol in the prevention of chronic diseases is discussed in relation to experimentally determined antioxidant activity [stoichiometric factor n and inhibition rate constants (k_{inh}/k_p)] and theoretical parameters (BDE, IP, and ω), which were calculated using a density functional theory (DFT) method [3, 9, 14, 19–24]. The biological activity of eugenol in animals and humans was also investigated by a review of the literature.

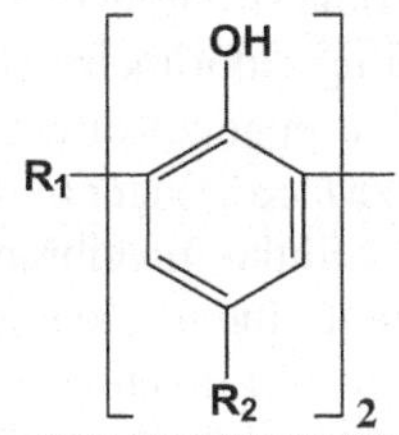

dimer	R_1	R_2
Eugenol	Methoxy	Allyl
MMP	Methoxy	Methyl
BHA	2-*t*-Butyl	Methoxy
Magnolol	H	Allyl
2,2'-Biphenol	H	H

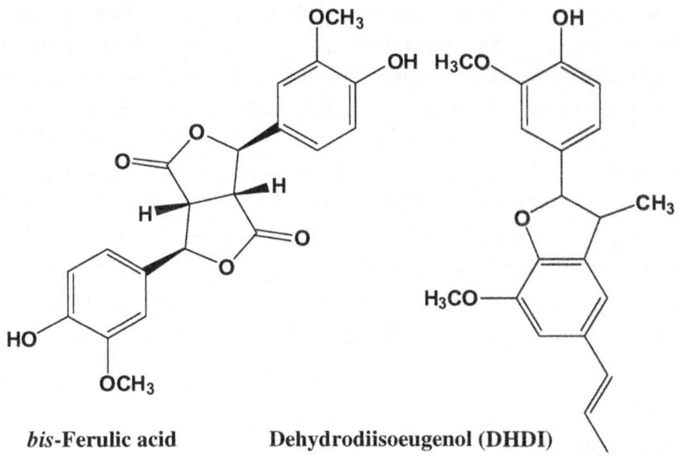

***bis*-Ferulic acid** **Dehydrodiisoeugenol (DHDI)**

Fig. 1 Structure of dimers

2 Physicochemical Properties of Eugenol

2.1 Chemistry and Metabolites

Eugenol is generally well soluble in organic solvents and sparingly soluble in water (log $P = 2.49$). Since the environments inside most living organisms are heterogeneous, a certain degree of hydrophobicity is necessary in order for antioxidants to penetrate cellular membranes. Eugenol lowers the phase transition temperature and decreases the enthalpy (ΔH) of L-α-dipalmitoylphosphatidylcholine (DPPC) liposomes in a biomembrane model and also shows little diffusion from eugenol/DPPC liposomes (1:4 molar ratio) due to its strong hydrophobic interaction with DPPC, as determined by differential scanning calorimetry (DSC) and NMR studies, respectively [25, 26]. This indicates that eugenol directly penetrates the lipid bilayer of liposomes, and exists on the surface. Eugenol is able to prevent free radical-mediated lipid peroxidation in cellular membranes containing unsaturated fatty acids by acting as an antioxidant. Indeed, eugenol has been shown to inhibit non-enzymatic peroxidation in liver mitochondria [27]. Also, eugenol binds to proteins such as serum albumin through hydrophobic interaction [28]. On the other hand, eugenol can also act as a prooxidant. Under alkaline conditions at pH 9.5, eugenol produces a phenoxyl radical at room temperature with a half-life of about 3.5 min, as determined by electron spin resonance spectroscopy (ESR), suggesting that the eugenol phenoxyl radical can exist for relatively long time in cellular systems [6]. Eugenol is converted to eugenol quinone methide (QM) via the one-electron oxidation pathway, and eugenol-QM intermediates bind to thiols such as glutathione (GSH). In the formation of oxidized GSH, oxygen consumption is increased, and a thiyl radical becomes detectable. GSH then reacts with the eugenol-QM, resulting in the formation of a eugenol-GSH conjugate [29]. The metabolism of eugenol leads to the production of cytotoxic compounds, particularly involving two pathways: a peroxidation reaction and a reaction catalyzed by P-450 microsomal enzymes [29]. This may lead to production of the 2′,3′-oxide of eugenol. Another study has revealed that the anti-DPPH radical activity of eugenol shows slow kinetics, whereas that of isoeugenol shows rapid kinetics [30]. This suggests that eugenol produces a phenoxyl radical, whereas isoeugenol produces a benzyl radical [13]. In humans, eugenol is rapidly absorbed and metabolized after oral administration, and almost completely excreted into urine as 4-hydroxy-3-methoxyphenyl-propane, isoeugenol, and other compounds [31].

2.2 *Antioxidant Activity (Stoichiometric Factor* N *and* K_{inh}/K_p*)*

Antioxidants have two forms [32]: peroxide-decomposing (preventive) antioxidants and conventional chain-breaking antioxidants. In biological systems, a variety of enzymes (such as superoxide dismutase (SOD), catalase, GSH peroxidase, GSH reductase), scavenge reactive oxygen species (ROS, comprising the hydroxyl radical OH^-, nitric oxide NO, the peroxy radical $ROO^{\cdot}$, and the alkyl radical $R^{\cdot}$), and mediate cellular events such as induction of apoptosis and necrosis. Biological systems can generate high amounts of ROS following an oxidant challenge, such as the presence of LPS, bacterial fimbriae, pro-inflammatory cytokines, or chemical and physical factors [3, 4]. Enzymes such as antioxidants prevent the generation of radicals indirectly, whereas eugenol-related compounds scavenge the radicals directly and are known as chain-breaking antioxidants. In general, the reproducibility of lipid peroxidation by free radicals in biological systems is poor because of auto-oxidation initiated by minute and highly variable quantities of impurities (e.g., peroxide and transition metal ions). Therefore, some kinetic studies have examined the use of ROO˙ or R˙ radicals. The induction period (IP_t) method has been generally applied for evaluating the inhibition rate constant (k_{inh}) of various phenols and amines in the chlorobenzene/styrene-azoinitiator system [32] and also in linoleic acid/sodium dodecyl sulfate micelles initiated by the water-soluble azoinitiator system under O_2 at 760 torr [33]. However, these studies were carried out in air, and some compounds were not detectable because their indicated induction period was too small to measure using this system [33]. By contrast, we have previously proposed the use of DSC and the induction period method in a methyl methacrylate (MMA)–benzoyl peroxide (BPO) system under nearly anaerobic conditions. This IP_t method has proved to be reliable for evaluating the activity of phenolic compounds because the DSC technique is very sensitive and extraordinarily precise [3, 6–9]. Also, living organisms have a low oxygen tension (15 torr) [32] and cancer cells are well known to exhibit anaerobic metabolism (i.e., they do not utilize oxygen). Although such initiators employed in chemical studies are not present in biological systems, data obtained in kinetic studies are useful for interpreting the mechanisms of free radical-mediated biological activities. The antioxidant activities of 23 eugenol-related compounds are shown in Table 1.

The n value (the number of free radicals trapped by one mole of phenolic antioxidant moiety) is calculated from the IP_t in the presence of inhibitors [IH] as follows:

$$n = (R_i \times [IP_t])/[IH] \tag{1}$$

where R_i is the rate of initiator BPO decomposition at 70 °C, i.e., 2.28×10^{-6} mol l^{-1} s^{-1} in this work [8, 9].

k_{inh}/k_p can be calculated using the following equation:

$$k_{inh}/k_p = [MMA]/([IP_t] \times [\,Rp_{inh}]) \tag{2}$$

where Rp_{inh} is the rate constant for chain propagation in the presence of an inhibitor. [MMA] is the concentration of methyl methacrylate and is 9.4 mol/l.

The n value of 10 monophenols and 2 polyphenols (hesperatin and hesperidin) declined in the following order: 4-hydroxyanisole (2.4) > BHA (2.2) > 2,6-di-*t*-butyl-4-methoxyphenol, DTBMP (2.00 as a control) > isoeugenol (1.7) > ferulic acid ≈ MMP (1.6) > eugenol (1.4) > guaiacol (1.1) > hesperetin (0.9) > DHDI (0.8) > vanillin (0.2) > hesperidin (0.04). In general, a monofunctional phenol reacts with two ROO˙ radicals to give a product that is stable, giving an n of 2. If the products themselves become inhibitors, this monophenol would lead to higher n values ($n > 2$), which would vary according to the nature of the second reaction, and this was the case for BHA and 4-hydroxy anisole with substituted OCH_3 at the *para* position. By contrast, the n value of eugenol, ferulic acid, MMP, and isoeugenol was reduced to 1.3–1.7 and that of guaiacol, DHDI, and hesperetin to

Table 1 Antioxidant activities and theoretical parameters (IP and BDE) for eugenol-related compounds

ID	Compound, CAS No.	IPM		Anti-DPPH·	IP	BDE
		n[a]	k_{inh}/k_p[b]	IC_{50} (mM)[c]	eV	kJ mol^{-1}
	(A) Guaiacol group					
1	Eugenol, 97-53-0	1.4	7.07	0.082	5.45	346.8
2	Eugenol-dimer, 4433-08-3	2.3	6.71	0.042	5.19 (5.46)	336.5 (354.0)
3	Isoeugenol, 97-54-1	1.7	9.0	0.055	5.18	339.2
4	α-diisoeugenol	2.7	5.87	0.05	5.28 (5.30)	343.2 (347.2)
5	DHDI, 2680-81-1	0.8	18.29	1.3	5.2	–
6	Vanillin, 21-33-5	0.2	101.1	27.4	6.08	361.9
7	Guaiacol, 90-05-1	1.1	15.71	0.108	5.53	364.6
8	MMP, 93-51-6	1.6	8.96	0.09	5.38	344.1
9	MMP-dimer	2.4	6.26	0.02	5.11 (5.02)	338.1 (338.2)
10	Curcumin, 458-37-7	3.9	4.89	0.043	5.27 (5.37)	344.0 (347.0)
11	THC, 36062-04-1	3.2	5.04	0.035	–	–
12	Ferulic acid, 537-98-4	1.6	10.56	0.145	5.7	355.7
13	*bis*-Ferulic acid	–	–	3.16[d]	5.77 (5.89)[d]	360.2 (360.9)[d]
14	Hesperetin, 520-33-2	0.9	18	–	–	–
15	Hesperidin, 520-26-3	0.02	362	–	–	–
	(B) Biphenol group					
16	Honokiol, 35354-74-6	3.2	4.77	–	5.87 (5.53)	396.4 (403.3)
17	Magnolol, 528-43-8	2.2	6.71[d]	–	5.51 (5.47)	392.4 (405.1)
18	2,2′-biphenol, 1806-29-7	0.8	32.19	–	5.97 (5.67)	287.3 (449.1)
19	4,4′-biphenol, 92-88-6	2.4	10.21	–	5.35 (5.44)	346.1 (346.1)
	(C) Anisole group					
20	4-hydroxyanisole, 150-76-5	2.4	8.16	–	5.35	343.6[e]
21	BHA, 121-00-6	2.15	6.53[d]	–	5.3	325
22	BHA-dimer	2.1	6.65	0.012	5.38 (5.15)	312.8 (319.7)
23	DTBMP, 489-01-0	(2.00)	8.21[d]	0.09	–	327.3[e]

IPM Induction period method; *IP* Ionization potential according to Koopman's theorem; *BDE* Phenolic O–H bond dissociation enthalpy

[a]Stoichiometric factor n: the number of free radicals trapped by one mole of phenolic antioxidant moiety

[b]The ratio of the rate constant of inhibition to propagation, k_{inh}/k_p

[c]The amount of inhibition necessary to decrease to the initial DPPH concentration by 50 %, DPPH 0.1 mM

[d]This work

[e]Taken from [37]; ( ), 2nd oxidation value (see the text)

Note that IDs 1–10 and 21–22 were taken from [8, 9]. IDs 11, 12, and 20 were taken from [14, 21, 24], respectively. IDs 16 and 17 from [23]. IDs 18 and 19 from [22]

approx. 1. Such a reduction is probably due to the strong hydrogen bond between the phenolic O–H and OCH_3 substituents on the benzene ring, and compounds having an *n* value of less than 2 would undergo dimerization due to the *ortho–ortho* coupling reactions derived from antioxidant phenoxyl radicals [30, 34]. The free radical coupling reaction of the guaiacol non-enzymatically leads to the formation of dimeric intermediates [35]. For the *n* values of the guaiacol group see Table 1. By contrast, the *n* value for vanillin, a guaiacol group, was 0.2, making it a very weak antioxidant, which may be explained by the presence of electron-withdrawing CHO substituent at the *para* position. For phenol dimers, the *n* values of curcumin, THC, honokiol, and α-diisoeugenol were 3–4 and they were strong antioxidants. In contrast, the *n* values of 4,4′-biphenol and magnolol and the dimers of eugenol, BHA, and MMP were 2.1–2.4 and these compounds were weak antioxidants. Interestingly, the *n* value of 2,2′-biphenol, a stereoisomer of 4,4′-biphenol, was about 1, suggesting the formation of a dimeric compound from 2,2′-biphenol molecules. Note that the *n* value of fully oxidized phenol dimers should be 4.

The anti-DPPH˙ radical activity of eugenol-related compounds is also shown in Table 1. The activity of vanillin was poor. The IC_{50} value of DHDI and *bis*-ferulic acid was 1.3 and 3.2 mM, respectively, indicating that these compounds were considerably weak antioxidants. By contrast, the IC_{50} values for curcumin, THC, α-diisoeugenol, eugenol-dimer, MMP-dimer, and BHA-dimer were 0.02–0.05 mM, their antioxidant activity being higher than that of DHDI, *bis*-ferulic acid, or the corresponding monophenols.

The k_{inh}/k_p values for a series of 23 selected eugenol-related compounds determined by the IP_t are also shown in Table 1. Hesperidin and hesperetin are polyphenols, but are grouped as monophenols because they have one hydroxyl substituent in the B ring. The k_{inh}/k_p values of monophenols declined in the following order: hesperidin (362) > vanillin (101) > DHDI (18) ≈ hesperetin (18) > guaiacol (16) > ferulic acid (11) > MMP ≈ isoeugenol (9) > DTBMP ≈ 4-hydroxyanisole (8) > BHA (7) ≈ eugenol (7). By contrast, the k_{inh}/k_p values of the dimers declined in the order 2,2′-biphenol (32) > 4,4′-biphenol (10) > magnolol ≈ eugenol-dimer ≈ BHA-dimer (7) > MMP-dimer ≈ α-diisoeugenol (6) > THC ≈ honokiol ≈ curcumin (5). For monophenols, the k_{inh}/k_p values for eugenol and BHA were the smallest, followed by 4-hydroxy anisole. BHA and 4-hydroxy anisole are well known to be polymerization inhibitors. Eugenol and BHA were the most efficient radical scavengers. Among the dimers, honokiol, THC, and curcumin were the most potent antioxidants. In the present study, there was a good significant relationship between anti-DPPH radical activity (IC_{50}) and the k_{inh}/k_p value for compounds classified as guaiacols ($n = 15$, $r^2 = 0.98, p < 0.01$); the IC_{50} value increased along with the k_{inh}/k_p value. However, there was a weak relationship between the IC_{50} and the stoichiometric factor *n* value ($n = 15, r^2 = 0.30, p < 0.05$). Considering the effectiveness of the *n* and k_{inh}/k_p values, the *n* value may be useful for estimation of intermediates and by-products produced during the IP_t.

To clarify the co-oxidation mechanism of thiols, the radical-scavenging activity of eugenol, isoeugenol, and curcumin in the presence of mercaptomethylimidazole (MMI), a thiol, was investigated using the IP_t method in the BPO-MMA system.

MMI was used as a representative thiol, since attempts to use *N*-acetylcysteine (NAC) and GSH-bearing SH groups were unsuccessful because of the fact that NAC and GSH show only limited solubility in MMA. The IP_t for the combination of curcumin, isoeugenol, or eugenol with MMI was compared to that without MMI. The curcumin/MMI (1:1 molar ratio) and isoeugenol/MMI (1:1) complex, particularly the former, showed a decrease in IP_t, indicating an antagonistic effect between the antioxidant and MMI. Conversely, the eugenol/MMI complex (1:1) showed an increase in the IP_t, indicating a synergistic effect [7]. Therefore, it was assumed that MMI reacted with the eugenol phenoxyl radical and reduced it back to the parent eugenol compound. Such a synergistic (recycling) effect and the formation of eugenol conjugates have been reported previously [29].

2.3 *Theoretical Parameters (BDE and IP) Versus* K_{inh}/K_p

In recent years, theoretical methods in combination with physical organic chemistry theory have found broad applications in studies of antioxidants. Theoretical calculation can offer a deep insight into differences in radical-scavenging mechanisms and antioxidant activities among various phenolic compounds with a wide range of structures [36]. The BDE, the lowest unoccupied molecular orbital (LUMO) energy (E_{LUMO}), the highest occupied molecular orbital (HOMO) energy (E_{HOMO}), the IP value according to Koopman's theorem (absolute HOMO value), and the η, χ, and ω values for eugenol-related compounds were taken from our previous reports [3, 8, 9, 14, 19–24], and all calculations were performed using the density function theory (DFT)Becke-3-LYP (B3LYP)/ 6-31G* method [8, 9].

BDE is the most widely used parameter of radical-scavenging activity for phenolic antioxidants and is also correlated well with the logarithm of the inhibition (radical-scavenging) rate constant (k_{inh}) for chain-breaking antioxidants. From a kinetics viewpoint, the thermodynamically preferred mechanism accords with the following equation [36, 37]:

$$-\text{RT} \ln k_{\text{inh}} = \Delta G^0_{\#} \approx \text{BDE} \qquad (3)$$

where $\Delta G^0_{\#}$ is the activation free energy. Equation 3 indicates a certain correlation between the k_{inh}/k_p and BDE values. Note that k_p is a propagation rate constant for MMA. The relationship between the k_{inh}/k_p and BDE values for 17 selected eugenol-related compounds was investigated. Except for magnolol and honokiol, a significant linear relationship in terms of BDE (note, however, that the BDE for dimers is $\text{BDE}_{2\text{nd}}$, a second H atom abstraction from the phenoxyl radical) was observed as follows:

$$\text{Log}\, k_{\text{inh}}/k_p = -1.14(\pm 0.28) + 0.01\,(\pm 0.08)\,\text{BDE} \quad (n = 17,\ r^2 = 0.33,\ p < 0.05,\ p = 0.015) \tag{4}$$

As the BDE increased, the k_{inh}/k_p also increased. Thus, the BDE of eugenol-related compounds probably plays a key role in the determination of antioxidant activity, reflecting the importance of hydrogen atom (H) transfer for radical scavenging.

Another report has demonstrated a good relationship between the k_{inh}/k_p and BDE or IP value of 2-methoxyphenols in each descriptor ($n = 5$, $r^2 = 0.95$, $p < 0.01$) [8]. Also, in the present study, a significant relationship between the k_{inh}/k_p and IP values of 23 eugenol-related compounds was observed, but the r^2 value was smaller than that of the BDE in Eq. (4). Although there was a significant relationship between the antioxidant activity and the BDE or IP value for eugenol-related compounds, the molecular mechanism regulating the antioxidant activity may be more complex than hydrogen (H)-atom abstraction, electron transfer, or proton transfer [38].

3 Modulation of Cell Signaling Pathways by Eugenol

Chronic inflammatory diseases are mediated by oxidative stress, which can activate a variety of transcription factors including NF-κB, activator protein-1 (AP-1), p53, hypoxia-inducible factor-1α (HIF-1α), peroxisome proliferator-activated receptor-γ (PPAR-γ), β-catenin/Wnt, and nuclear factor erythroid 2-related factor 2 (Nrf2) and other factors. Activation of these transcription factors can lead to the expression of over 500 different genes, including those of growth factors, inflammatory cytokines, chemokines, cell cycle regulatory molecules, and anti-inflammatory molecules [4]. The anti-proliferative and anti-inflammatory activities of eugenol and its related compounds are described in the following paragraphs.

3.1 Anti-proliferative Activity

A number of studies have investigated the mechanism responsible for the antioxidant activity of eugenol. In the HSG (human submandibular) cell line, the cytotoxicity of eugenol determined by the MTT method was one order of magnitude lower than that of isoeugenol (CC_{50}: eugenol, 0.395 mM; isoeugenol, 0.052 mM), and production of ROS (determined by carboxy-2′,7′ dichlorofluorescein diacetate (CDF) staining) was induced significantly by isoeugenol, but not by eugenol. In the presence of H_2O_2 plus horseradish peroxidase, or under visible light irradiation (which induces oxidative stress), eugenol triggered biphasic ROS production that was enhanced at lower concentrations (5–10 μM) and decreased at higher concentrations (500 μM). In contrast, isoeugenol enhanced ROS production over a wide range of concentrations (5–500 μM). Isoeugenol at cytotoxic high concentrations of 1000 μM was reduced to below the detectable levels. The high cytotoxicity of isoeugenol may be attributed to its induction of high ROS production and low GSH levels [13]. The decrease in the ROS level at higher concentrations of eugenol may be responsible for its ROS scavenging activity. Indeed, eugenol scavenged hydroxyl radicals (OH^-) effectively and also trapped OH^- directly, as determined by the electron spin resonance (ESR) spectroscopy, and was subsequently metabolized to the dimer in vitro [39]. Thus, ROS at high concentrations may have been scavenged by eugenol, and therefore, cell viability was not altered. This action of eugenol appears to be greatly different from that of isoeugenol. In general, elevated levels of ROS lead to oxidation of proteins, lipids, and nucleic acids. ROS are the main products of cellular redox processes and exert a dual effect; a low concentration of ROS can be beneficial for cellular redox signaling and immune function, but a high concentration may result in oxidative stress and subsequent damage to cell function and structure [40]. As an antioxidant, eugenol may be a substance that can scavenge harmful free radicals such as ROS and help reduce the incidence of damage due to oxidative stress, thus helping to maintain cellular redox balance.

With regard to the kinetics of their antioxidant action, cloves, eugenol and isoeugenol, are known to produce dimeric compounds and other metabolites, which probably have cell-type specificity. It has been reported that the CC_{50} values of isoeugenol for HL-60 cells, human gingival fibroblasts (HGF), and human pulp cells (HPC) were 30, 32, and 37 μM, respectively, whereas those of eugenol were 178, 232, and 214 μM, respectively. By contrast, the corresponding values of eugenol-dimer were 105, 666, and 369 μM, respectively [8]. The cytotoxicity of isoeugenol for all cell types was one order greater than that of eugenol, and interestingly, eugenol-dimer was active on HL-60 cells. In another study, eugenol-dimer was more toxic than eugenol to HL-60 cells, and DNA fragmentation was induced most strongly by eugenol-dimer, followed in order by eugenol, MMP, and MMP-dimer. Furthermore, in HL-60 cells, the expression of mRNAs for manganese (Mn) SOD and copper (Cu)/zinc (Zn) SOD, particularly the latter, was inhibited by eugenol at 1 mM and the inhibition was strongly potentiated by the addition of GSH [11]; eugenol suppressed Cu/Zn SOD activity and increased the intracellular superoxide concentration, possibly acting as an inhibitor of cytosolic (Cu, Zn) at higher concentration through its action as a metal-ion chelator. In another study using HL-60 cells, eugenol treatment reduced the mitochondrial membrane potential and also resulted in reduction of bcl_2, release of cytochrome *c*, and activation of caspase-9 and caspase-3 [41]. On the other hand, some dimeric forms of eugenol (C2-symmetric structure, as shown in Fig. 1) showed anti-proliferative activity against melanoma cells, indicating that eugenol-dimer has mild activity, whereas curcumin and a racemic mixture of brominated biphenyl have potent activities. Some synthesized curcumin-related hydroxylated biphenyls have been reported to show higher anti-proliferative activities than curcumin itself [42]. In another study, eugenol at a concentration of 0.5 μM inhibited the growth of

SBC12 primary melanoma cells and VM3211 cells in radial growth phase by 50 %, whereas isoeugenol did not inhibit melanoma cell growth up to a concentration of 0.5 μM. Eugenol, but not isoeugenol, inhibits the proliferation of melanoma cells by arresting them in S-phase of the cell cycle and inducing apoptosis [43].

In another context, where interleukin (IL)-1β-stimulated HGF cells and periodontal ligament fibroblasts have been reported to produce large amounts of IL-8, treatment with eugenol stimulated the production of IL-8 [44]. In HPC cells, eugenol inhibited IL-8 production at a higher concentration [44]. Also, in HSC-2 cells (human oral squamous cancer cell), eugenol induced non-apoptotic cell death [45]. Taken together, these results imply that eugenol is probably capable of manipulating the equilibrium between pro- and anti-apoptotic proteins [46] and also has cell-type specificity.

There are some stereoisomers among eugenol-related compounds. The mechanism responsible for the cytotoxicity of isomers and stereoisomers is complex. In studies using RAW264.7 cells, magnolol, honokiol, 2,2′-biphenolm and 4,4′-biphenol were tested for their potential cytotoxicity, and the data indicated that magnolol was more cytotoxic than honokiol, and 4,4′-biphenol was more cytotoxic than 2,2′-biphenol [22, 23]. Magnolol and 2,2′-biphenol had lower IP values than the corresponding stereoisomer, and the lower IP value enhanced the cytotoxicity. A low IP may enhance prooxidant activity via direct transfer of an electron to oxygen [47].

Phenol-induced cytotoxicity is related to the phenoxyl radical, an oxygen-centered radical; this radical may interact with redox-sensitive cysteines in DNA-binding domains of transcription factors, or it may represent a slightly enhanced transport of the phenoxyl radical in a cellular environment. The strong correlation between the IP and BDE values suggests that phenol-induced cytotoxicity might be attributable to the radical-mediated mechanism [48]. A significant linear relationship between cytotoxicity (log $1/CC_{50}$) to HSG or HGF cells and the k_{inh}/k_p value was observed for both 2-methoxy- and 2-*t*-butyl-phenols ($n = 13$, $r^2 = 0.5, p < 0.01$) [9]. This suggests that the cytotoxicity of these compounds may also be related to the BDE value, resulting from Eq. (4). In general, compounds with higher BDE (or IP) values were less toxic. For phenolic compounds, electron-donating groups reduce their BDE and IP value, whereas electron-withdrawing groups have opposite effects [47]. These findings indicate that eugenol induced cytotoxicities, toxicities, and anticancer activities are probably related to its intermediates, including antioxidant-derived radicals.

3.2 *Cox-2 Inhibition*

Cox-2 is a major contributor to increases in the spinal level of prostaglandin E_2, which augments the processing of nociceptive stimuli following inflammation. We therefore focused on the Cox-2-inhibitory activity of selected eugenol-related compounds. The inhibitory effects of eugenol-related compounds in macrophage cell lines activated with LPS or Pg. fimbriae have been investigated in our laboratory in order to develop more effective chemopreventive agents and to elucidate their mechanism of action [10–24], and the results are shown in Table 2.

The 50 % inhibitory concentration of COX-2 (IC_{50}, μM) declined in the following order: eugenol (500 <) > MMP (308) > eugenol-dimer (287) > hesperetin (256) > hesperidin (254) > MMP-dimer (250) > guaiacol (205) > vanillin (125) > ferulic acid (52) > THC (24) > isoeugenol (23) > honokiol ≈ magnolol (20) > 4-hydroxyanisole (15) > *bis*-ferulic acid (10) > BHA-dimer (9.2) > 2,2′-biphenol (7) > curcumin (6) > DHDI (0.1). The Cox-2-inhibitory activity of DHDI was the highest, followed by curcumin. NF-κB is a signaling molecule acting upstream of Cox-2 expression and also regulates the production of pro-inflammatory cytokines such as IL-6, tumor necrosis factor (TNF)-α, and prostaglandin E_2. The inhibitory effect of eugenol-related compounds on NF-κB activation is also shown in Table 2.

Table 2 Anti-inflammatory activities of eugenol-related compounds

Compound	COX-2 IC_{50} value (stimulated RAW264.7 cell) (μM)	NF-κB inhibition (stimulated RAW264.7 cell) (μM)	References
Eugenol	>500	−(500)	[10, 11]
Eugenol-dimer	286.8	++(500)	[10, 11]
Isoeugenol	23.4	ne	This work
DHDI	0.1	++(0.1)	[16]
α-diisoeugenol	>10	ne	[16]
MMP	307.9	ne	[11]
MMP-dimer	250	ne	[11]
Hesperetin	256.2	ne	[15]
Hesperidin	254.1	ne	[15]
Ferulic acid	52.1	ne	[14, 19]
bis-Ferulic acid	9.8	++(10)	[14, 19]
Guaiacol	205	−(250)	[20]
Vanillin	125	++(250)	[20]
2,2′-biphenol	6.9	++(10)	[22]
4,4′-biphenol	>10	ne	[22]
4-hydroxyanisole	15.3	+(10)	[24]
BHA	>10	−(10)	[17, 18]
BHA-dimer	9.2	++(10)	[17, 18]
Curcumin	5.8	++(10)	This work
THC	23.6	+(20)	[21]
Magnolol	20.2	++(40)	[23]
Honokiol	20.4	++(40)	[23]

++, 75 % inhibition <; +, 50 % inhibition ≫; −, no inhibition; ne, no experiment

In drug screening, it is generally considered that if the concentration of drug required for 50 % inhibition of COX-2 (IC_{50}) is less than 3 μM, this compound can be regarded as a strong enzyme inhibitor. When carrying out screening based on the activation of the Cox-2 pathway by serum-free stimulation of the human lung cancer cell line, A549, the IC_{50} threshold for candidate compounds should be less than 10 μM [49]. As has already been reported, eugenol demonstrated slightly higher Cox-2-inhibitory activity when assayed at a concentration of 1000 μM [50]. In the present study, the IC_{50} value of Cox-2 inhibition by eugenol was >500 μM. The IC_{50} values of vanillin and hesperidin, with a lower antioxidant activity, were 125 and 260 μM, respectively. The values of eugenol-dimer, MMP, and MMP-dimer were 250–300 μM, respectively. The IC_{50} values of magnolol, honokiol, and THC were approx. 20 μM, and these compounds were placed in a moderate activity group. Screening of 20 different analogs of curcumin at 50 μM showed that the inhibitory activity of curcumin on TNF-induced NF-κB-dependent reporter gene expression was most potent, followed in order by eugenol and zingerone [51]. The most effective curcumin is a compound with an aromatic *o*-methoxy phenolic group, α, β-unsaturated β-diketo moiety, and a seven-carbon linker, which is a C4-symmetric guaiacol dimer. As descried above, magnolol and honokiol without an *o*-methoxy group, 4-allylphenol dimers, showed the moderate activity; however, 4-allylphenol did not show Cox-2 inhibition at a concentration of 50 μM [52]. In another report, the IC_{50} values of honokiol and magnolol were relatively smaller concentration of approx. 15 μM [53]. Interestingly, the anti-inflammatory activity of C2-symmetric dimers, eugenol-, MMP-, BHA-, 4-allylphenol, and phenol-dimer (Fig. 1) was higher than that for the corresponding monophenols. The C2-symmetric dimers, with structural conformation, enhanced Cox-2 inhibition as well as antioxidant activity. Molecules having two symmetric potential binding moieties bearing a flexible unit of suitable length and nature would enhance binding affinity providing higher activity than those lacking these elements. The Cox-2-inhibitory activity of ferulic acid was weak, and notably, its dimer (*bis*-ferulic acid) with two symmetric potential binding moieties (Fig. 1) showed potent activity. Some kind of bioactive dimeric compound of ferulic acid should be produced via intracellular radical oxidation, as estimated from the n value of 1.6 for ferulic acid. Also, ferulic acid has been reported to interfere with the biological pathways involved in apoptosis induced by oxidative stress and inflammation caused by misfolding and aggregation of the amyloid-β peptide (Aβ) [54]. These beneficial effects may be enhanced by the formation of bioactive dimeric compounds.

The inhibitory effect of DHPI, an isoeugenol-dimer on NF-κB activation, was the most potent, followed by curcumin, *bis*-ferulic acid, and BHA-dimer.

Quantum chemical calculation might provide a closer insight into the molecular mechanisms of anti-inflammatory activity. The electronegativity ($\chi = -(E_{HOMO} + E_{LUMO})/2$) and chemical hardness ($\eta = (E_{LUMO} - E_{HOMO})/2$) principle can be applied at the level of ligand-receptor binding in order to predict the genotoxicity and carcinogenicity of various chemicals [55]. The molecular χ is first equalized with that of the receptor, leading to selection of a molecular fragment with χ

complementary to that of the receptor, or adjustment of the receptor pocket to fit with the ligand χ. From these hypotheses, it is assumed that the Cox-2 enzyme and NF-κB proteins activated by pro-inflammatory stimuli such as LPS, ROS, and bacterial fimbriae may be controlled by the χ value of phenolic antioxidants such as biphenols and polyphenols. In a similar context, the ω value ($\omega = \chi^2/2\eta$) in particular has been used for electrophilic ranking of reactive compounds, as it seems to be related to both biological effects and the reactivity of unsaturated compounds with nucleophilic additions [56, 57]. Therefore, the ω value may be highly applicable for estimating the inhibitory effect of eugenol-related compounds on Cox-2 expression [3]. The ω value may be related to the anti-inflammatory activity of these compounds because χ and η are key indicators of the overall reactivity of the molecules.

For monophenols, the ω values for eugenol, isoeugenol, guaiacol, MMP, BHA, 4-allylphenol, and DHDI were 1.13, 1.66, 1.16, 1.12, 1.40, 0.95, and 1.64 eV, respectively, whereas those for eugenol-dimer, MMP-dimer, and BHA-dimer were 1.69, 1.62, and 2.15 eV, respectively, and those for curcumin, magnolol, honokiol, and 2,2′-biphenol were 4.65, 2.36, 2.45, and 2.10 eV, respectively [3, 9, 23]. Note that the ω values for monophenols lie within the one-electron oxidation pathway, whereas those for dimers lie within the two-electron oxidation pathway. Curcumin had the largest ω value, followed in order by magnolol, honokiol, BHA-dimer, and 2.2′-biphenol. Curcumin with the highest ω value showed efficient anti-inflammatory activity. However, despite the potent anti-inflammatory activity of DHDI, this compound did not have a high ω value, and therefore, the activity of DHDI may be attributable to other factors such as the formation of dimeric compounds. Further studies to clarify the molecular mechanism of DHDI will be necessary.

4 Role of Eugenol in Chronic Diseases

Extensive research has demonstrated the mechanism by which persistent oxidative stress can lead to chronic inflammation, which in turn could cause many chronic diseases such as cancer, type-2 DM, stroke, obesity, arthritis, and others. Oxidative stress is defined as a disturbance in the balance between the production of ROS and antioxidant defenses through elimination by protective mechanisms [4]. ROS play a central role both upstream and downstream of the NF-κB and TNF-α pathways, which are located at the center of the inflammatory response. Chronic diseases are radical-mediated, and eugenol and its related compounds scavenge free radicals and help reduce the incidence of oxidative stress-induced damage, thus preventing chronic inflammatory diseases. We have been actively searching for phytophenol antioxidants that might have preventive effects against chronic periodontal disease (PD) and other oral diseases, including cancers, in view of the possible link between such oral diseases and systemic diseases.

For this purpose, we have investigated the anti-inflammatory activity of eugenol and its related compounds in vitro using RAW264.7 cells stimulated with LPS or Pg. fimbriae. Chronic PD is induced by an inflammatory host immune response to Pg pathogenic bacteria. LPS and Pg fimbriae produce large amounts of ROS and damage both the gingival tissue and alveolar bone [58]. Eugenol at relatively high concentrations inhibited Cox-2 expression in RAW264.7 cells stimulated with LPS or Pg fimbriae, and some eugenol-related compounds exerted potent anti-inflammatory activity at relatively low concentrations (Table 2). In another study, eugenol dose-dependently inhibited the receptor activator of NF-κB ligand (RANKL)-induced formation of multinucleated osteoclasts and tartrate-resistant acid phosphatase (TRAP) activity in RAW264.7 macrophages [59]. The therapeutic role of eugenol for chronic inflammatory diseases will be discussed in the following sections.

5 Biological Activities of Eugenol in Animal Models

Studies to demonstrate the chemopreventive efficacy of eugenol against free radical-mediated chronic diseases in vivo have been limited [60]. Some anticancer studies using chemically induced tumor models have been reviewed. Skin tumors were initiated by the application of 7,12-dimethylbenzanthracene (DMBA) and promoted by 12-*o*-tetradecanoylphorbol-13-acetate (TPA). Initiation with DMBA led to significant upregulation of p53 expression with a concomitant increase in p21 (WAF1) levels in epidermal cells, indicating induction of DNA damage. However, pretreatment with eugenol led to overexpression of these genes, which probably helped stimulate apoptosis of the damaged cells. Eugenol inhibited the activation of NF-κB and markedly protected against chemically induced skin cancer [61].

Also, eugenol exhibited chemopreventive effects against *N*-methyl-N′-nitro-N-nitrosoguanidine (MNNG)-induced gastric carcinogenesis in Wistar rats, as determined by the analysis of markers of apoptosis, invasion, and angiogenesis. Administration of eugenol induced apoptosis via the mitochondrial pathway by modulating the Bcl-2 family proteins, Apaf-1, cytochrome *c*, and caspases, and by inhibiting invasion and angiogenesis, as evidenced by changes in the activities of their markers. Administration of eugenol significantly reduced the incidence of MNNG-induced gastric tumors by suppressing NF-κB activation and modulating the expression of NF-κB target genes that regulate cell proliferation and survival. Eugenol is an attractive candidate for the prevention of tumor progression [46]. Another report has indicated that thioacetamide (TA)-induced hepatic injury in adult Wistar rats was suppressed by eugenol. Eugenol pretreatment prevented liver injury by decreasing cytochrome P4502E1 (CYP2E1) activity, lipid peroxidation indices, protein oxidation, and inflammatory markers. Eugenol pretreatment prevented DNA strand breaks induced by TA. Increased expression of the Cox-2 gene induced by TA was also abolished by eugenol [62]. These studies demonstrated that eugenol inhibits the upstream signaling molecule, NF-κB and NF-κB-regulated genes, and markedly protects against chemically induced breast, skin, gastric, or hepatic cancer, possibly by virtue of its anti-proliferative, anti-inflammatory, and antioxidant activities.

On the other hand, both transition metals and radicals are well known to play key roles in a number of chronic diseases. Many natural products such as, ascorbic acid, α-tocopherol, and GSH are also known to possess both metal-chelating and radical-scavenging properties. Eugenol can also bind the transition metal ion, Zn^{2+} [3]. Zn is an essential component of numerous proteins involved in defense against oxidative stress, and deficiency of Zn may enhance DNA damage via impairment of DNA repair mechanisms. Additionally, Zn has an impact on the immune system and possesses neuroprotective properties [63]. Zn insufficiency has been associated with vulnerability to development of many tumors, whereas conversely, Zn treatment can inhibit tumor development. The fact that eugenol efficiently inhibits chemically induced tumorigenesis in animal models may be related to its simultaneous metal-chelating and radical-scavenging properties. Intrinsically, eugenol with Zn may be incorporated into the cellular bilayer due to the high liphophilic activity of eugenol. Pretreatment and administration of eugenol may help to protect the cells, tissues, and organs from damage due to tumor invasion and angiogenesis.

It has been reported that in male C57BL/6 J mice with hyperglycemia induced by a high-fat diet (HFD), eugenol significantly inhibited glucagon-induced glucose production and enhanced adenosine monophosphate (AMP)-activated protein kinase (AMPK) phosphorylation in HepG2 cells and primary rat hepatocytes. In an animal study, plasma glucose and insulin levels of eugenol-treated mice were decreased by 31–63 % in comparison with HFD controls. Eugenol effectively ameliorates hyperglycemia through inhibition of hepatic gluconeogenesis by modulating the calcium calmodulin kinase kinase (CAMKK)-c-AMP-response element-binding protein (AMPK-CREB) signaling pathway [64].

It has been considered that dehydrodiisoeugenol (DHDI) may effectively ameliorate hyperglycemia [65]. Type-2 DM is caused by a combination of insulin resistance and pancreatic β cell insufficiency. One of the receptor targets for the treatment of Type-2 DM is peroxisome PPARγ, which is a master ligand-activated transcription factor belonging to the nuclear receptor family. One potent anti-DM drug is a high-affinity agonist of PPARγ [66], bearing hydrogen bond donor and acceptor groups for interacting with threonine (Thr) 473. Thus, Thr 473 might be a critical site of interaction between the PPARγ ligand-binding domains and its agonists. A molecular modeling study has shown that DHDI exerts anti-DM activity in vitro [65].

Eugenol is well known to have antimicrobial, antinociceptive, and antiviral activities [1] and is effective for prophylaxis and treatment of vaginal and oral candidiasis in immunosuppressed rats [67, 68]. Thus, eugenol exerts anti-tumorigenic, anti-hyperglycemic, or immunosuppressive activity against chronic diseases in animal models. However, no well-controlled clinical studies of eugenol in human patients with various chronic diseases have yet been performed.

6 Biological Activities of Eugenol in Humans

Eugenol in cloves has been used to prevent infection and reduce pain and was approved in monographs of the expert panel German Commission E published between 1983 and 1993. Eugenol is widely used as the liquid constituent of zinc oxide eugenol (ZOE) chelate cement and 2-ethoxybenzoic acid (EBA)-modified ZOE cement in dentistry. ZOE has been used for pulp capping, root canal filling, and as an impression and surgical pack material. ZOE has been used as standard cement for fillings in dental work [3]. Although early evidence suggests that ZOE has promise for use in dentistry, its use as an impression material and surgical pack material is limited due to its weak allergenicity [69]. Eugenol is generally non-allergenic, although in sensitized individuals it may cause a range of tissue reactions from low-grade local to systemic. Low concentrations of eugenol are well known to exert local anti-inflammatory, antiseptic, and anesthetic effects on dental pulp. A eugenol-containing zinc oxide gel has been used as an intra-pocket delivery system for treatment of periodontitis. The gel can release eugenol into the gingival pocket at a very low concentration to prevent bacterial infection [70]. Also, eugenol may have antibacterial effects that are beneficial for dental hygiene, being included in materials such as toothpastes and mouthwashes. Since isoeugenol has potent allergenicity, isoeugenol-related compounds were evaluated by patch testing in 2262 patients, demonstrating a high degree of concomitant reactivity [71]. Reduction of sensitization potency achieved by dimerization of isoeugenol may lead to development of safer cosmetic ingredients. In the guinea pig maximization test, isoeugenol, the dimer beta-O-4-dilignol, and another dimer DHDI were classified as having extreme, weak, and moderate allergenicity, respectively [72]. These dimers may be promising candidates for cosmetic ingredients with a low sensitization risk, but no clinical trials have yet been performed. By contrast, isoeugenol acetate is present in perfumes, aftershaves, etc., but may cause contact allergy in isoeugenol-sensitized individual [73]. Many eugenol-related compounds are allergenic themselves, but are activated in the skin (e.g., metabolically) or before skin contact (e.g., via air oxidation) to form skin sensitizers [74]. Although many studies have investigated the use of eugenol for preventing chronic diseases in in vitro and animal models, the therapeutic use of eugenol in humans still remains unexplored.

7 Conclusions

We have presented the results of our experiments to determine the antioxidant, anti-proliferative, and anti-inflammatory activities of eugenol and its related compounds and discussed the molecular basis of their action when used for the prevention of chronic diseases on the basis of experimental antioxidant parameters and theoretical parameters with reference to the recent literature. Eugenol and its related compounds prevent free radical-induced chronic diseases due to their efficient antioxidant activities (as a chain-breaking antioxidant). Also, eugenol exerts anti-inflammatory activities in in vitro and animal models through suppression of pro-inflammatory cytokines such as NF-κB, TNF-α, and ILs. Eugenol and its related compounds, particularly their dimers, may have beneficial effects in the prevention of various chronic diseases.

Acknowledgments We are grateful to Toshiko Atsumi, Mariko Ishihara, Hiroshi Sakagami, Yoshinori Kadoma and Shigeru Ito for their valuable support.

References

1. Cortés-Rojas DF, de Souza CR, Oliveira WP (2014) Clove (*Syzygium aromaticum*): a precious spice. Asian Pac J Trop Biomed 4:90–96. doi:10.1016/S2221-1691(14)60215-X
2. Prakash P, Gupta N (2005) Therapeutic uses of *Ocimum sanctum* Linn (Tulsi) with a note on eugenol and its pharmacological actions: a short review. Indian J Physiol Pharmacol 49:125–131
3. Kadoma Y, Murakami Y, Atsumi T, Ito S, Fujisawa S (2009) Cloves (Eugenol). In: Aggarwal BB, Kunnumakkara AB (eds) Molecular targets and therapeutic uses of species: modern uses for ancient medicine. World Scientific, Singapore, pp 117–148
4. Reuter S, Gupta SC, Chaturvedi MM, Aggarwal BB (2010) Oxidative stress, inflammation, and cancer: how are they linked? Free Radic Biol Med 49:1603–1616. doi:10.1016/j.freeradbiomed.2010.09.006
5. Carreras A, Mateos-Martín ML, Velázquez-Palenzuela A, Brillas E, Sánchez-Tena S, Cascante M, Juliá L, Torres JL (2012) Punicalagin and catechins contain polyphenolic substructures that influence cell viability and can be monitored by radical chemosensors sensitive to electron transfer. J Agric Food Chem 60:1659–1665. doi:10.1021/jf204059x
6. Fujisawa S, Atsumi T, Kadoma Y, Sakagami H (2002) Antioxidant and prooxidant action of eugenol-related compounds and their cytotoxicity. Toxicology 177:39–54
7. Fujisawa S, Atsumi T, Murakami Y, Kadoma Y (2005) Dimerization, ROS formation and biological activity of *o*-mrthoxyphenols. Arch Immunol Ther Exp (Warsz) 53:28–38
8. Kadoma Y, Ito S, Atsumi T, Fujisawa S (2009) Mechanisms of cytotoxicity of 2- or 2,6-di-tert-butylphenols and 2-methoxyphenols in terms of inhibition rate constant and a theoretical parameter. Chemosphere 74:626–632. doi:10.1016/j
9. Fujisawa S, Kadoma Y (2012) Relationship between phenol-induced cytotoxicity and experimental inhibition rate constant or a theoretical parameter. Mini Rev Med Chem 12:477–490
10. Murakami Y, Shoji M, Hanazawa S, Tanaka S, Fujisawa S (2003) Preventive effect of *bis*-eugenol, a eugenol ortho dimer, on lipopolysaccharide-stimulated nuclear factor kappa B activation and inflammatory cytokine expression in macrophages. Biochem Pharmacol 66:1061–1066
11. Okada N, Hirata A, Murakami Y, Shoji M, Sakagami H, Fujisawa S (2005) Induction of cytotoxicity and apoptosis and inhibition of cyclooxygenase-2 gene expression by eugenol-related compounds. Anticancer Res 25:3263–3269
12. Atsumi T, Murakami Y, Shibuya K, Tonosaki K, Fujisawa S (2005) Induction of cytotoxicity and apoptosis and inhibition of cyclooxygenase-2 gene expression, by curcumin and its analog, alpha-diisoeugenol. Anticancer Res 25:4029–4036
13. Atsumi T, Fujisawa S, Tonosaki K (2005) A comparative study of the antioxidant/prooxidant activities of eugenol and isoeugenol with various concentrations and oxidation conditions. Toxcol In Vitro 19:1024–1033. doi:10.1016/j.tiv.2005.04.012

14. Hirata A, Murakami Y, Atsumi T, Shoji M, Ogiwara T, Shibuya K, Ito S, Yokoe I, Fujisawa S (2005) Ferulic acid dimer inhibits lipopolysaccharide-stimulated cyclooxygenase-2 expression in macrophages. In Vivo 19:849–853
15. Hirata A, Murakami Y, Shoji M, Kadoma Y, Fujisawa S (2005) Kinetics of radical-scavenging activity of hesperetin and hesperidin and their inhibitory a ctivity on COX-2 expression. Anticancer Res 25:3367–3374
16. Murakami Y, Shoji M, Hirata A, Tanaka S, Yokoe I, Fujisawa S (2005) Dehydrodiisoeugenol, an isoeugenol dimer, inhibits lipopolysaccharide-stimulated nuclear factor kappa B activation and cyclooxygenase-2 expression in macrophages. Arch Biochem Biophys 434:326–332
17. Murakami Y, Shoji M, Hirata A, Tanaka S, Hanazawa S, Yokoe I, Fujisawa S (2006) An ortho dimer of butylated hydroxyanisole inhibits nuclear factor kappa B activation and gene expression of inflammatory cytokines in macrophages stimulated by *Porphyromonas gingivalis* fimbriae. Arch Biochem Biophys 449:171–177
18. Murakami Y, Shoji M, Ogiwara T, Tanaka S, Yokoe I, Fujisawa S (2006) Preventive effect of ortho dimer of butylated hydroxyanisole on activator protein-1 activation and cyclooxygenase-2 expression in macrophages stimulated by fimbriae of *Porphyromonas gingivalis*, an oral anaerobe. Anticancer Res 26:2915–2920
19. Hirata A (2006) Inhibitory effects of ortho-methoxyphenol-related compounds on lipopolysaccharide-stimulated cyclooxygenase-2 expression in macrophages. J Meikai Dent Med 35:42–52 (Japanese)
20. Murakami Y, Hirata A, Ito S, Shoji M, Tanaka S, Yasui T, Machino M, Fujisawa S (2007) Re-evaluation of cyclooxygenase-2-inhibiting activity of vanillin and guaiacol in macrophages stimulated with lipopolysaccharide. Anticancer Res 27:801–807
21. Murakami Y, Ishii H, Takada N, Tanaka S, Machino M, Ito S, Fujisawa S (2008) Comparative anti-inflammatory activities of curcumin and tetrahydrocurcumin based on the phenolic O–H bond dissociation enthalpy, ionization potential and quantum chemical descriptor. Anticancer Res 28:699–707
22. Murakami Y, Ishii H, Hoshina S, Takada N, Ueki A, Tanaka S, Kadoma Y, Ito S, Machino M, Fujisawa S (2009) Antioxidant and cyclooxygenase-2-inhibiting activity of 4,4′-biphenol, 2,2′-biphenol and phenol. Anticancer Res 9:2403–2410
23. Murakami Y, Kawata A, Seki Y, Koh T, Yuhara K, Maruyama T, Machino M, Ito S, Kadoma Y, Fujisawa S (2012) Comparative inhibitory effects of magnolol, honokiol, eugenol and *bis*-eugenol on cyclooxygenase-2 expression and nuclear factor-kappa B activation in RAW264.7 macrophage-like cells stimulated with fimbriae of *Porphyromonas gingivalis*. In Vivo 26:941–950
24. Murakami Y, Kawata A, Ito S, Katayama T, Fujisawa S (2014). Inhibitory of *p*-cresol and *p*-hydroxy anisole dimers on expression of the cyclooxygenase-2 gene and lipopolysaccharide-stimulated activation of nuclear factor-κB in RAW264.7 cells. In Vivo 28:719–725
25. Fujisawa S, Kadoma Y, Masuhara E (1987) A calorimetric study of the interaction of synthetic phospholipid liposomes with lipid-soluble small molecules used as dental materials and devices. Biomed Mater Res 21:89–98
26. Fujisawa S, Kadoma Y, Komoda Y (1988) 1H and 13C NMR studies of the interaction of eugenol, phenol, and triethyleneglycol dimethacrylate with phospholipid liposomes as a model system for odontoblast membranes. J Dent Res 67:1438–1441
27. Nagababu E, Lakshmaiah N (1994) Inhibition of microsomal lipid peroxidation and monooxygenase activities by eugenol. Free Radic Res 20:253–266
28. Fujisawa S, Masuhara E (1981) Binding of eugenol and *o*-ethoxybenzoic acid to bovine serum albumin. J Dent Res 60:860–864
29. Thompson D, Norbeck K, Olsson LI, Constantin-Teodosiu D, Van der Zee J, Moldéus P (1989) Peroxidase-catalyzed oxidation of eugenol: formation of a cytotoxic metabolite(s). J Biol Chem 264:1016–1021
30. Bondet V, Brand-Williams W, Berset C (1997) Mechanism of antioxidant activity using DPPH· free radical method. Lebensm-Wiss u-Technol 30:609–615

31. Fischer IU, von Unruh GE, Dengler HJ (1990) The metabolism of eugenol in man. Xenobiotica 20:209–222
32. Burton GW, Ingold KU (1984) beta-Carotene: an unusual type of lipid antioxidant. Science 224:569–573
33. Pryor WA, Stricland T, Church DF (1988) Comparison of the efficiency of several natural and synthetic antioxidants in aqueous sodium dodecyl sulfate micelle solutions. J Am Chem Soc 110:2224–2229. doi:10.1021/ja00215a036
34. Horswill EC, Howard JA, Ingold KU (1966) The oxidation of phenol. III. The stoichiometries for the oxidation of some substituted phenols with peroxy radicals. Can J Chem 44:985–991
35. Simmons KE, Minard RD, Bollag JM (1988) Oxidative coupling and polymerization of guaiacol, a lignin derivative. Soil Sci Soc Am J 52:1356–1360. doi:10.2136/sssaj1988.03615995005200050028x
36. Zhang H-Y (2005) Structure-activity relationships and rational design strategies for radical-scavenging antioxidants. Curr Comput Aided Drug Des 1:257–273. doi:10.2174/1573409054367691
37. Amorati R, Ferroni F, Pedulli GF, Valgimigli L (2003) Modeling the co-antioxidant behavior of monofunctional phenols. Applications to some relevant compounds. J Org Chem 68:9654–9658. doi:10.1021/jo0351825.14656091
38. Cheng Z, Ren J, Yan G, Li Y, Chang W, Chen Z (2003) Quantitative elucidation of the molecular mechanisms of hydroxyl radical quenching reactivity of phenolic compounds. Bioorg Chem 31:149–162
39. Ogata M, Hoshi M, Urano S, Endo T (2000) Antioxidant activity of eugenol and related monomeric and dimeric compounds. Chem Pharm Bull (Tokyo) 48:1467–1469
40. Di Carlo M, Giacomazza D, Picone P, Nuzzo D, San Biagio PL (2012) Are oxidative stress and mitochondrial dysfunction the key players in the neurodegerative diseases? Free Radic Res 46:1327–1338. doi:10.3109/10715762.2012.714466
41. Yoo CB, Han KT, Cho KS, Ha J, Park HJ, Nam JH, Kil UH, Lee KT (2005) Eugenol isolated from the essential oil of Eugenia caryophyllata induces a reactive oxygen species-mediated apoptosis in HL-60 human promyelocytic leukemia cells. Cancer Lett 225:41–52
42. Pisano M, Pagnan G, Loi M, Mura ME, Tilocca GM, Palmieri G, Fabbri D, Dettori MA, Delogu G, Ponzoni M, Rozzo C (2007) Antiproliferative and pro-apoptotic activity of eugenol-related biphenyls on malignant melanoma cells. Mol Cancer 6:8. doi:10.1186/1476-4598-6-8
43. Ghosh R, Nadiminty N, Fitzpatrick JE, Alworth WL, Slaga TJ, Kumar AP (2005) Eugenol causes melanoma growth suppression through inhibition of E2F1 transcriptional activity. J Biol Chem 280:5812–5819
44. Koh T, Murakami Y, Tanaka S, Machino M, Sakagami H (2013) Re-evaluation of anti-inflammatory potential of eugenol in IL-1β-stimulated gingival fibroblast and pulp cells. In Vivo 27:269–273
45. Koh T, Murakami Y, Tanaka S, Machino M, Onuma H, Kaneko M, Sugimoto M, Soga T, Tomita M, Sakagami H (2013) Changes of metabolic profiles in an oral squamous cell carcinoma cell line induced by eugenol. In Vivo 27:233–243
46. Manikandan P, Vinothini G, Vidya Priyadarsini R, Prathiba D, Nagini S (2011) Eugenol inhibits cell proliferation via NF-κB suppression in a rat model of gastric carcinogenesis induced by MNNG. Invest New Drugs 29:110–117. doi:10.1007/s10637-009-9345-2
47. Wright JS, Erin R. Johnson ER, DiLabio GA (2001) Predicting the activity of phenolic antioxidants: theoretical method, analysis of substituent effects, and application to major families of antioxidants. J Am Chem Soc 123:1173–1183. doi:10.1021/ja002455u
48. Selassie CD, DeSoyza TV, Rosario M, Gao H, Hansch C (1998) Phenol toxicity in leukemia cells: a radical process? Chem Biol Interact 113:175–190. doi:10.1016/S0009-2797(98)00027-1
49. Yao JC, Duan WG, Yun Y, de Liu Q, Yan M, Jiang ZZ, Zhang LY (2007) Screening method for nonsteroidal antiinflammatory drugs based on the cyclooxygenase 2 pathway activated by serum-free stimulation in A549 cells. Yakugaku Zasshi 127:527–532

50. Kelm MA, Nair MG, Strasburg GM, DeWitt DL (2000) Antioxidant and cyclooxygenase inhibitory phenolic compounds from Ocimum sanctum Linn. Phytomedicine 7–13
51. Aggarwal S, Ichikawa H, Takada Y, Sandur SK, Shishodia S, Aggarwal BB (2006) Curcumin (diferuloylmethane) down-regulates expression of cell proliferation and antiapoptotic and metastatic gene products through suppression of IkappaBalpha kinase and Akt activation. Mol Pharmacol 69:195–206
52. Murakami Y, Kawata A, Ito S, Katayama T, Fujisawa S (2015) The radical scavenging activity and cytotoxicity of resveratrol, orcinol and 4-allylphenol and their inhibitory effects on Cox-2 gene expression and Nf-κB activation in RAW264.7 cells stimulated with *Porphyromonas gingivalis*-fimbriae. In Vivo 29:341–349
53. Lee J, Jung E, Park J, Jung K, Lee S, Hong S, Park J, Park E, Kim J, Park S, Park D (2005) Anti-inflammatory effects of magnolol and honokiol are mediated through inhibition of the downstream pathway of MEKK-1 in NF-kappaB activation signaling. Planta Med 71:338–343
54. Sgarbossa A, Giacomazza D, di Carlo M (2015) Ferulic acid: a hope for Alzheimer's disease therapy from plants. Nutrients 5764–5782. doi:10.3390/nu7075246
55. Putz MV, Ionaşcu C, Putz AM, Ostafe V (2011) Alert-QSAR. Implications for electrophilic theory of chemical carcinogenesis. Int J Mol Sci 12:5098–5134
56. Enoch SJ, Madden JC, Cronin MT (2008) Identification of mechanisms of toxic action for skin sensitisation using a SMARTS pattern based approach. SAR QSAR Environ Res 19:555–578. doi:10.1080/10629360802348985
57. LoPachin RM, Barber DS, Gavin T (2008) Molecular mechanisms of the conjugated alpha, beta-unsaturated carbonyl derivatives: relevance to neurotoxicity and neurodegenerative diseases. Toxicol Sci 104:235–249
58. Chapple IL (1996) Role of free radicals and antioxidants in the pathogenesis of inflammatory periodontal diseases. Clin Mol Pathol 49:247–255
59. Deepak V, Kasonga A, Kruger MC, Coetzee M (2015) Inhibitory effects of eugenol on RANKL-induced osteoclast formation via attenuation of NF-κB and MAPK pathways. Connect Tissue Res 56:195–203. doi:10.3109/03008207.2014.989320
60. Jaganathan SK, Supriyanto E (2012) Antiproliferative and molecular mechanism of eugenol-induced apoptosis in cancer cells. Molecules 17:6290–6304. doi:10.3390/molecules17066290
61. Kaur G, Athar M, Alam MS (2010) Eugenol precludes cutaneous chemical carcinogenesis in mouse by preventing oxidative stress and inflammation and by inducing apoptosis. Mol Carcinog 49:290–301. doi:10.1002/mc.20601
62. Yogalakshmi B, Viswanathan P, Anuradha CV (2010) Investigation of antioxidant, anti-inflammatory and DNA-protective properties of eugenol in thioacetamide-induced liver injury in rats. Toxicology 268:204–212. doi:10.1016/j.tox.2009.12.018
63. Jomova K, Valko M (2011) Advances in metal-induced oxidative stress and human disease. Toxicology 283:65–87. doi:10.1016/j.tox.2011.03.001
64. Jeong KJ, Kim do Y, Quan HY, Jo HK, Kim GW, Chung SH (2014) Effects of eugenol on hepatic glucose production and AMPK signaling pathway in hepatocytes and C57BL/6 J mice. Fitoterapia 93:150–162. doi:10.1016/j.fitote.2013.12.023
65. Saptarini NM, Saputri FA, Levita J (2014) Molecular modeling study of PPARr agonists: dehydro-di-isoeugenol, macelignan, pioglitazone, netoglitazone, and rosiglitazone as antidiabetic. Inter J Chem 6. http://dx.doi.org/10.5539/ijc.v6n2p48
66. Willson TM, Brown PJ, Sternbach DD, Henke BR (2000) The PPARs: from orphan receptors to drug discovery. J Med Chem 43:527–550
67. Chami N, Chami F, Bennis S, Trouillas J, Remmal A (2004) Antifungal treatment with carvacrol and eugenol of oral candidiasis in immunosuppressed rats. Braz J Infect Dis 8:217–226
68. Chami F, Chami N, Bennis S, Trouillas J, Remmal A (2004) Evaluation of carvacrol and eugenol as prophylaxis and treatment of vaginal candidiasis in an immunosuppressed rat model. J Antimicrob Chemother 54:909–914
69. Natsch A, Haupt T (2013) Utility of rat liver S9 fractions to study skin-sensitizing prohaptens in a modified KeratinoSens assay. Toxicol Sci 135:356–368. doi:10.1093/toxsci/kft160

70. Mahadlek J, Charoenteeraboon J, Phaechamud T (2010) Zinc Oxide Gels for periodontitis treatment. J Metal Mater Mineral 20:159–163
71. Tanaka S, Royds C, Buckley D, Basketter DA, Goossens A, Bruze M, Svedman C, Menné T, Johansen JD, White IR, McFadden JP (2004) Contact allergy to isoeugenol and its derivatives: problems with allergen substitution. Contact Dermatitis 51:288–291
72. Takeyoshi M, Iida K, Suzuki K, Yamazaki S (2008) Skin sensitization potency of isoeugenol and its dimers evaluated by a non-radioisotopic modification of the local lymph node assay and guinea pig maximization test. J Appl Toxicol 28:530–534
73. Rastogi SC, Johansen JD (2008) Significant exposures to isoeugenol derivatives in perfumes. Contact Dermatitis 58:278–281. doi:10.1111/j.1600-0536.2007.01283.x
74. Karlberg AT, Bergström MA, Börje A, Luthman K, Nilsson JL (2008) Allergic contact dermatitis–formation, structural requirements, and reactivity of skin sensitizers. Chem Res Toxicol 21:53–69

Catechins and Its Role in Chronic Diseases

Yohei Shirakami, Hiroyasu Sakai, Takahiro Kochi, Mitsuru Seishima and Masahito Shimizu

Abstract The mechanisms of action of polyphenols have attracted much attention. Catechins are generally known as tea polyphenols. Researchers have extensively investigated the molecular mechanisms of these substances, especially (−)-epigallocatechin gallate of green tea catechin, and have provided new insights in the prevention and therapy for chronic diseases. This chapter summarizes catechins and their effects on chronic diseases, including metabolic syndromes, cardiovascular diseases, neurodegenerative diseases, and cancer, focusing on the effects of green tea catechins.

Keywords Catechin · Green tea · Cancer · Chemoprevention · Obesity · Metabolic syndrome · Cardiovascular disease · Neurodegenerative disease

1 Introduction

Catechins are generally known as tea polyphenols. Tea, produced from the plant *Camellia sinensis* and brewed from its dried leaves, is one of the most widely consumed beverages throughout the world; three major types of tea are consumed globally: green, black, and Oolong teas. Green tea is usually consumed in Asian countries, while black tea is dominant in Western countries. Green, black, and Oolong teas are processed differently during manufacturing. Green tea is produced by drying and steaming fresh green tea leaves by hot steam to inactivate oxidation

Y. Shirakami (✉) · M. Seishima
Department of Informative Clinical Medicine, Graduate School of Medicine, Gifu University, 1-1 Yanagido, Gifu 501-1194, Japan
e-mail: ys2443@gifu-u.ac.jp

Y. Shirakami · H. Sakai · T. Kochi · M. Shimizu
Department of Gastroenterology, Graduate School of Medicine, Gifu University, Gifu 501-1194, Japan

S.C. Gupta et al. (eds.), *Drug Discovery from Mother Nature*,
Advances in Experimental Medicine and Biology 929,
DOI 10.1007/978-3-319-41342-6_4

of polyphenols and to prevent fermentation. Therefore, green tea is known as "non-fermented" tea. Tea leaves from black or Oolong teas are fully or partially fermented, respectively [1]. Compared to black and Oolong teas, green tea possesses a large amount of green tea catechins (GTCs), which are major polyphenols in green tea [2]. A cup of green tea with 2 g of tea leaves in 200 mL of hot water usually contains 500–700 mg of dry materials, of which 30–40 % are catechins [3]. The four major catechins are (−)-epigallocatechin gallate (EGCG), (−)-epigallocatechin (EGC), (−)-epicatechin gallate (ECG), and (−)-epicatechin (EC) [4].

Inflammation and oxidative stress are considered to be major causes of various chronic diseases [5, 6]. Various epidemiological studies have demonstrated that tea exerts beneficial effects on human health and that consumption of tea is related to decreased incidence of various chronic diseases [7]. Reported health benefits of tea consumption include antioxidation, anti-inflammation, prevention of cancer, prevention of obesity, and reduced risk of heart disease. Various experimental studies in animal models have also indicated that tea, especially green tea, or its constituents suppress the development of various diseases [8]. Therefore, the possible effects of tea on health promotion have received much attention and are still being extensively examined.

This chapter summarizes catechins and their effects in chronic diseases, focusing on the effects of GTCs, especially EGCG, on metabolic syndromes, cardiovascular diseases, neurodegenerative diseases, and cancer.

2 Physicochemical Properties of Catechins

Among the four major catechins, EGCG is the most abundant, accounting for approximately 70 % of the total catechins in tea, followed by EGC, ECG, and EC [4]. Figure 1 shows the structures of EGCG. There are smaller quantities of GTCs, including gallocatechin gallate, gallocatechin, catechin gallate, catechin, epigallocatechin digallates, epicatechin digallate, 3-*O*-methyl EC, 3-*O*-methyl EGC, and

Fig. 1 Chemical structure of (–)-epigallocatechin-3-gallate (EGCG)

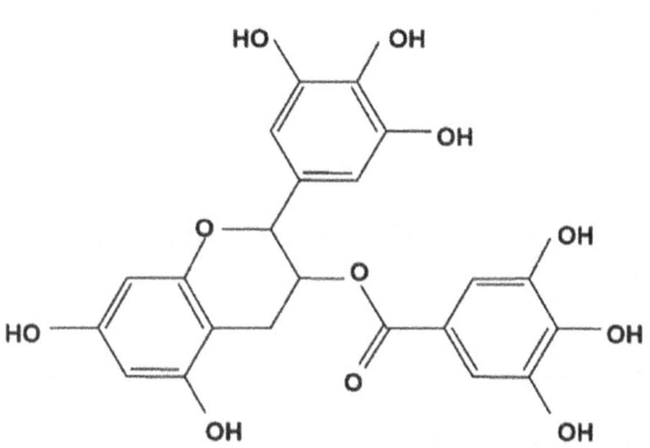

afzelechin. Flavonols and caffeine are also present in tea [9, 10]. Catechins possess antioxidant activities because of their ability to neutralize free radicals. Among tea catechins, ECG has the strongest potency as a radical scavenger, followed by EGCG, EGC, EC, and catechin [11, 12]. The metal-chelating properties of GTCs also contribute to the antioxidant effects [11]. The antioxidant properties are attributable to the phenolic groups, the molecular structures of which are sensitive to oxidation and can generate quinones. The antioxidative activity is enhanced by the presence of the trihydroxyl structure in the D-ring in EGCG [13, 14].

As a large number of natural phenolic compounds exhibit antioxidant and cell protective effects in cell culture models, the antioxidant property of catechins is considered to be highly beneficial to human health [15, 16] as it increases the activities of important detoxifying enzymes [17]. Reactive oxygen species (ROS) are markers for oxidative stress and are key agents in regulating cell signaling by acting as secondary messengers [18]. Generation of ROS plays an important role in physiological processes and can activate endogenous defense systems, while excess production of ROS induces cytotoxicity and various diseases and conditions, including arteriosclerosis, cancer, and aging.

Catechins appear to be able to generate as well as scavenge free radicals and show their beneficial effects due to a combination of both mechanisms [19, 20]. Previous studies have reported the oxidative effects of catechins, indicating that catechins possess a dual function of antioxidation and pro-oxidation, depending on the dose, administration duration, and interaction with other dietary contents [11]. The pro-oxidant activity is thought be attributable to the catechin–quinone redox system. The antioxidant efficacy of catechins is exerted through various mechanisms: scavenging ROS, chelating metal ions, inducing antioxidant enzymes, inhibiting pro-oxidant enzymes, and producing phase II detoxification enzymes and antioxidant enzymes [21].

GTCs are absorbed in the small intestine, but large quantities of catechins reach the large intestine because of the low absorption rate of the small intestine. Previous reports have indicated that less tea constituents were observed in the plasma compared to the total amount ingested orally. This has been investigated in a study where only 0.2–2.0 % of the ingested amount of tea catechin was detected in the plasma [22]. The low bioavailability of catechins may be owing to their short half-life, which ranges from 1.87 to 4.58 h for a dose of 50–1600 mg (approximately 0.7–23 mg/kg body weight, based on a body weight of 70 kg) [23]. The pharmacokinetics of catechins, including EGCG, have been revealed in several clinical investigations in healthy subjects. The serum level of EGCG reaches 1 μM after consumption of a cup of green tea [24]. Orally administered 1600 mg of EGCG led plasma concentrations higher than 1 μM, with peak concentrations from 1.3 to 2.2 h. The plasma kinetics and safety of multiple-dose administration of EGCG mixed with other green tea catechins, called polyphenon E, was evaluated by Chow et al. [25]. In this study, 400 and 800 mg of EGCG were administered once and twice a day for more than four weeks; the results indicated that peak plasma concentrations of EGCG was at a high nano-molar range and that chronic intake increases bioavailability. Varied responses are obtained to EGCG or other catechins in different human populations because of genetic polymorphisms in the enzymes involved in polyphenol metabolism.

3 Modulation of Cell Signaling Pathways by Catechins

In previous investigations, a number of specific phytochemicals, including catechins, have been identified to exert anticancer effects in experimental systems [26]. Various mechanisms of action of catechins against cancers have been extensively examined, including anti-inflammatory and antioxidation, induction of drug metabolizing and detoxifying enzymes, promotion of DNA repair, and modulation of tumor suppressor genes [27]. In addition, recent studies have revealed that GTCs, especially EGCG, exert an anticancer effect by regulating several types of receptor tyrosine kinases (RTKs) and their downstream signaling pathways, which are associated with gene expressions involved in cell proliferation, angiogenesis, and apoptosis [8, 26, 28, 29]. In this section, catechin-modulated cell signaling pathways are summarized focusing on signaling against cancer. Among them, major signaling pathways are shown in Fig. 2. Other pathways altered by catechins are also described.

GTCs, especially EGCG, have been extensively investigated and are reported to exhibit various anticancer effects, such as induction of apoptosis and cell-cycle arrest, inhibition of NF-κB, suppression of cyclooxygenase-2 (COX-2) overexpression, and inhibition of the activation of various types of RTKs [15, 30–36]. Regulation of the apoptotic process is a critical step in the prevention or treatment of cancer. Apoptosis is known to play a significant role in eliminating precancerous and cancer cells and function as protective mechanisms against cancer [37]. Cell experiment researches have shown that EGCG is capable of inhibiting the growth of various types of mouse and human cancer cells through induction of apoptosis [38, 39]. Shanker et al. [40] have reported that treatment of human pancreatic cancer cells with EGCG induces apoptosis through ROS generation and activation of caspase-3 and caspase-9 and that EGCG also regulates the expressions of cyclin D1, cdk4, $p21^{CIP1}$, and $p27^{KIP1}$, which induce cell-cycle arrest during the G1 phase. EGCG in combination with other tea polyphenols has also been reported to inhibit

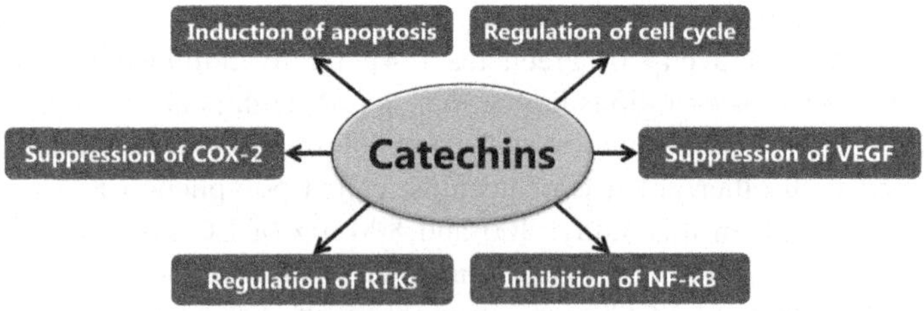

Fig. 2 Modulation of cell signaling pathways by catechins

cellular growth via cell-cycle arrest at the G2/M phase in human lung cancer cells [41]. In addition, it is reported that EGCG treatment increases the proportion of cancer cells during the G1 phase, decreases cyclin D1, and increases $p21^{CIP1}$ and $p27^{KIP1}$ in head and neck squamous cell carcinoma (HNSCC) cell lines [32]. In another study using human colon cancer cells, treatment with EGCG increases the number of cells in the G1 phase, decreases cyclin D1 and Bcl-xL, and increases caspase-3 and caspase-9 activities [35]. Moreover, an in vivo-based examination employing azoxymethane (AOM)-induced colon carcinogenesis model has demonstrated that orally administered EGCG decreases the level of cyclin D1 protein in colonic mucosa, leading to a significant suppression of colon precancerous lesions [42].

Cyclooxygenase-2 (COX-2) expression is controlled by many factors, including mitogens, tumor promoters, cytokines, and growth factors, and overexpression of COX-2 has been noticed in a variety of premalignant and malignant conditions [43]. Previous studies have indicated that EGCG suppresses mitogen-stimulated COX-2 expression in human prostate carcinoma cells [44] and decreases the expression of COX-2 in human mammary and colon cancer cells [34, 45]. In addition, Peng et al. have found that the suppressive effects of EGCG on COX-2 expression may be due to the down-regulation of COX-2 promoter activity through inhibition of nuclear factor kappa B (NF-κB) activation [46].

NF-κB, known as a nuclear transcriptional factor, is considered to be closely associated with inflammation and cancer development [47]. EGCG treatment can inhibit NF-κB activation in human HNSCC and breast cancer cells [30]. Treatment with EGCG also down-regulates NF-κB by inducing kinase expression in human lung cancer cells [48]. Nuclear translocation of NF-κB induces the activation of NF-κB, which is associated with the suppression of cellular apoptosis and induction of proliferation, invasion, transformation, metastasis, and inflammation. Gupta et al. [49] have reported that EGCG is capable of reducing nuclear translocation of NF-κB in epidermoid carcinoma cells in a dose- and time-dependent manner. EGCG is also shown to inhibit nuclear translocation of NF-κB p65 subunit and degradation of IκB-α [50].

Receptor tyrosine kinases (RTKs) play essential roles in various fundamental cellular processes. Their overexpression or constitutive activation is observed in various types of diseases, including cancers. Previous studies have revealed that RTKs and their downstream signaling, such as Ras/ERK and PI3K/Akt signaling pathways, regulate the expression of various target genes associated with cellular proliferation and apoptosis [51, 52]. Premalignant and malignant cells tend to exhibit inappropriate activation of RTKs through mutation or overexpression [53, 54]. Among the RTK superfamily, the epidermal growth factor receptor (EGFR) family includes four members: EGFR (erbB1), HER2 (neu/erbB2), HER3 (neu/erbB3), and HER4 (neu/erbB4). Insulin-like growth factor-1 receptor (IGF-1R) and vascular endothelial growth factor receptor (VEGFR) are also involved in other RTK subgroups. Abnormalities in certain RTKs, especially EGFR, IGF-1R, and VEGFR2, are thought to be significantly associated with the acquisition of malignant properties [53–55]. Recently, RTKs are considered to be possible targets of GTCs against malignancy [15, 28]. A previous important study has been carried out to observe the effects of EGCG on the activation of receptor HER2 in human HNSCC and breast cancer cells, indicating that treatment with EGCG inhibits tyrosine phosphorylation of HER2 and cellular growth [31]. Another study has been performed to investigate the effects of EGCG on the receptor HER2-overexpressing breast cancer cells, and the findings show that EGCG decreases the activation of basal HER2 and reduces downstream signaling pathways [56]. EGCG treatment inhibits the activation of EGFR and HER3 as well as HER2 and their downstream signaling in various human cancer cell lines [30, 32, 35]. The researchers have also reported that treatment with EGCG, alone or combination with other GTCs, reduces phosphorylation of EGFR and HER2, leading to decreased downstream signaling pathways, such as ERK and Akt [35]. The effect of GTCs, including EGCG, on other RTKs family has also been well examined and documented. The development of prostate cancer and its metastatic lesions are suppressed by the administration of GTCs, at a 0.1 % concentration in drinking water, in a rodent prostate cancer model [57]. This treatment induces decreased IGF-1 levels and restoration of IGF binding protein-3 (IGFBP-3) levels, which are associated with reduced levels of PI3K and phosphorylated forms of Akt and ERK [57, 58]. Other in vivo experimental results reported by Shimizu et al. showed that drinking EGCG decreases serum IGF-1 levels and increases serum IGFBP-3 levels in AOM-induced colon carcinogenesis model, which appears to suppress the development of colon precancerous lesions [42]. In this study, the researcher also showed down-regulated levels of both total and activated IGF-1R in colonic mucosa. Decreased levels of IGF-1 and IGF-1R by EGCG treatment are demonstrated in a cell experiment as well using human colon cancer and hepatoma cells. These studies have together shown that EGCG exerts an inhibitory effect on the IGF/IGF-1R axis [33, 59].

The effects of EGCG on the VEGF/VEGFR axis have also been studied. Masuda et al. [30] have indicated that in human cancer cell lines, VEGF production is suppressed by treatment with EGCG through down-regulating activation of signal transducer and activator of transcription (STAT)-3 and NF-κB. Other studies have been carried out to determine that EGCG reduces VEGF expression and activation of VEGFR2, ERK, and Akt, leading to the suppression of xenograft growth in mice generated from human cancer cells [60, 61]. In addition, EGCG treatment inhibits phosphorylation of both VEGFR1 and VEGFR2 and induces apoptosis in B cell chronic lymphocytic leukemia cells [62].

The mechanism action of EGCG on cell signaling pathways has not been completely characterized and elucidated. As one possible mechanism, the 67-kDa laminin receptor has identified as a cell surface receptor for EGCG, which responds to EGCG in various cancer cells during physiological concentrations [63]. Detergent-insoluble ordered plasma membrane domains have also identified as another promising target of EGCG for its activity, especially those associated with RTKs. The membrane domains are known as "lipid rafts," which play a vital role as signal processing hubs of RTKs. Adachi et al. [64, 65] have demonstrated that EGCG alters the lipid organization in the cell membrane, induces internalization of

EGFR into endosomes, and prevents ligands from binding to EGFR. The degradation of EGFR following its internalization is induced by the phosphorylation of the receptor at serine 1046/1047, which is associated with the activation of p38 MAPK caused by EGCG [66]. Because most RTKs function on lipid rafts, this suggested mechanism for EGCG activity is considered to account for the ubiquitous effects of EGCG in the regulation of the expressions and signaling pathways of various types of RTKs.

GTCs are also known to have anti-obesity potential, which have been investigated in cell culture, animal, and human subjects. The activities of catechins against obesity may be as follows: inhibition of pre-adipocyte differentiation, decrease in lipogenesis and adipocyte proliferation, and promotion of lipolysis and adipocyte apoptosis [67]. Peroxisome proliferator-activated receptor gamma (PPAR-γ) and CCAAT/enhancer-binding protein alpha (C/EBPα) are two key regulators of adipocyte differentiation, which regulate the expression of genes related to adipogenesis and lipogenesis. The expression levels of PPAR-γ and C/EBPα are inhibited by EGCG treatment; this may be due to the activation of adenosine monophosphate-activated protein kinase (AMPK) in 3T3L1 adipocytes [68]. EGCG has also been reported to induce G2/M growth arrest in mature 3T3L1 adipocytes [68] and to up-regulate the levels of uncoupling protein-2, a key protein for thermogenesis [69].

4 Biological Activities of Catechins in Animal Models

EGCG is the most abundant catechin in green tea infusions and possesses highest antioxidant activity compared to other catechins [70]. Therefore, EGCG has attracted the most attentions among catechins in the medical chemistry field. This section summarizes animal studies and the inhibitory effects of catechins, especially EGCG on metabolic syndrome, tumorigenesis, cardiovascular disease, and neurodegenerative diseases. These are shown in Table 1.

Metabolic syndrome consists of abdominal obesity, hyperglycemia, elevated blood pressure, and dyslipidemia. EGCG have been shown to exert preventive effects against such disorders. Bose et al. [71] have publicized that supplementation with dietary EGCG treatment of high-fat-diet-fed mice for 16 weeks reduces body weight and percent body fat and visceral fat weight compared to control mice, accompanied by increased fecal lipids, attenuated insulin resistance, plasma cholesterol, and monocyte chemoattractant protein concentrations. It has been reported that administration of EGCG has prevented the progression to glucose intolerance in genetically obese and diabetic C57BL/KsJ-*db/db* (db/db) mice via preservation of the islet structure [72]. In a rat model, Snoussi et al. [73] have reported that the EGCG decoction improved glucose tolerance and reduced weight gain of high-fat-induced obesity due to reduction in intestinal SGLT1/GLUT2 ratio, which is indicative of the regulation of glucose absorption in enterocytes and enhancement of adipose GLUT4. The preventive role of EGCG against obesity and

Table 1 Biological activities of catechins in animal models

Activities for	Catechins	Dose	Animal model	Major effect	Reference
Metabolic syndrome	EGCG	3.2 g/kg diet	High-fat-induced obese mice	Reducing body weight gain, percent body fat, and visceral fat weight	[71]
	EGCG	10 g/kg diet	Obese and diabetic *db/db* mice	Improving glucose tolerance and increasing glucose-stimulated insulin secretion	[72]
	EGCG	550 mg/500 mL (drinking)	Rats fed high-cholesterol and/or high-sucrose diet	Reducing body weight, cholesterol and LDL and lowering serum glucose and insulin levels	[74]
	EGCG	200 mg/kg/day (by gavage)	Hypertensive SHR rats	Lowering systolic blood pressure, improving insulin sensitivity, and raising plasma adiponectin	[75]
Cardiovascular diseases	Green tea polyphenol	(drinking)	Stroke-prone hypertensive SHRSP rats	Lowering blood pressure	[93]
	Green tea extract	0.8 g/L (drinking)	Apoprotein E-deficient mice fed an atherogenic diet	Preventing atherosclerosis development	[94]
	EGCG	0.02, 0.04, or 0.08 % (drinking)	Aorta-constricted rats	Attenuating cardiac hypertrophy	[95]
	EGCG	5 μM	Isolated rat hearts	Protecting ischemic/reperfusion injury	[96]
Neurogenerative diseases	Green tea catechins	0.02 % (drinking)	Aged mice with accelerated senescence (SAMP10)	Suppressing memory regression	[99]
	EGCG	25 or 50 mg/kg i. p.	Gerbil with occluded common carotid arteries	Reducing hippocampal neuronal damage	[103]
	EGCG	1.5 or 3 mg/kg body weight (drinking)	Mice with intracerebroventricular administration of 0.5 μg β-amyloid peptide	Reducing β-amyloid peptide -induced memory dysfunction	[104]
	EGCG	3 mg/kg body weight (drinking)	Genetically developed preseniline 2 (PS2) mutant Alzheimer's disease mice	Enhancing memory function	[104]

(continued)

Table 1 (continued)

Activities for	Catechins	Dose	Animal model	Major effect	Reference
Cancer	Green tea	6 mg tea solids/ml (drinking)	7,12-Dimethylbenz[a]anthracene (DMBA)-induced oral cancer in hamsters	Decreasing the number of tumors and the tumor volume	[78]
	Decaffeinated green tea	6 mg tea solids/ml (drinking)	*N*-nitrosomethylbenzylamine (NMBzA)-induced esophageal tumors in rats	Reducing esophageal papilloma incidence and multiplicity	[79]
	EGCG	0.05 % (drinking)	*N*-methyl- *N*'-nitro- *N*-nitrosoguanidine (MNNG)-induced gastric tumors in rats	Reducing gastric tumor incidence	[80]
	EGCG	0.08 or 0.16 % (drinking)	Apc (min/+) mice (a mouse model for human intestinal cancer)	Decreasing small intestinal tumor formation	[81]
	EGCG or Polyphenon E	0.01 or 0.1 % (drinking)	Colon cancer induced by AOM and dextran sodium sulfate (DSS) in mice	Suppressing the multiplicity and volume of colonic neoplasms	[82]
	EGCG	0.01 or 0.1 % (drinking)	AOM-induced colonic premalignant lesions in *db/db* mice	Decreasing the number of aberrant crypt foci, colonic premalignant lesions	[42]
	EGCG	0.1 % (drinking)	Diethylnitrosamine (DEN)-induced liver tumorigenesis in *db/db* obese mice	Inhibiting the development of liver cell adenomas	[86]
	Green tea infusion	0.63 or 1.25 % (drinking)	N-nitrosodiethylamine (NDEA)-induced pulmonary tumors in mice	Decreasing tumor incidence and the tumor multiplicity	[87]
	Green tea	6 mg tea solids/ml (drinking)	Skin tumors in UVB-pretreated SKH-1 mice	Decreasing the number of tumors per mouse	[89]
	Green tea catechins	0.3 % (drinking)	Prostate cancer in transgenic adenocarcinoma mouse prostate (TRAMP) mice	Preventing prostate tumor progression	[90]
	Green tea leaves	3.0 % powdered green tea in diet	*N*-butyl- *N*-(4-hydroxybutyl)-nitrosamine (BBN)-induced bladder tumors in rats	Preventing the growth of urinary bladder tumors	[91]

its related disorders, especially hypercholesterolemia and hyperglycemia, is also described [74]. In addition, the beneficial properties of EGCG against hypertension have been reported using spontaneously hypertensive rats, where EGCG improved endothelial function and insulin sensitivity and reduced blood pressure through nitric oxide (NO) production from the endothelium using PI-3-kinase pathway [75].

Inhibition of tumorigenesis at different organ sites, including the oral cavity, esophagus, stomach, small intestine, colon, liver, lung, skin, prostate, and bladder, has been reported in many laboratories worldwide and has been previously reviewed [76, 77]. Reports have demonstrated that green tea suppresses chemically induced oral carcinogenesis in a hamster model [78], esophageal tumorigenesis in a rat model [79], and that EGCG inhibits carcinogen-induced tumorigenesis in rat stomach [80]. In $Apc^{Min/+}$ mice that develop a number of adenomas in the intestine by the same mechanism or process as seen in humans, EGCG inhibits intestinal tumorigenesis through increase in E-cadherin levels in the cell plasma membrane as well as decrease in nuclear β-catenin, c-Myc, phosphorylated-Akt and phosphorylated-Erk levels in tumors [81]. Shirakami et al. [82] have reported that administration of EGCG and polyphenon E, a mixture of GTCs, attenuate inflammation-related mouse colon carcinogenesis induced by AOM and dextran sodium sulfate. Kochi et al. [83] demonstrated that supplementation of EGCG suppressed colitis-associated colon carcinogenesis using Kyoto Apc Delta rat, a novel adenomatous polyposis coli mutant rat strain.

Recently, metabolic syndrome has been recognized as major risk factors for the development of certain carcinoma including the colon and liver [84, 85]. Shimizu and colleagues have shown that EGCG is available to attenuate obesity-related carcinogenesis using *db/db* mice in the colon [42] and liver [86]. Consumption of green tea has also shown to inhibit chemically induced lung carcinogenesis in A/J mice [87] and hamsters [88]. Oral administration of tea suppresses UVB-induced skin tumorigenesis, which is closely associated with lowered level of tissue fat in SKH-1 hairless mice [89]. In transgenic mice, which spontaneously develop prostate cancer, supplementation with GTCs prevents prostate tumor progression accompanied by clusterin overexpression [90]. Moreover, the preventive effects of GTCs on chemically induced urinary bladder tumorigenesis in Wister rats have been documented [91].

GTCs have been shown to exert preventive effects against cardiovascular diseases. Oxidative stress and ROS are involved in endothelial dysfunction and progression to atherosclerosis and injury in sustained myocardial infarctions [92]. The major vasoprotective molecule produced by endothelial cells is NO, which is involved in the relaxation of blood vessels. The effects of GTC on the modulation of the production of endothelial NO synthase (eNOS) and NO in in vivo experiments are demonstrated. In stroke-prone spontaneous hypertensive rats, consuming green tea polyphenols attenuates increase in blood pressure through attenuation of oxidative stress [93]. The oxidation of LDL and subsequent infiltration into the subendothelium is the initial event in the generation of atherosclerotic plaques. In ApoE-deficient mice that show accumulation of cholesterol-rich remnants in the plasma and arteriosclerosis, administration of EGCG prevents the development of atherosclerosis and decreases aortic cholesterol and triglyceride levels [94]. In addition, EGCG is capable of attenuating cardiac hypertrophy, increasing left ventricular systolic dimensions, and deterioration in systolic functions in an aorta-constricted rat model [95]. Moreover, EGCG has shown to exert protective effects on ischemic/reperfusion injury in isolated rat hearts via antioxidant anti-apoptotic activities [96].

Oxidative stress and ROS are implicated in senescence and related dysfunctions [97]. GTCs have been shown to exert suppressive effects against morphologic and functional regression in the brain [98] and memory regression in aged mice with accelerated senescence [99]. Oxidative stress is also strongly related to ischemic stroke [100]. Although it is not fully elucidated whether catechins pass through the blood-brain barrier or not, EGCG has been reported to exert protective effects against neuronal damage after ischemia using gerbils [101–103]. It has also been documented that inhibitory effects of EGCG on β-amyloid, involved in Alzheimer's disease, induce cognitive dysfunction in ICR mice and modulate amyloid precursor protein cleavage and reduce cerebral amyloidosis in Tg APPsw mice [104].

5 Biological Activities of Catechins in Humans

Tea polyphenols are basic tea constituents and have physiological properties, including antioxidant and anti-inflammatory activities [105, 106]. In particular, GTCs, the major polyphenolic components of green tea, have strong antioxidant activity and prevent ROS formation [107]. In addition, the anti-inflammatory property of GTCs has been demonstrated in recent experimental animal studies [82, 108–110], which are also described in a previous section. Here, the oxidative stress and inflammation are thought to be associated with the pathogenesis of chronic diseases, including metabolic syndrome (MetS), cardiovascular diseases (CVDs), neurodegenerative diseases [111], and malignant diseases [5, 6], indicating that GTCs can improve or prevent these chronic disorders. Accumulating evidence from clinical studies has demonstrated that the consumption of green tea, the most optimal source of catechins among the food products [112], yielded beneficial effects on metabolism, cardiovascular system, neurodegenerative diseases [113, 114], and cancer [5, 6]. In this section, we summarize the beneficial role of catechins, especially GTCs, on chronic human diseases by reviewing recent clinical studies.

Obesity is serious health problems worldwide and leads to various obesity-related disorders, including diabetes mellitus and MetS [115], indicating that obesity is a critical therapeutic target for the prevention of these metabolic disorders. The effects of green tea consumption on body weight and biomarkers of MetS have been studied in many randomized controlled trials (RCTs) during the past decade. A meta-analysis of 11 randomized trials has reported the beneficial effects of green tea consumption in improving obesity and the features of MetS

[116]. A recent RCT with 35 obese subjects has indicated that daily supplementation of 870 or 928 mg of GTCs for 8 weeks significantly reduces body weight and lipid peroxidation compared to the control group [117]. In other RCTs, GTC supplementation to obese individuals reduces not only body weight but also the waist circumference [118–121]. Moreover, a retrospective cohort study of 17,413 Japanese adults has reported that daily consumption of more than six cups of green tea lower the incidence of diabetes by 33 % [122]. Thus, a number of clinical studies have reported the beneficial effects of GTCs in the improvement of obesity and its related metabolic disorders, including diabetes and MetS. However, not all human studies have demonstrated positive results for obesity-related measures. In contrast to the above-mentioned beneficial effects, several clinical trials have reported that the consumption of green tea or GTCs does not cause changes in body weight, body mass index, fat mass, energy and fat metabolism, and LDL cholesterol levels [123–126]. Therefore, the effects of GTCs on human obesity remain controversial. The discrepancies among these clinical studies may result from differences in the length of the study and characteristics of the study subjects, such as extent of obesity, dietary intake, physical activity intensity, genetic background of the populations, body composition, and dietary habits [115]. Therefore, more well-controlled, long-term human studies are needed to confirm the positive effects of GTCs on obesity in humans.

It is reported that obesity and MetS are one of the risk factors for CVDs [127, 128]. As demonstrated above, recent clinical studies have reported that the consumption of green tea or GTCs not only reduces body weight, abdominal fat mass, and LDL cholesterol levels, but also improves hypertension and insulin resistance [129, 130], indicating that GTCs may prevent the emergence of CVDs. A large cohort study in Japan (n = 40,530) has reported that CVD-related death are decreased dose-dependently by green tea consumption [131]. Besides, in another trial with 76,979 Japanese adults, green tea consumption is associated with lower mortality in patients with CVDs [132]. Thus, drinking green tea is considered to be beneficial for the prevention of CVDs. Interestingly, a meta-analysis of 18 clinical trials has demonstrated that a reduced risk of coronary artery disease observed in subjects treated with green tea is not confirmed in subjects treated with black tea [133]. Moreover, it is reported that only higher consumption of green tea (at least 7 cups per day) may have a prophylactic effect on CVDs [134]. Here, green tea contains more catechins compared to black tea [134]. Furthermore, GTCs are known to be the major polyphenolic components in green tea. Therefore, it is considered that GTCs may have a beneficial effect in the prevention of CVDs.

Alzheimer's disease (AD) and Parkinson's disease (PD), which are neurodegenerative diseases, are the leading causes of mortality in the USA [135]. A recent publication has demonstrated that oxidative stress and its related ROS generation play a key role in the pathogenesis of neurodegenerative diseases [136]. Considering the antioxidative activity of GTCs, the consumption of green tea, especially GTCs, may protect the neurons from excess oxidative stress, resulting in the inhibition of neurodegenerative diseases. Indeed, a cross-sectional study has revealed that green tea consumption significantly reduced the risk of AD [137]. Moreover, a population study has reported that long-term consumption of tea has an inverse correlation with the onset of PD [138]. Therefore, a number of clinical studies have reported the beneficial effects of tea catechins in neurodegenerative diseases. As shown by an epidemiological study [139], however, higher GTC intake than the recommended daily allowance is needed for these beneficial effects.

Many researchers have extensively examined the effects of drinking green tea on the risk of cancer, including lung, esophagus, stomach, liver, pancreas, colon, breast, and prostate. Only some of these investigations, however, have demonstrated a protective effect of green tea against cancer. In addition, epidemiological studies have not yet provided conclusive findings in order to confirm the chemoprevention of cancer by green tea consumption [76]. For instance, a meta-analysis investigating the relationship between green tea intake and the risk for colorectal cancer has reported that several case–control studies showed an inverse relationship between green tea consumption and colorectal cancer risk, while other cohort studies found no association [140]. On the other hand, cell experimental and animal carcinogenesis studies have consistently indicated that GTCs, especially EGCG, exert anticancer efficacy in a large number of malignant cases.

Several clinical trials have been conducted to investigate the cancer chemopreventive effects of tea catechins and EGCG. Among them, a double-blinded trial has revealed that oral administration of mixed tea products for 6 months causes a marked decrease in the size of leukoplakia, a precancerous lesion of the oral mucosa [141]. Another randomized, double-blind, placebo-controlled study has found that oral administration of 600 mg/day of GTCs for 12 months is able to suppress the progression from high-grade prostate intraepithelial neoplasia to prostate cancer [142]. On the other hand, no evidence of beneficial effects of tea catechins has been provided in other interventional studies to examine the efficacy of green tea against prostate cancer [143–145]. In a pilot study, the effects of administration of green tea extracts (GTEs) on the development of colorectal adenoma, a precancerous lesion in the colorectum, are investigated [146]. The participants are patients who have undergone polypectomy for removal of colorectal adenomas. Researchers have found that administration of 1.5 g/day of GTEs for 1 year successfully inhibits the development of metachronous colorectal adenoma in comparison with an untreated control group (Fig. 3). The study has also demonstrated that the size of recurrent adenomas in the green tea extract-administered group was significantly smaller than that in the untreated control group, and no adverse events are observed in the treatment group. A similar clinical trial that is currently being planned and conducted with a large sample size and longer observation period will provide convincing evidence on the effect of GTE on recurrence of colorectal adenomas [147].

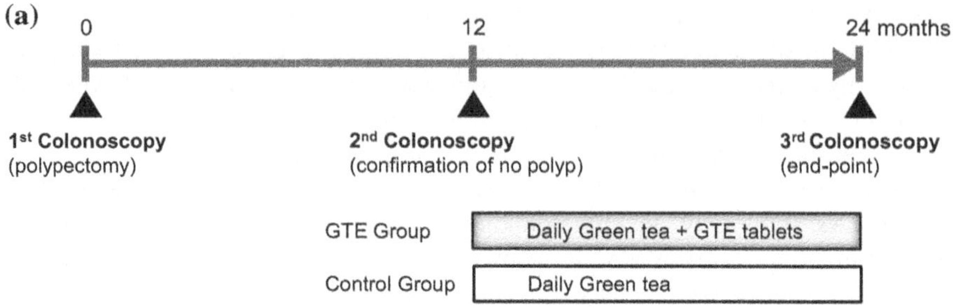

(b)

Characteristic	GTE Group	Control Group	*P*
Total no. of patients	60	65	–
No. of patients with metachronous adenomas (%)	9 (15)	20 (31)	< 0.05
Size of relapsed adenomas (mm), mean ±SD	3.0 ± 1.0	4.0 ± 1.3	< 0.001

Fig. 3 A pilot study investigating the chemopreventive effects of green tea extracts (GTEs) on metachronous adenomas after endoscopic polypectomy. **a** Study protocol. The study included 136 participants who underwent endoscopic resection of colorectal adenomas. The participants received another total colonoscopy in 12 months to confirm the absence of the remaining detectable adenoma. Then the participants were randomized into two groups: The GTE group ($n = 71$) was given three GTE tablets per day for 12 months, and the control group ($n = 65$) received no supplement. After 12 months of GTE administration, a follow-up (end-point) colonoscopy was conducted in 125 patients (60 in the GTE group and 65 in the control group) to examine the presence of new adenomas. One tablet of GTE (500 mg), which contains 52.5 mg EGCG, 58 mg of other types of GTCs, and 15.7 mg caffeine, is equivalent to approximately two Japanese-size cups of green tea. **b** Effects of GTE supplementation on the incidence and size of metachronous adenomas at the end-point observation by colonoscopy

6 Conclusions

In the research field for human diseases, the mechanisms of action of plant-derived natural agents, such as polyphenols, have gained considerable attention. Researchers have extensively investigated the molecular mechanisms of these substances, especially EGCG of GTC, and have provided new insights in the prevention and therapy for chronic diseases, including metabolic syndrome (MetS), cardiovascular diseases (CVDs), neurodegenerative diseases, and malignant diseases.

Although preventive and/or therapeutic efficacy of catechins on various diseases is demonstrated in a number of cell experimental and animal studies, epidemiological and interventional examinations do not always produce consistent results of the effects of GTCs and EGCG. As described in previous sections, the bioavailability and plasma concentration of GTCs following tea consumption are relatively low, and researchers should consider this when reviewing the findings of in vivo experimental and human clinical studies on the absorption, distribution, and metabolism of tea catechins [148]. In fact, the concentrations of EGCG required to exert biological effects are significantly higher in many cellular experiments than the detected levels in plasma and tissue in human trials or experimental animal studies [149]. Therefore, it still needs to be clarified whether the results obtained from in vitro studies using EGCG can be directly extrapolated to those in experimental animal and human studies. For obtaining higher serum concentrations of GTCs, several trials have been carried out using increased doses of tea catechins in non-traditional forms, such as pills and capsules [150]. Although there have been case reports of adverse events by supplemented catechins, which include increased gas production, nausea, heartburn, stomachache, abdominal pain, dizziness, and hepatotoxicity [25, 150], GTCs can be considered as relatively safe phytochemicals based on the long consumption history.

In order to understand the molecular mechanisms and recognized and newly discovered effects of catechins on human diseases, future research should be conducted to investigate the effect of GTCs in the prevention and treatment of human chronic diseases in various organ sites. For the clinical application of catechins as preventive and therapeutic agents, a greater number of well-designed epidemiological and interventional studies should be performed to elucidate the activity and mechanism in human subjects.

References

1. Cabrera C, Gimenez R, Lopez MC (2003) Determination of tea components with antioxidant activity. J Agric Food Chem 51(15):4427–4435. doi:10.1021/jf0300801
2. Basu A, Lucas EA (2007) Mechanisms and effects of green tea on cardiovascular health. Nutr Rev 65(8 Pt 1):361–375
3. Wang S, Noh SK, Koo SI (2006) Green tea catechins inhibit pancreatic phospholipase A(2) and intestinal absorption of lipids in ovariectomized rats. J Nutr Biochem 17(7):492–498. doi:10.1016/j.jnutbio.2006.03.004
4. Chen Z, Zhu QY, Tsang D, Huang Y (2001) Degradation of green tea catechins in tea drinks. J Agric Food Chem 49(1):477–482
5. Majumder K, Mine Y, Wu J (2015) The potential of food-protein derived anti-inflammatory peptides against various chronic inflammatory diseases. J Sci Food Agric. doi:10.1002/jsfa.7600
6. Zhang YJ, Gan RY, Li S, Zhou Y, Li AN, Xu DP, Li HB (2015) Antioxidant phytochemicals for the prevention and treatment of chronic diseases. Molecules 20(12):21138–21156. doi:10.3390/molecules201219753
7. Yang CS, Wang ZY (1993) Tea and cancer. J Natl Cancer Inst 85(13):1038–1049
8. Khan N, Afaq F, Saleem M, Ahmad N, Mukhtar H (2006) Targeting multiple signaling pathways by green tea polyphenol (-)-epigallocatechin-3-gallate. Cancer Res 66(5):2500–2505. doi:10.1158/0008-5472.CAN-05-3636
9. Chiu FL, Lin JK (2005) HPLC analysis of naturally occurring methylated catechins, 3' '- and 4' '-methyl-epigallocatechin gallate, in various fresh tea leaves and commercial teas and

their potent inhibitory effects on inducible nitric oxide synthase in macrophages. J Agric Food Chem 53(18):7035–7042. doi:10.1021/jf0507442
10. Mukhtar H, Ahmad N (1999) Green tea in chemoprevention of cancer. Toxicol Sci Official J Soc Toxicol 52(2 Suppl):111–117
11. Zaveri NT (2006) Green tea and its polyphenolic catechins: medicinal uses in cancer and noncancer applications. Life Sci 78(18):2073–2080. doi:10.1016/j.lfs.2005.12.006
12. Zheng LT, Ryu GM, Kwon BM, Lee WH, Suk K (2008) Anti-inflammatory effects of catechols in lipopolysaccharide-stimulated microglia cells: inhibition of microglial neurotoxicity. Eur J Pharmacol 588(1):106–113. doi:10.1016/j.ejphar.2008.04.035
13. Lambert JD, Elias RJ (2010) The antioxidant and pro-oxidant activities of green tea polyphenols: a role in cancer prevention. Arch Biochem Biophys 501(1):65–72. doi:10.1016/j.abb.2010.06.013
14. Mukhtar H, Ahmad N (2000) Tea polyphenols: prevention of cancer and optimizing health. Am J Clin Nutr 71(6 Suppl):1698S–1702S; discussion 1703S–1694S
15. Shimizu M, Shirakami Y, Moriwaki H (2008) Targeting receptor tyrosine kinases for chemoprevention by green tea catechin, EGCG. Int J Mol Sci 9(6):1034–1049. doi:10.3390/ijms9061034
16. Tachibana H (2009) Molecular basis for cancer chemoprevention by green tea polyphenol EGCG. Forum Nutr 61:156–169. doi:10.1159/000212748 000212748[pii]
17. Chedea VS, Braicu C, Chirila F, Ogola HJ, Pelmus RS, Calin LG, Socaciu C (2014) Antioxidant/prooxidant and antibacterial/probacterial effects of a grape seed extract in complex with lipoxygenase. BioMed Res Int 2014:313684. doi:10.1155/2014/313684
18. Groeger G, Quiney C, Cotter TG (2009) Hydrogen peroxide as a cell-survival signaling molecule. Antioxid Redox Sig 11(11):2655–2671. doi:10.1089/ARS.2009.2728
19. Oliveira-Marques V, Marinho HS, Cyrne L, Antunes F (2009) Role of hydrogen peroxide in NF-kappaB activation: from inducer to modulator. Antioxid Redox Sig 11(9):2223–2243. doi:10.1089/ARS.2009.2601
20. Valko M, Leibfritz D, Moncol J, Cronin MT, Mazur M, Telser J (2007) Free radicals and antioxidants in normal physiological functions and human disease. Int J Biochem Cell Biol 39(1):44–84. doi:10.1016/j.biocel.2006.07.001
21. Youn HS, Lee JY, Saitoh SI, Miyake K, Kang KW, Choi YJ, Hwang DH (2006) Suppression of MyD88- and TRIF-dependent signaling pathways of Toll-like receptor by (-)-epigallocatechin-3-gallate, a polyphenol component of green tea. Biochem Pharmacol 72 (7):850–859. doi:10.1016/j.bcp.2006.06.021
22. Nakagawa K, Okuda S, Miyazawa T (1997) Dose-dependent incorporation of tea catechins, (-)-epigallocatechin-3-gallate and (-)-epigallocatechin, into human plasma. Biosci Biotechnol Biochem 61(12):1981–1985
23. Ullmann U, Haller J, Decourt JP, Girault N, Girault J, Richard-Caudron AS, Pineau B, Weber P (2003) A single ascending dose study of epigallocatechin gallate in healthy volunteers. J Int Med Res 31(2):88–101
24. Van het Hof KH, Wiseman SA, Yang CS, Tijburg LB (1999) Plasma and lipoprotein levels of tea catechins following repeated tea consumption. In: Proceedings of the society for experimental biology and medicine society for experimental biology and medicine, vol 220, no 4, pp 203–209
25. Chow HH, Cai Y, Hakim IA, Crowell JA, Shahi F, Brooks CA, Dorr RT, Hara Y, Alberts DS (2003) Pharmacokinetics and safety of green tea polyphenols after multiple-dose administration of epigallocatechin gallate and polyphenon E in healthy individuals. Clin Cancer Res 9(9):3312–3319
26. Surh YJ (2003) Cancer chemoprevention with dietary phytochemicals. Nat Rev Cancer 3 (10):768–780
27. Hanausek M, Walaszek Z, Slaga TJ (2003) Detoxifying cancer causing agents to prevent cancer. Integr Cancer Ther 2(2):139–144. doi:10.1177/1534735403002002005
28. Shimizu M, Weinstein IB (2005) Modulation of signal transduction by tea catechins and related phytochemicals. Mutat Res 591(1–2):147–160

29. Wang J, Eltoum IE, Lamartiniere CA (2004) Genistein alters growth factor signaling in transgenic prostate model (TRAMP). Mol Cell Endocrinol 219(1–2):171–180. doi:10.1016/j.mce.2003.12.018
30. Masuda M, Suzui M, Lim JT, Deguchi A, Soh JW, Weinstein IB (2002) Epigallocatechin-3-gallate decreases VEGF production in head and neck and breast carcinoma cells by inhibiting EGFR-related pathways of signal transduction. J Exp Ther Oncol 2(6):350–359
31. Masuda M, Suzui M, Lim JT, Weinstein IB (2003) Epigallocatechin-3-gallate inhibits activation of HER-2/neu and downstream signaling pathways in human head and neck and breast carcinoma cells. Clin Cancer Res 9(9):3486–3491
32. Masuda M, Suzui M, Weinstein IB (2001) Effects of epigallocatechin-3-gallate on growth, epidermal growth factor receptor signaling pathways, gene expression, and chemosensitivity in human head and neck squamous cell carcinoma cell lines. Clin Cancer Res 7(12):4220–4229
33. Shimizu M, Deguchi A, Hara Y, Moriwaki H, Weinstein IB (2005) EGCG inhibits activation of the insulin-like growth factor-1 receptor in human colon cancer cells. Biochem Biophys Res Commun 334(3):947–953
34. Shimizu M, Deguchi A, Joe AK, McKoy JF, Moriwaki H, Weinstein IB (2005) EGCG inhibits activation of HER3 and expression of cyclooxygenase-2 in human colon cancer cells. J Exp Ther Oncol 5(1):69–78
35. Shimizu M, Deguchi A, Lim JT, Moriwaki H, Kopelovich L, Weinstein IB (2005) (-)-Epigallocatechin gallate and polyphenon E inhibit growth and activation of the epidermal growth factor receptor and human epidermal growth factor receptor-2 signaling pathways in human colon cancer cells. Clin Cancer Res 11(7):2735–2746
36. Yang CS, Maliakal P, Meng X (2002) Inhibition of carcinogenesis by tea. Annu Rev Pharmacol Toxicol 42:25–54
37. Shankar S, Ganapathy S, Hingorani SR, Srivastava RK (2008) EGCG inhibits growth, invasion, angiogenesis and metastasis of pancreatic cancer. Front Biosci J Virtual Libr 13:440–452
38. Barthelman M, Bair WB 3rd, Stickland KK, Chen W, Timmermann BN, Valcic S, Dong Z, Bowden GT (1998) (-)-Epigallocatechin-3-gallate inhibition of ultraviolet B-induced AP-1 activity. Carcinogenesis 19(12):2201–2204
39. Gupta S, Ahmad N, Nieminen AL, Mukhtar H (2000) Growth inhibition, cell-cycle dysregulation, and induction of apoptosis by green tea constituent (-)-epigallocatechin-3-gallate in androgen-sensitive and androgen-insensitive human prostate carcinoma cells. Toxicol Appl Pharmacol 164(1):82–90. doi:10.1006/taap.1999.8885
40. Shankar S, Suthakar G, Srivastava RK (2007) Epigallocatechin-3-gallate inhibits cell cycle and induces apoptosis in pancreatic cancer. Front Biosci J Virtual Libr 12:5039–5051
41. Fujiki H, Suganuma M, Okabe S, Sueoka N, Komori A, Sueoka E, Kozu T, Tada Y, Suga K, Imai K, Nakachi K (1998) Cancer inhibition by green tea. Mutat Res 402(1–2):307–310
42. Shimizu M, Shirakami Y, Sakai H, Adachi S, Hata K, Hirose Y, Tsurumi H, Tanaka T, Moriwaki H (2008) (-)-Epigallocatechin gallate suppresses azoxymethane-induced colonic premalignant lesions in male C57BL/KsJ-*db/db* mice. Cancer Prev Res (Phila) 1(4):298–304. doi:10.1158/1940-6207.CAPR-08-0045 1/4/298 [pii]
43. Aggarwal BB, Kumar A, Bharti AC (2003) Anticancer potential of curcumin: preclinical and clinical studies. Anticancer Res 23(1A):363–398
44. Hussain T, Gupta S, Adhami VM, Mukhtar H (2005) Green tea constituent epigallocatechin-3-gallate selectively inhibits COX-2 without affecting COX-1 expression in human prostate carcinoma cells. Int J Cancer (Journal international du cancer) 113 (4):660–669. doi:10.1002/ijc.20629
45. Kundu JK, Na HK, Chun KS, Kim YK, Lee SJ, Lee SS, Lee OS, Sim YC, Surh YJ (2003) Inhibition of phorbol ester-induced COX-2 expression by epigallocatechin gallate in mouse skin and cultured human mammary epithelial cells. J Nutr 133(11 Suppl 1):3805S–3810S

46. Peng G, Wargovich MJ, Dixon DA (2006) Anti-proliferative effects of green tea polyphenol EGCG on Ha-Ras-induced transformation of intestinal epithelial cells. Cancer Lett 238 (2):260–270. doi:10.1016/j.canlet.2005.07.018 S0304-3835(05)00666-X [pii]
47. Ahmad N, Feyes DK, Nieminen AL, Agarwal R, Mukhtar H (1997) Green tea constituent epigallocatechin-3-gallate and induction of apoptosis and cell cycle arrest in human carcinoma cells. J Natl Cancer Inst 89(24):1881–1886
48. Okabe S, Fujimoto N, Sueoka N, Suganuma M, Fujiki H (2001) Modulation of gene expression by (-)-epigallocatechin gallate in PC-9 cells using a cDNA expression array. Biol Pharm Bull 24(8):883–886
49. Gupta S, Hastak K, Afaq F, Ahmad N, Mukhtar H (2004) Essential role of caspases in epigallocatechin-3-gallate-mediated inhibition of nuclear factor kappa B and induction of apoptosis. Oncogene 23(14):2507–2522. doi:10.1038/sj.onc.1207353
50. Cai Y, Yu SS, Chen TT, Gao S, Geng B, Yu Y, Ye JT, Liu PQ (2013) EGCG inhibits CTGF expression via blocking NF-kappaB activation in cardiac fibroblast. Phytomedicine Int J Phytotherapy Phytopharmacology 20(2):106–113. doi:10.1016/j.phymed.2012.10.002
51. Lemmon MA, Schlessinger J (2010) Cell signaling by receptor tyrosine kinases. Cell 141 (7):1117–1134. doi:10.1016/j.cell.2010.06.011 S0092-8674(10)00665-3 [pii]
52. Schlessinger J (2000) Cell signaling by receptor tyrosine kinases. Cell 103(2):211–225. doi:10.1016/S0092-8674(00)00114-8 [pii]
53. Hynes NE, Lane HA (2005) ERBB receptors and cancer: the complexity of targeted inhibitors. Nat Rev Cancer 5(5):341–354. doi:10.1038/nrc1609 nrc1609[pii]
54. Pollak MN, Schernhammer ES, Hankinson SE (2004) Insulin-like growth factors and neoplasia. Nat Rev Cancer 4(7):505–518. doi:10.1038/nrc1387 nrc1387 [pii]
55. Ellis LM, Hicklin DJ (2008) VEGF-targeted therapy: mechanisms of anti-tumour activity. Nat Rev Cancer 8(8):579–591. doi:10.1038/nrc2403 nrc2403[pii]
56. Pianetti S, Guo S, Kavanagh KT, Sonenshein GE (2002) Green tea polyphenol epigallocatechin-3 gallate inhibits Her-2/neu signaling, proliferation, and transformed phenotype of breast cancer cells. Cancer Res 62(3):652–655
57. Gupta S, Hastak K, Ahmad N, Lewin JS, Mukhtar H (2001) Inhibition of prostate carcinogenesis in TRAMP mice by oral infusion of green tea polyphenols. Proc Natl Acad Sci U S A 98(18):10350–10355. doi:10.1073/pnas.171326098
58. Adhami VM, Siddiqui IA, Ahmad N, Gupta S, Mukhtar H (2004) Oral consumption of green tea polyphenols inhibits insulin-like growth factor-I-induced signaling in an autochthonous mouse model of prostate cancer. Cancer Res 64(23):8715–8722. doi:10.1158/0008-5472.CAN-04-2840 64/23/8715 [pii]
59. Shimizu M, Shirakami Y, Sakai H, Tatebe H, Nakagawa T, Hara Y, Weinstein IB, Moriwaki H (2008) EGCG inhibits activation of the insulin-like growth factor (IGF)/IGF-1 receptor axis in human hepatocellular carcinoma cells. Cancer Lett 262(1):10–18
60. Shimizu M, Shirakami Y, Sakai H, Yasuda Y, Kubota M, Adachi S, Tsurumi H, Hara Y, Moriwaki H (2010) (-)-Epigallocatechin gallate inhibits growth and activation of the VEGF/VEGFR axis in human colorectal cancer cells. Chem Biol Inter 185(3):247–252. doi:10.1016/j.cbi.2010.03.036 S0009-2797(10)00199-7 [pii]
61. Shirakami Y, Shimizu M, Adachi S, Sakai H, Nakagawa T, Yasuda Y, Tsurumi H, Hara Y, Moriwaki H (2009) (-)-Epigallocatechin gallate suppresses the growth of human hepatocellular carcinoma cells by inhibiting activation of the vascular endothelial growth factor-vascular endothelial growth factor receptor axis. Cancer Sci 100(10):1957–1962. doi:10.1111/j.1349-7006.2009.01241.x CAS1241 [pii]
62. Lee YK, Bone ND, Strege AK, Shanafelt TD, Jelinek DF (2003) Kay NE (2004) VEGF receptor phosphorylation status and apoptosis is modulated by a green tea component, epigallocatechin-3-gallate (EGCG), in B-cell chronic lymphocytic leukemia. Blood 104 (3):788–794. doi:10.1182/blood-2003-08-2763 08-2763 [pii]
63. Umeda D, Yano S, Yamada K, Tachibana H (2008) Green tea polyphenol epigallocatechin-3-gallate signaling pathway through 67-kDa laminin receptor. J Biol Chem 283(6):3050–3058. doi:10.1074/jbc.M707892200 M707892200 [pii]

64. Adachi S, Nagao T, Ingolfsson HI, Maxfield FR, Andersen OS, Kopelovich L, Weinstein IB (2007) The inhibitory effect of (-)-epigallocatechin gallate on activation of the epidermal growth factor receptor is associated with altered lipid order in HT29 colon cancer cells. Cancer Res 67(13):6493–6501. doi:10.1158/0008-5472.CAN-07-0411 67/13/6493 [pii]
65. Adachi S, Nagao T, To S, Joe AK, Shimizu M, Matsushima-Nishiwaki R, Kozawa O, Moriwaki H, Maxfield FR, Weinstein IB (2008) (-)-Epigallocatechin gallate causes internalization of the epidermal growth factor receptor in human colon cancer cells. Carcinogenesis 29(10):1986–1993. doi:10.1093/carcin/bgn128 bgn128 [pii]
66. Adachi S, Shimizu M, Shirakami Y, Yamauchi J, Natsume H, Matsushima-Nishiwaki R, To S, Weinstein IB, Moriwaki H, Kozawa O (2009) (-)-Epigallocatechin gallate downregulates EGF receptor via phosphorylation at Ser 1046/1047 by p38 MAPK in colon cancer cells. Carcinogenesis 30(9):1544–1552. doi:10.1093/carcin/bgp166 bgp166 [pii]
67. Wang S, Moustaid-Moussa N, Chen L, Mo H, Shastri A, Su R, Bapat P, Kwun I, Shen CL (2014) Novel insights of dietary polyphenols and obesity. J Nutr Biochem 25(1):1–18. doi:10.1016/j.jnutbio.2013.09.001
68. Chan CY, Wei L, Castro-Munozledo F, Koo WL (2011) (-)-Epigallocatechin-3-gallate blocks 3T3-L1 adipose conversion by inhibition of cell proliferation and suppression of adipose phenotype expression. Life Sci 89(21–22):779–785. doi:10.1016/j.lfs.2011.09.006
69. Lee MS, Kim Y (2009) (-)-Epigallocatechin-3-gallate enhances uncoupling protein 2 gene expression in 3T3-L1 adipocytes. Biosci Biotechnol Biochem 73(2):434–436. doi:10.1271/bbb.80563
70. Rice-Evans C (1999) Implications of the mechanisms of action of tea polyphenols as antioxidants in vitro for chemoprevention in humans. In: Proceedings of the society for experimental biology and medicine society for experimental biology and medicine, vol 220, no 4, pp 262–266
71. Bose M, Lambert JD, Ju J, Reuhl KR, Shapses SA, Yang CS (2008) The major green tea polyphenol, (-)-epigallocatechin-3-gallate, inhibits obesity, metabolic syndrome, and fatty liver disease in high-fat-fed mice. J Nutr 138(9):1677–1683
72. Ortsater H, Grankvist N, Wolfram S, Kuehn N, Sjoholm A (2012) Diet supplementation with green tea extract epigallocatechin gallate prevents progression to glucose intolerance in *db/db* mice. Nutr Metab 9:11. doi:10.1186/1743-7075-9-11
73. Snoussi C, Ducroc R, Hamdaoui MH, Dhaouadi K, Abaidi H, Cluzeaud F, Nazaret C, Le Gall M, Bado A (2014) Green tea decoction improves glucose tolerance and reduces weight gain of rats fed normal and high-fat diet. J Nutr Biochem 25(5):557–564. doi:10.1016/j.jnutbio.2014.01.006
74. Ahmad RS, Butt MS, Sultan MT, Mushtaq Z, Ahmad S, Dewanjee S, De Feo V, Zia-Ul-Haq M (2015) Preventive role of green tea catechins from obesity and related disorders especially hypercholesterolemia and hyperglycemia. J Transl Med 13:79. doi:10.1186/s12967-015-0436-x
75. Potenza MA, Marasciulo FL, Tarquinio M, Tiravanti E, Colantuono G, Federici A, Kim JA, Quon MJ, Montagnani M (2007) EGCG, a green tea polyphenol, improves endothelial function and insulin sensitivity, reduces blood pressure, and protects against myocardial I/R injury in SHR. Am J Physiol Endocrinol Metab 292(5):E1378–E1387. doi:10.1152/ajpendo.00698.2006
76. Shirakami Y, Shimizu M, Moriwaki H (2012) Cancer chemoprevention with green tea catechins: from bench to bed. Curr Drug Targets 13(14):1842–1857
77. Yang CS, Wang H, Li GX, Yang Z, Guan F, Jin H (2011) Cancer prevention by tea: evidence from laboratory studies. Pharmacol Res 64(2):113–122. doi:10.1016/j.phrs.2011.03.001
78. Li N, Chen X, Liao J, Yang G, Wang S, Josephson Y, Han C, Chen J, Huang MT, Yang CS (2002) Inhibition of 7,12-dimethylbenz[a]anthracene (DMBA)-induced oral carcinogenesis in hamsters by tea and curcumin. Carcinogenesis 23(8):1307–1313

79. Wang ZY, Wang LD, Lee MJ, Ho CT, Huang MT, Conney AH, Yang CS (1995) Inhibition of *N*-nitrosomethylbenzylamine-induced esophageal tumorigenesis in rats by green and black tea. Carcinogenesis 16(9):2143–2148
80. Yamane T, Takahashi T, Kuwata K, Oya K, Inagake M, Kitao Y, Suganuma M, Fujiki H (1995) Inhibition of *N*-methyl- *N*'-nitro- *N*-nitrosoguanidine-induced carcinogenesis by (-)-epigallocatechin gallate in the rat glandular stomach. Cancer Res 55(10):2081–2084
81. Ju J, Hong J, Zhou JN, Pan Z, Bose M, Liao J, Yang GY, Liu YY, Hou Z, Lin Y, Ma J, Shih WJ, Carothers AM, Yang CS (2005) Inhibition of intestinal tumorigenesis in Apcmin/ + mice by (-)-epigallocatechin-3-gallate, the major catechin in green tea. Cancer Res 65 (22):10623–10631. doi:10.1158/0008-5472.CAN-05-1949 65/22/10623 [pii]
82. Shirakami Y, Shimizu M, Tsurumi H, Hara Y, Tanaka T, Moriwaki H (2008) EGCG and Polyphenon E attenuate inflammation-related mouse colon carcinogenesis induced by AOM plus DDS. Mol Med Rep 1:355–361
83. Kochi T, Shimizu M, Shirakami Y, Yoshimi K, Kuramoto T, Tanaka T, Moriwaki H (2015) Utility of Apc-mutant rats with a colitis-associated colon carcinogenesis model for chemoprevention studies. Eur J Cancer Prev Official J Eur Cancer Prev Organ 24(3):180–187. doi:10.1097/CEJ.0000000000000063
84. Ishino K, Mutoh M, Totsuka Y, Nakagama H (2013) Metabolic syndrome: a novel high-risk state for colorectal cancer. Cancer Lett 334(1):56–61. doi:10.1016/j.canlet.2012.10.012
85. Jinjuvadia R, Patel S, Liangpunsakul S (2014) The association between metabolic syndrome and hepatocellular carcinoma: systemic review and meta-analysis. J Clin Gastroenterol 48 (2):172–177. doi:10.1097/MCG.0b013e3182a030c4
86. Shimizu M, Sakai H, Shirakami Y, Yasuda Y, Kubota M, Terakura D, Baba A, Ohno T, Hara Y, Tanaka T, Moriwaki H (2011) Preventive effects of (-)-epigallocatechin gallate on diethylnitrosamine-induced liver tumorigenesis in obese and diabetic C57BL/KsJ-*db/db* mice. Cancer Prev Res (Phila) 4(3):396–403. doi:10.1158/1940-6207.CAPR-10-0331 4/3/396 [pii]
87. Wang ZY, Hong JY, Huang MT, Reuhl KR, Conney AH, Yang CS (1992) Inhibition of *N*-nitrosodiethylamine- and 4-(methylnitrosamino)-1-(3-pyridyl)-1-butanone-induced tumorigenesis in A/J mice by green tea and black tea. Cancer Res 52(7):1943–1947
88. Schuller HM, Porter B, Riechert A, Walker K, Schmoyer R (2004) Neuroendocrine lung carcinogenesis in hamsters is inhibited by green tea or theophylline while the development of adenocarcinomas is promoted: implications for chemoprevention in smokers. Lung Cancer 45(1):11–18. doi:10.1016/j.lungcan.2003.12.007
89. Lu YP, Lou YR, Lin Y, Shih WJ, Huang MT, Yang CS, Conney AH (2001) Inhibitory effects of orally administered green tea, black tea, and caffeine on skin carcinogenesis in mice previously treated with ultraviolet B light (high-risk mice): relationship to decreased tissue fat. Cancer Res 61(13):5002–5009
90. Caporali A, Davalli P, Astancolle S, D'Arca D, Brausi M, Bettuzzi S, Corti A (2004) The chemopreventive action of catechins in the TRAMP mouse model of prostate carcinogenesis is accompanied by clusterin over-expression. Carcinogenesis 25(11):2217–2224. doi:10.1093/carcin/bgh235
91. Sato D, Matsushima M (2003) Preventive effects of urinary bladder tumors induced by *N*-butyl- *N*-(4-hydroxybutyl)-nitrosamine in rat by green tea leaves. Int J Urol Official J Japan Urol Assoc 10(3):160–166
92. Sugamura K, Keaney JF Jr (2011) Reactive oxygen species in cardiovascular disease. Free Radic Biol Med 51(5):978–992. doi:10.1016/j.freeradbiomed.2011.05.004
93. Negishi H, Xu JW, Ikeda K, Njelekela M, Nara Y, Yamori Y (2004) Black and green tea polyphenols attenuate blood pressure increases in stroke-prone spontaneously hypertensive rats. J Nutr 134(1):38–42
94. Miura Y, Chiba T, Tomita I, Koizumi H, Miura S, Umegaki K, Hara Y, Ikeda M, Tomita T (2001) Tea catechins prevent the development of atherosclerosis in apoprotein E-deficient mice. J Nutr 131(1):27–32

95. Hao J, Kim CH, Ha TS, Ahn HY (2007) Epigallocatechin-3 gallate prevents cardiac hypertrophy induced by pressure overload in rats. J Vet Sci 8(2):121–129
96. Piao CS, Kim DS, Ha KC, Kim HR, Chae HJ, Chae SW (2011) The Protective Effect of Epigallocatechin-3 Gallate on Ischemia/Reperfusion Injury in Isolated Rat Hearts: An ex vivo Approach. Korean J Physiol Pharm Official J Korean Physiol Soc Korean Soc Pharm 15(5):259–266. doi:10.4196/kjpp.2011.15.5.259
97. Sasaki T, Unno K, Tahara S, Shimada A, Chiba Y, Hoshino M, Kaneko T (2008) Age-related increase of superoxide generation in the brains of mammals and birds. Aging Cell 7(4):459–469. doi:10.1111/j.1474-9726.2008.00394.x
98. Unno K, Takabayashi F, Kishido T, Oku N (2004) Suppressive effect of green tea catechins on morphologic and functional regression of the brain in aged mice with accelerated senescence (SAMP10). Exp Gerontol 39(7):1027–1034. doi:10.1016/j.exger.2004.03.033
99. Unno K, Takabayashi F, Yoshida H, Choba D, Fukutomi R, Kikunaga N, Kishido T, Oku N, Hoshino M (2007) Daily consumption of green tea catechin delays memory regression in aged mice. Biogerontology 8(2):89–95. doi:10.1007/s10522-006-9036-8
100. Allen CL, Bayraktutan U (2009) Oxidative stress and its role in the pathogenesis of ischaemic stroke. Int J Stroke Official J Int Stroke Soc 4(6):461–470. doi:10.1111/j.1747-4949.2009.00387.x
101. Inanami O, Watanabe Y, Syuto B, Nakano M, Tsuji M, Kuwabara M (1998) Oral administration of (-)catechin protects against ischemia-reperfusion-induced neuronal death in the gerbil. Free Radical Res 29(4):359–365
102. Lee H, Bae JH, Lee SR (2004) Protective effect of green tea polyphenol EGCG against neuronal damage and brain edema after unilateral cerebral ischemia in gerbils. J Neurosci Res 77(6):892–900. doi:10.1002/jnr.20193
103. Lee S, Suh S, Kim S (2000) Protective effects of the green tea polyphenol (-)-epigallocatechin gallate against hippocampal neuronal damage after transient global ischemia in gerbils. Neurosci Lett 287(3):191–194
104. Lee JW, Lee YK, Ban JO, Ha TY, Yun YP, Han SB, Oh KW, Hong JT (2009) Green tea (-)-epigallocatechin-3-gallate inhibits beta-amyloid-induced cognitive dysfunction through modification of secretase activity via inhibition of ERK and NF-kappaB pathways in mice. J Nutr 139(10):1987–1993. doi:10.3945/jn.109.109785
105. Rauf A, Khan R, Raza M, Khan H, Pervez S, De Feo V, Maione F, Mascolo N (2015) Suppression of inflammatory response by chrysin, a flavone isolated from Potentilla evestita Th. Wolf. In silico predictive study on its mechanistic effect. Fitoterapia 103:129–135. doi:10.1016/j.fitote.2015.03.019
106. Weerawatanakorn M, Lee YL, Tsai CY, Lai CS, Wan X, Ho CT, Li S, Pan MH (2015) Protective effect of theaflavin-enriched black tea extracts against dimethylnitrosamine-induced liver fibrosis in rats. Food Funct 6(6):1832–1840. doi:10.1039/c5fo00126a
107. Sang S, Lambert JD, Ho CT, Yang CS (2011) The chemistry and biotransformation of tea constituents. Pharmacol Res 64(2):87–99. doi:10.1016/j.phrs.2011.02.007
108. Byun JK, Yoon BY, Jhun JY, Oh HJ, Kim EK, Min JK, Cho ML (2014) Epigallocatechin-3-gallate ameliorates both obesity and autoinflammatory arthritis aggravated by obesity by altering the balance among CD4 + T-cell subsets. Immunol Lett 157(1–2):51–59. doi:10.1016/j.imlet.2013.11.006
109. Okuda MH, Zemdegs JC, de Santana AA, Santamarina AB, Moreno MF, Hachul AC, dos Santos B, do Nascimento CM, Ribeiro EB, Oyama LM (2014) Green tea extract improves high fat diet-induced hypothalamic inflammation, without affecting the serotoninergic system. J Nutr Biochem 25(10):1084–1089. doi:10.1016/j.jnutbio.2014.05.012
110. Qin B, Polansky MM, Harry D, Anderson RA (2010) Green tea polyphenols improve cardiac muscle mRNA and protein levels of signal pathways related to insulin and lipid metabolism and inflammation in insulin-resistant rats. Mol Nutr Food Res 54(Suppl 1):S14–S23. doi:10.1002/mnfr.200900306

111. Afzal M, Safer AM, Menon M (2015) Green tea polyphenols and their potential role in health and disease. Inflammopharmacology 23(4):151–161. doi:10.1007/s10787-015-0236-1
112. Cabrera C, Artacho R, Gimenez R (2006) Beneficial effects of green tea–a review. J Am Coll Nutr 25(2):79–99
113. Hernandez Figueroa TT, Rodriguez-Rodriguez E, Sanchez-Muniz FJ (2004) The green tea, a good choice for cardiovascular disease prevention? Arch Latinoam Nutr 54(4):380–394
114. Yang CS, Hong J (2013) Prevention of chronic diseases by tea: possible mechanisms and human relevance. Annu Rev Nutr 33:161–181. doi:10.1146/annurev-nutr-071811-150717
115. Huang J, Wang Y, Xie Z, Zhou Y, Zhang Y, Wan X (2014) The anti-obesity effects of green tea in human intervention and basic molecular studies. Eur J Clin Nutr 68(10):1075–1087. doi:10.1038/ejcn.2014.143
116. Hursel R, Viechtbauer W, Westerterp-Plantenga MS (2009) The effects of green tea on weight loss and weight maintenance: a meta-analysis. Int J Obes (Lond) 33(9):956–961. doi:10.1038/ijo.2009.135
117. Basu A, Sanchez K, Leyva MJ, Wu M, Betts NM, Aston CE, Lyons TJ (2010) Green tea supplementation affects body weight, lipids, and lipid peroxidation in obese subjects with metabolic syndrome. J Am Coll Nutr 29(1):31–40
118. Chantre P, Lairon D (2002) Recent findings of green tea extract AR25 (Exolise) and its activity for the treatment of obesity. Phytomed Int J Phytotherapy Phytopharmacology 9 (1):3–8. doi:10.1078/0944-7113-00078
119. Kovacs EM, Lejeune MP, Nijs I, Westerterp-Plantenga MS (2004) Effects of green tea on weight maintenance after body-weight loss. Br J Nutr 91(3):431–437. doi:10.1079/BJN20041061
120. Maki KC, Reeves MS, Farmer M, Yasunaga K, Matsuo N, Katsuragi Y, Komikado M, Tokimitsu I, Wilder D, Jones F, Blumberg JB, Cartwright Y (2009) Green tea catechin consumption enhances exercise-induced abdominal fat loss in overweight and obese adults. J Nutr 139(2):264–270. doi:10.3945/jn.108.098293
121. Nagao T, Hase T, Tokimitsu I (2007) A green tea extract high in catechins reduces body fat and cardiovascular risks in humans. Obesity 15(6):1473–1483. doi:10.1038/oby.2007.176
122. Iso H, Date C, Wakai K, Fukui M, Tamakoshi A, Group JS (2006) The relationship between green tea and total caffeine intake and risk for self-reported type 2 diabetes among Japanese adults. Ann Inter Med 144 (8):554–562
123. Diepvens K, Kovacs EM, Nijs IM, Vogels N, Westerterp-Plantenga MS (2005) Effect of green tea on resting energy expenditure and substrate oxidation during weight loss in overweight females. Br J Nutr 94(6):1026–1034
124. Hill AM, Coates AM, Buckley JD, Ross R, Thielecke F, Howe PR (2007) Can EGCG reduce abdominal fat in obese subjects? J Am Coll Nutr 26(4):396S–402S
125. Hsu CH, Tsai TH, Kao YH, Hwang KC, Tseng TY, Chou P (2008) Effect of green tea extract on obese women: a randomized, double-blind, placebo-controlled clinical trial. Clin Nutr 27(3):363–370. doi:10.1016/j.clnu.2008.03.007
126. Mielgo-Ayuso J, Barrenechea L, Alcorta P, Larrarte E, Margareto J, Labayen I (2014) Effects of dietary supplementation with epigallocatechin-3-gallate on weight loss, energy homeostasis, cardiometabolic risk factors and liver function in obese women: randomised, double-blind, placebo-controlled clinical trial. Br J Nutr 111(7):1263–1271. doi:10.1017/S0007114513003784
127. Eckel RH, Krauss RM (1998) American Heart Association call to action: obesity as a major risk factor for coronary heart disease. AHA Nutr Committee Circ 97(21):2099–2100
128. Isomaa B, Almgren P, Tuomi T, Forsen B, Lahti K, Nissen M, Taskinen MR, Groop L (2001) Cardiovascular morbidity and mortality associated with the metabolic syndrome. Diab Care 24(4):683–689
129. Hartley L, Flowers N, Holmes J, Clarke A, Stranges S, Hooper L, Rees K (2013) Green and black tea for the primary prevention of cardiovascular disease. Cochrane Datab Syst Rev 6: CD009934. doi:10.1002/14651858.CD009934.pub2

130. Munir KM, Chandrasekaran S, Gao F, Quon MJ (2013) Mechanisms for food polyphenols to ameliorate insulin resistance and endothelial dysfunction: therapeutic implications for diabetes and its cardiovascular complications. Am J Physiol Endocrinol Metab 305(6): E679–E686. doi:10.1152/ajpendo.00377.2013
131. Kuriyama S, Shimazu T, Ohmori K, Kikuchi N, Nakaya N, Nishino Y, Tsubono Y, Tsuji I (2006) Green tea consumption and mortality due to cardiovascular disease, cancer, and all causes in Japan: the Ohsaki study. JAMA 296(10):1255–1265. doi:10.1001/jama.296.10.1255
132. Mineharu Y, Koizumi A, Wada Y, Iso H, Watanabe Y, Date C, Yamamoto A, Kikuchi S, Inaba Y, Toyoshima H, Kondo T, Tamakoshi A, Group Js (2011) Coffee, green tea, black tea and oolong tea consumption and risk of mortality from cardiovascular disease in Japanese men and women. J Epidemiol Community Health 65(3):230–240. doi:10.1136/jech.2009.097311
133. Wang ZM, Zhou B, Wang YS, Gong QY, Wang QM, Yan JJ, Gao W, Wang LS (2011) Black and green tea consumption and the risk of coronary artery disease: a meta-analysis. Am J Clin Nutr 93(3):506–515. doi:10.3945/ajcn.110.005363
134. Wierzejska R (2014) Tea and health—a review of the current state of knowledge. Przeglad Epidemiologiczny 68(3):501–506, 595–509
135. Alzheimer's A (2015) 2015 Alzheimer's disease facts and figures. Alzheimer's Dement J Alzheimer's Assoc 11(3):332–384
136. Halliwell B (2001) Role of free radicals in the neurodegenerative diseases: therapeutic implications for antioxidant treatment. Drugs Aging 18(9):685–716
137. Kuriyama S, Hozawa A, Ohmori K, Shimazu T, Matsui T, Ebihara S, Awata S, Nagatomi R, Arai H, Tsuji I (2006) Green tea consumption and cognitive function: a cross-sectional study from the Tsurugaya Project 1. Am J Clin Nutr 83(2):355–361
138. Kandinov B, Giladi N, Korczyn AD (2009) Smoking and tea consumption delay onset of Parkinson's disease. Parkinsonism Relat Disord 15(1):41–46. doi:10.1016/j.parkreldis.2008.02.011
139. Mak JC (2012) Potential role of green tea catechins in various disease therapies: progress and promise. Clin Exp Pharmacol Physiol 39(3):265–273. doi:10.1111/j.1440-1681.2012.05673.x
140. Sun CL, Yuan JM, Koh WP, Yu MC (2006) Green tea, black tea and colorectal cancer risk: a meta-analysis of epidemiologic studies. Carcinogenesis 27(7):1301–1309. doi:10.1093/carcin/bgl024
141. Li N, Sun Z, Han C, Chen J (1999) The chemopreventive effects of tea on human oral precancerous mucosa lesions. In: Proceedings of the society for experimental biology and medicine society for experimental biology and medicine, vol 220, no 4, pp 218–224
142. Bettuzzi S, Brausi M, Rizzi F, Castagnetti G, Peracchia G, Corti A (2006) Chemoprevention of human prostate cancer by oral administration of green tea catechins in volunteers with high-grade prostate intraepithelial neoplasia: a preliminary report from a one-year proof-of-principle study. Cancer Res 66(2):1234–1240
143. Choan E, Segal R, Jonker D, Malone S, Reaume N, Eapen L, Gallant V (2005) A prospective clinical trial of green tea for hormone refractory prostate cancer: an evaluation of the complementary/alternative therapy approach. Urol Oncol 23(2):108–113. doi:10.1016/j.urolonc.2004.10.008
144. Jatoi A, Ellison N, Burch PA, Sloan JA, Dakhil SR, Novotny P, Tan W, Fitch TR, Rowland KM, Young CY, Flynn PJ (2003) A phase II trial of green tea in the treatment of patients with androgen independent metastatic prostate carcinoma. Cancer 97(6):1442–1446. doi:10.1002/cncr.11200
145. McLarty J, Bigelow RL, Smith M, Elmajian D, Ankem M, Cardelli JA (2009) Tea polyphenols decrease serum levels of prostate-specific antigen, hepatocyte growth factor, and vascular endothelial growth factor in prostate cancer patients and inhibit production of hepatocyte growth factor and vascular endothelial growth factor in vitro. Cancer Prev Res (Phila) 2(7):673–682. doi:10.1158/1940-6207.CAPR-08-0167 1940-6207.CAPR-08-0167[pii]

146. Shimizu M, Fukutomi Y, Ninomiya M, Nagura K, Kato T, Araki H, Suganuma M, Fujiki H, Moriwaki H (2008) Green tea extracts for the prevention of metachronous colorectal adenomas: a pilot study. Cancer Epidemiol Biomarkers Prev 17(11):3020–3025
147. Stingl JC, Ettrich T, Muche R, Wiedom M, Brockmoller J, Seeringer A, Seufferlein T (2011) Protocol for minimizing the risk of metachronous adenomas of the colorectum with green tea extract (MIRACLE): a randomised controlled trial of green tea extract versus placebo for nutriprevention of metachronous colon adenomas in the elderly population. BMC Cancer 11:360. doi:10.1186/1471-2407-11-360
148. Lee MJ, Wang ZY, Li H, Chen L, Sun Y, Gobbo S, Balentine DA, Yang CS (1995) Analysis of plasma and urinary tea polyphenols in human subjects. Cancer Epidemiol Biomarkers Prev 4(4):393–399
149. Yang F, de Villiers WJ, McClain CJ, Varilek GW (1998) Green tea polyphenols block endotoxin-induced tumor necrosis factor-production and lethality in a murine model. J Nutr 128(12):2334–2340
150. Jimenez-Saenz M, Martinez-Sanchez Mdel C (2006) Acute hepatitis associated with the use of green tea infusions. J Hepatol 44(3):616–617 S0168-8278(05)00816-0 [pii]/j.jhep.2005.11.041

Capsaicin and Its Role in Chronic Diseases

E.S. Fernandes, A.R.A. Cerqueira, A.G. Soares and Soraia K.P. Costa

Abstract A significant number of experimental and clinical studies published in peer-reviewed journals have demonstrated promising pharmacological properties of capsaicin in relieving signs and symptoms of non-communicable diseases (chronic diseases). This chapter provides an overview made from basic and clinical research studies of the potential therapeutic effects of capsaicin, loaded in different application forms, such as solution and cream, on chronic diseases (e.g. arthritis, chronic pain, functional gastrointestinal disorders and cancer). In addition to the anti-inflammatory and analgesic properties of capsaicin largely recognized via, mainly, interaction with the TRPV1, the effects of capsaicin on different cell signalling pathways will be further discussed here. The analgesic, anti-inflammatory or apoptotic effects of capsaicin show promising results in arthritis, neuropathic pain, gastrointestinal disorders or cancer, since evidence demonstrates that the oral or local application of capsaicin reduce inflammation and pain in rheumatoid arthritis, promotes gastric protection against ulcer and induces apoptosis of the tumour cells. Sadly, these results have been paralleled by conflicting studies, which indicate that high concentrations of capsaicin are likely to evoke deleterious effects, thus suggesting that capsaicin activates different pathways at different concentrations in both human and rodent tissues. Thus, to establish effective capsaicin doses for chronic conditions, which can be benefited from capsaicin therapeutic effects, is a real challenge that must be pursued.

Keywords Red pepper · Capsaicin · Chronic diseases · Respiratory diseases · Pain relief · Cancer

E.S. Fernandes
Programa de Pós-Graduação, Universidade Ceuma, São Luís-MA, Brazil

E.S. Fernandes
Vascular Biology Section, Cardiovascular Division, King's College London, London, UK

A.R.A. Cerqueira · A.G. Soares · S.K.P. Costa (✉)
Department of Pharmacology, Institute of Biomedical Sciences (ICB), University of São Paulo (USP), Av. Prof. Lineu Prestes, 1524 - Room 326, Butantan, São Paulo 05508-900, SP, Brazil
e-mail: scosta@icb.usp.br

S.C. Gupta et al. (eds.), *Drug Discovery from Mother Nature*,
Advances in Experimental Medicine and Biology 929,
DOI 10.1007/978-3-319-41342-6_5

1 Introduction

1.1 Physico-Chemical Properties of Capsaicin

In parallel to the popular use of red and green chilli peppers as spices and/or additives in food, over the last 70 years, at least 12,000 Medline reports have assigned the pharmacological and physiological contribution of capsaicin, an alkaloid isolated from chillies as a medicinal plant, to treat pain, cough [222, 224] and other host conditions, such as cancer (vide review: 47), allergic [228] and gastro-intestinal diseases [235]. It is believed that the gates were opened to the field of neurogenic inflammation with the work produced by Jancsó et al. in the mid-60s [121]; however, the effects of capsaicin on heat regulation stem from the early 50s [116, 117].

Along with studies dating back to the 40s, the chemistry and biology of capsaicin, the major alkaloid found in chilli (*Capsicum* sp.) has been extensively explored (for review see: [187]). It is believed that *Capsicum* species are native from Central or South America. Nowadays, it is known that at least 20 *Capsicum* species are endemic or are already cultivated in distinct regions worldwide, including tropical America, Central and South America (e.g. Mexico and Colombia swamps, and in Bolivia and Peru highlands), Southern Europe, all Asian countries and Africa [79, 234].

Capsaicin chemical structure (8-Methyl-N-vanillyl-trans-6-nonenamide) was first identified by Tresh in 1876, but its molecular structure was only described more than 20 years later by Dawson, in 1919 (Fig. 1; for review see: [187]). Since then, structure–activity relationship studies (SARs) based on capsaicin structure were carried out, leading to the discovery, in chilli peppers, of at least ten unsaturated and saturated amides, named capsaicinoids, as well as the production of synthetic analogues [137], which displayed some similarities or more potent responses than capsaicin [9, 153, 211]; for review see: [187]. The capsaicinoids nordihydrocapsaicin, homodihydrocapsaicin and homocapsaicin exhibit only half of the pungency (spicy flavour) of capsaicin and dihydrocapsaicin. On the other hand, the naturally occurring chemical found in resin spurge (*Euphorbia resinifera*), named Resiniferatoxin (RTX), is an ultrapotent (100–10,000 fold) analogue of capsaicin (for review see: [210]).

Based on SARs studies, capsaicin molecule can be divided into three regions: aromatic, amide bond and hydrophobic side chain. It has two hydrogen-bond donors, three hydrogen-bond acceptors, nine rotatable bonds, Log P of $\sim$3.0, a polar surface of 58.6 Å, a melting point of 65 °C, a boiling point of 210–220 °C at 0.01 mm Hg, sublimates at 115 °C and presents a spectral point for UVmax at 227, 281 nm (ε = 7000, 2500). Changes in capsaicin primary structure (e.g. replacing positions in the aromatic ring, and groups in the hydrophobic side chain) are essential to affect either its agonist activity or potency [18, 130]. The properties of hydrogen bonds (donor and acceptor) of the phenol group of capsaicin and analogues/agonists also contribute to the potent biological activities [130]. Thus,

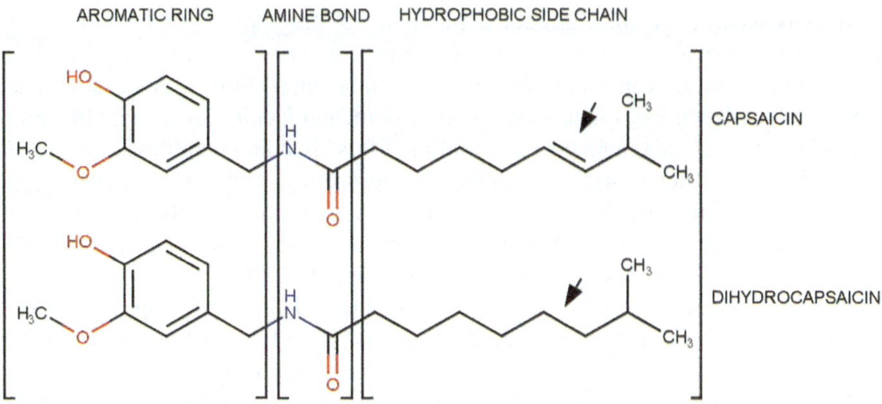

Fig. 1 Capsaicin and dyhidrocapsaicin chemical structures differing among the removal on the double bond on the 6th carbon position for the latter, which increase the degree of its flexibility. Both capsaicin and dyhidrocapsaicin chemical structures comprise a lateral chain with 8-carbon long lateral chain, an aromatic region (I), amide bond (II) and the hydrophobic side chain (III). Changes in the capsaicinoids ring will reflect in changes in their potency, mainly in the 3 and 4 ring positions

changes in the number of both hydrogen- and rotatable bonds may interfere with drug distribution, making these compounds more or less lipophilic.

In order to display maximum potency at molecular target transient receptor potential vanilloid 1 (TRPV1), capsaicin and capsaicinoids structures might possess a specific aromatic A-ring configuration, the presence of a hydrogen bond-donating group in the B region, and a hydrophobic hydrocarbon C-region tail of 8–12 carbons [5, 233]. Commercially available, capsaicin is presented as a crystalline hydrophobic and colourless alkaloid highly volatile with a pungent odour but freely soluble in alcohol, ether or benzene. Its burning taste when placed into the oral cavity can be detectable in 1 part in 100,000 ([182]; for review see: [187]; International Union of Pure and Applied Chemistry-IUPAC). Although capsaicin presents *cis/trans* isomerism, the *trans* isomer is the most stable structure as a consequence of the steric hindrance between the isopropyl group [–$CH(CH_3)_2$] and the long hydrocarbon chain in the *cis* isomer (Fig. 1; for review see: [11, 187]).

At least two distinct pathways are involved in the synthesis of capsaicinoids: one related to the formation of the aromatic molecule and another to the hydrophobic side chain, and both are joined by an amine bond. Capsaicin can be synthesized in vivo by two pathways: (i) phenylpropanoid, involved in the synthesis of the aromatic ring; and (ii) fatty acid metabolic, which determines its fatty acids [11, 178]. In the event of a reduction of the capsaicin in the acyl chain, the molecule is turned into dihydrocapsaicin (Fig. 1; see review: [187]). Such changes might be processed by the action of enzyme family dehydrogenase/reductase. ETR (2-noyl thioester reductase) reduces the hydrophobic chain converting capsaicin in dihydrocapsaicin. Interfering with the acyl formation before the complete formation of the molecule might have a similar effect with less energy expenditure [4, 14, 41, 230].

Increased capsaicin concentration is paralleled by fruit development, and it peaks 40–50 days later after development [51]. Different types of chilli vary widely in their heat. Likewise, capsaicin biosynthesis and accumulation in vivo varies from plant to plant depending on genetic and environmental factors, such as hydric stress [102, 187]. In fact, augmented concentration of this alkaloid in chillies is commonly seen following water shortage (via the phenylpropanoid pathway) and augmented activity of enzymes involved in capsaicin production, such involved in capsaicin production, such as phenylalanine ammonia lyase (PAL), cinnamic acid 4-hydroxylase (Ca4H) and capsaicinoid synthetase (CS) [80, 207].

In the cayenne pepper (*Capsicum* annuum L.), both capsaicin (MW 305.41 g/mol) and dihydrocapsaicin (MW 307.42 g/mol) comprise 79 % to 90 % of the existing capsaicinoids [19]. Capsaicin and dihydrocapsaicin chemical and molecular structures are identical, differing only in the saturation of an acyl group (Fig. 1). In terms of activity, capsaicin and dihydrocapsaicin appear to promote, but evidence shows that on different cell lines, such as human colon cancer (HCT116), breast cancer (MCF-7), normal lung epithelial and fibroblast cells (WI38), the latter, at high concentrations, evokes a more pronounced effect on cell viability than the former [179]. Likewise, short-lasting treatment with dihydrocapsaicin on human lung carcinoma cell line (A549) induced a marked acute response compared with capsaicin [99, 179].

The implication of *Pal*, *Ca4h*, *Comt*, *Kas*, *Acl* and *Fat* genes on capsaicin metabolism has been suggested elsewhere [7, 60]. In particular, *Pun1* locus (product of *Pun1*) participates in the development of vesicles, where the capsaicinoids are stored, and the relative spiciness of the chilli [11].

1.1.1 Activities and Modulation of Cell Signalling Pathways by Capsaicin

A significant number of scientific studies have described the biological and toxicological actions of capsaicin in different systems. In spite of capsaicin's popular therapeutic property being officially described over 150 years ago [227], an endogenous target for capsaicin effects was only proposed in the 70s by Szolcsányi and Gábor [218]. In addition, in the early 90s, binding studies using an specific [3H]RTX provided the first and indirect evidence of a specific membrane recognition site, named vanilloid receptor, thought to be expressed almost exclusively by primary sensory neurons, involved in nociception and neurogenic inflammation [211]. It was suggested that the vanilloid receptor structure was very complex (size around 270 $\pm$ 25 kDa) and could only be recognized by the homovanillic acid present in capsaicinoids and RTX. The affinity order to both RTX and capsaicin binding to vanilloid receptors in rat tissues is higher for RTX [209, 212].

It was not established until the mid-90s, whether endogenous ligands would regulate the activity of the vanilloid receptor, nor whether this receptor belonged to the TRPs family [209]. Soon after, numerous evidence arose to suggest that the vanilloid receptor is not only a single receptor but rather a family of receptors, capable of recognizing RTX, capsaicin and related structural analogues among others, thus suggesting that new specific vanilloid receptor subtype compounds should be synthesized exempt from the detrimental side effects of capsaicin [213]. During that period, evidences suggested that resiniferatoxin is only similar to capsaicin in potency for induction of pain; however, it is much more effective to provoke desensitization [214].

In the later 90s, structure–activity analysis in whole animal experiments provided further evidence for biologic dissociation, strongly arguing for the existence of vanilloid receptor subclasses. In fact, studies by Biró et al. [25] showed that whereas multiple high-affinity vanilloid receptor subclasses mediate vanilloid responses, the subclass of vanilloid receptors sensitive to resiniferatoxin does not seem to be the voltage-independent, cation-nonselective ion channel. In the same period, Caterina et al. [38] cloned a capsaicin receptor from C-fibre small-diameter sensory neurons and named it as vanilloid-gated nonselective cation channel (VR1) due to its structural relationship (six transmembrane domains and a short, pore-forming hydrophobic stretch between the fifth and sixth transmembrane domains) with members of the transient receptor potential (TRP) channel family, first identified as a component of the *Drosophila* phototransduction pathway [170].

Soon after VR1 was later named as TRPV1, and , an avalanche of studies began to explore its expression and signalling mechanisms. This receptor was found to be also expressed in a variety of non-neuronal cells [185, 225, 245]; for review see: Fernandes et al. [82]. Differences in the magnitude of agonist responses to the VR1 were described to animal species and population expression in tissues, thus showing some intra- and inter-species heterogeneity for this receptor [126].

In parallel, a significant number of unrelated vanniloid substances or stimuli, such as increase in temperature in the noxious range (>43 °C; Caterina et al. [38]), low pH [23], voltage dependence [199], lipids [255] and animal toxins isolated from spider, snake and wasp venom, seem to display a capsaicin like effect on sensory nerve fibres [53–58, 61, 63, 201, 250].

1.1.2 Capsaicin Effects on Neuronal and Non-neuronal Cells

To date, the best studied effects of capsaicin are related to sensory neurons. The binding of capsaicin to TRPV1, expressed on sensory neurons, may trigger extracellular Ca^{+2}influx, a response that becomes usually desensitized upon continuous stimulation with capsaicin [38, 150, 247]. Desensitization has been associated with the availability of extracellular Ca^{+2} [38]. Interestingly, capsaicin sensitizes TRPV1 to endogenous and exogenous agonists, even at concentrations unable to induce cation influx [111]. Capsaicin effects might be amplified following cell exposure to other stimuli known to activate TRPV1, e.g. pH and heat <43 °C [38, 191].

It is well known that capsaicin given to newborn rats, at high concentration, induces selective degeneration (death) of a distinct population of primary sensory neurones in vivo [119], via a mechanism dependent on excessive ion influx and, perhaps necrosis rather than apoptosis of sensory neurons [24]. However, capsaicin, at low concentration (nM range), induces apoptosis in cultured rat cortical and in dorsal root ganglion (DRG) cells [200, 237]. These effects are suggested to be TRPV1-mediated [24, 200] and to involve the downstream activation of kinases [200]. Interestingly, Guo et al. [96] showed that capsaicin protects rat hippocampal neurons from hypoxia-reoxygenation-induced apoptosis via phosphorylation of Akt and phosphoinositide 3-kinase (PI3K), independently of TRPV1-mediated capsaicin actions.

Capsaicin is a lipophilic compound and evidence accounts to suggest that capsaicin binding site on TRPV1 is intracellular [91, 127]; for review see: Rosenbaum and Simon [190]. Indeed, capsaicin binds to the residues Arg114 and Glu761 in the intracellular N- and C-termini, respectively [128], and to the residues Tyr511, Ser512 and Thr550 in the third and fifth TRPV1 transmembrane domains [91, 126]. Either in vitro or in vivo studies on cellular and molecular mechanisms show that TRPV1 activation by capsaicin is followed by downstream phosphorylation of protein kinase (ERK) in small-diameter DRG neurons [62]. Either the p38 mitogen-activated protein kinase [167] or ERK5 [166] plays a similar role in TRPV1-mediated capsaicin effects in small- and medium-sized DRG rat neurons. To sense nociceptive effects, it has been shown that TRPV1 activation by capsaicin followed by downstream phosphorylation of ERK, p38 and ERK5 is mandatory [62, 166, 167].

Countless studies have demonstrated the ability of capsaicin to trigger neuropeptides release, such as substance P (SP) and calcitonin-gene-related peptide (CGRP), from sensory neurons in a Ca^{+2}-depending manner, which in turn commonly leads to neurogenic inflammation [55, 84, 90, 109, 192]. Most of these neuropeptide-mediated responses were later shown to be resultant on TRPV1 activation by capsaicin [76, 83, 196]. More recently, it has been shown that activation of PKC following capsaicin-induced TRPV1 activation is essential for neuropeptide release from sensory neurons [243]. In fact, previous studies by the same authors show that TRPV1 mRNA and protein levels in skin sensory neurons are rapidly increased via a PKC-dependent mechanism, which involves capsaicin-mediated TRPV1 activation in vivo [242]. Likewise, PAR-4 mRNA levels were significantly increased in DRG neurons exposed to capsaicin [42]. This finding is of relevance as it may amplify TRPV1-mediated responses by exogenous and, in special, by endogenous agonists.

Although a number of supporting evidences have shown that capsaicin actions on sensory neurons are mediated by TRPV1, an emerging intriguing finding by Yang et al. [246] shows an inhibitory effect of capsaicin on voltage-gated potassium channels in cultured trigeminal ganglions, independently of TRPV1 activation, but dependently on protein kinase A (PKA) activation on these cells.

In addition to the related actions of capsaicin on neuronal cells, a group of evidence has emerged in the 70s, showing capsaicin effects on peripheral target tissues. These evidences were based on the fact that TRPV1 was found to be functionally expressed on non-neuronal cells [82, 119, 129]. This has highlighted the importance of understanding capsaicin effects on others structures, which may be mediated or not by TRPV1.

As previously described for sensory neurons, capsaicin, at μM concentrations, produces toxicity in non-neuronal cells in vitro, including different cancer cell lines: HeLa, ovarian carcinoma, mammary adenocarcinoma, HL-60 cells [154, 155, 171], HepG2 human hepatoma cells [132, 145] and pancreatic cancer cells [251, 252]. The capsaicin-induced apoptosis in cancer cells is thought to be mediated through reactive oxygen species (ROS) generation, such as hydrogen peroxide, which is linked to cell cycle arrest and activation of apoptosis-related molecules such as caspase-3 and p53. An important capsaicin-induced endoplasmic reticulum (ER) stress-dependent apoptosis was also described [149]. Nonetheless, a significant number of studies do not show clear evidence for capsaicin-induced apoptosis in cancer cells via TRPV1, as they required high concentrations of capsaicin (μM) to evoke its effects [134, 175]. In agreement, the pretreatment of pancreatic cancer cells with capsazepine, a non-selective TRPV1 antagonist, failed to prevent capsaicin-induced apoptosis [251, 252]. Accordingly, at high but not low concentrations, capsaicin evokes toxic effects in human keratinocytes [136], normal human epidermal keratinocytes and HaCaT cells [183]. Of note, at nM concentrations, capsaicin evokes apoptosis in neurons [183].

Capsaicin effects on cancer cells have been associated with increases in intracellular Ca^{+2} [110, 155], thus suggesting that it is possible that although TRPV1 may be implicated in Ca^{+2} influx in these cells, its activation does not influence ROS generation and apoptosis. Besides TRPV1 was shown to be functionally expressed on normal human epidermal keratinocytes [115]; the effects resultant from high concentrations of capsaicin on these cells have been suggested to be TRPV1-independent [13, 126, 183]. The in vivo intra tumoural injection of capsaicin into a mouse fibro sarcoma [22] or mouse with pancreatic cancer induced tumour apoptosis [149].

Interestingly, capsaicin also evoked toxicity in both the cultured human epidermal fibroblasts [136] and human lung epithelial fibroblast cells (WI38 cells), in addition to promoting cell death at high doses [180]. Exposure of human lung fibroblasts to capsaicin led to different levels of p53, associated with ER stress, which induced cell cycle arrest and subsequent apoptosis [180]. Capsaicin when incubated with fibroblast-like SW982 cell line, at 1 μM range, triggers ROS production in a TRPV1-dependent manner [236]. Moreover, both mRNA and protein expressions of TRPV1 at cultured human synovial fibroblasts have been shown elsewhere [108, 138, 139, 236].

Capsaicin may also present different effects on other cell types depending on the stimuli. When incubated with HUVEC cells, high concentrations of capsaicin protect these cells against oxLDL-induced apoptosis, via inhibition of oxidative stress, reduction of caspase-3 expression and increase of the anti-apoptotic protein Bcl-2 [40]. Conversely, capsaicin further increases anandamide-induced death in HUVEC cells via TRPV1 [244]. Capsaicin effects on endothelial cells go beyond cell survival. Indeed, capsaicin at a relatively low concentration induces endothelial-dependent relaxation in pig coronary arteries by activation of TRPV1, and downstream production of nitric oxide via eNOS and opening of K^+ channels [33]. Similarly, a study by Kark et al. [129] showed that capsaicin (up to 10 nM) causes relaxation of rat muscle arterioles by acting on endothelial cells. These findings were later supported by a study in which mice were fed with capsaicin diet for 7 months [245]. In the latter study, dietary capsaicin increased the activation of PKA and eNOS, triggering release of NO and subsequent relaxation, via TRPV1 activation. Additionally to its effects on endothelial cells, capsaicin is also able to evoke responses in smooth muscle cells. The same study by Kark et al. [129] presented evidence of a constrictor effect for high concentrations of capsaicin. This effect was dependent on TRPV1 expression and activation on smooth muscle cells.

Recently, studies have shown the expression of TRPV1 on mouse and human adipocytes. Indeed, capsaicin was shown to reduce adipogenesis in 3T3-L1-preadipocytes, via TRPV1, and to increase its expression in vitro [253]. As for other cell types, high concentrations of capsaicin reduced the viability of 3T3-L1-preadipocytes [107]. However, incubation of these cells with lower concentrations of this compound did not alter cell survival [146]. The same study showed that capsaicin stimulates lipolysis in adipocytes, possibly due to the suppression of protein expression of the adipogenic transcription factors, peroxisome proliferator-activated receptor-g (PPAR-γ) and CCAAT enhancer-binding protein-α (C/EBP-α) during the stage of adipocyte differentiation [107]. Capsaicin also increases the mRNA expression of HSL, CPT-Iα and UCP2, involved in lipid catabolism in adipocytes [146]. Interestingly, in vivo topical application of 0.075 % capsaicin cream in the mouse abdominal skin for 8 weeks reduced mesenteric and epididymal adipose tissue as lipid accumulation in adipocytes was diminished in mice fed with high-fat diet [147]. Analysis of their mesenteric adipose tissue demonstrated lower levels of tumour necrosis factor-α (TNF-α) and interleukin-6 (IL-6) levels in comparison with obese control animals. This was accompanied by increased mRNA expression of adipokines and genes related to lipid metabolism: adiponectin, adipsin, visfatin, lipoproteinlipase (LPL), PPAR(α, β/δ, γ), UCP2, fatty acid-binding protein 4(FABP4), fatty acid transporter 1 and acyl-CoA synthetase long-chain family member 1 (ACSL1) [147]. Novel evidence in vivo showed that capsaicin only prevents lipid accumulation at lower doses, while at higher doses it enhances accumulation of lipids [15]. The same study suggests that capsaicin inhibitory actions on adipocyte differentiation are TRPV1-mediated.

Altogether the evidence accounts to suggest that capsaicin (and its TRPV1 receptor) represents a potential alternative therapeutic class to treat a range of inflammatory diseases, including those related to chronic stage.

1.1.3 Do Capsaicin and Its TRPV1 Receptor Represent a Target for Multiple Chronic Diseases Therapy?

Chronic diseases, also named as Non-Communicable Diseases (NCD), as they do not pass from one person to another, are usually of difficult diagnosis, long duration (>3 months) and generally slow progression. They can be defined as any pathology that has no cure and, regardless of being caused by genetic or environmental factors, the chronic diseases cannot be pharmacologically prevented, but can be controlled, thus improving the life quality of patients [35]. According to medical criteria, chronic diseases require frequent medical appointments, examinations and treatments and, in particular, are potential causes of early disability or significant reduction of life expectancy.

Among the chronic diseases, some are highlighted by the World Health Organization (241), including cardiovascular diseases (CVD), diabetes, arthritis and related pain process, chronic obstructive pulmonary diseases, gastrointestinal diseases and cancer. They are the leading causes of mortality and by far can be blamed for 60 % of all deaths worldwide [238, 241]. These diseases promote high healthcare expenditures and are associated with high morbidity rates and disabilities, leading to loss of work and depression [32, 77, 181, 238].

The current therapy may not effectively control the progress of chronic diseases; thus, the search for alternative treatments is still the subject of intense research. In this context, over the last thirty years, scientific database research, such as Medline and Embase, has retrieved more than 19,000 articles on the therapeutic potential of capsaicin to treat pain, and a range of non-communicable diseases. Of these, at least 55 % are related to basic research, and a minor percentage (3 %) is correlated with capsaicin and clinical studies (Fig. 2). The vast majority of these capsaicin studies focus on chronic pain (1598), followed by cancer research (1289), arthritis (517) and others.

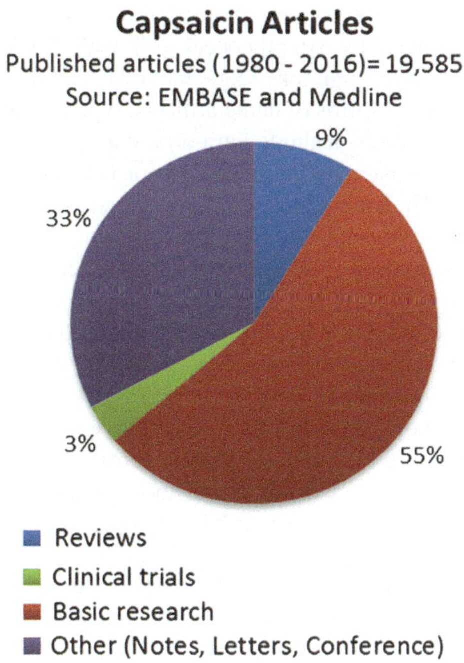

Fig. 2 Displays the cumulative number (19,585) and corresponding percentage of capsaicin studies assigned to chronic diseases in basic and clinical science in PubMed (Medline) database from 1980 to Jan 2016. Embase database contains approximately the same number

1.1.4 Effects of Capsaicin on Arthritis

Arthritis is a common word to refer to an inflammatory response on one or more joints that causes pain and stiffness, which commonly leads to disability. There are at least 100 types of arthritis, commonly known as the connective tissue disorders that can affect individuals of all ages, sexes and races; however, there is significant evidence to suggest that both the elderly and women are more affected [202].

Among different types of arthritis, the degenerative arthritis (osteoarthritis—OA) and inflammatory arthritis, such as rheumatoid arthritis (RA), are the leading cause of disability worldwide [74, 156, 202].

Rheumatoid arthritis (RA) is a systemic inflammatory autoimmune disease, characterized by impairment of the synovial membrane of peripheral joints, whereas OA is a progressive disorder of the joints caused by gradual loss of cartilage, thus leading to bony spurs and cysts development at the margins of the joints. In the USA, one in five adults (22.7 %) develops arthritis [35]. Likewise, arthritis is the greatest cause (10 million people) of disability in the UK, whose most prevalent forms are RA and OA, affecting approximately seven thousand and eight million people, respectively [125, 172, 202].

By comparison, animal models of arthritis were developed in the last 50 years in rodents, in addition to a variety of animal strains and genetically modified animals introduced in recent years, which have greatly helped rheumatologists and researchers to achieve a better understanding of inflammatory joint diseases and thus, develop new treatments for arthritic conditions [6]. Arthritis models share some similarities with the different forms of arthritis in humans, including innate and adaptive immunological characteristics. There are animal models of RA induced by streptococcal cell wall (SCW), collagen (CIA), Freund's complete adjuvant antigen (e.g. methylated bovine serum albumin—mBSA) injection. Several forms of acute arthritis, typically monoarticular, are widely used and can be induced by a single intra-articular injection of carrageenan (CGN) CFA, and kaolin, administered simultaneously or isolated [12, 34, 36, 67, 78, 85].

Of note, it seems that the first report on the protective effect of capsaicin in experimental arthritis was shown more than thirty years ago [50, 75, 193]. According to Colpaert et al. [50], capsaicin (20–80 mg/kg) injected s.c. reduced significantly *Mycobacterium butyricum*-induced inflammatory articular response in the rat, and this effect lasted longer than 20 days, being reproducible prior or post the onset of inflammation, as well as when inflammatory response peaked. Using an animal model of Complete Freund's adjuvant (CFA)-induced arthritis, the same authors observed that treatment with capsaicin reduced levels of substance P in neuronal tissues, suggesting a role for substance P in CFA-induced arthritis manifestations. Corroborating these findings, the involvement of substance P and its peripheral tachykinin NK1 receptor was later shown in a CGN model of arthritis in the rat temporomandibular joint (TMJ; Denadai-Souza [67]). Indeed, Carleson et al. [37] showed previously the pretreatment of animals with capsaicin or the denervation of the mandibular branch of the trigeminal nerve prevented the arthritis evoked by unilateral injection of a suspension containing heat-killed

Mycobacterium butyricum into the TMJ of female Lewis rats, as well as significantly lowered the levels of substance P-LI in the trigeminal ganglia and TMJ. Together, these findings show a close relationship between sympathetic neurones and neuropeptide release from sensory this model.

Further, Inman et al. [114] observed that capsaicin concomitantly administered with mBSA into the rat knee markedly reduced the severity of arthritis in comparison with the contralateral inflamed knee treated with vehicle, supporting a protective role for capsaicin in reducing the severity of antigen-induced arthritis in felines. Likewise, by injecting uric acid or Freund's complete adjuvant into the rat knee, a severe model of monoarthritis associated with long-lasting hyperalgesia was developed. Either uric acid or Freund's complete adjuvant-induced arthritis exhibited a high and dose-dependent sensitivity to capsaicin (s.c.), similar to that produced by the non-steroid anti-inflammatory agents, indomethacin and ibuprofen, [64]. Barton et al. [20] suggest that TRPV1 channels were involved in the mechanism of joint inflammation and mechanical hypersensitivity seen in CFA-induced arthritis.

Considering that the research into capsaicin-mediated amelioration of experimental arthritis has advanced, it has become clear that this alkaloid could also exert a protective effect against different forms of arthritis and pain-related processes in humans. Deal and co-workers [65], in 1991, demonstrated possibly for the first time in a double-blind randomized study the efficacy of capsaicin cream 0.025 %, four times a day, in reducing 57 % the painful knees in patients with OA ($n = 70$) and RA ($n = 31$). Soon after, McCarthy and McCarty [162] suggest, in a 4-week double-blind study, that topical capsaicin in higher concentration, 0.075 %, was more effective in reducing the painful joints in both RA and OA patients than that response with capsaicin at smaller concentration.

Interestingly, clinical research continued to provide new insights into a novel cream formulation containing glyceryl trinitrate (1.33 %) and small concentrations of capsaicin (0.025 %), which applied daily over the affected joint during 6-week period, produced a superior analgesic effect in painful OA compared to capsaicin alone [163]. Importantly, this association reduced the patient tolerance to capsaicin. Later on, Kosuwon et al. showed that capsaicin gel (0.0125 %) was markedly effective for treating mild to moderate degrees of OA in the elderly patient compared with placebo gel. Three years later, the same authors reported that this therapeutic scheme using capsaicin gel not only promoted the desired therapeutic effect, but also increased patient adherence to the treatment [140]. Soon after this study, Schnitzer et al. [194] showed that civamide, a capsaicin analogue (cis isomer of capsaicin), at 0.075 % in a topical cream formulation exhibited great therapeutic efficacy in the treatment of OA symptoms and, more importantly, exhibited low toxicity even during long term therapy.

Recently, a meta-analysis study concluded that topical capsaicin treatment applied during long periods and at a frequency of four times a day evokes moderate analgesic effect in addition to being well tolerated up to 20 weeks in patients with moderate pain or OA [144]. In contrast, a previous computer-assisted search of the Cochrane Central Register of Controlled Trials (CENTRAL) in 2010, revealed that topical capsaicin appears modestly effective compared to placebo in reducing pain in patients with RA (Richards et al. [188]).

Despite these conflicting studies on the role of capsaicin, clinical trials in progress continue trying to demonstrate the superiority of capsaicin in promoting analgesic effect, patient quality of life and satisfaction with the pain management with several other classic analgesics (NCT02403687).

1.1.5 Management of Chronic Pain by Capsaicin

It is well established that pain is a defensive mechanism in humans or contextually speaking, the painful sensation will act as a signalling mechanism to the body in response to a potential or aversive stimulus present in the environment that can cause damage to the body. In contrast to acute pain, chronic pain by definition has been recognized as a process that persists past normal healing time [30], and it is often characterized as a persistent pain process lasting longer than 3–6 months. Unlike acute pain form, chronic pain has no protective character, and its establishment entails marked psychological damage to the affected individual [161, 226]. In animals, the painful sensation induced by skin contact with a very hot surface, a sharp object or evoked by a chemical compound evokes learning behaviours of protection against such stimuli.

It is estimated that 10.1–55.2 % of the world population suffers from some type of chronic pain [101]. According to WHO, at least 1 in 10 adult individuals is diagnosed with chronic pain each year and, more importantly, 1 in five individuals worldwide suffers from moderate to severe chronic pain, thus leading to significant disruption of social lifestyle and depression with suicidal thoughts ([113]; for review see: Goldberg and McGee [92]).

Despite the huge impact and relevance of chronic pain, the exact mechanisms involved in the establishment of this framework are not fully understood. It is known that short- and long-term changes in parts of the central nervous system (CNS) and peripheral nervous system are involved in this process, which are very often caused by diseases (e.g. cancer and different types of arthritis such as RA and osteoarthritis), long-term tissue damage (e.g. nociceptive pain) or nerve fibres lesions (neuropathic pain), as stated elsewhere [48, 161]. In addition, the severity of the painful picture may even be graduated based on its intensity, pain-related distress and functional impairment [226].

Of recent interest a new International Classification of Diseases (ICD) version for chronic pain, that comprises 7 types of most common clinically relevant disorders, has been proposed by pain specialists and reviewed by the WHO Steering Committee, and they are as follows: (1) chronic primary pain, (2) chronic cancer pain, (3) chronic posttraumatic and postsurgical pain, (4) chronic neuropathic pain, (5) chronic headache and orofacial pain, (6) chronic visceral pain and (7) chronic musculoskeletal pain [226, 239].

Despite the analgesic effectiveness of NSAIDS and opioids, in many cases the chronic pain process is, resistant to these therapies. Thus, the search for therapeutic alternatives and better understanding of the mechanisms involved remain targets of intense research. In this review, due to the nature and complexity of chronic pain diseases, this article will address the role of capsaicin treatment in general models, including neuropathic pain (e.g. peripheral nerve injury, traumatic spinal cord injury (SCI), chemotherapeutic drug-induced (paclitaxel; see review: Jaggi et al. [118]) and related clinical neuropathies.

The protective or detrimental effect of capsaicin to chronic pain responses has been extensively explored. To date, the PubMed search tool for the term "capsaicin" retrieved more than 19,000 references and, when this search was performed with both terms capsaicin and "chronic pain", retrieved about 170 references for animal models and 21 references for clinical trials (see Fig. 2). We have decided not to include all, but mainly the original and directly relevant experimental and clinical references related to chronic pain and capsaicin.

Capsaicin has been historically used a pharmacological tool since the mid-60s to inhibit or induce neurogenic inflammation and some nociceptive responses. Historically, the literature suggests that a possible first contribution of capsaicin in the pain field was proposed in a work by Baraz et al. in the mid-60s, which demonstrated the stimulatory effects of capsaicin on receptors and sensory fibres of the cat small intestine [16, 17]. In parallel, Jancsó et al. showed the direct evidence that the denervation of primary sensory neurons by capsaicin treatment during neonatal period prevented neurogenic inflammation [121], potentially via depletion of neuropeptides (e.g. substance P) and changes in peripheral processes running in that and other nerves, including cranial and vagus nerve [90, 120, 121].

From the end of the 70s and during the 80s, an avalanche of experimental studies employing capsaicin was launched, some conflicting, but most have suggested and reinforced the importance of capsaicin in the control of anti-nociceptive processes. In this context, Jancsó et al. [120] showed that capsaicin applied to the peripheral nerve evoked long-lasting impairment of C fibres function in response to noxious heat or chemical induced-pain response [120]. Previously, Szolcsányi and co-workers, in 1975, demonstrated the long-lasting desensitizing ability of local or systemic treatment with capsaicin in certain nerve endings of the rat cornea, which was not reversed by pretreatment with actinomycin-D, 8-azaguanine, 6-azauracil, aminopterin, mannomustin or cycloheximide; however, either the alkaloid colchicine or the chemotherapy vinblastine potentiated the capsaicin action time, suggestive of axonal flow inhibition. Soon after this finding, the same author concluded, by using different pharmacological approaches, that capsaicin is a selective sensory blocking agent, acting firstly by stimulation and, subsequently, can lead to sensory blockage of polymodal nociceptors and warm receptors [216]. Jancsó and Jancsó-Gábor [120] observed that the treatment of adult rat with capsaicin attenuated substantially the analgesic effect of morphine, whereas capsaicin pretreatment during the neonatal period (2nd day of life) did not affect morphine analgesia. These authors suggest that only adult, but not selective neonatal capsaicin treatment, can account to induce impairment of determined hypothalamic preoptic neurones, known as an important region involved in endogenous pain control [120]. Furthermore, Szolcsányi [217], by using new technique approaches of nociceptive responses concluded that polymodal-type nociceptors, in addition to the interaction of other nociceptors and secondary dynamic changes in these structures, play a role in the anti-nociceptive effect of capsaicin.

Capsaicin, applied for a long period, at a topical range of 0.75 and 1 %, neither affected levels of neuropeptides nor caused cell death, but produced a transient nociceptive response followed by a decrease in sensitivity of the rat C fibres [164], reduced sensitivity to noxious stimuli (e.g. mechanical or heat) of primate spinothalamic neurons [46] and reduced sensitivity to mechanical hyperalgesia, but not cold allodynia evoked by spinal nerve transection [133]. Likewise, local long-lasting topical application of capsaicin produced a significant therapeutic effect in different types of neuropathic pain, such as peripheral neuropathy induced by loose ligation of the sciatic nerve with chromic gut suture [249], diabetic (streptozotocin-induced) neuropathy [26, 86, 203] and nerve injury-induced neuropathic pain in mice [186].

In addition, capsaicin receptor TRPV1 has been shown to act as a target to mediate nociceptive responses. In this way, the intrathecal injection of a siRNA against the TRPV1 suppressed cold allodynia in rat with mononeuropathic pain and diminished spontaneous visceral pain behaviour induced by capsaicin application to the rectum of mice [45]. The per sciatic injection of the mixture QX-314 and capsaicin greatly increased the mechanical and thermal withdrawal thresholds in rat with nerve constriction-induced neuropathic pain, thus suggesting that TRPV1 expressing in nociceptors contribute to neuropathic pain [198].

Interestingly, the use of nanotechnology in drug delivery has been shown to reduce toxicity and side effects of drugs among other risks to the patient. Due to capsaicin pungency and cytotoxicity, when applied in high concentration, nanoformulation containing capsaicin has been satisfactorily developed [44, 204, 254], which have been demonstrated to enhance and prolong the intestinal absorption of capsaicin in addition to reduced gastric mucosal irritation, thus supporting the idea that capsaicin can be loaded in nanoformulations for improved oral bioavailability, and thus be used as an effective p.o. drug for the treatment of neuropathic pain.

Based on advances in understanding the protective mechanisms of capsaicin in different animal models of chronic pain, scientific and clinical pioneering studies began over 20 years ago to show evidences supporting the use of capsaicin in topical formulation in chronic pain, mainly of neuropathic origin [69] for chronic neuropathic pain in adults. Cochrane Database Syst Rev 2013 [195].

In fact, in 1991, the topical effect of capsaicin cream 0.075 % was evaluated in the pain associated with diabetic neuropathy during a multicenter study [223]. In agreement with the data obtained in experimental studies, this study revealed that applying capsaicin cream 0.075 % a frequency of four times a day during 8 weeks relieves significantly the neuropathic pain-associated process, and importantly, at least 69 % of the patients exhibited pain improvement based on the global evaluation scale (the capsaicin study group; PMID 1953227). In contrast, the results from a

20-week double-blind crossover randomized study with patients suffering from painful diabetic neuropathy (PDN) showed that the topical administration of capsaicin gel, in a smaller concentration (0.024 %) for 8 weeks, with a washout period of 4 weeks between the two treatments, did not induce significant pain relief in patients with PDN, even though the treatment was well tolerated by the patients [141]. The discrepancies between both the earlier and the later studies suggest that applying capsaicin cream at higher not low concentration, is effective to ameliorate/control the PND. In the same period, a clinical trial involved 1044 patients with peripheral neuropathic pain and showed that the application of a cutaneous patch containing capsaicin 8 % is effective and safe to treat different neuropathic conditions; however, this study missed out showing a paired control group [157]. Using the same pharmaceutic form (patch), but in a smaller concentration of capsaicin (5 %), another more recent trial in a multicenter, randomized (1:1) blinded study performed in patients with peripheral neuropathic pain revealed that the application of a capsaicin patch 5 % in addition to previous treatment with the local anaesthetic lidocaine (4 %) or the opioid tramadol (50 mg;—30 min, p.o.) improved the peripheral neuropathic pain. Curiously, this therapeutic manoeuvre made the capsaicin patch 8 % much more tolerable and thus should be considered as an alternative pretreatment option in patients receiving long-lasting topical capsaicin treatment [124]. On the other hand, soon after this finding, Kern et al. [131] criticized the need of lidocaine or opioid in addition to the capsaicin patch 8 % for the treatment of peripheral neuropathic pain; as according to the survey made by the authors, the application of capsaicin a patch 8 % is overall tolerable and associated with a minor and short-lived discomfort. Furthermore, capsaicin patch 8 % by itself evokes similar efficacy and tolerability compared to capsaicin associated with lidocaine treatment [131].

In recent studies, the efficacy of a capsaicin 8 % patch has been compared with pregabalin, a GABA analogue used as a current standard therapy in peripheral neuropathic pain, which revealed that, similarly to pregabalin, the 8 % capsaicin patch produced equal pain relief with a faster onset of action, fewer systemic side effects [98] and a better cost-benefit in patients with peripheral neuropathic pain who have failed previous systemic treatments [159]. Likewise, a comparative clinical study to evaluate the cost-effectiveness of the 8 % capsaicin patch and existing therapies for post-herpetic neuralgia revealed that capsaicin patch had superior effective rates than the oral agents, and its cost-effective analysis was within an accepted cost compared to the oral products [10].

1.2 Effects of Capsaicin on Functional Gastrointestinal Disorders

Digestive diseases or the functional gastrointestinal disorders (FGIDs), by definition, are a heterogeneous group of chronic or recurrent gastrointestinal conditions that do not have an identified underlying pathophysiology that account for the symptoms [52, 73]. According to the Rome diagnostic criteria, these GI diseases can be into oesophageal, gastroduodenal, bowel, biliary, anorectal and abdominal pain subcategories [72].

Among these GI disorders, the best known is the chronic inflammatory bowel disease (IBD), defined as a complex inflammatory disease associated with an altered systemic immune response of unknown aetiology, which comprehends ulcerative colitis (UC), Crohn's disease (CD) and a very uncommon intermediate form of both. Whereas the UC is restricted to the colon, CD may affect any part of the digestive tract, from the mouth to the anus; however, the terminal ileum is the main disease site.

The incidence of IBD varies greatly worldwide, and a high incidence is seen in North America, mainly in the USA (e.g. up to 1.4 million people), and Europe (e.g. 250,000 people in the UK), whereas in developing countries, such as Africa and Asia, the incidence is still low [151, 169, 176], but recent evidences have suggest that these diseases are becoming more common in these countries [106, 176]. On the other hand, there is still no effective treatment or medical cure.

For the past six decades, controversial research on the protective effects of capsaicin and its receptor (TRPV1) on gastrointestinal disorders has been shown elsewhere [81, 105, 152, 184]. In fact, since ancient times, the popular use of capsaicin in culinary worldwide has been paralleled with discrepant experimental findings, showing GI disturbances caused by capsaicin or hot chilli, the source of this alkaloid [66, 220, 232]. For instance, in a pioneering experimental study, Makara et al. [158] showed that capsaicin application into the rat stomach led to aggravation of gastric ulceration in these animals [158]. In agreement, Szolcsányi and Barthó [221] revealed, possibly for the first time, in a series of experiments in which gastric ulcers were developed by either pylorus ligation or by acid distension, that prior treatment of rats (via s.c.) with capsaicin led to a marked blockage of capsaicin-sensitive nerve-ending function and a subsequent gastro-protection impairment, thus indicating that these fibres play an important role in the occurrence of peptic ulcers. A few years later, Szolcsányi and Mózsik [215] observed that lesion formation in response to intragastric application of distinct noxious stimuli (e.g. 96 % ethanol, 0.6 M HCl, 0.2 M NaOH or 25 % NaCl) was not prevented by capsaicin-induced nerve desensitization, apart from reducing the severity of the mucosal neurogenic inflammation/damage.

Corroborating previous studies, Szolcsányi et al. [104] observed that the chemical depletion of sensory neuron contents by capsaicin during the neonate period exacerbated indomethacin-induced ulcer, independently of the local concentration of prostaglandin E2 (PGE_2), a known endogenous mediator involved in gastro-protection. In addition, a significant concentration of calcitonin-gene-related peptide (CGRP), a potent vasodilator, has been found in the GI-surrounding tissue of control but capsaicin-pretreated rat suggesting that this neuropeptide played a neuroprotective role in GI tissues [205, 219]. Of note, the gastro-protective mechanism regulated by subepithelial microcirculation increment is unlikely to be the same as the one observed for epithelial cells cytoprotection, in which PGE_2 plays an important role [189].

Besides establishing that chemical ablation of primary afferent sensory neurons by neonatal capsaicin treatment exacerbates gastric inflammation in the rodent mucosa as stated above, it is worth mentioning that the sole stimulation of the afferent nerve endings by intragastric administration of capsaicin has produced a significant protection against ethanol-induced gastric mucosa damage [103]. It has been suggested that both the C- and Aδ polymodal nociceptor groups of primary afferent neurons are involved in capsaicin-sensitive visceral sense [219].

Reinforcing the protective role of capsaicin in GI disorders, Bass et al. [21], using a rabbit model of esophagitis produced by ethanol 50 %, showed that the pretreatment of animals with capsaicin (1 %) produced a marked GI mucosa protection. Furthermore, others demonstrated that the intragastric application of capsaicin, at high and low doses, produced differential protective responses in experimental gastric ulcer evoked by intragastric taking aspirin, ethanol or HCl 0.6 M in rats. Whereas higher doses of capsaicin induced mucosal damage, lower doses of this alkaloid promoted gastric protection against ulcer or did not affect the mucosa [1].

In addition to being widely used as a pharmacological tool to elucidate and the physiopathology of both the inflammatory and nociceptive events, growing interest in the actions of capsaicin on GI diseases has led to the clinical research into the protective effects of capsaicin against chronic GI manifestations. Similarly to experimental studies, controversial findings on the protective role of capsaicin have also been shown.

For instance, almost 30 years ago, an interesting double-blind study evaluated the effects of intragastric administration of test meals containing high concentrations of red and black pepper and compared the effects in healthy individuals taking aspirin (655 mg). The analysis for both red pepper and black pepper groups revealed that in addition to mucosal microbleeding a significant increase in parietal secretion, pepsin secretion, potassium loss and gastric cell exfoliation was found in gastric washes, which did not significantly differ from aspirin responses in any of the studied parameter [173]. In contrast, soon after, the same group carried out a diagnostic clinical study, using video endoscopy images, which revealed severe gastric erosions in individuals taking aspirin and having eaten blended meal after 24 h and, in contrast, no significant mucosal damage was observed in healthy individuals taking spicy Mexican meal, thus ruling out the association of chilli food (capsaicin) ingestion and development of gastric mucosal injury in healthy individuals [95]. Yeoh et al. [248] demonstrated other controversial findings, in which they observed that the oral ingestion of chilli (20 g) reduced the aspirin-induced gastric mucosal injury score, thus supporting a gastro-protective effect of chilli in human subjects.

After nearly fifteen years, a more refined clinical study by Mózsik et al. [174] designed to employ capsaicin as a tool to investigate the human gastrointestinal physiology, pathology and pharmacology, reinforced the protective role of capsaicin in GI disorders and revealed that the administration of capsaicin has reduced the gastric basal output and enhanced the nonparietal component of gastric secretory responses, gastric emptying and glucagon release. Furthermore, the gastric mucosal injury (microbleeding) evoked by both indomethacin and ethanol intake was significantly inhibited in individuals taking concomitantly capsaicin, and capsaicin itself enhanced the gastric transmucosal potential difference [174]. In addition, with the aid of immunohistochemical investigation the varied expression of TRVP1 (and neuropeptides CGRP and SP) in the GI mucosa of patients with distinct acute and chronic GI disorders has been shown elsewhere [39, 174].

Interestingly, randomized, double-blinded and crossover study on patients with diarrhoea-predominant irritable bowel syndrome (IBS) suggests that chronic ingestion of chilli (capsaicin source) desensitizes TRPV1 in the proximal gut and rectum, thus leading to decrease of IBS-D symptoms, such as postprandial abdominal burning and increased rectal sensory threshold [8]. On the other hand, when capsaicin was applied via rectal mucosa in patients with IBS and visceral hypersensitivity to rectal distension, no benefits were recorded and these patients experienced an increased pain perception to rectal application of capsaicin, as well as an increased anxiety response, associated with absence of TRPV1 upregulation in rectal biopsies [235]. Of note, Bortolotti and Porta [31], evaluated the chronic effect of rectal administration of red pepper powder loaded in enteric-coated pills on IBS symptoms and observed a significant reduction of IBS symptoms (e.g. intensity of abdominal pain and bloating) compared with the placebo group.

The positive influence of capsaicin-containing red pepper sauce suspension on upper gastrointestinal motility, thus leading to a faster transit through the small bowel, has been shown in healthy volunteers [43, 94], but this response has failed in patients with Barrett's oesophagus [135] or IBS [197]. In parallel, the effects of capsaicin on gut pain and hyperalgesia have been shown by several studies in healthy individuals [71, 93] as well as in individuals with GI diseases, such as IBS, known to exhibit lower rectal sensitivity threshold [2, 93, 235]. The results obtained in these studies are discrepant, as some have shown that capsaicin intake or administrated via rectal in healthy patients led to increased mechanical hyperalgesia and rectal pain threshold and, in contrast, did not increment this response in individuals with IBS. Others observed the opposite, whereas the ingestions of chilli in meals by IBS patients exerted a pronounced pain and burning sensation; the same treatment did not evoke similar effects in healthy volunteers. It should be stated that the decrease of abdominal pain and burning sensation in IBS patients submitted long-lasting use of capsaicin, which in turn causes neuronal desensitizing effect.

1.3 Capsaicin and Cancer

Cancer is a serious disease of high incidence, in which abnormal cells divide without control, and usually invade nearby tissues. According to the recent estimates from the International Agency for Research on Cancer available at GLOBOCAN database, in [89], at least 14.1 million people were diagnosed with some type of cancer and there were more than 32 million people living with cancer within 5 years of diagnosis. In addition, more than 8 million cancer deaths were reported worldwide, of which the incidence was higher (57 %) in developing countries (WHO 2012).

By comparison, the literature exhibits an increasing number of controversial studies showing the beneficial properties or potential dietary risk of phytochemicals, such as capsaicin. In addition, the pharmacological potential of capsaicin (and the role played by its receptor TRPV1) on human and experimental cancer types, acting in different steps of the growing tumour cells, such as survival, proliferation, invasion, angiogenesis and metastasis has been shown elsewhere (see reviews: [27, 29, 47, 97).

Among the topics addressed, perhaps this topic contains the most controversial evidence of the protective and harmful actions of capsaicin. Therefore, here, we have attempted to summarize evidences related to the effects of capsaicin on carcinogenesis steps, as the number of available information, sometimes using the same technical approach, show a role for capsaicin as pro-, co- or anti-carcinogenic.

The in vivo study by LaHann [143] was possibly the first to evaluate the effects of capsaicin treatment in a mouse model of skin tumorigenesis induced by the phorbol ester, known as TPA (phorbol 12-myristate 13-acetate), which is derived from croton seed, a well-known tumour promoter. However, capsaicin failed to affect the incidence and rate of TPA-induced skin papillomas and instead, it optimized the tumour growth time. Parallel to these findings, Agrawal et al. [3] reinforced this evidence showing a co-promoter effect of chilli extract in both the DMN-OAc (methyl(acetoxymethyl)nitrosamine)-induced stomach tumours and BHC (Lindane)-induced mouse liver carcinogenesis. In addition, Bode et al. [28] showed that TPA-induced skin carcinogenesis is markedly enhanced in capsaicin receptor (TRPV1) knockout (KO) mice compared with wild-type (WT) mice, thus indicating that the blockade or absence of TRPV1 may cause severe consequences in existing tumour cells or perhaps increase the risk of cancer development (Bode et al. [28]).

Curiously, and, in a mechanistic study by Hwang et al. [112] it was shown that the co-carcinogenic effect of capsaicin on TPA-induced skin tumorigenesis in vivo occurs through the epidermal growth factor receptor (EGFR), and independently of TRPV1, since TRPV1 KO mice exhibited more incidence and larger skin tumours associated with increased COX-2 expression than in TRPV1 WT. These conclusions were also based on in vitro studies, in which they observed that the inhibition of EGFR/MEK signalling pathway in vitro led to the suppression of TPA/capsaicin-induced increased COX-2 expression in fibroblast obtained from TRPV1 KO mice. This indicates a role for EGFR (and related downstream signalling) for COX-2 increment. Recently, additional mechanistic findings for capsaicin co-carcinogenic effects show that up-regulation of phosphorylated NF-κB, Erk, p38 and both inflammation-related factors COX-2 and iNOS are implicated in the mouse skin model of DMBA-initiated and TPA-promoted larger skin tumours, hyperplasia and tumour proliferation compared to mice without capsaicin pretreatment.

Furthermore, in a pulmonary adenoma model developed in newborn NIH (GP) mice by s.c. injection of polycyclic aromatic hydrocarbons, benzo(a)pyrene (BP) or 9,10-demethyl-1,2-benzanthracene (DMBA), the authors show that long-lasting administration of capsaicin 0.01 % given in the diet caused a significant inhibitory effect on the incidence and tumour rate, which was more pronounced in the female group [122]. Shortly after, Surh et al. [208] suggest that the in vitro chemoprotective effects of capsaicin on vinyl carbamate (VC)- and N-nitrosodimethylamine (NDMA)-induced mutagenesis or tumorigenesis in *Salmonella typhimurium* TA100 are partially dependent on the inhibition of cytochrome P-450 IIE1 [208].

More recently, the inhibitory capsaicin properties in vivo on cell growth were evaluated in combination with genistein, a phytoestrogen belonging to the isoflavones family, in a mature female Sprague–Dawley rat model of mammary glands cancer and in vitro in a human mammary cancer cell line (MCF-7 human breast cancer cell line). In fact results show that the topical application of TPA, as shown before, led to inflammation/carcinogenesis, breast cancer cell, proliferation [165] and increased COX-2 expression in either the animal skin or breast cancer cell cultures. These effects were suppressed by the association of capsaicin and genistein, through the modulation of AMPK and COX-2 expression [110]. A further study using a gastric cancer cell line HGC-27 demonstrated that capsaicin exhibits a marked ability against the cell line HGC-27, thus reinforcing a role for capsaicin as potential medicine to be used for treating gastric carcinoma.

Likewise, using an in vivo murine model of prostate cancer, which resembles the human prostate disease (TRAMP), Venier et al. [229] showed that the oral treatment of mice with capsaicin associated with radiotherapy (RT) resulted in a marked growth delay and reduction in the tumour growth rate compared with either capsaicin or RT treatment alone, possibly via reduction in proliferation and NFκB expression. These authors suggest that capsaicin can be used as a radio-sensitizing agent, capable of sensitizing tumour cells to the lethal effects of radiotherapy (RT), thus allowing lower doses of radiation paralleled to reduced side effects of RT to normal tissues.

1.4 Capsaicin and Asthma

Chronic respiratory diseases are those affecting the airways and other lung-related structures. Among them, special highlights have been given to asthma and chronic obstructive pulmonary diseases (COPD). It is estimated that at least 235 million people suffer from asthma worldwide, which incidence occurs independently of the level of countries development [240].

Asthma is a chronic disease characterized by recurrent attacks of breathlessness and wheezing, which may vary in severity and frequency from person to person. Common asthma hallmarks in both human and experimental animal models include bronchoconstriction, bronchospasm and mucus secretion. It can be triggered by infections microorganisms, pollutants and other environmental allergens, non-specific stimuli and inflammatory process (see reviews: [59, 168]). A high parasympathetic tone leading to bronchoconstriction and neurogenic inflammation may occur in the asthmatic lung, thus leading to the release of neuropeptides (e.g. neurokinin A, substance P and CGRP) from sensory nerves, which in turn contributes to evoke muscular constriction and increased vascular permeability [70]; for review see: [59].

Over 300 articles have been published in scientific databases showing a conflicting relationship between protective and deleterious effects of capsaicin on asthma. Additionally, capsaicin has been widely used as a tool in diagnosis for asthmatic individuals, as capsaicin challenge evokes airway hypersensitivity [59, 70, 177]. Previously, Collier and Fuller [49] showed that short exposure of humans to inhaled capsaicin (at μM increasing concentrations) produces a significant and rapid (in sec) dose-dependent coughing in both healthy and mild asthmatic volunteers; besides it does not evoke breathlessness feeling or changes in the forced expiratory flow. Also, the cough response was not altered by sodium cromoglycate, a mast cell stabilizer, but it was significantly affected by the local anaesthetic lidocaine, thus suggesting that stimulation of sensory nerve terminals in the larynx might be involved in capsaicin-induced cough.

As stated elsewhere, dose-dependent cough response evoked by capsaicin nebulization has been widely used as a pharmacological approach in experimental asthma models and in patients [87, 88, 100, 148]. Curiously, Ventresca et al. [231] showed that inhaled furosemide inhibits cough induced by a solution containing low chloride concentration, but not by capsaicin. In contrast, a recent study shows that the ingestion of capsaicin capsules during four weeks, followed by placebo capsules, for further 4 weeks significantly decreased the cough sensitivity and symptoms, thus indicating that persistent TRPV1 activation might lead to receptor desensitization [222].

2 Conclusive Remark and Future Direction

The analgesic, anti-inflammatory and the apoptotic effects of capsaicin has showed promising effects in non-communicable disease studies, such as arthritis, neuropathic pain, gastrointestinal disorders and cancer, since the oral or topical application of capsaicin reduces inflammation and pain associated with rheumatoid arthritis, promotes gastric protection against ulcer and induces apoptosis of tumour cells. While the capsaicin anti-inflammatory and analgesic properties have been recognized, via interactions with the TRPV1, the effects of capsaicin-induced apoptosis in cancer cells are thought to be mediated through reactive oxygen species (ROS) generations, such as hydrogen peroxide, which in turn result in cell cycle arrest and activation of apoptosis-related molecules, such as caspase-3. This chapter provides an overview made from capsaicin basic and clinical research studies of the potential therapeutic effects of capsaicin, loaded in different application forms, on five chronic diseases (e.g. arthritis, chronic pain, functional gastrointestinal disorders, cancer and asthma). This has been paralleled by conflicting capsaicin studies on the same subject, which support the idea that high concentrations of capsaicin are likely to evoke deleterious effects, thus suggesting that capsaicin activates different pathways at different concentrations in both the human and the rat tissues. Therefore, to establish the effective dose for use in the various pathologies that can benefit from the therapeutic action of capsaicin is a challenge that must be pursued.

References

1. Abdel Salam OM, Mozsik G, Szolcsanyi J (1995) Studies on the effect of intragastric capsaicin on gastric ulcer and on the prostacyclin-induced cytoprotection in rats. Pharmacol Res 32:209–15
2. Agarwal MK, Bhatia SJ, Desai SA, Bhure U, Melgiri S (2002) Effect of red chillies on small bowel and colonic transit and rectal sensitivity in men with irritable bowel syndrome. Indian J Gastroenterol 21(5):179–182
3. Agrawal RC, Wiessler M, Hecker E, Bhide SV (1986) Tumour-promoting effect of chilli extract in BALB/c mice. Int J Cancer 38(5):689–95
4. Airenne TT, Torkko JM, Van den plas S, Sormunen RT, Kastaniotis AJ, Wierenga RK, Hiltunen JK (2003) Structure-function analysis of enoyl thioester reductase involved in mitochondrial maintenance. J Mol Biol 327(1):47–59
5. Alberti A, Galasso V, Kovac B, Modelli A, Pichierri F (2008) Probing the molecular and electronic structure of capsaicin: a spectroscopic and quantum mechanical study. J Phys Chem A 112:5700–5711
6. Allen KD, Adams SB, Setton LA (2010) Evaluating intra-articular drug delivery for the treatment of osteoarthritis in a rat model. Tissue Eng Part B Rev 16(1):81–92. doi:10.1089/ten.teb.2009.0447
7. Aluru MR, Mazourek M, Landry LG, Curry J, Jahn M, O'Conell MA (2003) Differential expression of fatty acid synthase genes, Acl, Fat and Kas, in Capsicum fruit. J Exp Bot 54:1655–1664
8. Aniwan S, Gonlachanvit S (2014) Effects of chilli treatment on gastrointestinal and rectal sensation in diarrhea-predominant irritable bowel syndrome: a randomized, double-blinded, crossover study. J Neurogastroenterol Motil 20:400–406
9. Appendino G, De Petrocellis L, Trevisani M, Minassi A, Daddario N, Moriello AS, Gazzieri D, Ligresti A, Campi B, Fontana G, Pinna C, Geppetti P, Di Marzo V (2005) Development of the first ultra-potent "capsaicinoid" agonist at transient receptor potential vanilloid type 1 (TRPV1) channels and its therapeutic potential. J Pharmacol Exp Ther 312:561–570
10. Armstrong EP, Malone DC, McCarberg B, Panarites CJ, Pham SV (2011) Cost-effectiveness analysis of a new 8 % capsaicin patch compared to existing therapies for postherpetic neuralgia. Curr Med Res Opin 27(5):939–50. doi:10.1185/03007995.2011.562885 Epub 2011 Mar 4
11. Arora R, Gill NS, Chauhan G, Rana AC (2011) An overview about versatile molecule capsaicin. Int J Pharm Sci Drug Res 3:280–286
12. Asquith DL, Miller AM, McInnes IB, Liew FY (2009) Animal models of rheumatoid arthritis. Eur J Immunol 39(8):2040–4. doi:10.1002/eji.200939578
13. Athanasiou A, Smith PA, Vakilpour S, Kumaran NM, Turner AE et al (2007) Vanilloid receptor agonists and antagonists are mitochondrial inhibitors: how vanilloids cause non-vanilloid receptor mediated cell death. Biochem Biophys Res Commun 354:50–55

14. Aza-González C, Núñez-Palenius HG, Ochoa-Alejo N (2011) Molecular biology of capsaicinoid biosynthesis in chilli pepper (*Capsicum* spp.). Plant Cell Rep 30(5):695–706. doi:10.1007/s00299-010-0968-8 Epub 2010 Dec 14
15. Baboota RK, Singh DP, Sarma SM, Kaur J, Sandhir R, Boparai RK, Kondepudi KK, Bishnoi M (2014) Capsaicin induces "brite" phenotype in differentiating 3T3-L1 preadipocytes. PLoS ONE 9(7):e103093
16. Baraz LA, Khayutin VM, Molnár J (1968) Effects of capsaicin upon the stimulatory action of potassium chloride in the visceral branches of spinal afferents of the cat. Acta Physiol Acad Sci Hung 33(2):237–246
17. Baraz LA, Khayutin VM, Molnár J (1968) Analysis of the stimulatory action of capsaicin on receptors and sensory fibres of the small intestine in the cat. Further contribution to the problem of pain. Acta Physiol Acad Sci Hung 33(2):225–35
18. Barbero GF, Molinillo JMG, Varela RM, Palma M, Macias FA, Barroso CG (2010) Application of Hansch′s model to capsaicinoids and capsinoids: a study using the quantitative structure-activity relationship. A novel method for the synthesis of capsinoids. J Agric Food Chem 58:3342–3349
19. Barbero GF, Ruiz AG, Liazid A, Palma M, Vera JC, Barroso CG (2014) Evolution of total and individual capsaicinoids in peppers during ripening of the Cayenne pepper plant (*Capsicum* annuum L.). Food Chem 15(153):200–6. doi:10.1016/j.foodchem.2013.12.068
20. Barton NJ, McQueen DS, Thomson D, Gauldie SD, Wilson AW, Salter DM, Chessell IP (2006) Attenuation of experimental arthritis in TRPV1R knockout mice. Exp Mol Pathol 81 (2):166–70 Epub 2006 Jun 16
21. Bass BL, Trad KS, Harmon JW, Hakki FZ (1991) Capsaicin-sensitive nerves mediate esophageal mucosal protection. Surgery 110:419–425; discussion 425–426
22. Beltran J, Ghosh AK, Basu S (2007) Immunotherapy of tumors with neuroimmune ligand capsaicin. J Immunol 178(5):3260–3264
23. Bevan S, Geppetti P (1994) Protons: small stimulants of capsaicin-sensitive sensory nerves. Trends Neurosci 17:509–12
24. Bevan S, Szolcsanyi J (1990) Sensory neuron-specific actions of capsaicin: mechanisms and applications. Trends Pharmacol Sci 11:330–333
25. Biro T, Acs G, Acs P, Modarres S, Blumberg PM (1997) Recent advances in understanding of vanilloid receptors: a therapeutic target for treatment of pain and inflammation in skin. J Investig Dermatol Symp Proc 2:56–60
26. Bishnoi M, Bosgraaf CA, Abooj M, Zhong L, Premkumar LS (2011) Streptozotocin-induced early thermal hyperalgesia is independent of glycemic state of rats: role of transient receptor potential vanilloid 1(TRPV1) and inflammatory mediators. Mol Pain 27(7):52. doi:10.1186/1744-8069-7-52
27. Bley K, Boorman G, Mohammad B, McKenzie D, Babbar S (2012) A comprehensive review of the carcinogenic and anticarcinogenic potential of capsaicin. Toxicol Pathol. 40(6):847–73
28. Bode AM, Cho Y-Y, Zheng D, Zhu F, Ericson ME, Ma WY, Yao K, Dong Z (2009) Transient Receptor Potential Type Vanilloid 1 Suppresses Skin Carcinogenesis. Cancer Res 69(3):903–905
29. Bode AM, Dong Z. (2015) Toxic phytochemicals and their potential risks for human cancer. Cancer Prev Res (Phila) 8(1):1–8
30. Bonica JJ (ed) (1953) The management of pain. Lea & Febiger, Philadelphia
31. Bortolotti M, Porta S (2011) Effect of red pepper on symptoms of irritable bowel syndrome: preliminary study. Dig Dis Sci 56(11):3288–3295
32. Brand CA, Ackerman IN, Tropea J (2014) Chronic disease management: improving care for people with osteoarthritis. Best Pract Res Clin Rheumatol 28(1):119–142. doi:10.1016/j.berh.2014.01.011
33. Bratz IN, Dick GM, Tune JD, Edwards JM, Neeb ZP, Dincer UD, Sturek M (2008) Impaired capsaicin-induced relaxation of coronary arteries in a porcine model of the metabolic syndrome. Am J Physiol Heart Circ Physiol 294(6):H2489–H2496

34. Brown DH, Bruin J, Lewis AJ, McNeillie A, Smith WE (1978) The effect of gold salts in kaolin-induced paw oedema and adjuvant-induced arthritis in the rat (proceedings). Br J Pharmacol 64(3):462p–463p. 23;381(9871):970–972. doi:10.1016/S0140-6736(13)60188-9. Epub 2013 Mar 5
35. CDC: Centers for Disease Control and Prevention—Prevalence of doctor-diagnosed arthritis and arthritis-attributable activity limitation–United States, 2010–2012 (2013). MMWR Morb Mortal Wkly Rep 62(44):869–873
36. Camargo LL, Denadai-Souza A, Yshii LM, Mesquita FP, Soares AG, Lima C, Schenka A, Grant A, Fernandes E, Muscará MN, Costa SK (2015) Peripheral neurokinin-1 receptors contribute to kaolin-induced acute monoarthritis in rats. NeuroImmunomodulation 22 (6):373–384. doi:10.1159/000381549
37. Carleson J, Kogner P, Bileviciute I, Theodorsson E, Appelgren A, Appelgren B, Kopp S, Yousef N, Lundeberg T (1997) Effects of capsaicin in temporomandibular joint arthritis in rats. Arch Oral Biol 42(12):869–76
38. Caterina MJ, Schumacher MA, Tominaga M, Rosen TA, Levine JD, Julius D (1997) The capsaicin receptor: a heat-activated ion channel in the pain pathway. Nature 389(6653):816–24
39. Chan CL, Facer P, Davis JB, Smith GD, Egerton J, Bountra C, Williams NS, Anand P (2003) Sensory fibres expressing capsaicin receptor TRPV1 in patients with rectal hypersensitivity and faecal urgency. Lancet 361:385–391
40. Chen KS, Chen PN, Hsieh YS, Lin CY, Lee YH, Chu SC (2015) Capsaicin protects endothelial cells and macrophage against oxidized low-density lipoprotein-induced injury by direct antioxidant action. Chem Biol Interact 228:35–45
41. Chen ZJ, Pudas R, Sharma S, Smart OS, Juffer AH, Hiltunen JK, Wierenga RK, Haapalainen AM (2008) Structural enzymological studies of 2-enoyl thioester reductase of the human mitochondrial FAS II pathway: new insights into its substrate recognition properties. J Mol Biol 379(4):830–844. doi:10.1016/j.jmb.2008.04.041
42. Chen D, Wang Z, Zhang Z, Zhang R, Yu L (2013) Capsaicin up-regulates protease-activated receptor-4 mRNA and protein in primary cultured dorsal root ganglion neurons. Cell Mol Neurobiol 33:337–46
43. Chen CL, Liu TT, Yi CH, Orr WC (2010) Effects of capsaicin-containing red pepper sauce suspension on esophageal secondary peristalsis in humans. Neurogastroenterol Motil 22 (11):1177–1182, e312–3. doi:10.1111/j.1365-2982.2010.01561.x
44. Choi AY, Kim CT, Park HY, Kim HO, Lee NR, Lee KE, Gwak HS (2013) Pharmacokinetic characteristics of capsaicin-loaded nanoemulsions fabricated with alginate and chitosan. J Agric Food Chem 61(9):2096–2102. doi:10.1021/jf3052708
45. Christoph T, Grünweller A, Mika J, Schäfer MK, Wade EJ, Weihe E, Erdmann VA, Frank R, Gillen C, Kurreck J (2006) Silencing of vanilloid receptor TRPV1 by RNAi reduces neuropathic and visceral pain in vivo. Biochem Biophys Res Commun 350(1):238–43
46. Chung JM, Paik KS, Kim JS, Nam SC, Kim KJ, Oh UT, Hasegawa T, Chung K, Willis WD (1993) Chronic effects of topical application of capsaicin to the sciatic nerve on responses of primate spinothalamic neurons. Pain 53(3):311–321
47. Clark R, Lee SH (2016) Anticancer Properties of Capsaicin Against Human Cancer. Anticancer Res 36(3):837-43
48. Coderre S, Mandin H, Harasym PH, Fick GH (2003) Diagnostic reasoning strategies and diagnostic success. Med Educ 37(8):695–703
49. Collier JG, Fuller RW (1984) Capsaicin inhalation in man and the effects of sodium cromoglycate. Br J Pharmacol 81:113–7
50. Colpaert FC, Donnerer J, Lembeck F (1983) Effects of capsaicin on inflammation and on the substance P content of nervous tissues in rats with adjuvant arthritis. Life Sci 32(16):1827–34
51. Contreras-Padilla M, Yahia EM (1998) Changes in capsaicinoids during development, maturation, and senescence of chile peppers and relation with peroxidase activity. J Agric Food Chem 46:2075–2079

52. Corazziari E (2004) Definition and epidemiology of functional gastrointestinal disorders. Best Pract Res Clin Gastroenterol 18(4):613–631
53. Costa SK, Brain SD, Antunes E, De Nucci G, Docherty RJ (2003) Phoneutria nigriventer spider venom activates 5-HT4 receptors in rat-isolated vagus nerve. Br J Pharmacol 139 (1):59–64
54. Costa SKP, Brain SD, Antunes E, De Nucci G, Docherty RJ (2003) Phoneutria nigriventer spider venom activates 5-HT4 receptors in rat-isolated vagus nerve. Br J Pharmacol 139:59–64
55. Costa SK, Esquisatto LC, Camargo E, Gambero A, Brain SD, De Nucci G, Antunes E (2001) Comparative effect of Phoneutria nigriventer spider venom and capsaicin on the rat paw oedema. Life Sci 69(13):1573–85
56. Costa SK, Moreno RA, Esquisatto LC, Juliano L, Brain SD, De Nucci G, Antunes E (2002) Role of kinins and sensory neurons in the rat pleural leukocyte migration induced by Phoneutria nigriventer spider venom. Neurosci Lett 318(3):158–62
57. Costa SK, De Nucci G, Antunes E (2000) Brain SD Involvement of vanilloid receptors and purinoceptors in the Phoneutria nigriventer spider venom-induced plasma extravasation in rat skin. Eur J Pharmacol 391(3):305–15
58. Costa SK, De Nucci G, Antunes E, Brain SD (2000) Involvement of vanilloid receptors and purinoceptors in the Phoneutria nigriventer spider venom-induced plasma extravasation in rat skin. Eur J Pharmacol 391(3):305–15
59. Couto M, de Diego A, Perpini M, Delgado L, Moreira A (2013) Cough reflex testing with inhaled capsaicin and TRPV1 activation in asthma and comorbid conditions. J Investig Allergol Clin Immunol 23:289–301
60. Curry J, Aluru M, Mendoza M, Nevarez J, Melendrez M, O'Connell MA (1999) Transcripts for possible capsaicinoid biosynthetic genes are differentially accumulated in pungent and nonpungent *Capsicum* spp. Plant Sci 148:47–57
61. Câmara PR, Esquisatto LC, Camargo EA, Ribela MT, Toyama MH, Marangoni S, De Nucci G, Antunes E (2003) Inflammatory oedema induced by phospholipases A2 isolated from Crotalus durissus sp. in the rat dorsal skin: a role for mast cells and sensory C-fibers. Toxicon 41(7):823–829
62. Dai Y, Iwata K, Fukuoka T, Kondo E, Tokunaga A, Yamanaka H, Tachibana T, Liu Y, Noguchi K (2002) Phosphorylation of extracellular signal-regulated kinase in primary afferent neurons by noxious stimuli and its involvement in peripheral sensitization. J Neurosci 22(17):7737–45
63. Dalmolin GD, Silva CR, Rigo FK, Gomes GM, Cordeiro Mdo N, Richardson M, Silva MA, Prado MA, Gomez MV, Ferreira J (2011) Antinociceptive effect of Brazilian armed spider venom toxin Tx3-3 in animal models of neuropathic pain. Pain 152(10):2224–2232. doi:10.1016/j.pain.2011.04.015
64. Davis A, Perkins MN (1993) The effect of capsaicin and conventional analgesics in two models of monoarthritis in the rat. Agents Actions 38 Spec No:C10–2
65. Deal CL, Schnitzer TJ, Lipstein E, Seibold JR, Stevens RM, Levy MD, Albert D, Renold F (1991) Treatment of arthritis with topical capsaicin: a double-blind trial. Clin Ther 13 (3):383–395
66. Deluca V Jr, Gray SJ, Schneider MA (1956) The effect of spice ingestion upon the stomach. Am J Gastroenterol 26(6):722–732
67. Denadai-Souza A, Camargo Lde L, Ribela MT, Keeble JE, Costa SK, Muscará MN (2009) Participation of peripheral tachykinin NK1 receptors in the carrageenan-induced inflammation of the rat temporomandibular joint. Eur J Pain 13(8):812–819. doi:10.1016/j.ejpain.2008.09.012
68. Derry S, Lloyd R, Moore RA, McQuay HJ (2009) Topical capsaicin for chronic neuropathic pain in adults. Cochrane Database Syst Rev Cd007393
69. Derry S, Sven-Rice A, Cole P, Tan T, Moore RA (2013) Topical capsaicin (high concentration) for chronic neuropathic pain in adults. Cochrane Database Syst Rev 2: CD007393. doi:10.1002/14651858.CD007393.pub3

70. Doherty MJ, Mister R, Pearson MG, Calverley PM (2000) Capsaicin responsiveness and cough in asthma and chronic obstructive pulmonary disease. Thorax 55:643–649
71. Drewes AM, Schipper KP, Dimcevski G, Petersen P, Gregersen H, Funch-Jensen P, Arendt-Nielsen L (2003) Gut pain and hyperalgesia induced by capsaicin: a human experimental model. Pain 104:333–341
72. Drossman DA, Corazziari E, Talley NJ et al (2000) Rome II functional gastrointestinal disorders. Degnon Associates, McLean, VA
73. Drossman DA, Funch-Jensen P, Janssens J et al (1990) Identification of subgroups of functional bowel disorders. Gastroenterol Int 3:159–172
74. Dubin A (2016) Managing osteoarthritis and other chronic musculoskeletal pain disorders. Med Clin North Am 100(1):143–150. doi:10.1016/j.mcna.2015.08.008
75. Dumonde DC, Glynn LE (1962) The production of arthritis in rabbits by an immunological reaction to fibrin. Br J Exp Pathol 43:373–83
76. Dux M, Sántha P, Jancsó G (2003) Capsaicin-sensitive neurogenic sensory vasodilatation in the dura mater of the rat. J Physiol 552:859–67
77. Dwarswaard J, Bakker EJ, van Staa A, Boeije HR (2016) Self-management support from the perspective of patients with a chronic condition: a thematic synthesis of qualitative studies. Health Expect 19(2):194–208. doi:10.1111/hex.12346 (Epub 2015 Jan 26. Review)
78. Ekundi-Valentim E, Santos KT, Camargo EA, Denadai-Souza A, Teixeira SA, Zanoni CI, Grant AD, Wallace J, Muscará MN, Costa SK (2010) Differing effects of exogenous and endogenous hydrogen sulphide in carrageenan-induced knee joint synovitis in the rat. Br J Pharmacol 159(7):1463–74. doi:10.1111/j.1476-5381.2010.00640.x
79. Eshbaugh WH, PG Smith, DL Nickrent (1983) Capsicum tovarii (Solanaceae), a new species of pepper from Peru. Brittonia 35:55–60
80. Estrada B, Pomar F, Díaz J, Merino F, Bernal MA (1999) Pungency levels in fruits of the pardon pepper with different water supply. Hort Sci 81:385–396
81. Evangelista S (2014) Capsaicin receptor as target of calcitonin gene-related peptide in the gut. Prog Drug Res 68:259–76
82. Fernandes ES, Fernandes MA, Keeble JE (2012) The functions of TRPA1 and TRPV1: moving away from sensory nerves. Br J Pharmacol 166(2):510–21
83. Fischer MJ, Reeh PW, Sauer SK (2003) Proton-induced calcitonin gene-related peptide release from rat sciatic nerve axons, in vitro, involving TRPV1. Eur J Neurosci 18(4):803–810
84. Franco-Cereceda A, Henke H, Lundberg JM, Petermann JB, Hökfelt T, Fischer JA (1987) Calcitonin gene-related peptide (CGRP) in capsaicin-sensitive substance P-immunoreactive sensory neurons in animals and man: distribution and release by capsaicin. Peptides 8 (2):399–410
85. Freeman PC, West GB (1972) Proceedings: resistance of rats to carrageenan and to adjuvant-induced arthritis. Br J Pharmacol 44(2):327P–328P
86. Fuchs D, Birklein F, Reeh PW, Sauer SK (2010) Sensitized peripheral nociception in experimental diabetes of the rat. Pain 151(2):496–505. doi:10.1016/j.pain.2010.08.010
87. Fujimura M, Sakamoto S, Kamio Y, Bando T, Kurashima K, Matsuda T (1993) Effect of inhaled procaterol on cough receptor sensitivity to capsaicin in patients with asthma or chronic bronchitis and in normal subjects. Thorax 48:615–618
88. Fuller RW, Karlsson JA, Choudry NB, Pride NB (1988) Effect of inhaled and systemic opiates on responses to inhaled capsaicin in humans. J Appl Physiol 65:1125–1130
89. GLOBOCAN (2012) Estimated cancer incidence, mortality and prevalence worldwide in 2012. http://globocan.iarc.fr/old/FactSheets/cancers/stomach-new.asp. Accessed 10 August 2016
90. Gamse R, Holzer P, Lembeck F (1980) Decrease of substance P in primary afferent neurones and impairment of neurogenic plasma extravasation by capsaicin. Br J Pharmacol 68(2):207–13

91. Gavva NR, Klionsky L, Qu Y, Shi L, Tamir R, Edenson S, Zhang TJ, Viswanadhan VN, Toth A, Pearce LV et al (2004) Molecular determinants of vanilloid sensitivity in TRPV1. J Biol Chem 279:20283–20295
92. Goldberg and McGee BMC Public Health (2011) 11:770. http://www.biomedcentral.com/1471-2458/11/770
93. Gonlachanvit S, Mahayosnond A, Kullavanijaya P (2009) Effects of chilli on postprandial gastrointestinal symptoms in diarrhoea predominant irritable bowel syndrome: evidence for capsaicin-sensitive visceral nociception hypersensitivity. Neurogastroenterol Motil 21:23–32
94. Gonzalez R, Dunkel R, Koletzko B, Schusdziarra V, Allescher HD (1998) Effect of capsaicin-containing red pepper sauce suspension on upper gastrointestinal motility in healthy volunteers. Dig Dis Sci 43(6):1165–71
95. Graham DY, Smith JL, Opekun AR (1988) Spicy food and the stomach. Evaluation by videoendoscopy. JAMA 260(23):3473–3475
96. Guo SY, Yang GP, Jiang DJ, Wang F, Song T, Tan XH, Sun ZQ (2008) Protection of capsaicin against hypoxia-reoxygenation-induced apoptosis of rat hippocampal neurons. Can J Physiol Pharmacol 86(11):785–792
97. Gupta SC, Kim JH, Prasad S, Aggarwal BB (2010) Regulation of survival, proliferation, invasion, angiogenesis, and metastasis of tumor cells through modulation of inflammatory pathways by nutraceuticals. Cancer Metastasis Rev 29(3):405–434
98. Haanpää M, Cruccu G, Nurmikko TJ, McBride WT, Docu Axelarad A, Bosilkov A, Chambers C, Ernault E, Abdulahad AK (2016) Capsaicin 8 % patch versus oral pregabalin in patients with peripheral neuropathic pain. Eur J Pain 20(2):316–328. doi:10.1002/ejp.731
99. Halme M, Pesonen M, Salo H, Soderstrom M, Pasanen M, Vahakangas K, Vanninen P (2016) Comparison of in vitro metabolism and cytotoxicity of capsaicin and dihydrocapsaicin. J Chromatogr B Analyt Technol Biomed Life Sci 1009–1010:17–24
100. Hansson L, Midgren B, Karlsson JA (1994) Effects of inhaled lignocaine and adrenaline on capsaicin-induced cough in humans. Thorax 49:1166–1168
101. Harstall C, Ospina M (2003) How prevalent is chronic pain? Pain Clin Updates XI(2). http://www.iasp-pain.org/PublicationsNews/NewsletterIssue.aspx?ItemNumber=2136. Accessed 10 Mar 2016
102. Harvell KP, Bosland PW (1998) The environment produces a significant effect on pungency of chiles. Hort Sci 32:1292
103. Holzer P, Lippe IT (1988) Stimulation of afferent nerve endings by intragastric capsaicin protects against ethanol-induced damage of gastric mucosa. Neuroscience 27:981–7
104. Holzer P, Sametz W (1986) Gastric mucosal protection against ulcerogenic factors in the rat mediated by capsaicin-sensitive afferent neurons. Gastroenterology 91:975–981
105. Holzer P, Schluet W, Lippe IT, Sametz W (1987) Involvement of capsaicin-sensitive sensory neurons in gastrointestinal function. Acta Physiol Hung 69:403–11
106. Hou JK, El-Serag H, Thirumurthi S (2009) Distribution and manifestations of inflammatory bowel disease in Asians, Hispanics, and African Americans: a systematic review. Am J Gastroenterol 104(8):2100–2109. doi:10.1038/ajg.2009.190
107. Hsu CL, Yen GC (2007) Effects of capsaicin on induction of apoptosis and inhibition of adipogenesis in 3T3-L1 cells. J Agric Food Chem 55:1730–1736
108. Hu F, Sun WW, Zhao XT, Cui ZJ, Yang WX (2008) TRPV1 mediates cell death in rat synovial fibroblasts through calcium entry-dependent ROS production and mitochondrial depolarization. Biochem Biophys Res Commun 369(4):989–993
109. Hua XY (1986) Tachykinins and calcitonin gene-related peptide in relation to peripheral functions of capsaicin-sensitive sensory neurons. Acta Physiol Scand Suppl 551:1–45
110. Huang SP, Chen JC, Wu CC, Chen CT, Tang NY, Ho YT, Lo C, Lin JP, Chung JG, Lin JG (2009) Capsaicin-induced apoptosis in human hepatoma HepG2 cells. Anticancer Res 29(1):165–74
111. Hui K, Liu B, Qin F (2003) Capsaicin activation of the pain receptor, VR1: multiple open states from both partial and full binding. J Gen Physiol 84:2957–2968

112. Hwang MK, Bode AM, Byun S, Song NR, Lee HJ, Lee KW, Dong Z (2010) Cocarcinogenic effect of capsaicin involves activation of EGFR signaling but not TRPV1. Cancer Res 70 (17):6859-69
113. IASP (2003) Pain clinical updates 2003. In: Carr DB (ed). International association for the study of pain (2003), vol XI, no.2. http://iasp.files.cms-plus.com/Content/ContentFolders/Publications2/PainClinicalUpdates/Archives/PCU03-2_1390265045864_38.pdf. Accessed 10 Aug 2016
114. Inman RD, Chiu B, Rabinovich S, Marshall W (1989) Neuromodulation of synovitis: capsaicin effect on severity of experimental arthritis. J Neuroimmunol 24(1–2):17–22
115. Inoue K, Koizumi S, Fuziwara S, Denda S, Inoue K, Denda M (2002) Functional vanilloid receptors in cultured normal human epidermal keratinocytes. Biochem Biophys Res Commun 291(1):124–9
116. Issekutz B Jr, Lichtneckert I, Nagy H (1950) Effect of capsaicin and histamine on heat regulation. Arch Int Pharmacodyn Ther 81(1):35–46
117. Issekutz B Jr, Lichtneckert I, Winter M (1950) Effect of histamine, capsaicine and procaine on heat-regulation. Arch Int Pharmacodyn Ther 83(2):319–326
118. Jaggi AS, Jain V, Singh N (2011) Animal models of neuropathic pain. Fundam Clin Pharmacol 25(1):1–28. doi:10.1111/j.1472-8206.2009.00801.x
119. Jancso G, Kiraly E, Jancso-Gabor A (1977) Pharmacologically induced selective degeneration of chemosensitive primary sensory neurons. Nature 270:741–743
120. Jancsó G, Jancsó-Gábor A (1980) Effect of capsaicin on morphine analgesia–possible involvement of hypothalamic structures. Naunyn Schmiedebergs Arch Pharmacol 311 (3):285–288
121. Jancsó N, Jancsó-Gábor A, Szolcsányi J (1967) Direct evidence for neurogenic inflammation and its prevention by denervation and by pretreatment with capsaicin. Br J Pharmacol Chemother 31(1):138–151
122. Jang JJ, Kim SH, Yun TK (1989) Inhibitory effect of capsaicin on mouse lung tumor development. In Vivo 3(1):49–53
123. Jarisch A (1940) Vom Herzen ausgehende Kreislaufreflexe. Arch Kreislaufforsch 7:260–274
124. Jensen TS, Høye K, Fricová J, Vanelderen P, Ernault E, Siciliano T, Marques S (2014) Tolerability of the capsaicin 8 % patch following pretreatment with lidocaine or tramadol in patients with peripheral neuropathic pain: a multicentre, randomized, assessor-blinded study. Eur J Pain 18(9):1240–1247. doi:10.1002/j.1532-2149.2014.00479.x Epub 2014 Mar 24
125. Jessop EG (2013) Health in the UK: could do even better? Lancet 381(9871):9970–2. doi:10.1016/S0140-6736(13)60188-9
126. Jordt SE, Julius D (2002) Molecular basis for species-specific sensitivity to "hot" chilli peppers. Cell 108(3):421–30
127. Jung J, Hwang SW, Kwak J, Lee SY, Kang CJ, Kim WB, Kim D, Oh U (1999) Capsaicin binds to the intracellular domain of the capsaicin-activated ion channel. J Neurosci 19:529–38
128. Jung J, Lee SY, Hwang SW, Cho H, Shin J, Kang YS, Kim S, Oh U (2002) Agonist recognition sites in the cytosolic tails of vanilloid receptor 1. J Biol Chem 277:44448–44454
129. Kark T, Bagi Z, Lizanecz E, Pásztor ET, Erdei N, Czikora A, Papp Z, Edes I, Pórszász R, Tóth A (2008) Tissue-specific regulation of microvascular diameter: opposite functional roles of neuronal and smooth muscle located vanilloid receptor-1. Mol Pharmacol 73(5):1405–12
130. Katritzky AR, Xu YJ, Vakulenko AV, Wilcox AL, Bley KR (2003) Model compounds of caged capsaicin: design, synthesis, and photoreactivity. J Org Chem 68:9100–9104
131. Kern KU, Nowack W, Poole C (2014) Treatment of neuropathic pain with the capsaicin 8 % patch: is pretreatment with lidocaine necessary? Pain Pract 14(2):E42–50. doi:10.1111/papr.12143 Epub 2013 Dec 1
132. Kim JA, Kang YS, Lee YS (2005) A phospholipase C-dependent intracellular Ca2+ release pathway mediates the capsaicin-induced apoptosis in HepG2 human hepatoma cells. Arch Pharm Res 28(1):73–80

133. Kim SM, Kim J, Kim E, Hwang SJ, Shin HK, Lee SE (2008) Local application of capsaicin alleviates mechanical hyperalgesia after spinal nerve transection. Neurosci Lett 433(3):199–204. doi:10.1016/j.neulet.2008.01.008 Epub 2008 Jan 11
134. Kim JP, Park JG, Lee MD, Han MD, Park ST, Lee BH, Jung SE (1985) Co-carcinogenic effects of several Korean foods on gastric cancer induced by N-methyl-N'-nitro-N-nitrosoguanidine in rats. Jpn J Surg 15:427–37
135. Király A, Süto G, Czimmer J, Horváth OP, Mózsik G (2001) Failure of capsaicin-containing red pepper sauce suspension to induce esophageal motility response in patients with Barrett's esophagus. J Physiol Paris 95(1–6):197–200
136. Ko F, Diaz M, Smith P, Emerson E, Kim YJ, Krizek TJ, Robson MC (1998) Toxic effects of capsaicin on keratinocytes and fibroblasts. J Burn Care Rehabil 19(5):409–413
137. Kobata K, Toyoshima M, Kawamura M, Watanabe T (1998) Lipase-catalyzed synthesis of capsaicin analogs using natural oils as an acyl donor. Biotechnol Lett 20:781–783
138. Kochukov MY, McNearney TA, Fu Y, Westlund KN (2006) Thermosensitive TRP ion channels mediate cytosolic calcium response in human synoviocytes. Am J Physiol Cell Physiol 291(3):C424–C432
139. Kochukov MY, McNearney TA, Yin H, Zhang L, Ma F, Ponomareva L, Abshire S, Westlund KN (2009) Tumor necrosis factor-alpha (TNF-alpha) enhances functional thermal and chemical responses of TRP cation channels in human synoviocytes. Mol Pain 20(5):49
140. Kosuwon W, Sirichatiwapee W, Wisanuyotin T, Jeeravipoolvarn P, Laupattarakasem W (2010) Efficacy of symptomatic control of knee osteoarthritis with 0.0125 % of capsaicin versus placebo. J Med Assoc Thai 93(10):1188–95
141. Kulkantrakorn K, Lorsuwansiri C, Meesawatsom P (2013) 0.025 % capsaicin gel for the treatment of painful diabetic neuropathy: a randomized, double-blind, crossover, placebo-controlled trial. Pain Pract 13(6):497–503. doi:10.1111/papr.12013 Epub 2012 Dec 10
142. Källner G (1998) Release and effects of calcitonin gene-related peptide in myocardial ischaemia. Scand Cardiovasc J Suppl 49:1–35
143. LaHann TR (1986) Effect of capsaicin on croton oil and TPA induced tumorigenesis and inflammation. Proc West Pharmacol Soc 29:145–9
144. Laslett LL, Jones G (2014) Capsaicin for osteoarthritis pain. Prog Drug Res 68:277–291
145. Lee YS, Kang YS, Lee JS, Nicolova S, Kim JA (2004) Involvement of NADPH oxidase-mediated generation of reactive oxygen species in the apototic cell death by capsaicin in HepG2 human hepatoma cells. Free Radic Res 38(4):405–412
146. Lee MS, Kim CT, Kim IH, Kim Y (2011) Effects of capsaicin on lipid catabolism in 3T3-L1 adipocytes. Phytother Res 25(6):935–939
147. Lee GR, Shin MK, Yoon DJ, Kim AR, Yu R, Park NH, Han IS (2013) Topical application of capsaicin reduces visceral adipose fat by affecting adipokine levels in high-fat diet-induced obese mice. Obesity (Silver Spring) 21(1):115–122. doi:10.1002/oby.20246
148. Leech J, Mazzone SB, Farrell MJ (2012) The effect of placebo conditioning on capsaicin evoked urge to cough. Chest 142:951–957
149. Lin S, Zhang J, Chen H, Chen K, Lai F, Luo J, Wang Z, Bu H, Zhang R, Li H, Tong H (2013) Involvement of endoplasmic reticulum stress in capsaicin-induced apoptosis of human pancreatic cancer cells. Evid Based Complement Alternat Med 2013:629750
150. Liu L, Simon SA (1994) A rapid capsaicin-activated current in rat trigeminal ganglion neurons. Proc Natl Acad Sci U S A 91:738–741
151. Loftus EV Jr (2004) Clinical epidemiology of inflammatory bowel disease: incidence, prevalence, and environmental influences. Gastroenterology 126(6):1504–17
152. Luo XJ, Liu B, Dai Z, Yang ZC, Peng J (2013) Stimulation of calcitonin gene-related peptide release through targeting capsaicin receptor: a potential strategy for gastric mucosal protection. Dig Dis Sci 58(2):320–325. doi:10.1007/s10620-012-2362-6
153. Luo XJ, Peng J, Li YJ (2011) Recent advances in the study on capsaicinoids and capsinoids. Eur J Pharmacol 650(1):1–7. doi:10.1016/j.ejphar.2010.09.074 Epub 2010 Oct 12

154. Macho A, Blázquez MV, Navas P, Muñoz E (1998) Induction of apoptosis by vanilloid compounds does not require de novo gene transcription and activator protein 1 activity. Cell Growth Differ 9(3):277–286
155. Macho A, Calzado MA, Muñoz-Blanco J, Gómez-Díaz C, Gajate C, Mollinedo F, Navas P, Muñoz E (1999) Selective induction of apoptosis by capsaicin in transformed cells: the role of reactive oxygen species and calcium. Cell Death Differ 6(2):155–65
156. Mahmood S, Lesuis N, van Tuyl LH, van Riel P, Landewé R (2015) Quality in rheumatoid arthritis care. Best Pract Res Clin Rheumatol 29(4–5):664–679. doi:10.1016/j.berh.2015.09.009 (Epub 2015 Nov 7. Review)
157. Maihofner C, Heskamp ML (2013) Prospective, non-interventional study on the tolerability and analgesic effectiveness over 12 weeks after a single application of capsaicin 8 % cutaneous patch in 1044 patients with peripheral neuropathic pain: first results of the QUEPP study. Curr Med Res Opin 29(6):673–683. doi:10.1185/03007995.2013.792246 Epub 2013 Apr 25
158. Makara GB, Csalay L, Frenkl R, Somfai Z, Szepeshazi K (1965) Effect of capsaicin on experimental ulcer in the rat. Acta Med Acad Sci Hung 21:213–216
159. Mankowski C, Patel S, Trueman D, Bentley A, Poole C (2016) Cost-effectiveness of capsaicin 8 % patch compared with pregabalin for the treatment of patients with peripheral neuropathic pain in scotland. PLoS ONE 11(3):e0150973. doi:10.1371/journal.pone.0150973
160. Marabini S, Ciabatti PG, Polli G, Fusco BM, Geppetti P (1991) Beneficial effects of intranasal applications of capsaicin in patients with vasomotor rhinitis. Eur Arch Otorhinolaryngol 248:191–194
161. Marchand F, Perretti M, McMahon SB (2005) Role of the immune system in chronic pain. Nat Rev Neurosci 6(7):521–532 (Review)
162. McCarthy GM, McCarty DJ (1992) Effect of topical capsaicin in the therapy of painful osteoarthritis of the hands. J Rheumatol 19(4):604–607
163. McCleane G (2000) The analgesic efficacy of topical capsaicin is enhanced by glyceryl trinitrate in painful osteoarthritis: a randomized, double blind, placebo controlled study. Eur J Pain 4(4):355–360
164. McMahon SB, Lewin G, Bloom SR (1991) The consequences of long-term topical capsaicin application in the rat. Pain 44(3):301–310
165. Meral O, Alpay M, Kismali G, Kosova F, Cakir DU, Pekcan M, Yigit S, Sel T (2014) Capsaicin inhibits cell proliferation by cytochrome c release in gastric cancer cells. Tumour Biol 35(7):6485–6492. doi:10.1007/s13277-014-1864-6 Epub 2014 Mar 30
166. Mizushima T, Obata K, Katsura H, Sakurai J, Kobayashi K, Yamanaka H, Dai Y, Fukuoka T, Mashimo T, Noguchi K (2007) Intensity-dependent activation of extracellular signal-regulated protein kinase 5 in sensory neurons contributes to pain hypersensitivity. J Pharmacol Exp Ther 321(1):28–34
167. Mizushima T, Obata K, Yamanaka H, Dai Y, Fukuoka T, Tokunaga A, Mashimo T, Noguchi K (2005) Activation of p38 MAPK in primary afferent neurons by noxious stimulation and its involvement in the development of thermal hyperalgesia. Pain 113(1–2):51–60
168. Moeller A, Carlsen KH, Sly PD, Baraldi E, Piacentini G, Pavord I, Lex C, Saglani S (2015) ERS task force monitoring asthma in children. Monitoring asthma in childhood: lung function, bronchial responsiveness and inflammation. Eur Respir Rev 24(136):204–215. doi:10.1183/16000617.00003914 (Review)
169. Molodecky NA, Soon IS, Rabi DM, Ghali WA, Ferris M, Chernoff G, Benchimol EI, Panaccione R, Ghosh S, Barkema HW, Kaplan GG (2012) Increasing incidence and prevalence of the inflammatory bowel diseases with time, based on systematic review. Gastroenterology 142(1):46–54. e42; quiz e30. doi:10.1053/j.gastro.2011.10.001
170. Montell C, Rubin GM (1989) Molecular characterization of the Drosophila trp locus: a putative integral membrane protein required for phototransduction. Neuron 2(4):1313–1323

171. Morré DJ, Chueh PJ, Morré DM (1995) Capsaicin inhibits preferentially the NADH oxidase and growth of transformed cells in culture. Proc Natl Acad Sci U S A 92(6):1831–1835
172. Murray CJ, Richards MA, Newton JN, Fenton KA, Anderson HR, Atkinson C, Bennett D, Bernabé E, Blencowe H, Bourne R, Braithwaite T, Brayne C, Bruce NG, Brugha TS, Burney P, Dherani M, Dolk H, Edmond K, Ezzati M, Flaxman AD, Fleming TD, Freedman G, Gunnell D, Hay RJ, Hutchings SJ, Ohno SL, Lozano R, Lyons RA, Marcenes W, Naghavi M, Newton CR, Pearce N, Pope D, Rushton L, Salomon JA, Shibuya K, Vos T, Wang H, Williams HC, Woolf AD, Lopez AD, Davis A (2013) UK health performance: findings of the global burden of disease study (2010). Lancet 381:997–1020
173. Myers BM, Smith JL, Graham DY (1987) Effect of red pepper and black pepper on the stomach. Am J Gastroenterol 82(3):211–214
174. Mózsik G, Szolcsányi J, Dömötör A (2007) Capsaicin research as a new tool to approach of the human gastrointestinal physiology, pathology and pharmacology. Inflammopharmacology 15(6):232–245. doi:10.1007/s10787-007-1584-2
175. Nagabhushan M, Bhide SV (1985) Mutagenicity of chilli extract and capsaicin in short-term tests. Environ Mutagen 7:881–888
176. Ng SC, Chan FK (2013) Infections and inflammatory bowel disease: challenges in Asia. J Dig Dis 14(11):567–573. doi:10.1111/1751-2980
177. Nieto L, de Diego A, Perpiñá M, Compte L, Garrigues V, Martínez E, Ponce J (2003) Cough reflex testing with inhaled capsaicin in the study of chronic cough. Respir Med 97(4):393–400
178. Ochoa-Alejo N, Gomez-Peralta JE (1993) Activity of enzymes involved in capsaicin biosynthesis in callus tissue and fruits of chilli pepper (*Capsicum* annuum L). J Plant Physiol 141:147–152
179. Oh SH, Kim YS, Lim SC, Hou YF, Chang IY, You HJ (2008) Dihydrocapsaicin (DHC), a saturated structural analog of capsaicin, induces autophagy in human cancer cells in a catalase-regulated manner. Autophagy 4:1009–19
180. Oh SH, Lim SC (2009) Endoplasmic reticulum stress-mediated autophagy/apoptosis induced by capsaicin (8-methyl-N-vanillyl-6-nonenamide) and dihydrocapsaicin is regulated by the extent of c-Jun NH2-terminal kinase/extracellular signal-regulated kinase activation in WI38 lung epithelial fibroblast cells. J Pharmacol Exp Ther 329:112–22
181. Oliver JE, Silman AJ (2009) Why are women predisposed to autoimmune rheumatic diseases? Arthritis Res Ther 11(5):252. doi:10.1186/ar2825 (Epub 2009 Oct 26. Review)
182. O'Neil MJ (2001) The merck index—an encyclopedia of chemicals, drugs, and biologicals. 13th edn. Whitehouse Station, NJ: Merck and Co., Inc., p 296
183. Pecze L, Szabo K, Szell M, Josvay K, Kaszas K, Kusz E, Letoha T, Prorok J, Koncz I, Toth A, Kemeny L, Vizler C, Olah Z (2008) Human keratinocytes are vanilloid resistant. PLoS ONE 3:e3419
184. Peng J, Li YJ (2010) The vanilloid receptor TRPV1: role in cardiovascular and gastrointestinal protection. Eur J Pharmacol 627(1–3):1–7. doi:10.1016/j.ejphar.2009.10.053
185. Pozsgai G, Bodkin JV, Graepel R, Bevan S, Andersson DA, Brain SD (2010) Evidence for the pathophysiological relevance of TRPA1 receptors in the cardiovascular system in vivo. Cardiovasc Res 87:760–8
186. Rashid MH, Inoue M, Kondo S, Kawashima T, Bakoshi S, Ueda H (2003) Novel expression of vanilloid receptor 1 on capsaicin-insensitive fibers accounts for the analgesic effect of capsaicin cream in neuropathic pain. J Pharmacol Exp Ther 304(3):940–8
187. Reyes-Escogido ML, Gonzalez-Mondragon EG, Vazquez-Tzompantzi E (2011) Chemical and pharmacological aspects of capsaicin. Molecules 16:1253–1270
188. Richards BL, Whittle SL, van der Heijde DM, Buchbinder R (2012) Efficacy and safety of neuromodulators in inflammatory arthritis: a cochrane systematic review. J Rheumatol Suppl 90:28–33

189. Robert A, Nezamis JE, Lancaster C, Hanchar AJ (1979) Cytoprotection by prostaglandins in rats. Prevention of gastric necrosis produced by alcohol, HCl, NaOH, hypertonic NaCl, and thermal injury. Gastroenterology 77(3):433–43
190. Rosenbaum T, Simon SA (2007) TRPV1 receptors and signal transduction. In: Liedtke WB, Heller S (eds) TRP Ion channel function in sensory transduction and cellular signaling cascades. CRC Press/Taylor & Francis, Boca Raton (FL) (Chapter 5)
191. Ryu S, Liu B, Qin F (2003) Low pH potentiates both capsaicin binding and channel gating of VR1 receptors. J Gen Physiol 122:45–61
192. Saria A, Lundberg JM, Hua X, Lembeck F (1983) Capsaicin-induced substance P release and sensory control of vascular permeability in the guinea-pig ureter. Neurosci Lett 41(1–2):167–172
193. Scheiffarth F, Baenkler HW, Schörg G (1970) Effect and storage of gold in experimental formalin arthritis of rats. Z Rheumaforsch 29(1):42–46
194. Schnitzer TJ, Pelletier JP, Haselwood DM, Ellison WT, Ervin JE, Gordon RD, Lisse JR, Archambault WT, Sampson AR, Fezatte HB, Phillips SB, Bernstein JE (2012) Civamide cream 0.075 % in patients with osteoarthritis of the knee: a 12-week randomized controlled clinical trial with a longterm extension. J Rheumatol 39(3):610–20. doi:10.3899/jrheum.110192 Epub 2011 Nov 15
195. Schumacher M, Pasvankas G (2014) Topical capsaicin formulations in the management of neuropathic pain. Prog Drug Res 68:105–28
196. Scotland RS, Chauhan S, Davis C, De Felipe C, Hunt S, Kabir J, Kotsonis P, Oh U, Ahluwalia A (2004) Vanilloid receptor TRPV1, sensory C-fibers, and vascular autoregulation: a novel mechanism involved in myogenic constriction. Circ Res 95 (10):1027–34
197. Shah SK, Abraham P, Mistry FP (2000) Effect of cold pressor test and a high-chilli diet on rectosigmoid motility in irritable bowel syndrome. Indian J Gastroenterol 19(4):161–164
198. Shen J, Fox LE, Cheng J (2012) Differential effects of peripheral versus central coadministration of QX-314 and capsaicin on neuropathic pain in rats. Anesthesiology 117(2):365–80. doi:10.1097/ALN.0b013e318260de41
199. Shimizu T, Janssens A, Voets T, Nilius B (2009) Regulation of the murine TRPP3 channel by voltage, pH, and changes in cell volume. Pflugers Arch 457:795–807
200. Shirakawa H, Yamaoka T, Sanpei K, Sasaoka H, Nakagawa T, Kaneko S (2008) TRPV1 stimulation triggers apoptotic cell death of rat cortical neurons. Biochem Biophys Res Commun 377(4):1211–1215
201. Siemens J, Zhou S, Piskorowski R, Nikai T, Lumpkin EA, Basbaum AI, King D, Julius D (2006) Spider toxins activate the capsaicin receptor to produce inflammatory pain. Nature 444(7116):208–212
202. Simple Tasks: Rheumatic conditions in the UK: The problem (2013) The impact. The answers. The British society for rheumatology. http://www.rheumatology.org.uk/includes/documents/cm_docs/2013/w/white_paper_report.pdf
203. Smith HS, Argoff CE (2011) Pharmacological treatment of diabetic neuropathic pain. Drugs 71(5):557–589. doi:10.2165/11588940-000000000-00000
204. Somagoni J, Boakye CH, Godugu C, Patel AR, Mendonca Faria HA, Zucolotto V, Singh M (2014) Nanomiemgel–a novel drug delivery system for topical application–in vitro and in vivo evaluation. PLoS ONE 9:e115952
205. Sternini C, Reeve JR Jr, Brecha N (1987) Distribution and characterization of calcitonin gene-related peptide immunoreactivity in the digestive system of normal and capsaicin-treated rats. Gastroenterology 93(4):852–862
206. Sun J, Zhao Y, Hu J (2013) Curcumin inhibits imiquimod-induced psoriasis-like inflammation by inhibiting IL-1beta and IL-6 production in mice. PLoS ONE 8:e67078
207. Sung Y, Chang YY, Ting NL (2005) Capsaicin biosynthesis in water-stressed hot pepper fruits. Bot Bull Acad Sin 46:35–42

208. Surh YJ, Lee RC, Park KK, Mayne ST, Liem A, Miller JA (1995) Chemoprotective effects of capsaicin and diallyl sulfide against mutagenesis or tumorigenesis by vinyl carbamate and N-nitrosodimethylamine. Carcinogenesis 16(10):2467–2471
209. Szallasi A (1994) The vanilloid (capsaicin) receptor: receptor types and species differences. Gen Pharmacol 25:223–243
210. Szallasi A, Blumberg PM (1989) Resiniferatoxin, a phorbol-related diterpene, acts as an ultrapotent analog of capsaicin, the irritant constituent in red pepper. Neuroscience 30:515–20
211. Szallasi A, Blumberg PM (1990) Resiniferatoxin and its analogs provide novel insights into the pharmacology of the vanilloid (capsaicin) receptor. Life Sci 47:1399–1408
212. Szallasi A, Blumberg PM (1991) Molecular target size of the vanilloid (capsaicin) receptor in pig dorsal root ganglia. Life Sci 48:1863–1869
213. Szallasi A, Blumberg PM (1996) Vanilloid receptors: new insights enhance potential as a therapeutic target. Pain 68:195–208
214. Szallasi A, Blumberg PM (1999) Vanilloid (Capsaicin) receptors and mechanisms. Pharmacol Rev 51(2):159–212
215. Szolcsányi J, Mozsik G (1984) Effects of capsaicin on the development of gastric mucosal damage by different necrotizing agents and of gastric cytoprotection by PGI2 atropine and cimetidine on rats. Acta Physiol Hung 64:287–291
216. Szolcsányi J (1977) A pharmacological approach to elucidation of the role of different nerve fibres and receptor endings in mediation of pain. J Physiol (Paris) 73(3):251–259
217. Szolcsányi J (1987) Capsaicin and nociception. Acta Physiol Hung 69(3–4):323–332
218. Szolcsányi J, Jancso-Gabor A (1975) JOO F. Functional and fine structural characteristics of the sensory neuron blocking effect of capsaicin. Naunyn Schmiedebergs Arch Pharmacol 287 (2):157–169
219. Szolcsányi J (1996) Capsaicin-sensitive sensory nerve terminals with local and systemic efferent functions: facts and scopes of an unorthodox neuroregulatory mechanism. Prog Brain Res 113:343–59 (Review)
220. Szolcsányi J (2014) Capsaicin and sensory neurones: a historical perspective. Prog Drug Res 68:1–37 (Review)
221. Szolcsányi J, Barthó L (1981) Impaired defense mechanism to peptic ulcer in the capsaicin-desensitized rat. In: Mózsik Gy, Hänninen O, Jávor T (Eds.), Gastrointestinal defense mechanism. Adv. Physiol. Sci., vol 29. Akadémiai Kiadó-Pergamon Press, Budapest, pp 39–51
222. Ternesten-Hasseus E, Johansson EL, Millqvist E (2015) Cough reduction using capsaicin. Respir Med 109:27–37
223. The Capsaicin Study Group (1991) Treatment of painful diabetic neuropathy with topical capsaicin. A multicenter, double-blind, vehicle-controlled study. Arch Intern Med 151 (11):2225–2229
224. Thresh JC (1876) Isolation of capsaicin. Pharm J Trans 3rd ser 6:941–947
225. Toth DM, Szoke E, Bolcskei K, Kvell K, Bender B, Bosze Z, Szolcsanyi J, Sandor Z (2011) Nociception, neurogenic inflammation and thermoregulation in TRPV1 knockdown transgenic mice. Cell Mol Life Sci 68:2589–2601
226. Treede RD, Rief W, Barke A, Aziz Q, Bennett MI, Benoliel R, Cohen M, Evers S, Finnerup NB, First MB, Giamberardino MA, Kaasa S, Kosek E, Lavand'homme P, Nicholas M, Perrot S, Scholz J, Schug S, Smith BH, Svensson P, Vlaeyen JW, Wang SJ (2015) A classification of chronic pain for ICD-11. Pain 156(6):1003–1007. doi:10.1097/j.pain.0000000000000160
227. Turnbull A (1850) Tincture of capsaicin as a remedy for chilblains and toothache, vol 1. Free Press, Dublin, pp 95–96
228. Van Gerven L, Alpizar YA, Wouters MM, Hox V, Hauben E, Jorissen M, Boeckxstaens G, Talavera K, Hellings PW (2014) Capsaicin treatment reduces nasal hyperreactivity and transient receptor potential cation channel subfamily V, receptor 1 (TRPV1) overexpression in patients with idiopathic rhinitis. J Allergy Clin Immunol 133:1332–1339, 1339.e1-3

229. Venier NA, Yamamoto T, Sugar LM, Adomat H, Fleshner NE, Klotz LH, Venkateswaran V (2015) Capsaicin reduces the metastatic burden in the transgenic adenocarcinoma of the mouse prostate model. Prostate 75(12):1300–1311. doi:10.1002/pros.23013 Epub 2015 Jun 5
230. Venkatesan R, Sah-Teli SK, Awoniyi LO, Jiang G, Prus P, Kastaniotis AJ, Hiltunen JK, Wierenga RK, Chen Z (2014) Insights into mitochondrial fatty acid synthesis from the structure of heterotetrameric 3-ketoacyl-ACP reductase/3R-hydroxyacyl-CoA dehydrogenase. Nat Commun 9(5):4805
231. Ventresca PG, Nichol GM, Barnes PJ, Chung KF (1990) Inhaled furosemide inhibits cough induced by low chloride content solutions but not by capsaicin. Am Rev Respir Dis 142:143–146
232. Viranuvatti V, Kalayasiri C, Chearani O, Plengvanit U (1972) Selective celiac angiography in carcinoma of liver and amebic liver abscess. Geriatrics 27(1):176–177
233. Walpole CS, Wrigglesworth R, Bevan S, Campbell EA, Dray A, James IF, Perkins MN, Reid DJ, Winter J (1993) Analogues of capsaicin with agonist activity as novel analgesic agents; structure-activity studies. 1. The aromatic "A-region". J Med Chem 36:2362–2372
234. Walsh BM, Hoot SB (2001) Phylogenetic relationships of capsicum (Solanaceae) using DNA sequences from two noncoding regions: the chloroplast atpB-rbcL spacer region and nuclear waxy introns. Int J Plant Sci 162(6):1409–1418. doi:10.1086/323273
235. van Wanrooij SJ, Wouters MM, Van Oudenhove L, Vanbrabant W, Mondelaers S, Kollmann P, Kreutz F, Schemann M, Boeckxstaens GE (2014) Sensitivity testing in irritable bowel syndrome with rectal capsaicin stimulations: role of TRPV1 upregulation and sensitization in visceral hypersensitivity? Am J Gastroenterol 109:99–109
236. Westlund KN, Kochukov MY, Lu Y, McNearney TA (2010) Impact of central and peripheral TRPV1 and ROS levels on proinflammatory mediators and nociceptive behavior. Mol Pain 6 (6):46
237. Wood JN, Winter J, James IF, Rang HP, Yeats J, Bevan S (1988) Capsaicin-induced ion fluxes in dorsal root ganglion cells in culture. J Neurosci 8:3208–3220
238. World Health Organization (2005) WHO global report 2005: preventing chronic diseases: a vital investment. http://www.who.int/chp/chronic_disease_report/full_report.pdf. Accessed 10 Aug 2016
239. World Health Organization (2011) WHO content model reference guide 2011 (11th). http://www.who.int/classifications/icd/revision/contentmodel/en/. Accessed 28 Feb 2016
240. World Health Organization (2013) WHO chronic respiratory diseases (asthma) 2013. http://www.who.int/mediacentre/factsheets/fs307/en/. Accessed 28 Feb 2016
241. World Health Organization (2014) Global status report on noncommunicable diseases 2014. http://apps.who.int/iris/bitstream/10665/148114/1/9789241564854_eng.pdf. Accessed 28 Feb 2016
242. Xu X, Wang P, Zou X, Li D, Fang L, Lin Q (2009) Increases in transient receptor potential vanilloid-1 mRNA and protein in primary afferent neurons stimulated by protein kinase C and their possible role in neurogenic inflammation. J Neurosci Res 87:482–494
243. Xu YP, Zhang JW, Li L, Ye ZY, Zhang Y, Gao X, Li F, Yan XS, Liu ZG, Liu LJ, Cao XH (2012) Complex regulation of capsaicin on intracellular second messengers by calcium dependent and independent mechanisms in primary sensory neurons. Neurosci Lett 517 (1):30–35
244. Yamaji K, Sarker KP, Kawahara K, Iino S, Yamakuchi M, Abeyama K, Hashiguchi T, Maruyama I (2003) Anandamide induces apoptosis in human endothelial cells: its regulation system and clinical implications. Thromb Haemost 89(5):875–884
245. Yang D, Luo Z, Ma S, Wong WT, Ma L, Zhong J, He H, Zhao Z, Cao T, Yan Z, Liu D, Arendshorst WJ, Huang Y, Tepel M, Zhu Z (2010) Activation of TRPV1 by dietary capsaicin improves endothelium-dependent vasorelaxation and prevents hypertension. Cell Metab 12(2):130–141
246. Yang R, Xiong Z, Liu C, Liu L (2014) Inhibitory effects of capsaicin on voltage-gated potassium channels by TRPV1-independent pathway. Cell Mol Neurobiol 34(4):565–576

247. Yeats JC, Docherty RJ, Bevan S (1992) Calcium-dependent and -independent desensitization of capsaicin-evoked responses in voltage-clamped adult rat dorsal root ganglion (DRG) neurones in culture. J Physiol (Lond) 446:390P
248. Yeoh KG, Kang JY, Yap I, Guan R, Tan CC, Wee A, Teng CH (1995) Chilli protects against aspirin-induced gastroduodenal mucosal injury in humans. Dig Dis Sci 40:580–583
249. Yoshimura M, Yonehara N (2001) Influence of capsaicin cream in rats with peripheral neuropathy. Pharmacol Res 44(2):105–111
250. Yshii LM, Souza GH, Camargo EA, Eberlin MN, Ribela MT, Muscará MN, Hyslop S, Costa SK (2009) Characterization of the mechanisms underlying the inflammatory response to Polistes lanio lanio (paper wasp) venom in mouse dorsal skin. Toxicon 53(1):42–52. doi:10.1016/j.toxicon.2008.10.006 Epub 2008 Oct 17
251. Zhang R, Humphreys I, Sahu RP, Shi Y, Srivastava SK (2008) In vitro and in vivo induction of apoptosis by capsaicin in pancreatic cancer cells is mediated through ROS generation and mitochondrial death pathway. Apoptosis 13(12):1465–1478
252. Zhang R, Humphreys I, Sahu RP, Shi Y, Srivastava SK (2008) In vitro and in vivo induction of apoptosis by capsaicin in pancreatic cancer cells is mediated through ROS generation and mitochondrial death pathway. Apoptosis 13(12):1465–1478
253. Zhang LL, Yan Liu D, Ma LQ, Luo ZD, Cao TB, Zhong J, Yan ZC, Wang LJ, Zhao ZG, Zhu SJ, Schrader M, Thilo F, Zhu ZM, Tepel M (2007) Activation of transient receptor potential vanilloid type-1 channel prevents adipogenesis and obesity. Circ Res 100(7):1063–1070
254. Zhu Y, Wang M, Zhang J, Peng W, Firempong CK, Deng W, Wang Q, Wang S, Shi F, Yu J, Xu X, Zhang W (2015) Improved oral bioavailability of capsaicin via liposomal nanoformulation: preparation, in vitro drug release and pharmacokinetics in rats. Arch Pharm Res 38(4):512–521. doi:10.1007/s12272-014-0481-7
255. Zygmunt PM, Petersson J, Andersson DA, Chuang H, Sørgård M, Di Marzo V, Julius D, Högestätt ED (1999) Vanilloid receptors on sensory nerves mediate the vasodilator action of anandamide. Nature 400(6743):452–457

Diallyl Sulfide and Its Role in Chronic Diseases Prevention

Shankar Suman and Yogeshwer Shukla

Abstract Diallyl sulfide ($C_6H_{10}S$, DAS) is one of the novel natural organosulfur compounds, which is mostly obtained from the genus *Allium* plants. Numerous studies have revealed several unique properties of DAS in terms of its health-promoting effects. DAS has proved to be anticancer, antimicrobial, anti-angiogenic, and immunomodulatory like unique functions as demonstrated by the multiple investigations. Diallyl sulfide can also impede oxidative stress and chronic inflammation as suggested by the literature. Studies also explored that DAS could thwart the development of chronic diseases like cancer, neuronal, cardiovascular disease through modulating mechanistic pathways involved in pathogenesis. In this book chapter, we have attempted to give the comprehensive view on DAS about the physiochemical and biological properties, and its preventive role in chronic diseases with a mechanistic overview.

Keywords Diallyl sulfide · Chronic disease · Signaling pathways · Biological activities

1 Introduction

Diallyl sulfide ($C_6H_{10}S$) is a lipophilic thioallyl-ether and one of the organosulfur compounds extracted most commonly from garlic (*Allium sativam* L.). From the late nineteenth century, organosulfur compounds are recognized as the pungent smelling material of garlic, and diallyl sulfide is one of the components of distilled garlic oil [1]. Diallyl sulfide is one among the dietary phytochemicals, which showed many beneficial health effects in various experimental studies [2–4]. There is a growing body of literature, where the implications of diallyl sulfide in various chronic diseases, including cancer, neuronal, cardiovascular, liver, and numerous

S. Suman · Y. Shukla (✉)
Food, Drug and Chemical Toxicology Division, CSIR-Indian Institute of Toxicology Research, 31, Vish Vigyan Bhawan, M.G. Marg, Lucknow 226001, UP, India
e-mail: yshukla@iitr.res.in

S.C. Gupta et al. (eds.), *Drug Discovery from Mother Nature*,
Advances in Experimental Medicine and Biology 929,
DOI 10.1007/978-3-319-41342-6_6

Table 1 Beneficial health effects of diallyl sulfide

Sr. No.	Effects	Studies	References
1	Antioxidant activities	Oral administration protects against pentachlorophenol-induced oxidative damage Modulate GSH-related antioxidant system reacting with free radical generated by UVC-activated hydrogen peroxide	[8, 91, 92]
2	Protection against coronary heart disease	Long-term administration inhibits platelet aggregation Protect LDL for oxidation and glycation	[9, 62]
3	Antimicrobial activity	Against gram-positive and gram-negative bacterial Against *Helicobacter pyroli* and *Pseudomonas aerogenosa*	[21, 93]
4	Antimutagenic activities	Reduce mutagenicity of styrene oxide and 4-nitroquinoline-1-oxide in Ames test Inhibited micronuclei formation Antimutagenic potential of cyclophosphamide-induced chromosomal aberration	[82, 84, 94]
5	Immunomodulatory Mechanism	Diallyl sulfide-modulated interleukin (IL)-1beta, and IL-6 and IL-10	[14]
6	Anticancer activities	Inhibit two-stage tumorigenesis in mouse skin tumorigenesis	[57]

other diseases have been reported [2, 5–7]. A plethora of studies revealed that diallyl sulfide possesses versatile medicinal properties, including antioxidant [8], cardioprotective [9], antihepatotoxic [10], immunomodulatory, and antineoplastic [11]. The details of its diverse health benefits of diallyl sulfide are mentioned in Table 1. In the present chapter, the characteristics and varied applications of diallyl sulfide are mentioned incorporating recent studies.

2 Diallyl Sulfide as an Important Ingredient of Garlic

The medicinal uses of garlic are used to recognize for ages, and it is well recognized for various biological activities for human health benefits against many diseases [2, 5, 12–15]. For example, diallyl sulfide has shown to be a selective inhibitor of cytochrome P450 2E1 (CYP2E1), a known enzyme for xenobiotic metabolism of a large number of compounds, such as alcohol and analgesic drugs in liver [3, 16, 17]. In the xenobiotic metabolism, reactive oxygen species (ROS) and reactive metabolites are produced, which damages DNA, protein, and lipid, hence impair liver. Additionally, not only diallyl sulfide is minimizing the cellular toxicity laid by alcohol and drug, but it may also thwart HIV protein and diabetes-mediated toxicities through inhibiting CYP2E1 selectively in multiple cell types [3]. Garlic extracts possess several of bioactive compounds, including sulfur compounds, amino acids, vitamins (A, B1, and C) as well as nutrients (germanium, calcium, copper, iron, selenium, zinc, potassium, magnesium) [2]. In a study, the range of organic sulfide recoveries is 77.1–99.8 % from garlic sprouts [18]. Various garlic extracts showed a therapeutic benefit for several diseases [19]. In the primary sulfur compounds, the major constituents are Y-glutamyl-*S*-alk(en)yl-L-cysteines, Y-glutamyl-*S*-alk(en)yl-L-cysteine sulfoxide, and alliin [20]. Whenever garlic is damaged by external factors (crushed, cut or chewed, pulverized or attacked by microbes), the vacuolar enzyme alliinase rapidly degrades allinin to cytotoxic and oliferous compound, including allicin [20]. Allicin and other sulfonates decompose instantly to hundred soluble organosulfur compounds, including diallyl sulfide, diallyl disulfide, diallyl trisulfide, diallyl tetrasulfide, allyl methyl sulfide, methyl allyl disulfide, methyl allyl trisulfide, dithin, and ajoene compounds [21]. Among all these compounds, diallyl sulfide is one of the important organosulfur compounds.

3 Physiochemical Properties of Diallyl Sulfide

Diallyl sulfide is the most commonly extracted compound from the distilled oil and sprouts of garlic. Moreover, it is also produced by the decomposition of allicin present in the plant of Alliaceae family. Diallyl sulfide is colorless, water insoluble, and possesses strong garlic odor (more details of physiochemical characteristics of diallyl sulfide are mentioned in Table 2). Diallyl sulfide has been also used as a synthetic food flavoring agent in many countries [22]. Diallyl sulfide has known to possess high chemical activities. For example, allyl sulfides, including diallyl sulfide, is one of the reactive substrates for olefin metathesis reaction (a chemical reaction involving the bimolecular process through exchange of bonds between the reacting chemical species) catalyzed by ruthenium and demonstrated as traceless promoters in relayed ring-closing metathesis reactions [23]. Diallyl sulfide

Table 2 Details of physical and chemical properties of diallyl sulfide

	Physical properties	References
Chemical formula	$C_6H_{10}S$	
Molecular weight	114.2086 g/mol	
Appearance	Colorless liquid	[95]
Density	0.888 at 27/4 °C	[96]
Boiling point and melting point	139 and −85 °C	[97]
Solubility	Soluble in ethanol and oils and insoluble in water alcohol, chloroform, ether, and carbon tetrachloride	[96]
Vapor pressure	9.22 mm Hg at 25° C	[98]

can be converted to diallyl sulfoxide (DASO) and diallyl sulfone (DASO2) by CYP2E1 in liver [24]. Furthermore, diallyl sulfide is chemically oxidized to allicin with hydrogen peroxide or peracetic acid [25]. Reaction of diallyl sulfide with liquid sulfur gives the mixture of diallyl polysulfides, which are useful materials for medicines and agriculture such as environmentally benign nematicides [26, 27].

4 Modulation of Cell Signaling Pathways by Diallyl Sulfide

The experimental observations from the various investigations revealed diallyl sulfide as potential compound to combat deadly diseases. Diallyl sulfide modulates cell signaling pathways related to the pathogenesis of several chronic diseases. In cancer, supplementation of diallyl sulfide retarded onset, multiplicity, growth in cancer cell lines, and chemically induced carcinogenic model [10, 28–30]. Diallyl sulfide is also found to modulate cell cycle regulators and apoptotic genes, indicating its potential function as an anticancer compound [4, 5, 7, 31, 32]. In tumorigenesis, a variety of signaling pathways are deregulated and garlic products showed their potential effect against these pathways in both in vitro and in vivo studies [5]. The important pathways modulated by diallyl sulfide are as follows.

4.1 Cell Cycle-Associated Pathways

Diallyl sulfide affects cell cycle regulation and apoptosis in many cancer types. In cervical cancer (Ca Ski) cells, it regulates cell cycle and apoptosis by increasing G0/G1 phase arrest and increasing expression of p21, p27, and p53 with decreasing expression of CDK2, CDK6, and CHK2 [31]. Flow cytometry assay indicated that diallyl sulfide promoted Ca^{2+} accumulation and lowering of mitochondrial membrane potential in Ca Ski cells and also revealed that diallyl sulfide might act as a chemotherapeutic agent for cervical cancer [31]. Wild-type p53 is understood as guardian or gatekeeper of the cell cycle, in the major cancer types, wild-type p53 expression is down-regulated, and mutant type p53 expression is increased in many cancers [33]. Studies from our laboratory showed that topical application of diallyl sulfide induces wild-type p53 expression and down-regulated the expression of mutant p53 in skin tumorigenic model, which may delay the skin tumorigenesis process [34]. Study also showed that liposomized diallyl sulfide formulations ensued upregulation of p53wt and p21/Waf1 and down-regulation of p53mut through which it acts as a chemopreventive agent against DMBA-induced skin papilloma animals [35]. Several other characteristics of allyl sulfides included their ability to suppress the proliferative pathways via depressing cell cycle progression and inducing apoptosis. Knowles et al. studied the effect of diallyl sulfide in reducing cell division concomitant with an increase of G2/M percentage in the cell cycle as an anticancer effect [32].

4.2 Cellular Mechanistic Pathways

Study has shown that diallyl sulfide increases heme oxygenase-1 (HO-1) protein and mRNA levels without toxicity in HepG2 cells in a dose- and time-dependent manner [36]. HO-1 plays an important role in the cellular defense mechanism during oxidative stress. Gong et al. revealed that diallyl sulfide induced HO-1 by increasing production of ROS, Nrf2, and MAPK (ERK and p38), and hence, diallyl sulfide-mediated HO-1 induction may show protective antioxidative effects [36]. From our laboratory, we observed the chemopreventive ability of diallyl sulfide together with pomegranate fruit extract either alone or in combination through which it decreased the expression of phosphorylated ERK1/2, JNK1, and activated the expression of NF-κB/p65, IKKα, phosphorylated IκBα in the mouse tumor model [37]. Our studies also revealed that diallyl sulfide increased the expression of pro-apoptotic protein (Bax) and led to the down-regulation of survivin and Bcl-2 [38]. It also modulates Ras oncoprotein, and associated signaling molecules like PI3K/Akt and MAPKs [38]. In the 7,12-dimethylbenz[a]anthracene (DMBA)-induced skin carcinoma, diallyl sulfide reduces PI3K/Akt and p38MAPK expression [38]. Diallyl disulfide activates mitochondrial biogenesis through NOS-Nrf2-Tfam pathways, which is defective in isoproterenol-induced cardiac hypertrophy in rats [39].

4.3 Inflammatory Pathways

Ho et al. studied that diallyl sulfide reduces TNF-α- and histamine-induced proinflammatory responses in rat aortic smooth muscle (A7r5) cells, and hence, they suggested that diallyl sulfide might prevent oxidative stress-induced inflammation [40]. Inflammatory pathways are governed by oxidation of low-density lipoprotein (Ox-LDL), which promotes majority of vascular dysfunctioning. The enhanced Ox-LDL level subsequently produces inflammatory mediators like tumor necrosis factor (TNF)-α, nitric oxide (NO), interleukin (IL)-6, arachidonic acid, which are associated with inflammatory pathways involved in several of chronic diseases, including atherosclerosis, cancer, cardiovascular diseases. Diallyl sulfide is also responsible to modulate the glutathione (GSH) redox cycle and inhibits nuclear factor kappa B (NF-κB) activation in human T cells [7]. Diallyl sulfide blocks the inflammatory response induced by monosodium urate and interleukin-1beta (IL-1β), through inhibiting Cox-2 and NF-κB. Further, these anti-inflammatory characteristics of diallyl sulfide may be useful for the treatment of joint inflammation [41]. Study also revealed the diallyl sulfide attenuated bleomycin-induced pulmonary fibrosis. The administration of bleomycin in Wistar rats reduces the catalase (CAT), superoxide dismutase (SOD), and glutathione peroxidase (GPx) activities in the lung tissues, which lead to an increase in the lipid peroxidase (LPO) and myeloperoxidase (MPO) activities and reduced glutathione (GSH) level [42]. Immunohistochemical analysis demonstrated that diallyl sulfide lowered the activation of inducible nitric oxide synthase (iNOS) and nuclear factor kappa B (NF-κB) as well as decreased the augmented levels of the early inflammatory cytokines, tumor necrosis factor (TNF)-α, and IL-1β in the lung tissues activated by bleomycin [42]. Ovalbumin is the key agent which induces allergic asthma, and Ho et al. studied that diallyl sulfide imparts protection to ovalbumin-induced pulmonary inflammation of allergic asthma in BALB/c mice by modulating microRNA-144,-34a, and -34b/c-based Nrf2 activation [43]. Intraperitoneal injection of diallyl sulfide is able to attenuate paraquat-induced acute lung injury in rats by minimizing pulmonary edema by inhibiting NF-KB and TNF-α expression in lung tissue [44]. Diallyl sulfide is useful to cure periodontal inflammation as it diminished *Porphyromonas gingivalis* lipopolysaccharide-stimulated cytokine expression and nuclear factor kappa B (NF-κB) activation in human gingival fibroblasts (HGFs) [45].

5 Protective Effects of Diallyl Sulfide in Various Diseases

Several in vitro and in vivo studies delineated variety of protective effects of diallyl sulfide in various chronic diseases based on the experimental evidences. These actions suggest the potential role of diallyl sulfide against several diseases by cellular protection as mentioned below (Fig. 1).

5.1 Neuronal Diseases

Diallyl sulfide displayed significant anti-neuroinflammatory activity in lipopolysaccharide (LPS)-stimulated BV2 microglia cells [46]. The neuroprotective effect of diallyl sulfide against ischemia or reperfusion injury is well demonstrated in recent studies. Lin et al. [46] demonstrated that diallyl sulfide protects against transient focal cerebral ischemia through anti-apoptotic mechanism in rats. Diallyl sulfide also acts as a potent inhibitor of CYP42E1 and potentiated selective dopamine neuron degeneration in C57/BL mice [47]. The treatment with diallyl sulfide induces apoptosis in human neuroblastoma cells (SY5Y cells) [48]. Furthermore, diallyl sulfide also reduces toxicity by inhibiting CYP2E1 [49], which is responsible for induction of oxidative stress and cytotoxicity in the glutathione-depleted cerebellar granule neurons, and thus, diallyl sulfide decreases risk of neuronal diseases [50]. Presence of diallyl sulfide decreases ROS production from ethanol through inhibiting of alcohol-inducible (CYP2E1) enzyme in rat neurons and thymocytes [51].

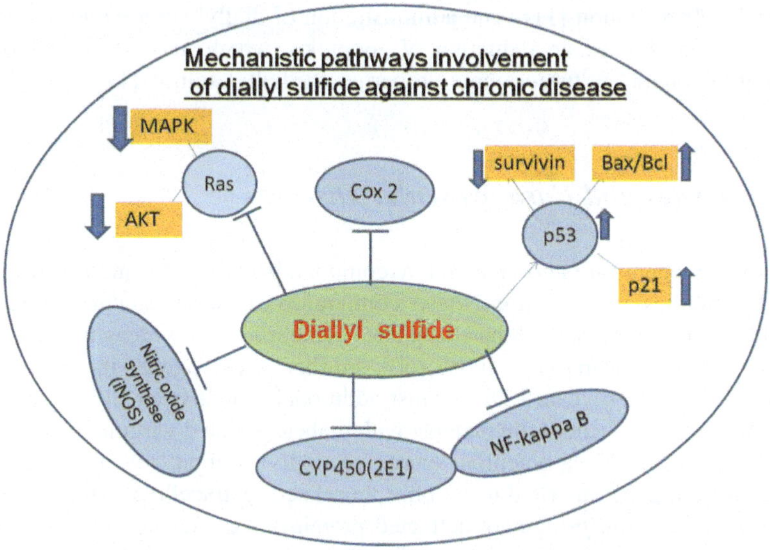

Fig. 1 Diallyl sulfide may target multiple signaling cascades, which are commonly involved in the various chronic diseases in including cancer and neuronal diseases

5.2 *Cancer Chemoprevention and Chemotherapeutic Properties*

Diallyl sulfide is involved in multiple signaling pathways for mediating apoptosis in mouse skin tumors [38]. *P*-glycoprotein is a key protein, which has major function as multiple drug resistance in cancer. Arora et al. [52] showed that diallyl sulfide can modulate this multidrug resistance protein. Diallyl sulfide was also found to inhibit the angiogenesis in Ehrlich ascites carcinoma bearing mice in a dose-dependent manner [53]. Study also suggested that diallyl sulfide had chemopreventive and chemotherapeutic properties with multiple mechanisms of actions [53]. Garlic organosulfur compounds are reported to inhibit proliferation and promotion of different types of cancer [11, 52, 54–57]. Studies also delineated that garlic constituents inhibit the growth of transplanted tumors and proliferative activity in a number of cancer types [52, 55]. Studies also suggested that diallyl sulfide inhibits the development of skin, and pulmonary cancer in experimental induced animals [11, 58]. Diallyl sulfide also showed an effective in modulating proliferative genes and apoptotic gene expression in non-small cell lung cancer cells [59]. Study demonstrates the induction of apoptosis with antiproliferative effect of diallyl sulfide in solid cancer as evident by flow cytometry analysis [11]. Terminal deoxynucleotidyl transferase-mediated dUTP nick end labeling (TUNEL) of the skin tumor-derived diallyl sulfide-supplemented animals showed an increase of apoptotic population compared to the control group that did not receive diallyl sulfide supplementation [11]. The administration of diallyl sulfide after carcinogen administration showed an induction of apoptosis, which may be the major contributing factor for antitumorigenic properties of diallyl sulfide [11].

5.3 Diabetes and Cardiovascular Diseases

Organosulfur agents are known as active compounds in diabetes and cardiovascular diseases. Studies revealed that these compounds increase catalase, glutathione peroxidase activities, and alpha-tocopherol retention of low-density lipoproteins (LDL) in blood plasma ($P < 0.05$) [60]. Further, these agents including diallyl sulfide oxidize and glycate LDL against additional oxidative or glycative deterioration, which might benefit the patients with diabetes-related vascular diseases [60]. Studies on garlic oil, a potential source of diallyl sulfide, revealed that it can significantly reduce interleukin-6, phosphorylated extracellular signal-regulated kinase-5, calcineurin, *p*-mitogen-activated protein kinase-5, nuclear factor of activated T-cell transcription factor, and p-GATA binding protein-4 in a hamster model [61]. Hence, garlic oil was suggested as an option for the treatment of hypertrophy-associated cardiovascular diseases [61]. Cardiovascular diseases are majorly associated with increased serum total cholesterol, LDL, LDL oxidation, platelet aggregation, and hypertension, and several of in vitro studies have revealed that garlic inhibits enzymes involved in lipid synthesis, platelet aggregation, lipid peroxidation of oxidized erythrocytes and LDL and angiotensin-converting enzyme as well as increased antioxidant capacity [7, 9, 61–63].

5.4 Lung Diseases

Diallyl sulfide has known its beneficial effects against several lung diseases. Study showed that intraperitoneal injection of diallyl sulfide can attenuate the extent of acute lung injury and ameliorate pathological changes in lung tissue of rats by paraquat poisoning [44]. Diallyl sulfide also acts against ovalbumin-induced allergic reaction, such as inflammatory cell infiltration and hyper-secretion of mucus in lung tissues of BALB/c mice [43]. Study has also revealed that diallyl sulfide attenuates the excessive collagen production and apoptosis in bleomycin-induced pulmonary fibrosis in the rat model through protease-activated receptor-2 (PAR-2) [43]. It is also showed that diallyl sulfide protects lung fibrosis through reducing bleomycin-induced activation of inducible nitric oxide synthase (iNOS) and nuclear factor kappa B (NF-κB) and early inflammatory cytokines such as tumor necrosis factor (TNF)-α and IL-1β, in the lung tissues [42]. The diallyl sulfide also activated the antioxidant enzymes in rat lungs, which prevent oxidative stress-induced lung injury in rats [64].

5.5 *Intestinal Disease*

Diallyl sulfide also showed the protective effects against intestinal diseases. The co-administration of diallyl disulfide reduces the severity of naproxen-induced small intestinal damage, inflammation, and bleeding in a dose-dependent manner [65]. Further, it also attenuated naproxen-induced cytotoxicity in bile on cultured enterocytes and prevented the naproxen-induced changes in the intestinal microbiota [65]. Ansar et al. [66] studied that diallyl sulfide attenuated ferric nitrilotriacetate (Fe-NTA)-induced renal toxicity, increase in LPO, hydrogen peroxide generation, and protein carbonyl formation in rats. Diallyl sulfide also ameliorates thioacetamide-induced hepatotoxicity and immunotoxicity in Sprague Dawley rats [16]. Study revealed that oral administration of 100, 200, and 400 mg/kg of diallyl sulfide for three consecutive days in as a corn oil formulation for three consecutive days, the activity of CYP 2E1-selective p-nitrophenol hydroxylase was suppressed in a dose-dependent manner. The treatment of diallyl sulfide induces CYP 2B-selective benzyloxyresorufin *O*-debenzylase and pentoxyresorufin-*O*-depentylase, which indicated that thioacetamide may activate to its toxic metabolite(s) by CYP 2E1, not by CYP 2B, in rats and mice [16].

5.6 *Hepatotoxicity and Liver Diseases*

Diallyl sulfide is also an important dietary phytochemical to reduce toxicity of various toxicant exposures in the animal model. Study revealed that pre-treatment with diallyl sulfide ameliorates several kinds of changes in biochemical parameters and has also shown that it effectively reduced thallium acetate (a cumulative poison)-induced liver toxicity in rat [67]. Study also revealed that allyl disulfide supplementation had a positive impact on liver regeneration and proliferation and against oxidative damage in an experimental hepatectomy model [68]. Diallyl sulfide also demonstrates its inhibitory effect in preneoplastic altered hepatic foci (AHF) in Wistar rats [30]. The supplementation of diallyl sulfide restores the normal enzyme level of glutathione S-transferase placental form, gamma-glutamyl transpeptidase, adenosine triphosphatase (ATPase), glucose-6-phosphatase, and alkaline phosphatase activity by exposing diethylnitrosamine (DEN)-initiated and 2-acetyl-aminofluorene (2-AAF)-promoted, two-stage carcinogenic process of AHF formation [30]. Hence, it has a protective role in rat hepatocarcinogenesis through suppressing DEN and 2-AAF-induced AHF development in Wistar rats [30]. Diallyl sulfide was also reported as a potent inhibitor in liver tumorigenesis and also revealed treatments with diallyl sulfide may protect most of the measured liver toxicity parameters, which is disturbed by liver tumorigenesis-promoting chemicals like *N*-nitrosodiethylamine (NDEA) [69]. Allyl sulfides from garlic have protective effect on arylamine *N*-acetyltransferase activity in Klebsiella pneumonia [70]. Diallyl sulfide has been reported to protect against DNA damage by alfatoxin B though increasing the glutathione S-transferase (GST) and glutathione peroxidase (GPx) activities [71].

6 Biological Activities of Diallyl Sulfide in Animal Models

Till date, a large number of animal models were utilized to study the biological effects of diallyl sulfide for numerous diseases. Diallyl sulfide studied as inhibitory agents of CYP2E1 participates in carcinogen as well as other xenobiotic metabolism [72]. Inflammatory bowel disease (IBD) is considered as incurable disease, which affects millions of people. Diallyl sulfide and diallyl disulfide exert high therapeutic effects in the dinitrobenzene sulfonic acid-induced colitis model [15]. These compounds can control the production of, IL-6, hydrogen sulfide or nitric oxide and STAT-1 expression in intestinal cells, which might explain the protective action of diallyl sulfide and diallyl disulfide in experimental IBD model [15]. Diabetes mellitus (DM) is understood as a risk factor for hepatocellular carcinoma (HCC); it is mainly due to metabolic reprogramming as DM directs glucose to sorbitol and fructose in polyol pathway (PP) [73, 74]. Co-induction of DM and HCC together in rats led to increase liver tissue lesion, serum alpha-fetoprotein, erythrocyte sorbitol, hepatocyte aldose reductase, and sorbitol dehydrogenase [73]. Treatment with diallyl sulfide and ascorbic acid lowered erythrocyte sorbitol by preventing hepatocyte aldose reductase activity in rats. Hence, diallyl sulfide and ascorbic acid combination showed promising results as chemopreventive and antidiabetic combination [73]. Studies from our laboratory revealed the chemopreventive properties of diallyl sulfide against several chemically induced carcinogenic models. The chemopreventive properties of diallyl sulfide possibly occurred by a number of mechanisms. We studied that diallyl sulfide administration leads to modulation of levels of p21/ras oncoprotein in the DMBA-induced rodent model [75]. The study on kindled rats, a common model for behavioral studies, showed that the use of diallyl sulfide with ketogenic diet (high-fat and low-carbohydrate diet used to treat neuronal disease like epilepsy) does not elevate amygdaloid after the discharge threshold (which is the discharge of neural impulses after terminating the initiation stimulus) in fully kindled rats, but the effect was not prominent by ketogenic diet only [76]. Ketogenic diet with diallyl sulfide also elevated the blood acetone level, while in the absence of diallyl sulfide, it was not changed significantly [76]. Diallyl sulfide is also well reported its protective effects in hepatic ischemia reperfusion injury in the rat model by reducing oxidative stress inducing heme oxygenase-1 and inhibiting CYP2E1 in rats [77]. Liposomal formulation of diallyl sulfide is reported to disseminate opportunistic fungal infections like Candidiasis albicans in a mice model [78].

6.1 Antioxidant Activity

Oxidative stress plays a vital role in pathophysiology of disease progression. Antioxidant activity has great significance as this activity suppresses chronic diseases. Diallyl sulfide decreases thiobarbituric acid-reactive substances (TBARS), and it acts as an effective antioxidant. It also plays a significant role in the defense against lipid peroxidation in trichinellosis [22]. Diallyl sulfide ameliorates gentamicin-induced nephrotoxicity as it increases the creatinine and urea in serum, *N*-acetyl-β-D-glucosaminidase, total protein, and necrosis of proximal tubular cell urinary secretion [79]. Diallyl sulfide inhibits CYP2E1-led bioactivation of acrylamide to glycidamide, a toxic product in liver [80]. Current ongoing investigations also revealed the several of diallyl sulfide analogs act as inhibitor CYP2E1 and also utilized against many of the diseases, including HIV and diabetes [3]. As mentioned above that diallyl sulfide is subsequently converted into diallyl sulfoxide, diallyl sulfones by action of CYP2E enzyme. These compounds can reduce the incidence of chemically induced tumors in animals [24]. It was found that the converted compounds impede phase I activation of carcinogens and may account for reduction of tumor incidence [24]. Despite these, compounds also reduce *N*-nitroso-dimethylamine, carbon tetrachloride, and acetaminophen-induced toxicity in rodent animals [24]. Study also revealed that diallyl sulfide and diallyl sulfone inhibit the bioactivation of 4-(methyl-nitrosamino)-1-(3-pyridyl)-1-butanone (NNK) and lung tumorigenesis in A/J mice. Yang et al. also reported that diallyl sulfide induced CYP and phase II enzymes, and decreases hepatic catalase activity [24]. In vivo study on diallyl sulfide showed that cyclophosphamide causes inflammation and dark coloration, whereas allyl sulfide-treated Swiss albino mice showed almost normal bladder morphology [6]. Histopathological analysis also showed that cyclophosphamide-treated group showed severe necrosis in tissues, but sulfur compounds showed normal bladder pathology [6]. Allyl sulfides, including diallyl sulfide, showed an effective action on the phase I and phase II drug-metabolizing enzymes with structure-function relationship [81].

6.2 Antigenotoxic Potential

Data from our group revealed that various compounds including diallyl sulfide possesses chemopreventive potential and minimizes the genotoxicity. The study revealed that these compounds reversed Salmonella typhimurium mutation and in vivo cytogenetic assays. The dietary constituent showed protective effects against Benzo(a) pyrene (BaP)- and cyclophosphamide (CP)-induced cytogenetic damage in mouse bone marrow cells [82]. Diallyl sulfide showed a significant reduction of micronucleus (MN) in human mesothelial cells (HMC) induced by exposing asbestos fibers [83]. Diallyl sulfide enhances phase II enzymes, including quinone reductase

(QR) activity and total and mu glutathione S-transferase activities, and reduces mutagenicity by mutagenicity of (+)-anti-7beta, 8-alpha-dihydroxy-9alpha,10-alpha-oxy-7,8,9,10-trahydrobenzo[a]pyrene (BPDE), and styrene oxide (SO) [84]. Despite these, diallyl sulfide inhibits arylamine *N*-acetyltransferase (NAT) activity and 2-aminofluorene-DNA adduct formation in human promyelocytic leukemia cells (HL-60) in a dose-dependent manner [85]. Diallyl sulfide also studied to protect diethylstilbestrol (DES)-induced DNA damage in normal breast cells, and it is reported as effective to recover cell viability, attenuation of DNA strand breaks, and lowering lipid peroxidation in MCF-10A cells [86].

6.3 Immunostimulation

Oral intake of garlic dose enhances immunomodulation in human health, and daily supplementation increases IL-12 level, which is a potent stimulator of T cell's immune response. In both garlic-treated groups, IL-8 and TNF-α were not significantly different from baseline and placebo levels in urine samples [13]. It was described that garlic oil derivatives differentially suppress the production of nitric oxide (NO) and prostaglandin E-2 (PGE2) in the activated macrophages. The results indicated that these garlic compounds possess a significant effects on the secretion of activated cytokines, such as inflammatory tumor necrosis factor (TNF)-α, interleukin (IL)-1β, and IL-6, and anti-inflammatory (IL-10) [14]. Diallyl sulfide inhibited the production of all stimulated cytokines in a concentration-dependent manner, which was closely associated with the suppression of NO and PGE2 production. DADS repressed the production of stimulated TNF-α and IL-10 as well as increased the production of activated IL-1β and IL-6 [14].

6.4 Antibacterial Activity

Garlic oil has reported for antibacterial activity, and it has been shown that different concentration of garlic oil inhibited the growth of *Staphylococcus aureus*, *Escherichia coli,* and *Bacillus subtilis* [87]. The diallyl sulfide possesses a potent bacteriocidal effect on the growth of *Klebsiella pneumoniae*. It also elicits strong antimicrobial activity against planktonic and sessile *Campylobacter jejuni* and hence application in reducing prevalence of these microbes in foods and biofilm reduction [88]. Diallyl sulfide as well possesses multiple protective functions against methicillin-resistant *Staphylococcus aureus* (MRSA) infection, in which diallyl sulfide could be considered as novel therapeutic agents for the treatment of MRSA infection [88].

6.5 *Anticarcinogenic Effects*

Diallyl sulfide inhibits cancer cell proliferation through multiple mechanisms of action. Allyl compounds are able to decreased level of cyclin-dependent kinase (Cdks)-Cdk7 protein levels, which arrest cell cycle to govern antiproliferative effects [4]. Gene expression analysis showed that diallyl sulfide inhibits arylamine *N*-acetyltransferase (NAT) activity (*N*-acetylation of 2-aminofluorene) in human colon cancer cell lines [28]. From our laboratory, we showed that diallyl sulfide possesses an antitumour activity in polycyclic aromatic hydrocarbon-induced mouse skin carcinogenesis model [56]. Diallyl sulfide also showed anticarcinogenic potential of diethylstilbestrol (DES) induces human cancer [10]. Study showed that diallyl sulfide inhibited DES-induced DNA adduct formation in a dose-dependent manner [10]. DES induces ROS through lipid peroxidation in breast tissue, and diallyl sulfide inhibits the production of ROS, which suggests that diallyl sulfide effectively inhibits DES bioactivation in female ACI rats [29]. Our study also showed that diallyl sulfide inhibits two-stage tumorigenesis in mouse skin tumorigenesis [57]. Guyonnet et al. [89] studied the anticancer effect on *N*-nitrosodiethylamine (NDEA) and phenobarbital-mediated hepatocarcinogenesis in rat. Morris et al. studied the mechanism of allyl sulfides and in vitro metabolism of esophageal carcinogen methyl-*N*-pentylnitrosamine (MPN) [90]. Diallyl sulfide plays a protective effect against NDEA-induced liver carcinogenesis [69].

7 Conclusions

In the contemporary, chronic diseases are the most common disease burden and emerged as a global concern for human health. Diallyl sulfide (organosulfur compound) is one of the dietary phytochemicals and acts as useful for preventing the incidence of chronic diseases, including cancer, diabetes, cardiovascular, and neuronal diseases. The protective effects of diallyl sulfide against chronic disease are due to possessing high antioxidant, antigenotoxic, and antiorganotoxic potential, etc. Studies from the laboratory and elsewhere revealed the mechanism of action of diallyl sulfide against chronic disease. Noticeably, diallyl sulfide has shown as a useful compound with high cancer chemopreventive potential against numerous cancer types. In overall, amalgamating research advancement of diallyl sulfide against chronic diseases has depicted a great significance of diallyl sulfide for human health benefits.

References

1. Reuter HD, Koch HP, Lawson LD (1996) Therapeutic effects and applications of garlic and its preparations. Garlic: the science and therapeutic applications of *Allium sativum* L. and related species. William and Wilkins, Baltimore, pp 135–212
2. Gebreyohannes G, Gebreyohannes M (2013) Medicinal values of garlic: a review. Int J Med Med Sci 5(9):401–408
3. Rao P et al (2015) Diallyl sulfide: potential use in novel therapeutic interventions in alcohol, drugs, and disease mediated cellular toxicity by targeting cytochrome P450 2E1. Curr Drug Metab 16(6):486–503
4. Wu CC et al (2004) Differential effects of allyl sulfides from garlic essential oil on cell cycle regulation in human liver tumor cells. Food Chem Toxicol 42(12):1937–1947
5. Cao HX et al (2014) Garlic-derived allyl sulfides in cancer therapy. Anticancer Agents Med Chem 14(6):793–799
6. Manesh C, Kuttan G (2002) Alleviation of cyclophosphamide-induced urotoxicity by naturally occurring sulphur compounds. J Exp Clin Cancer Res 21(4):509–517
7. Tapiero H, Townsend DM, Tew KD (2004) Organosulfur compounds from alliaceae in the prevention of human pathologies. Biomed Pharmacother 58(3):183–193
8. Wu CC et al (2001) Effects of organosulfur compounds from garlic oil on the antioxidation system in rat liver and red blood cells. Food Chem Toxicol 39(6):563–569
9. Ou CC et al (2003) Protective action on human LDL against oxidation and glycation by four organosulfur compounds derived from garlic. Lipids 38(3):219–224
10. Green M et al (2003) Inhibition of DES-induced DNA adducts by diallyl sulfide: implications in liver cancer prevention. Oncol Rep 10(3):767–771
11. Arora A, Shukla Y (2002) Induction of apoptosis by diallyl sulfide in DMBA-induced mouse skin tumors. Nutr Cancer 44(1):89–94
12. Abdullah TH et al (1988) Garlic revisited: therapeutic for the major diseases of our times? J Natl Med Assoc 80(4):439–445
13. Alma E et al (2014) The effect of garlic powder on human urinary cytokine excretion. Urol J 11(1):1308–1315
14. Chang HP, Huang SY, Chen YH (2005) Modulation of cytokine secretion by garlic oil derivatives is associated with suppressed nitric oxide production in stimulated macrophages. J Agric Food Chem 53(7):2530–2534
15. Fasolino I et al (2015) Orally administered allyl sulfides from garlic ameliorate murine colitis. Mol Nutr Food Res 59(3):434–442
16. Kim NH et al (2014) Protective effects of diallyl sulfide against thioacetamide-induced toxicity: a possible role of cytochrome P450 2E1. Biomol Ther (Seoul) 22(2):149–154
17. Sun Q et al (2015) Roles of CYP2e1 in 1,2-dichloroethane-induced liver damage in mice. Environ Toxicol. doi:10.1002/tox.22148
18. Hu Y et al (2015) In situ solvothermal growth of metal-organic framework-5 supported on porous copper foam for noninvasive sampling of plant volatile sulfides. Anal Chem 87 (1):406–412
19. Dethier B, Nott K, Fauconnier ML (2013) (Bio)synthesis, extraction and purification of garlic derivatives showing therapeutic properties. Commun Agric Appl Biol Sci 78(1):149–155
20. Lancaster JE, Shaw ML, Walton EF (2000) *S*-alk(en)yl-L-cysteine sulfoxides, alliinase and aroma in Leucocoryne. Phytochemistry 55(2):127–130
21. Fenwick GR, Hanley AB (1985) The genus Allium. Part 2. Crit Rev Food Sci Nutr 22(4):273–377
22. Grudzinski IP, Frankiewicz-Jozko A, Bany J (2001) Diallyl sulfide–a flavour component from garlic (*Allium sativum*) attenuates lipid peroxidation in mice infected with *Trichinella spiralis*. Phytomedicine 8(3):174–177

23. Edwards GA, Culp PA, Chalker JM (2015) Allyl sulphides in olefin metathesis: catalyst considerations and traceless promotion of ring-closing metathesis. Chem Commun (Camb) 51 (3):515–518
24. Yang CS et al (2001) Mechanisms of inhibition of chemical toxicity and carcinogenesis by diallyl sulfide (DAS) and related compounds from garlic. J Nutr 131(3s):1041S–1045S
25. Borlinghaus J et al (2014) Allicin: chemistry and biological properties. Molecules 19(8):12591
26. Wang K et al (2013) Liquid sulfur as a reagent: synthesis of polysulfanes with 20 or more sulfur atoms with characterization by UPLC-(Ag+)-coordination ion spray-MS. J Sulfur Chem 34(1–2):55–66
27. Anwar A (2009) Natural polysulfides-reactive sulfur species from Allium with applications in medicine and agriculture. Saarländische Universitäts- und Landesbibliothek, Saarbrücken
28. Chung JG et al (2004) Inhibition of *N*-acetyltransferase activity and gene expression in human colon cancer cell lines by diallyl sulfide. Food Chem Toxicol 42(2):195–202
29. Gued LR, Thomas RD, Green M (2003) Diallyl sulfide inhibits diethylstilbestrol-induced lipid peroxidation in breast tissue of female ACI rats: implications in breast cancer prevention. Oncol Rep 10(3):739–743
30. Singh A, Arora A, Shukla Y (2004) Modulation of altered hepatic foci induction by diallyl sulphide in Wistar rats. Eur J Cancer Prev 13(4):263–269
31. Chiu TH et al (2013) Diallyl sulfide promotes cell-cycle arrest through the p53 expression and triggers induction of apoptosis via caspase- and mitochondria-dependent signaling pathways in human cervical cancer Ca Ski cells. Nutr Cancer 65(3):505–514
32. Knowles LM, Milner JA (2001) Possible mechanism by which allyl sulfides suppress neoplastic cell proliferation. J Nutr 131(3s):1061S–1066S
33. Zilfou JT, Lowe SW (2009) Tumor suppressive functions of p53. Cold Spring Harb Perspect Biol 1(5):a001883
34. Arora A, Siddiqui IA, Shukla Y (2004) Modulation of p53 in 7,12-dimethylbenz[a] anthracene-induced skin tumors by diallyl sulfide in Swiss albino mice. Mol Cancer Ther 3 (11):1459–1466
35. Khan A et al (2007) Potential of diallyl sulfide bearing pH-sensitive liposomes in chemoprevention against DMBA-induced skin papilloma. Mol Med 13(7–8):443–451
36. Gong P, Hu B, Cederbaum AI (2004) Diallyl sulfide induces heme oxygenase-1 through MAPK pathway. Arch Biochem Biophys 432(2):252–260
37. George J et al (2011) Synergistic growth inhibition of mouse skin tumors by pomegranate fruit extract and diallyl sulfide: evidence for inhibition of activated MAPKs/NF-κB and reduced cell proliferation. Food Chem Toxicol 49(7):1511–1520
38. Kalra N, Arora A, Shukla Y (2006) Involvement of multiple signaling pathways in diallyl sulfide mediated apoptosis in mouse skin tumors. Asian Pac J Cancer Prev 7(4):556–562
39. Khatuaa TN et al (2015) Diallyl disulfide ameliorates isoproterenol induced cardiac hypertrophy activating mitochondrial biogenesis via eNOS-Nrf2-Tfam pathway in rats. Biochem Biophys Rep 5:77–88
40. Ho CY et al (2014) Diallyl sulfide as a potential dietary agent to reduce TNF-α-and histamine-induced proinflammatory responses in A7r5 cells. Mol Nutr Food Res 58(5):1069–1078
41. Lee HS et al (2009) Inhibition of cyclooxygenase 2 expression by diallyl sulfide on joint inflammation induced by urate crystal and IL-1beta. Osteoarthritis Cartilage 17(1):91–99
42. Kalayarasan S, Sriram N, Sudhandiran G (2008) Diallyl sulfide attenuates bleomycin-induced pulmonary fibrosis: critical role of iNOS, NF-κB, TNF-α and IL-1β. Life Sci 82(23–24):1142–1153
43. Ho CY et al (2015) Protective effects of diallyl sulfide on ovalbumin-induced pulmonary inflammation of allergic asthma mice by microRNA-144, -34a and -34b/c-modulated Nrf2 activation. J Agric Food Chem 64(1):151–160
44. Cao Y et al (2015) Inhibition of pulmonary nuclear factor -KappaB and tumor necrosis factor -alpha expression by diallyl sulfide in rats with paraquat poisoning. Zhonghua Wei Zhong Bing Ji Jiu Yi Xue 27(4):274–279

45. Fu E et al (2015) The effects of diallyl sulfide upon Porphyromonas gingivalis lipopolysaccharide stimulated proinflammatory cytokine expressions and nuclear factor-kappa B activation in human gingival fibroblasts. J Periodontal Res 50(3):380–388
46. Lin X et al (2012) Neuroprotective effects of diallyl sulfide against transient focal cerebral ischemia via anti-apoptosis in rats. Neurol Res 34(1):32–37
47. Viaggi C et al (2006) Cytochrome P450 and Parkinson's disease: protective role of neuronal CYP 2E1 from MPTP toxicity. J Neural Transm Suppl 70:173–176
48. Karmakar S et al (2007) Garlic compounds induced calpain and intrinsic caspase cascade for apoptosis in human malignant neuroblastoma SH-SY5Y cells. Apoptosis 12(4):671–684
49. Saldana-Ruiz S et al (2013) Reduced systemic toxicity and preserved vestibular toxicity following co-treatment with nitriles and CYP2E1 inhibitors: a mouse model for hair cell loss. J Assoc Res Otolaryngol 14(5):661–671
50. Valencia-Olvera AC et al (2014) CYP2E1 induction leads to oxidative stress and cytotoxicity in glutathione-depleted cerebellar granule neurons. Toxicol In Vitro 28(7):1206–1214
51. Huentelman MJ et al (1999) Ethanol has differential effects on rat neuron and thymocyte reactive oxygen species levels and cell viability. Comp Biochem Physiol C Pharmacol Toxicol Endocrinol 124(1):83–89
52. Arora A, Seth K, Shukla Y (2004) Reversal of *P*-glycoprotein-mediated multidrug resistance by diallyl sulfide in K562 leukemic cells and in mouse liver. Carcinogenesis 25(6):941–949
53. Shukla Y, Arora A, Singh A (2002) Antitumorigenic potential of diallyl sulfide in Ehrlich ascites tumor bearing mice. Biomed Environ Sci 15(1):41–47
54. Fukushima S et al (1997) Cancer prevention by organosulfur compounds from garlic and onion. J Cell Biochem Suppl 27:100–105
55. Pinto JT, Rivlin RS (2001) Antiproliferative effects of allium derivatives from garlic. J Nutr 131(3s):1058S–1060S
56. Singh A, Shukla Y (1998) Antitumour activity of diallyl sulfide on polycyclic aromatic hydrocarbon-induced mouse skin carcinogenesis. Cancer Lett 131(2):209–214
57. Singh A, Shukla Y (1998) Antitumor activity of diallyl sulfide in two-stage mouse skin model of carcinogenesis. Biomed Environ Sci 11(3):258–263
58. Kalayarasan S et al (2013) Diallylsulfide attenuates excessive collagen production and apoptosis in a rat model of bleomycin induced pulmonary fibrosis through the involvement of protease activated receptor-2. Toxicol Appl Pharmacol 271(2):184–195
59. Hong YS et al (2000) Effects of allyl sulfur compounds and garlic extract on the expression of Bcl-2, Bax, and p53 in non small cell lung cancer cell lines. Exp Mol Med 32(3):127–134
60. Huang CN, Horng JS, Yin MC (2004) Antioxidative and antiglycative effects of six organosulfur compounds in low-density lipoprotein and plasma. J Agric Food Chem 52 (11):3674–3678
61. Hsieh YL et al (2014) Effects of garlic oil on interleukin-6 mediated cardiac hypertrophy in hypercholesterol-fed hamsters. Chin J Physiol 57(6):320–328
62. Bordia A, Verma SK, Srivastava KC (1996) Effect of garlic on platelet aggregation in humans: a study in healthy subjects and patients with coronary artery disease. Prostaglandins Leukot Essent Fatty Acids 55(3):201–205
63. Mamas M et al (2011) The role of metabolites and metabolomics in clinically applicable biomarkers of disease. Arch Toxicol 85(1):5–17
64. Ho CY et al (2012) Effect of diallyl sulfide on in vitro and in vivo Nrf2-mediated pulmonic antioxidant enzyme expression via activation ERK/p38 signaling pathway. J Agric Food Chem 60(1):100–107
65. Blackler RW et al (2015) Hydrogen sulphide protects against NSAID-enteropathy through modulation of bile and the microbiota. Br J Pharmacol 172(4):992–1004
66. Ansar S, Iqbal M, AlJameil N (2014) Diallyl sulphide, a component of garlic, abrogates ferric nitrilotriacetate-induced oxidative stress and renal damage in rats. Hum Exp Toxicol 33 (12):1209–1216
67. Abdel-Daim MM, Abdou RH (2015) Protective effects of diallyl sulfide and curcumin separately against thallium-induced toxicity in rats. Cell J 17(2):379–388

68. Battal M et al (2015) Impact of allyl disulfide on oxidative damage and liver regeneration in an experimental hepatectomy model. Chirurgia (Bucur) 110(2):117–122
69. Ibrahim SS, Nassar NN (2008) Diallyl sulfide protects against *N*-nitrosodiethylamine-induced liver tumorigenesis: role of aldose reductase. World J Gastroenterol 14(40):6145–6153
70. Chen GW et al (1999) Effects of the garlic compounds diallyl sulphide and diallyl disulphide on arylamine *N*-acetyltransferase activity in Klebsiella pneumoniae. J Appl Toxicol 19(2):75–81
71. Sheen LY et al (2001) Effect of diallyl sulfide and diallyl disulfide, the active principles of garlic, on the aflatoxin B(1)-induced DNA damage in primary rat hepatocytes. Toxicol Lett 122(1):45–52
72. Wargovich MJ (2006) Diallylsulfide and allylmethylsulfide are uniquely effective among organosulfur compounds in inhibiting CYP2E1 protein in animal models. J Nutr 136(3 Suppl):832S–834S
73. Abdel-Hamid NM, Nazmy MH, Abdel-Bakey AI (2011) Polyol profile as an early diagnostic and prognostic marker in natural product chemoprevention of hepatocellular carcinoma in diabetic rats. Diabetes Res Clin Pract 92(2):228–237
74. Lorenzi M (2007) The polyol pathway as a mechanism for diabetic retinopathy: attractive, elusive, and resilient. Exp Diabetes Res 2007:61038
75. Arora A, Kalra N, Shukla Y (2006) Regulation of p21/ras protein expression by diallyl sulfide in DMBA induced neoplastic changes in mouse skin. Cancer Lett 242(1):28–36
76. Nylen K et al (2006) A ketogenic diet and diallyl sulfide do not elevate afterdischarge thresholds in adult kindled rats. Epilepsy Res 71(1):23–31
77. Shaik IH et al (2008) Protective effects of diallyl sulfide, a garlic constituent, on the warm hepatic ischemia-reperfusion injury in a rat model. Pharm Res 25(10):2231–2242
78. Maroof A, Farazuddin M, Owais M (2010) Potential use of liposomal diallyl sulfide in the treatment of experimental murine candidiasis. Biosci Rep 30(4):223–231
79. Pedraza-Chaverri J et al (2003) Protective effect of diallyl sulfide on oxidative stress and nephrotoxicity induced by gentamicin in rats. Mol Cell Biochem 254(1–2):125–130
80. Taubert D et al (2006) The garlic ingredient diallyl sulfide inhibits cytochrome P450 2E1 dependent bioactivation of acrylamide to glycidamide. Toxicol Lett 164(1):1–5
81. Fukao T et al (2004) The effects of allyl sulfides on the induction of phase II detoxification enzymes and liver injury by carbon tetrachloride. Food Chem Toxicol 42(5):743–749
82. Shukla Y, Arora A, Taneja P (2003) Antigenotoxic potential of certain dietary constituents. Teratog Carcinog Mutagen 23(Suppl 1):323–335
83. Lohani M et al (2003) Diallylsulfide attenuates asbestos-induced genotoxicity. Toxicol Lett 143(1):45–50
84. Guyonnet D et al (2001) Antimutagenic activity of organosulfur compounds from Allium is associated with phase II enzyme induction. Mutat Res 495(1–2):135–145
85. Lin JG et al (2002) Effects of garlic components diallyl sulfide and diallyl disulfide on arylamine *N*-acetyltransferase activity and 2-aminofluorene-DNA adducts in human promyelocytic leukemia cells. Am J Chin Med 30(2–3):315–325
86. McCaskill ML, Rogan E, Thomas RD (2014) Diallyl sulfide inhibits diethylstilbestrol induced DNA damage in human breast epithelial cells (MCF-10A). Steroids 92:96–100
87. Guo Y (2014) Experimental study on the optimization of extraction process of garlic oil and its antibacterial effects. Afr J Tradit Complement Altern Med 11(2):411–414
88. Tsao SM, Hsu CC, Yin MC (2003) Garlic extract and two diallyl sulphides inhibit methicillin-resistant *Staphylococcus aureus* infection in BALB/cA mice. J Antimicrob Chemother 52(6):974–980
89. Guyonnet D et al (2004) Post-initiation modulating effects of allyl sulfides in rat hepatocarcinogenesis. Food Chem Toxicol 42(9):1479–1485
90. Morris CR et al (2004) Inhibition by allyl sulfides and phenethyl isothiocyanate of methyl-n-pentylnitrosamine depentylation by rat esophageal microsomes, human and rat CYP2E1, and Rat CYP2A3. Nutr Cancer 48(1):54–63

91. Sai-Kato K et al (1995) Pentachlorophenol-induced oxidative DNA damage in mouse liver and protective effect of antioxidants. Food Chem Toxicol 33(10):877–882
92. Fanelli SL et al (1998) Mechanisms of the preventive properties of some garlic components in the carbon tetrachloride-promoted oxidative stress. Diallyl sulfide; diallyl disulfide; allyl mercaptan and allyl methyl sulfide. Res Commun Mol Pathol Pharmacol 102(2):163–174
93. Tsao S, Yin M (2001) In vitro activity of garlic oil and four diallyl sulphides against antibiotic-resistant *Pseudomonas aeruginosa* and *Klebsiella pneumoniae*. J Antimicrob Chemother 47(5):665–670
94. Marks HS, Anderson JL, Stoewsand GS (1992) Inhibition of benzo[a]pyrene-induced bone marrow micronuclei formation by diallyl thioethers in mice. J Toxicol Environ Health 37 (1):1–9
95. Lewis RJ (2001) Hawley's condensed chemical dictionary, 14th edn. Wiley & Sons, Inc., New York, p 38
96. O'Neil MJ (2001) The Merck index—an encyclopedia of chemicals, drugs, and biologicals, 13th edn. Merck and Co., Inc, Whitehouse Station, p 55
97. Lide DR, Milne GWA (eds) (1994) Handbook of data on organic compounds, 3rd edn, vol 5. CRC Press, Inc. Boca Raton, p 4531
98. Perry RH, Green D (1984) Perry's chemical handbook. Physical and chemical data, 6th edn. McGraw-Hill, NY

Lupeol and Its Role in Chronic Diseases

Fan-Shiu Tsai, Li-Wei Lin and Chi-Rei Wu

Abstract Lupeol belongs to pentacyclic lupane-type triterpenes and exhibits in edible vegetables, fruits and many plants. Many researches indicated that lupeol possesses many beneficial pharmacological activities including antioxidant, anti-inflammatory, anti-hyperglycemic, anti-dyslipidemic and anti-mutagenic effects. From various disease-targeted animal models, these reports indicated that lupeol has anti-diabetic, anti-asthma, anti-arthritic, cardioprotective, hepatoprotective, nephroprotective, neuroprotective and anticancer efficiency under various routes of administration such as topical, oral, subcutaneous, intraperitoneal and intravenous. It is worth mentioning that clinical trials of lupeol were performed to treat canine oral malignant melanoma and human moderate skin acne in Japan and Korea. The detailed mechanism of anti-inflammatory, anti-diabetic, hepatoprotective and anticancer activities was further reviewed from published papers. These evidence indicate that lupeol is a multi-target agent to exert diverse pharmacological potency with many potential targeting proteins such as α-glucosidase, α-amylase, protein tyrosine phosphatase 1B (PTP 1B) and TCA cycle enzymes and targeting pathway such as IL-1 receptor-associated kinase-mediated toll-like receptor 4 (IRAK-TLR4), Bcl-2 family, nuclear factor kappa B (NF-kB), phosphatidylinositol-3-kinase (PI3-K)/Akt and Wnt/β-catenin signaling pathways. This review also provides suggestion that lupeol might be a valuable and potential lead compound to develop as anti-inflammatory, anti-diabetic, hepatoprotective and anticancer drugs.

Keywords Lupeol · Triterpene · Anti-inflammatory · Anti-diabetic · Anticancer · Hepatoprotective · Cardioprotective · Nephroprotective

---

Fan-Shiu Tsai and Li-Wei Lin have equally contributed.

F.-S. Tsai · L.-W. Lin
School of Chinese Medicines for Post-Baccalaureate, I-Shou University, Kaohsiung 82445, Taiwan

C.-R. Wu (✉)
Department of Chinese Pharmaceutical Sciences and Chinese Medicine Resources, China Medical University, Taichung 40402, Taiwan
e-mail: crw@cmu.edu.tw

S.C. Gupta et al. (eds.), *Drug Discovery from Mother Nature*,
Advances in Experimental Medicine and Biology 929,
DOI 10.1007/978-3-319-41342-6_7

1 Introduction

Chronic diseases such as heart disease, stroke, cancer, liver disease, chronic respiratory diseases and diabetes comprise the leading cause of mortality in the world [101]. World Health Organization reports chronic non-communicable diseases to be by far the leading cause of mortality in the world, representing 35-million deaths in 2005 and over 60 % of all deaths. These diseases might be prevented by behavioral changes such as sport, using a healthy diet and keeping good living habit [139]. Triterpenes are natural components which are largely derived from vegetable oils, cereals and fruits. There are very large amounts of published data suggesting the effects of triterpenes for the treatment of many disease conditions [2, 74].

Lupeol (the structure shown in Fig. 1), also called as clerodol, farganasterol, fagarasterol, lupeol and monogynol B, belongs to one of the pentacyclic lupane-type triterpene compounds. Lupeol exists in many edible vegetables and fruits such as aloe plants, bitter root, black tea, carrot root, cucumber, date palm, figs, guava, ivy gourd, tomato, mango pulp, melon seeds, mulberries, pea, soy bean, strawberries red grapes, quebracho bark, uva ursi and white cabbage, pepper [26]. From quantitative analysis by high-performance liquid chromatography or gas chromatography, there are wide range of lupeol contents in microgram per gram of the above edible vegetables and fruits such as mango fruit (1.80 μg/g pulp), olive fruit (3 μg/g), ginseng oil (152 μg/g oil), Japanese pear (175 μg/g twig bark), aloe leaf (280 μg/g dry leaf) and elm plant (800 μg/g bark) [16, 45]. Lupeol has been also reported to be present in diverse species of plant families [21], but rare in fungal and animal kingdom (except for propolis) [46, 47, 99, 132, 141]. Lupeol is a principal active constituent of some medicinal herbs especially plants of Euphorbiaceae, Fabaceae and Rutaceae, [102, 113]. In Euphorbiaceae plants, *Emblica officinalis* is widely used in ayurvedic description and has anti-microbial, anti-inflammatory and antioxidant properties [35, 53, 145]. *Aegle marmelos* and *Zanthoxylum riedelianum* are two well-known lupeol-rich Rutaceae plants. *A. marmelos* is often used to treat chronic diarrhea and peptic ulcers in Indian, and

Fig. 1 Structure of lupeol

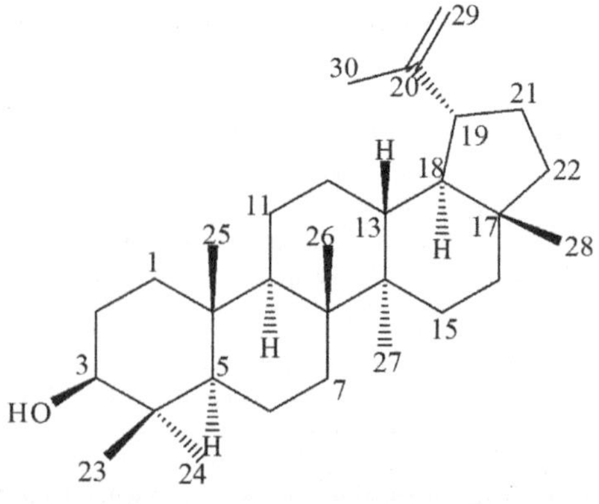

recent reports indicated that it possessed broad range of therapeutic effects such as anti-diabetic, anti-bacterial, anti-diarrheal, antioxidant, anti-viral, cardioprotective, gastroprotective, hepatoprotective and radioprotective effects [14, 31]. *Z. riedelianum* is mainly employed to relief tooth pain in Brazilian and possessed the anti-inflammatory and analgesic activity [60]. *Cajanus cajan, Cassia fistula, Glycine max, Glycyrrhiza glabra, Pisum sativum* and *Tamarindus indica* are the most frequently reported Fabaceae plants contain lupeol. Three Apocynaceae plants —*Aspidosperma nitidum, Hemidesmus indicus* and *Himatanthus sucuuba*—are used to treat reproductive tract inflammation, rheumatic arthritis, fever and malaria in the Amazon region. *Allanblackia monticola* (Guttiferae), *Bombax ceiba* (Malvaceae), *Careya arborea* (Barringtoniaceae), *Crataeva nurvala* (Capparidaceae), *Echinops echinatus* (Asteraceae) and *Leptadenia hastata* (Asclepiadaceae) are used in ayuverdic or other alterative therapy to treat reproductive system disorders, urolithiasis, tumors as well as an antidote to snake venom.

Triterpenes including lupeol are generally considered as secondary metabolites of plants to interrelate with their environment especially infection or external damage [18]. Many scientists have indicated that complete biosynthetic pathway of lupeol is considered as one of the most complex reactions occurring in nature and is orchestrated by triterpene synthases [89, 135]. The basic biosynthetic pathway of lupeol is quite well comprehended because lupeol is comprised of five, six-membered rings (ursanes and lanostanes) or four, six-membered rings and one, five-membered ring (lupanes and hopanes). Lupeol biosynthesis occurs in the cytosol and constitutes mevalonate (MVA) pathway, where a five-carbon unit isopentenyl pyrophosphate (IPP) and its allyl isomer dimethylallyl pyrophosphate (DMAPP) are formed from acetyl-CoA and sequentially catalyzed by farnesyl pyrophosphate synthase (FPS) to farnesyl pyrophosphate (FPP). Next, this precursor FPP is polymerized into squalene by squalene synthase (SQS). Squalene epoxidase (SQE) oxidizes squalene to 2, 3-oxidosqualene. Then, the last intermediate 2, 3-oxidosqualene is cyclized in a chair–chair–chair conformation by a member of the oxidosqualene cyclases family (OSCs) such as lupeol synthases (LUS) to form lupenyl cation through successive electrophilic additions, rearrangement and ring expansion. Finally, lupenyl cation is converted into lupeol by deprotonation of 29-methyl group (Fig. 2) [89, 135].

2 Physio-chemical Properties of Lupeol

The IUPAC name of lupeol is (1R,3aR,5aR,5bR,7aR,9S,11aR,11bR,13aR,13bR)-3a,5a,5b,8,8,11a-hexamethyl-1-prop-1-en-2-yl-1,2,3,4,5,6,7,7a,9,10,11,11b,12,13,13a,13b-hexadecahydrocyclopenta[a]chrysen-9-ol. Its chemical formula is $C_{30}H_{50}O$, and HPLC–MS studies show that the exact mass is 426.386 and a parent ion peak of olefinic moiety is identified at m/z 409 $(M + H - 18)^{(+)}$ [11, 102]. Lupeol, needle form recrystallized from alcohol or acetone, is very soluble in ethanol, acetone and chloroform, but is insoluble in dilute acid and alkalis. The

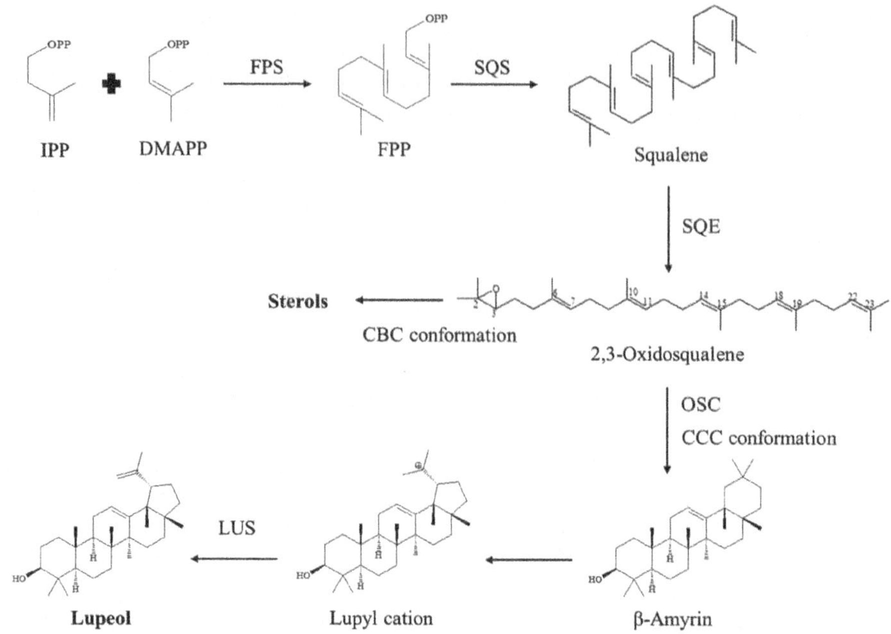

Fig. 2 Schematic representation of the critical steps of biosynthesis of lupeol in plants; *DMAPP* dimethylallyl pyrophosphate; *IPP* isopentenyl pyrophosphate; *FPS* farnesyl diphosphate synthase; *FPP* farnesyl pyrophosphate; *SQE* squalene epoxidase; *OSC* oxidosqualene cyclase; *LUS* lupeol synthase. Other abbreviations: *CBC* chair–boat–chair; *CCC* chair–chair–chair

melting point of lupeol is 212–216 °C, and the density is 0.9457 g/cm^3. The specific optical rotation of lupeol is +26.2° at 25 °C [29].

Because lupeol belongs to pentacyclic lupane-type triterpene, its olefinic moiety can be identified by infrared spectrum and NMR spectrum. The infrared spectrum of lupeol shows the presence of an olefinic moiety and a hydroxyl group at a spectrum of 1639 and 3326 cm^{-1} [102]. The ^{1}H and ^{13}C NMR spectrum of lupeol shows the typical signals of a pentacyclic lupane-type triterpene with olefinic protons/carbons at 4.69 and 4.57 (brs, H-29)/109.3 and 151.0 (C-29 and 20, respectively), the hydroxymethine proton/carbon at 3.19 (dd, 4.8 and 11.6 Hz, H-3)/79.0 (C-3) and seven singlet signals assigned to the tertiary methyl groups at 0.77, 0.80, 0.84, 0.95, 0.97, 1.03, 1.20/28.4, 15.8, 16.5, 16.3, 14.9, 18.9, 19.7 (H/C-23–28 and 30, respectively) [11, 29]. On the other hand, the crystal structure of lupeol was elucidated on the basis of X-ray diffraction analysis with the space group $P4_3$ and the stereochemistry specified by biosynthesis [22].

Due to the lower solubility of lupeol, its absorption and bioavailability are widely questioned. Siddique et al. [112] reported that serum lupeol levels were only 3.08 and 5.22 μM at 4 and 8 h after single treatment of lupeol (200 mg/kg) in mice. If treatment with lupeol (40 mg/kg) for 8-week, serum lupeol levels were only 10 and 20 μM at 4 week and 8 week administration, respectively. Fortunately, lupeol has a valuable bioactive lupane-type skeleton which not only possesses a high number of natural stereogenic centers, but also can be easily functionalized at two positions C-3 and C-20. Thus, some derivatives of lupeol were isolated from natural plants or synthesized to be as prodrugs improving the water solubility, absorption, distribution, metabolism, excretion (ADME), bioavailability and potency of lupeol. Firstly, lupeol esters such as acetate, palmitate, cinnamate, succinate or linoleate at C-3 position are usually found to be accompanied with lupeol in natural plants [5, 19, 20, 29, 30, 65, 78, 91, 136]. These natural derivatives especially lupeol linoleate were observed to exhibit more pharmacological efficacy than lupeol in the anti-inflammatory, anti-oxidative, anti-urolithic, cardioprotective hepatoprotective and nephroprotective effects [33, 119–124, 127, 130]. Lupeol acetate was found to exhibit inhibitory effect on melanoma cell growth [39]. In addition, C-3 esterification of lupeol by long-chain alkanoic acid or fatty acid also possessed more anti-fungal, anti-bacterial and anti-malarial activities than lupeol [29, 30, 91]. In fact, some researchers have demonstrated that esterification of triterpenes enhanced the efficiency of parent drug by increasing its penetration and retention ability into the cell membrane and improving the oral bioavailability [78, 83]. Besides, further C-3 esterification of lupeol was carried out by subjecting various aromatic and aliphatic acids. Reddy et al. [86] found that lupeol esters by adding nicotinic acid or 2 (pyridin-2-yl) acetic acid to C-3 position possessed the better anti-hyperglycemic and anti-dyslipidemic activity. However, adding aliphatic groups leads to the loss of anti-hyperglycemic activity of lupeol [50]. Srivastava et al. [117] also indicated that lupeol-derived chalcones by adding NO_2-substitued or halogen-substituted chalcones to C-2 and C-3 positions of lupeol possessed more anti-dyslipidemic and antioxidant activities. The addition of alkyl- and halogen-substituted indole to C-2 and C-3 positions of lupeol enhanced the inhibitory effect on TNF-α release [17]. The dicarboxyl group such as succinyl substitution at C-3 position helps to strengthen anti-tumor activities of lupeol [59]. For modification at the other functional position C-20, the terminal double bond between C-20 and C-30 in lupeol is very necessary in its anticancer activities [59] and the insertion of α,β-unsaturated carbonyl carbon between C-20 and C-30 in lupeol increases the potency of glucose uptake stimulation [50].

3 Modulation of Cell Signaling Pathways by Lupeol

3.1 Cell Signaling Pathways of Anti-inflammatory Mechanism

Lupeol, a major constituent of *Pimenta racemosa* var. ozua (Myrtaceae), reduced the inflammation in 12-o-tetradecanoylphorbol acetate (TPA)-treated mice through the reduction in myeloperoxidase (MPO) activity [27] and it also reduced prostaglandin E_2 (PGE_2) and cytokines (tumor necrosis factor (TNF)-α and interleukin (IL)-1β) production in A23187-stimulated or lipopolysaccharide (LPS)-treated

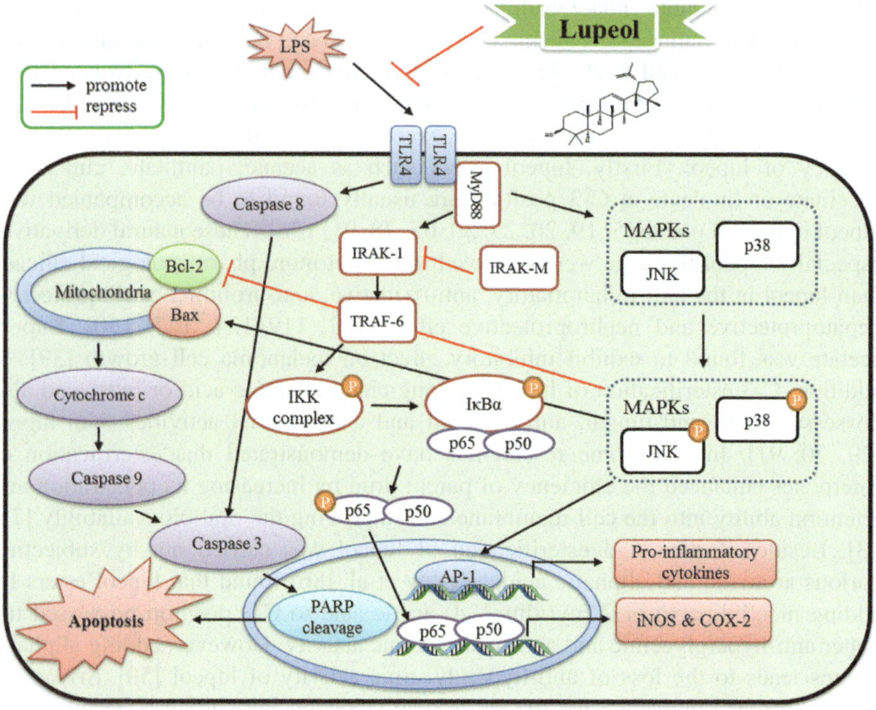

Fig. 3 Flowchart represents the anti-inflammatory mechanism of action of lupeol

macrophages [28]. The anti-inflammatory effect of lupeol probably relates to the opioid system, as indicated by complete blockade of opioid antagonist naloxone. In addition, lupeol reduced the number of inducible nitric oxide synthase (iNOS) cells and its anti-inflammatory effect was potentiated by TNF-α inhibitor pentoxifylline (PTX), indicating the participation of pro-inflammatory cytokines (such as TNF-α and IL-1β) and nitric oxide (NO) system [65]. However, lupeol was unable to inhibit the matrix metalloproteinase (MMP)-9 and cyclooxygenase (COX)-2 expression increased by phorbol 12-myristate 13-acetate (PMA) in cells [9]. Therefore, published studies provided evidence that the anti-inflammatory efficacy of lupeol may be mediated to modulate the expression or activity of pro-inflammatory cytokines IL-2, IL-4, IL-5, IL-β, TNF-α via nuclear factor kappa B (NF-kB) pathway (Fig. 3) [128].

3.2 *Cell Signaling Pathways of Hepatoprotective Effects*

Acetaminophen induces hepatotoxicity results in formation of the reactive oxygen species (ROS) and modulation of antioxidant status including glutathione

(GSH) depletion triggering the pathway of cell death. Acetaminophen downregulates Bcl-2 and upregulates Bax level in hepatocytes and simultaneously promotes binding of the pro-apoptotic protein Bax with the outer mitochondrial membrane involving oxidant/antioxidant imbalance and causes mitochondrial permeability transition. It enables the loss of mitochondrial membrane potential and release of cytochrome c from intermembrane compartment to cytosol. Further, activation of caspase-9/3 initiates self-digestion of cells and nuclear DNA fragmentation, eventually leading to cell death. Lupeol was found to effectively inhibit the key steps in this mechanism of cell death and provide protection against acetaminophen-mediated hepatotoxicity in vitro [54, 55]. In 7,12-dimethylbenz(a)anthracene (DMBA)-treated mice, down-regulation of anti-apoptotic Bcl-2 and upregulation of pro-apoptotic Bax and caspase 3 in liver were observed. These alterations were restored by lupeol, indicating inhibition of apoptosis [93]. Lupeol also improved survival rate and alleviation of liver injury induced by D-galactosamine (GalN) and lipopolysaccharide (LPS) through inhibition of IL-1 receptor-associated kinase (IRAK)-mediated toll-like receptor (TLR)4 signaling pathway, which may inhibit the expression of inflammatory cytokines [52]. Thus, the hepatoprotective mechanism of lupeol might be combined with upregulation of anti-apoptotic Bcl-2, downregulation of pro-apoptotic Bax and inhibition of the IRAK-mediated TLR4 signaling pathway via its antioxidant and anti-inflammatory activities.

3.3 *Cell Signaling Pathways of Anticancer Effects*

1. **Melanoma cell**

From 2000 to 2015, there were thirteen reports demonstrated that the anticancer effects of lupeol in melanoma cells and tumors mainly contained four levels: cell cycle arrest, apoptosis induction, survival inhibition and differentiation induction. Lupeol caused cell cycle arrest in G1–S phase in human metastatic 451Lu and non-metastatic WM35 melanoma cells by decreasing the expression level of cyclin-dependent kinase (cdk)-2 and cyclin D1 to modulate cyclin D1/cdk2/p21 complex. Lupeol also induced apoptosis in 451Lu and WM35 melanoma cells via downregulation of Bcl-2 and upregulation of Bax, following the activation of caspase-3 and the induction of poly(ADP-ribose)polymerase (PARP) cleavage [107]. Mitogen-activated protein kinase (MAPK) cascade including extracellular signal-regulated kinase (ERK) 1/2, p38 kinase and c-Jun N-terminal protein kinases (JNK) was demonstrated to be involved in the cell survival, proliferation and differentiation. Lupeol induced morphological differentiation (rearrangement of the actin cytoskeleton and dendrite formations) through inhibition of Rho signaling on short-term (8 h) treatment in B16 2F2 cell, and functional differentiation (activation of tyrosinase and melanogenesis) through activation of p38 signaling via cAMP-PKA pathway on long-term (48 h) exposure [39, 40, 82]. Wnt/β-catenin signaling pathway is known to play an important role in surviving, proliferating, and acquiring highly aggressive characteristics of various malignancies including melanoma, colorectal and prostate cancer because the translocation of β-catenin–TCF-4 complex to nucleus leads to transcriptional activation of target genes such as c-myc, MMP-2 and cyclin D1. Lupeol decreased the growth of Mel 928 cell with constitutive activation of Wnt/β-catenin signaling pathway via the restriction in the translocation of β-catenin from the cytoplasm to the nucleus and sequence the decrease in the expression of Wnt target genes c-myc and cyclin D1. Furthermore, they also found that lupeol decreased the ratios of MMP-9/TIMP1 and MMP-2/TIMP2 to regulate the angiogenesis [134]. In addition, lupeol inhibited DMBA-induced alterations on skin cell proliferation via G2/M-phase cell cycle arrest (induction in p21/WAF1 expression and inhibition in cyclin B1/cdc25C/cdc2 activation) and induction of mitochondria-mediated apoptosis (downregulation in Bcl-2 and survivin expression, and upregulation in Bax and caspase-3 expression) in mouse. Thus, the anticancer mechanism of lupeol on melanoma included cell cycle arrest via increasing p53 expression to induce p21 expression and inhibit cyclins/cdc2 activation, cell apoptosis via activating mitochondria-mediated apoptosis pathway and modulating Wnt/β-catenin signaling pathway, and cell differentiation via activating cAMP-PKA-p38 pathway (Fig. 4).

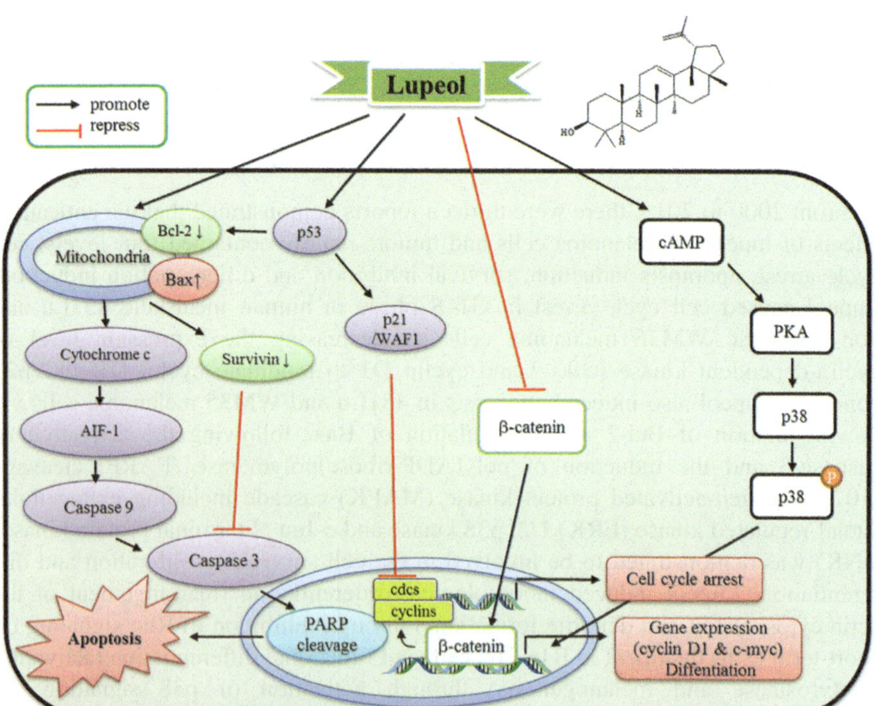

Fig. 4 Flowchart represents the anticancer mechanism of lupeol in melanoma

2. Prostate cancer

Published studies provide evidence that lupeol may have a potential to be an effective agent against prostate cancer. The serial studies of Saleem et al. [106, 108, 109] indicated lupeol in a dose-dependent manner activated the Fas receptor-mediated apoptotic pathway (including the initiator caspases (caspases-8 and caspase-9) activation, PARP cleavage and FADD protein expression) in androgen-sensitive prostate cancer LNCaP and CWR22Rυ1 cells. Lupeol also inhibited cell proliferation through decreasing the stabilized β-catenin by restoring the levels of active glycogen synthase kinase (GSK)-3β–axin protein complex to inhibit the transcription of proliferation-associated genes in prostate cancer LNCaP and DU145 cells. Lupeol further induced G2/M cell cycle arrest through decreasing the levels of cyclins and cdk-2, and disrupted microtubule assembly via decreasing the levels of microtubule regulatory proteins such as stathmin and survivin in prostate cancer LNCaP and DU145 cells. Thus, lupeol is suggested as an androgen receptor inhibitor, microtubule targeting agent and potent inhibitor of β-catenin signaling pathway to have numerous beneficial effects against the development, growth and progression of early (androgen dependent) as well as advanced stage (androgen independent) of prostate cancer in humans (Fig. 5).

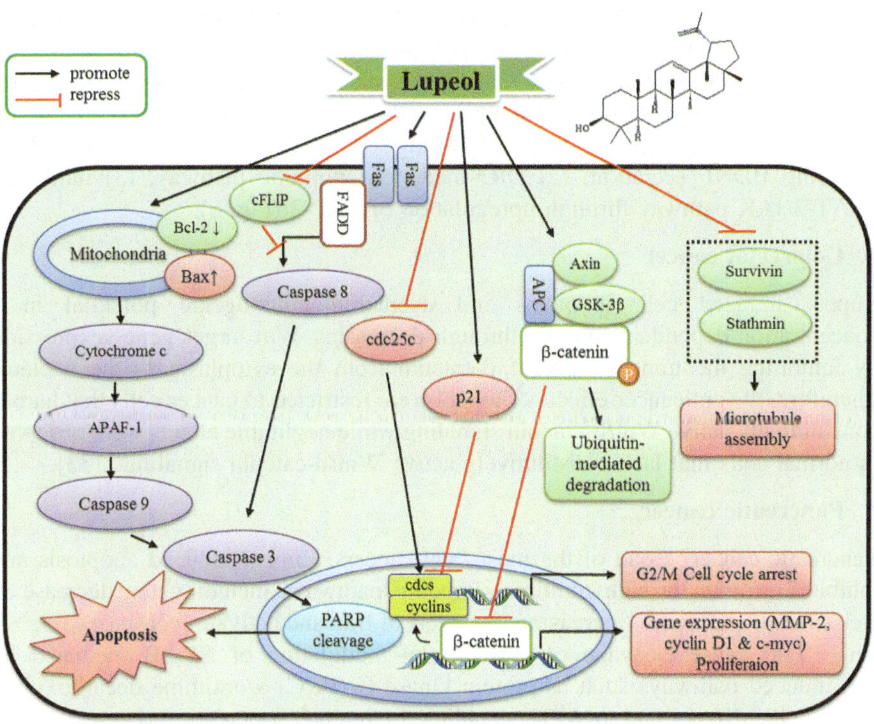

Fig. 5 Flowchart represents the anticancer mechanism of lupeol in prostate cancer

3. **Hepatocellular carcinoma**

Hepatocellular carcinoma (HCC) is the most common liver malignant tumor and primarily develops from chronic infections caused by hepatitis B and hepatitis C viruses, alcoholic injury. Lupeol induced apoptosis in HCC SMMC7721 cells by downregulation of death receptor 3 (DR3)-mediated apoptotic pathway to cause caspase-3 activation and PARP cleavage, but not by Fas-mediated apoptotic pathway [42, 149]. Siveen et al. [114] found that lupeol can negatively regulate signal transducer and activator of transcription signaling 3 (STAT3) activation through the suppression of upstream kinases (c-Src, JAK1 and JAK2) and induction of protein tyrosine phosphatase SHP-2 to exert its anticancer potency in HCC cell lines. They further indicated that lupeol induced apoptosis and cell cycle accumulation at sub-G1 phase via downregulation of the expression of Bcl-2, Bcl-xL and survivin, processing of caspase-8 and caspase-9, activation of caspase-3 and cleavage of PARP. Brain-derived neurotrophic factor (BDNF) has been confirmed to induce cell invasion via binding tropomysin-related kinase B (TrkB) and trigger downstream signaling molecules such as phosphatidyl inositol 3-kinase (PI3-K)/Akt, which regulates cell survival, cell cycle progression and apoptosis. Lupeol induced cell death and suppressed proliferation, which associated with a marked decrease in the protein expression of BDNF and GSK-3β, with concomitant suppression of PI3-K/Akt1, β-catenin, c-myc and cyclin D1 mRNA expression in HCC cells. Lupeol also inhibits LiCl-induced activation of Wnt/β-catenin signaling pathway via activating GSK-3β and exerts anti-invasive activity in Huh-7cells [148]. These results demonstrate that lupeol can inhibit tumor progress by (1) reversing the dysregulation of GSK-3β protein and suppressing Wnt/β-catenin signaling pathway, which is mediated through PI3-K/Akt inactivation caused by declining BDNF secretion; (2) DR3-mediated apoptotic pathway, (3) inhibiting STAT-3/JAK pathway through upregulation of SHP-2 (Fig. 6).

4. **Colorectal cancer**

Lupeol induced cell apoptosis and decreased colonogenic potential in a concentration-dependent manner through decreasing Wnt target genes expression by inhibiting the translocation of β-catenin from the cytoplasm to the nucleus. Therefore, the anticancer effects of lupeol were restricted to cancer cells that harbor constitutively active Wnt/β-catenin signaling while negligible effects were observed in normal cells that lack constitutively active Wnt/β-catenin signaling [133].

5. **Pancreatic cancer**

Pancreatic cancer is one of the most fatal cancers. Lupeol induced apoptosis and inhibited growth through multiple signaling pathways including the decrease in Bcl-2 family pathways (increasing the levels of Bax and activating caspases −3, −8, and −9 to cause cleavage of PARP), the modulation of NF-kB mediated by Ras-induced pathways such as protein kinase C (PKC)-α/ornithine decarboxylase (ODC), PI3-K/Akt and MAPK signaling in human pancreatic adenocarcinoma AsPC-1 cell [105] and through the decrease in the levels of *p*-AKT and *p*-ERK in

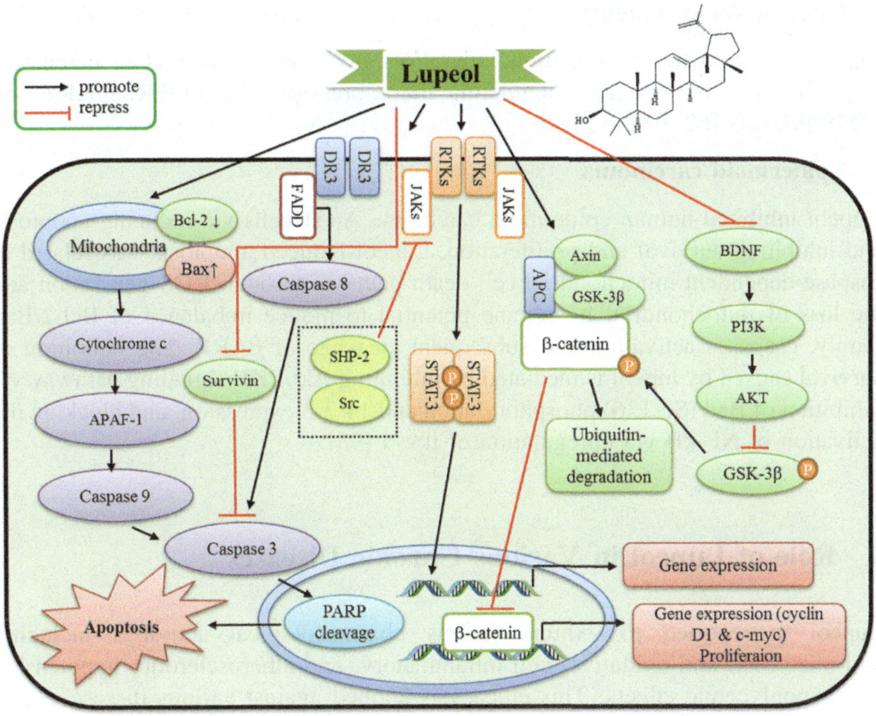

Fig. 6 Flowchart represents the anticancer mechanism of lupeol in hepatocellular carcinoma

human pancreatic cancer proliferating cell nuclear antigen 1 (PCNA-1) cells [64]. Lupeol also inhibited the proliferation of PCNA-1 cells and arrested cell cycle in G0/G1 phase by upregulating p21 and p27 and downregulating cyclin D1.

6. **Lung cancer**

Present study clearly demonstrates that lupeol induces cell death in A549 lung cancer cells in a time- and dose-dependent manner and the predominant process of cell death is autophagy rather than apoptosis and necrosis. Furthermore, the mechanism of lupeol-induced cell death is mediated by accumulating ROS, upregulation of Beclin 1 and inhibition of mTOR signaling pathway [37].

7. **Gastric cancer**

Lupeol inhibited the proliferation of gastric cancer cell lines BGC823, N87 and HGC27 through increasing the proliferation and the killing effect of NK cells. These promoting effects of lupeol on NK cells might be related to increase the expression of pore-forming protein (PFP), IFN-γ and CD107a via the activation of PI3-K/Akt and Wnt/β-catenin signaling pathways [140].

8. **Gallbladder carcinoma**

Lupeol inhibited the proliferation, migration, invasion of gallbladder carcinoma GBC-SD cells through downregulating the expression of *p*-EGFR, *p*-AKT and MMP-9 levels [62, 63].

9. **Epidermoid carcinoma**

Lupeol inhibited human epidermoid carcinoma A431 cells via inducing apoptosis and inhibiting survival and proliferation. Lupeol-induced apoptosis was related to caspase-dependent mitochondrial cell death pathway through ROS generation and the loss of mitochondrial membrane potential to induce imbalance of Bcl-2/Bax family, caspases activation and subsequent cleavage of PARP. The inhibition of survival caused by lupeol is mediated by inhibiting Akt/PKB signaling pathway via inhibition of Bad (Ser136) phosphorylation and 14-3-3 expression, and blocking the activation of NF-kB via upregulation of Ikk-α [95].

4 Role of Lupeol in Various Chronic Diseases

Lupeol is reported to exhibit various pharmacological activities including anti-microbial, anti-oxidative, anti-inflammatory, anti-atherosclerotic, hypotensive and hypoglycemic effects. This efficacy is applied against various disease conditions which include microbial infections, inflammatory and oxidative stress-related disorders such as arthritis, hepatotoxicity, renal disorder and cancer, and metabolic disorders such as cardiovascular ailments, diabetes and dyslipidemia (Fig. 7) [8, 10, 13, 23, 32, 36, 48, 51, 52, 55, 56, 61, 92, 103, 117, 125–127, 137, 146, 148].

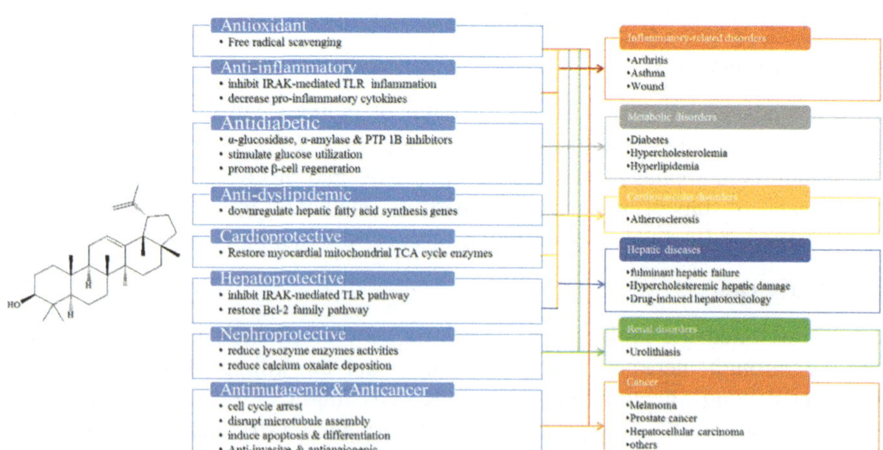

Fig. 7 Diagram represents the pharmacological effects of lupeol and its application in several chronic diseases

4.1 *Oxidative Stress-Related Disorders*

Physiologically, normal metabolic processes of body produce significant amounts of ROS. The damaging effects brought by ROS are being counteracted by the cellular antioxidant defense system which consists of enzymatic (such as superoxide dismutase, catalase and thioredoxin reductase) and non-enzymatic components (such as ascorbic acid and thioredoxin). However, oxidative stress is triggered due to the imbalance between the production of ROS and the antioxidant systems at certain conditions [115]. Oxidative stress is related to high-risk health conditions such as cardiovascular disease, neurodegenerative diseases, diabetes, cancer and inflammation [97]. Lupeol, isolated from many natural plants, may be responsible for the exhibited antioxidant property of these plants. Santiago and Mayor [110] showed that lupeol provided 34.4 % protection against low-density lipoprotein oxidation in vitro.

4.2 *Inflammatory Disorders Including Arthritis, Asthma and Wound*

Inflammation is a part of complex biological response of body tissues to harmful stimulation, and it happens as a response to either injurious agents or foreign materials such as chemical irritants, toxins and pathogens [69]. The immune response occurs when immunologically competent cells are activated in response to foreign organisms or antigenic substances liberated during acute or chronic inflammatory response. The outcome of the immune response for the host may be beneficial, as when it causes invading organisms to be phagocytosed or neutralized. On the other hand, the outcome may be deleterious if it leads to chronic inflammation without resolution of the underlying injurious process [49].

Some medicinal plants such as Compositae plants, *A. monticola*, *H. sucuuba*, *Mortonia greggii* and *P. racemosa* possessed anti-inflammatory effects in TPA-induced ear edema or carrageenan-induced paw edema via their major constituents such as lupeol [6, 24, 27, 75, 98]. Then, topical administration of lupeol (0.5 and 1 mg/ear) suppressed ear edema induced by TPA via preventing the production of some pro-inflammatory mediators in mice [28]. Lupeol (9.37 mg/kg, po) showed maximum reduction (about 57.14 %) in paw edema at 0.5 h after carrageenan injection [75]. Lucetti et al. [65] also found that lupeol possessed the anti-inflammatory effect on formalin-, carrageenan- and dextran-induced inflammation and paw edema via the opioid system, as indicated by complete blockade of the opioid antagonist naloxone. Furthermore, this effect was related to the inhibition of pro-inflammatory cytokines and the NO system, which PTX (a TNF-α inhibitor) potentiated it and the number of iNOS cells was decreased [12, 17]. Oral administration of lupeol at 12.5–200 mg/kg suppressed the cytotoxic (CD8) and helper (CD4) T cells to inhibit the secretion of pro-inflammatory cytokines such as TNF-α, IFN-γ, IL-2, and IL-4 in Balb/c mice [15]. However, [3] indicated that lupeol

(25–100 mg/kg, po) decreased exudate volume in carrageenan-induced pleurisy and the levels of TNF-α, IFN-γ and IL-2 but not IL-4 in the pleural exudate with the most significant effect at 100 mg/kg. In particular, lupeol does not exhibit any antinociceptive and ulcerogenic actions in arthritic animals when compared to well-known anti-inflammatory drugs indomethacin and aspirin, suggesting that the anti-inflammatory mechanism of lupeol is different from nonsteroidal anti-inflammatory drugs [33, 96].

Furthermore, Geetha et al. [32–34] found that lupeol (50 mg/kg, po) for 8 days decreased the destruction of structural macromolecules and modulated the generation of inflammatory factors such as collagen in adjuvant-induced arthritic inflammation. Saratha and Subramanian [111] further indicated that lupeol (50 mg/kg, po) for 4 weeks decreased the confusion of hematological parameters and the levels of pro-inflammatory cytokines in adjuvant-induced arthritic inflammation. Lupeol (60 mg/kg, po) also reduced cellularity and eosinophils in the bronchoalveolar lavage fluid, overall inflammation in the lung, and Th2-associated cytokines (IL-4, IL-5 and IL-13) levels in an allergic airway inflammation model induced by ovalbumin [137]. Therefore, lupeol is known to be a potential anti-inflammatory agent to exert anti-arthritic and anti-asthma activity.

In excision, incision and dead space wound models in rodents, topical application of lupeol had higher rate of wound contraction, lesser macrophages and shorter period in epithelization, and induced collagenization [38]. Lupeol not only protected polymorphonuclear cells, peripheral blood mononuclear cells and platelets from *E. carinatus* venom-induced oxidative stress, but also against *E. carinatus* venom-induced proteolytic cleavage of integrin α2β1, GP VI, DDR1 and CX3CR1 receptors present on these inflammatory cells [48]. Hence, this study has proved that lupeol is possible to be one of the potent wound healing and anti-inflammatory agents. Lupeol could promote the binding of collagen with collagen or integrin receptors to relieve inflammatory response and promote tissue repair.

4.3 Cardiovascular Disorders

Cyclophosphamide, a drug used in the treatment of cancer and autoimmune disorders, causes cardiotoxicology via free radicals attack generated from metabolites of cyclophosphamide such as phosphoramide mustard and acrolein. Lupeol (50 and 200 mg/kg) restored myocardial permeability, the activities of myocardial mitochondrial TCA cycle enzymes such as succinate dehydrogenase, malate dehydrogenase, and isocitrate dehydrogenase [125, 127]. Lupeol also preserved lysosomal integrity to decrease cardiac damage caused by cyclophosphamide [126]. Lupeol (50 mg/kg) prevented the hypertrophic cardiac histology and restored the normal ultrastructural architecture by minimizing the lipid abnormalities and abnormal biochemical changes induced by high-cholesterol diet in rats [121]. To normalize, lipid profiles by lupeol might be downregulated the mRNA level of hepatic fatty synthesis genes including 3-hydroxy-3-methylglutaryl-CoA reductase, fatty acid synthase, acetyl-CoA carboxylase and sterol response element binding protein 2

[10]. Thus, some researchers suggested that lupeol has cardioprotective activity due to its ability to ameliorate lipidemic–oxidative abnormalities in the early stage of hypocholesterolemic atherosclerosis in rats.

4.4 Hepatic Injury

Early studies indicated that lupeol (100–150 mg/kg, po) for 1, 3 or 7 days decreased the higher levels of serum AST and ALT levels caused by acetaminophen, cadmium or aflatoxin B1 via increasing intracellular antioxidant defense systems in rats [96, 130]. Kumari and Kakkar [54, 55] explored the cytoprotective potential of lupeol against acetaminophen-induced toxicity in vitro and in vivo. Lupeol exerted its cytoprotective effect on acetaminophen-induced hepatic injury through multiple pathways including modulation of hepatic redox homeostasis (induction of antioxidant capacity and suppression of ROS formation) and disruption of mitochondria-mediated apoptotic pathway (upregulating intracellular Bcl-2 levels, downregulating Bax level, and subsequently preventing caspase-9/3 activation and DNA damage). In the hypercholesterolemic serial studies of [123], lupeol (50 mg/kg, po) for 15 days also afforded protection against the hepatic abnormalities and lipoprotein peroxidation in rats. DMBA is metabolized by cytochrome P4501A1 and cytochrome P4501B1 in liver microsomes to form diol epoxides and other toxic ROS and then causes oxidative damage in hepatic liver. Lupeol (25 mg/kg, po) for 7 days reduced DMBA-induced hepatotoxicology via decreasing oxidative stress-induced cell apoptosis in mice. GalN and LPS-induced hepatic failure, similar to acute hepatic failure in the clinic, is a widely used animal model of liver injury. The GalN/LPS model causes improper activation of cytokine cascade and then leads to hepatocyte death. Kim et al. [52] found that lupeol (100 mg/kg, po) protected against fulminant hepatic failure induced by GalN and LPS through inhibiting IRAK-mediated TLR4 inflammatory signaling. In short, lupeol shows the hepatoprotective effect partially through the antioxidant and anti-inflammatory activities.

4.5 Urolithiasis and Renal Disorders

Lupeol (40 mg/kg, po) for 15 days protected renal damage caused by chronic cadmium exposure via reversing renal antioxidant status [72]. The association between hypercholesterolemia and kidney damage has been well known for the past few decades, hypercholesterolemic condition upregulates the oxidative stress and inflammatory responses to cause renal injury. Sudhahar et al. [119] found that lupeol (50 mg/kg, po) for 15 days restored the activities of renal marker enzymes such as alkaline phosphatase (ALP) and γ-glutamyl transferase (γ-GT), decreased renal lysosomal acid hydrolase or xanthine oxidase activities, and reversed the renal antioxidant defense levels to ameliorate the renal injury induced by high-cholesterol diet in rats. The generation of free radicals under oxalate overloading caused the alteration of renal anti-oxidative status and then damaged renal tissue. Sudhahar et al. [124] also reported that lupeol (50 mg/kg, po) for 15 days restored renal abnormal antioxidant status to reach its nephroprotective effect.

Several researchers have indicated that oral administration of lupeol (25 mg/kg for 15 days or 35 mg/kg for 21 days) inhibited calcium oxalate crystal aggregation and deposition and then reduced the extent of renal tubular damage caused by 2 % ammonium oxalate solution or pyridoxine-deficient diet containing 3 % glycolic acid in rats [66, 138]. Manjula et al. [67] found that lupeol (50 and 100 mg/kg, po) for 28 days decreased the levels of serum creatinine, uric acid, calcium and phosphate and reduced calcium oxalate deposition in the kidney induced by 0.75 % of ethylene glycol. Thus, lupeol at 25–100 mg/kg possessed the anti-urolithic and nephroprotective effects by restoring antioxidant status, increasing the solubility of calcium oxalate crystal deposits and then restoring normal renal tubules

4.6 Pancreatitis

Pancreatitis, a serious and complicated disease, is initiated in two phases. Firstly, intracellular enzyme activation occurs, which results in acinar cell injury. Then, a pancreatic inflammatory response occurs. Lupeol (10–50 mg/kg, ip) attenuated pancreatic edema and neutrophil infiltration caused by cerulein. In addition, lupeol inhibited elevation of digestive enzymes and cytokine levels such as TNF-α, IL-1 and IL-6. In conclusion, this result suggests that lupeol exhibits protective effects on cerulein-induced pancreatitis in mice [51].

4.7 Diabetic Mellitus and Dyslipidemia

Some medicinal plants for example *A. marmelos*, *Cenostigma macrophyllum*, *Eysenhardtia platycarpa*, *Rhizophora apiculata*, *Solanum xanthocarpum* and *Tournefortia hartwegiana*, which used by traditional physicians in treating diabetes, possessed anti-diabetic effects in alloxan-induced or streptozotocin-induced diabetic rodents via their major constituents such as lupeol [31, 57, 73, 84, 90]. In vitro and in vivo studies evidenced pentacyclic lupane-type triterpenoids such as lupeol and lupenone display anti-diabetic activity partially via inhibit the α-amylase, α-glucosidase and protein tyrosine phosphatase 1B (PTP 1B) activity [7, 25, 71, 74, 80, 84, 88]. Reddy et al. [86] found that lupeol (100 mg/kg) lowered the blood glucose levels by 17.8 and 19.6 % at 5 and 24 h in streptozotocin-induced diabetic rats, respectively. Administration of lupeol (20–100 mg/kg) for 21 days reduced serum glucose and glycated hemoglobin levels in streptozotocin-induced diabetic rats, with a concomitant increase in serum insulin level [36]. Khan et al. [50] and

Pereira et al. [88] showed that the anti-diabetic efficacy of lupeol might reduce blood glucose, at least in part, through stimulating glucose utilization by skeletal muscles or adipocytes. Gandhi et al. [31] also found that lupeol increased insulin levels through promoting β-cell regeneration or preventing β-cell damage, which decreasing the oxidative stress in β-cell.

On the other hand, lupeol supplement (50 mg/kg/day) for 15 days modulated the abnormalities of serum lipid status in high-cholesterol diet-induced hypercholesterolemic rats [122]. Lupeol (100 mg/kg, po) also decreased plasma levels of total cholesterol and triacylglycerol (about 11 %) in Triton-induced hyperlipidemic rats [117]. As in vitro anti-diabetic efficacy from its α-amylase, α-glucosidase and PTP 1B inhibitor, lupeol at 20–100 mg/kg possessed the anti-hyperglycemic activities in streptozotocin-induced diabetes. While at the same dose range, lupeol also possessed anti-dyslipidemic activity in high-cholesterol diet-induced hypercholesterolemia or Triton-induced hyperlipidemia.

4.8 *Neurodegenerative Disorders*

There is a close relationship between neuroinflammation and neurodegeneration such as Alzheimer's disease, Parkinson's disease and Huntington's disease. LPS is known to be a potent stimulator of brain macrophages. LPS attaches to the TLR4/CD14 receptor complex and initiates the generation of ROS and pro-inflammatory cytokines such as IL-1β and TNF-α via MAPK or NF-kB pathway, which results in neuronal apoptosis. Lupeol (50 mg/kg, ip) inhibited LPS-induced release of inflammatory markers such as TNF-α, IL-1β and NO via the P38-MAPK and JNK pathways and decreased the neuronal apoptosis in mice [13]. Therefore, lupeol has the potential to attenuate LPS-induced neuroinflammation and neurodegeneration.

4.9 *Mutagenesis and Cancer*

Substantial epidemiological data on populations indicate there is a close association between cancers and environmental carcinogens such as exposure to harmful UV irradiation and potent mutagens/carcinogens. Thus, anti-mutagenic and anticancer effects of lupeol were evidenced from two-type experimental models: carcinogen-induced mutants or cancers, and xenograft-implanted cancers. Benzo[a] pyrene (B[a]P), benzoyl peroxide (BPO), DMBA, TPA and N-butyl-N-(4-hydroxybutyl) nitrosamine (BBN) are usually used to induce DNA or chromosome mutation, genotoxicity and cancer. Lupeol has also been investigated for its strong anti-mutagenic activity in vitro and in vivo (Table 1). Earlier reports have

Table 1 Studies of lupeol on carcinogen-induced mutagenesis or toxicology

Lupeol treatment	Carcinogen	Effect and mechanism	References
2 μmol prior to TPA treatment	Initiated with DMBA (50 μg) to ICR mouse back and then with TPA (1 μg, twice weekly)	1. Inhibit tumor promotion	Yasukawa et al. [142]
0.75–1 mg prior to BPO	Topical with BPO (20 mg) to Swiss mice	1. Inhibit tumor promotion 2. Inhibit ODC activity and DNA synthesis 3. Decrease free radical mediated damage to the cellular macromolecules	Saleem et al. [104], Sultana et al. [129]
1–2 mg 30 min prior to TPA treatment	TPA (3.2 nmol) to dorsal side of CD-1 mouse skin	1. Modulate NF-kB and PI3-K/Akt pathways	Saleem et al. [103]
25 mg/kg (po) for 1 week after DMBA	DMBA (50 mg/kg, po) to Swiss mice	1. Restore antioxidant enzyme activities and mitochondria function 2. Downregulate the expression of Bcl-2 3. Upregulate the expression of Bax and Caspase 3	Prasad et al. [93]
50–200 μg prior or post to DMBA treatment	DMBA (100 μg) to interscapular region of Swiss mice	1. Inhibit DNA alkylation damage	Nigam et al. [77]
1 mg/animal (po) for 1 week	B[a]P (100 mg/kg, ip) to Swiss mice	1. Increase mitotic index 2. Decrease micronuclei	Prasad et al. [94]
50 mg/kg (po) 1 week before DMBA treatment	0.5 % DMBA (0.5 %, third weekly) for 14 weeks on buccal pouches of golden Syrian hamsters	1. Decrease the expression of p53 and Bcl-2 2. Increase the expression of Bax 3. Increase the activities of caspase 3 and 9 4. Modulate phase I and II xenobiotic metabolizing enzymes	Manoharan et al. [68], Palanimuthu et al. [85]
50 mg/kg (po) post to BBN treatment for 28 weeks	BBN (150 mg, twice weekly) for 8 weeks and then DMA (100 ppm) for 28 weeks to Wistar rats	1. Inhibit tumor growth 2. Increase PTEN expression 3. Decrease COX-2 levels and the expression of NF-kB and TNF-α	Prabhu et al. [92]

shown that lupeol inhibited BPO-induced DNA damage in vitro conditions [129]. Lupeol (50–200 μg/mouse) showed the preventive effects in DMBA-induced DNA strand breaks in dose-dependent manner. Lupeol (1 mg/mouse) supplement inhibited the induction of chromosomal aberration (42.4 %) and micronuclei (48.6 %) caused by B[a]P. Lupeol (0.75 and 1.5 mg/mouse) also showed a significant inhibition of BPO-induced cutaneous ODC activity and a significant reduction in BPO-enhanced [^{3}H] thymidine uptake in cutaneous DNA [104]. Topical application of lupeol (1–2 mg/mouse) also afforded significant inhibition against TPA-mediated increase in skin edema or DMBA-mediated neoplastic events [76]. Further study indicated that lupeol (50 mg/kg, po) for 14–16 weeks completely inhibited the formation of oral tumors in DMBA-induced oral carcinogenesis [68, 85]. Lupeol (2 μmol/mouse) for 20 weeks decreased tumor formation (96 %) by TPA in DMBA-initiated mice [142]. Lupeol treatment (50 mg/kg, po) for 28 weeks showed the inhibition of bladder carcinogenesis induced by BBN [92]. Therefore, these results showed that lupeol reduced the incidence of DNA and chromosome mutation and inhibited tumor promotion induced by carcinogens.

Recently, lupeol was reported to inhibit the growth of several cancer types by modulating key molecular pathways, which are involved in proliferation, survival and apoptosis (Table 2). In tumorigenicity studies, lupeol (1 mg/mouse, 3 times/week, ip) treatment for 12 weeks reduced tumor growth and serum prostate-specific antigen levels in athymic nude mice implanted with CWR22Rυ1 cells [106]. At the same treatment for 7 weeks, lupeol also reduced tumor growth and modulated the expression of proliferation markers in athymic nude mice implanted with 451Lu cells [107]. Lupeol (40 mg/kg, 3 times/week, ip) treatment for 9 weeks reduced Mel 928-implanted tumor volume (35 %), Mel 928-implanted tumor burden (50 %) and AsPC-1-implanted tumor growth in athymic nude mice [70, 134]. At later study of Siddique et al. [112], lupeol treatment for 56 days also reduced tumor volume in athymic nude mice implanted with ADPC (LNCaP) or CRPC (C4-2b) cells. He et al. [42] also found that lupeol (80 mg/kg, 3 times/week, ip) treatment for 30 days inhibited the growth of transplanted HCC tumors (SMMC7721 cells). Lupeol (30 and 60 mg/kg, iv) for 7–10 days reduced PCNA-1-implanted tumor volume (37.71 and 58.25 %) or GBC-SD-implanted tumor volume (337.75 and 56.91 %) in Balb/c nude mice [63, 64]. In melanoma-bearing mouse model, systemic administration of lupeol inhibits the growth and proliferation of highly aggressive human metastatic melanoma cells by inducing apoptosis in C57BL/6 mice [79]. Therefore, these findings showed lupeol possessed the anticancer efficacy against some tumor cells implantation in nude mice. The most noticeable observation is that lupeol did not display any toxic effect on normal human cells at the dose which it kills cancer cells [70]. Furthermore, lupeol could target liver tumor-initiating cells and increase the sensitization of chemotherapeutic agents or radiotherapy to HCC cells through phosphatase and tensin homolog (PTEN)-Akt-ABCG2 pathway [44, 58].

Table 2 Studies of lupeol on tumor growth, proliferation and differentiation in vitro and in vivo (2010–2015)

Cancer model	Tumor cell	Effect and mechanism	References
In vitro melanoma and in vivo xenograft-implanted athymic mice	Mel 928, Mel 1011 and Mel 1241 melanoma cells	1. Decrease cell viability 2. Induce cell apoptosis 3. Decrease clonogenic potential 4. Decrease the activity of Wnt/β-catenin pathway 5. Inhibit the tumorigenicity	Tarapore et al. [134]
In vitro hepatocellular carcinoma and in vivo xenograft-implanted athymic mice	SMMC7721 and HepG2 cells	1. Decrease cell viability 2. Induce cell apoptosis via inducing caspase-3 activity 3. Inhibit the tumorigenicity via TRAIL pathway	He et al. [42]
In vitro hepatocellular carcinoma and in vivo xenograft-implanted athymic mice	MHCC-LM3, Huh-7 and PLC-8024 cells	1. Inhibited the self-renewal ability of liver T-ICs 2. Inhibit the tumorigenicity 3. Sensitize HCC cells to chemotherapeutic agents through PTEN–Akt–ABCG2 pathway	Lee et al. [58]
In vitro prostate cancer and in vivo xenograft-implanted athymic mice	LAPC4, LnCaP and C4-2b cells	1. Inhibit cell growth 2. Inhibit the activity of transcript factor AR and the expression of PSA 3. Compete with androgen for AR 4. Block the binding of AR-responsive genes 5. Inhibit the recruitment of RNA Pol II to target genes 6. Inhibit the tumorigenicity	Siddique et al. [112]
In vivo xenograft-implanted C57BL/6 mice	B16 2F2 melanoma cells	1. Inhibit the tumorigenicity 2. Decrease the percentage of Ki 67 and PCNA-positive areas in the tumor tissues	Nitta et al. [79]
In vitro colorectal cancer	DLD 1 and HCT 116 cells	1. Decrease cell viability 2. Induce cell apoptosis 3. Decrease clonogenic potential 4. Decrease the activity of Wnt/β-catenin pathway	Tarapore et al. [133]
In vitro gastric cancer	BGC823, N87 and HGC27 cells	1. Inhibit cancer cell proliferation 2. Increase the killing effect of NK cells via upregulating the expression of PFP, IFN-γ and CD107a. Wnt/β-catenin signaling pathway and PI3-K/Akt signaling pathway	Wu et al. [140]
In vitro gallbladder cancer and in vivo xenograft-implanted Balb/c mice	GBC-SD cells	1. Decrease cell proliferation 2. Induce cell apoptosis 3. Inhibit cell migration and invasion via suppressing the activation of EGFR and MMP-9 4. Inhibit the tumorigenicity	Liu et al. [63]

(continued)

Table 2 (continued)

Cancer model	Tumor cell	Effect and mechanism	References
In vitro hepatocellular carcinoma	HepG2, C3A, PLC/PRF5, HUH-7 and Hep3B cells	1. Inhibit cell proliferation via downregulating JAK-STAT3 cascades and increasing the expression of SHP-2 2. Inhibit angiogenesis though suppressing the expression of STAT3-regulated gene products 3. Decrease the binding of STAT3 to VEGF promoter 4. Induce cell apoptosis	Siveen et al. [114]
In vitro pancreatic cancer and in vivo xenograft-implanted Balb/c mice	PCNA-1 cells	1. Cell cycle arrest in G0/G1 phase by upregulating P21 and P27 and downregulating cyclin D1 2. Induce cell apoptosis by decreasing Akt and ERK pathway 3. Inhibit the tumorigenicity	Liu et al. [62, 64]
In vitro hepatocellular carcinoma	HCCLM3 and HepG2 cells	1. Suppress cell proliferation by inhibiting BDNF secretion and phosphorylation of GSK-3β, cooperated with blockade of Akt/PI3-K and Wnt signaling pathway 2. Induce cell apoptosis by caspase 3 pathway	Zhang et al. [148]

5 Biological Activities of Lupeol in Humans

Although these above review described diverse pharmacological activities of lupeol in vitro and in vivo, only topical or subcutaneous treatment of lupeol is further evaluated its efficacy in melanoma and acne of canine or human. For first time about clinical utility of lupeol in treating diseases, lupeol (0.75–1.5 mg per site) was topically injected to seven cases canine with spontaneous melanoma [41]. In cases I III (injected at metastatic sites), lupeol induced disappearance or differentiation of metastatic melanoma cell (the increase in melanosomes). In cases IV (injected at primary sites), lupeol induced the focal lysis of tumor tissues. In cases V–VII, lupeol an adjuvant therapeutic agent was combined with hyperthermia and immunotherapy to treat melanoma. They also found that lupeol combination induced disappearance of metastatic melanoma cell. This study concluded that topical administration of lupeol was successful treatment in 6 out of 7 canine with malignant melanomas. They further indicated that lupeol possessed the differentiation-inducing and anti-proliferative activities for oral malignant melanoma in canine [81]. Moreover, lupeol (10 mg/kg, sc) at various times after surgery prevented local tumor progression (no local recurrence) and distant metastasis [144]. Furthermore, they also found that combination with lupeol and other alternative therapeutic methods such as hyperthermia and dendritic cell therapy had the potential to prolong the life span and maintain an excellent life quality for canine suffering melanoma [43]. Therefore, they suggested that lupeol may be a novel adjuvant treatment for oral malignant melanoma, and a higher dose and/or repeated injection of lupeol appeared to be more effective in treating the melanoma [81]. These serial studies in canine oral malignant melanoma give more opportunity for preclinical studies and clinical trials to validate the usefulness of lupeol on diverse pharmacological activities, especially anti-inflammatory, anticancer and hepatoprotective effects. Recent clinical trials were conducted by Dr. Dae Hun Suh in Seoul National University Hospital, which 2 % lupeol cream was applied to treat patients suffering mild–moderate face acne twice daily for 4 or 8 weeks. However, regarding to the intervals of administration, the dosage design of lupeol and interspecies differences from animal studies must be further investigated and attention.

6 Conclusions

From in vitro and in vivo results, we demonstrated that lupeol possessed anti-oxidative, anti-inflammatory, anticancer, anti-hyperglycemic and anti-dyslipidemic activities. Hence, we further reviewed the preclinical toxicological and pharmacokinetic reports of lupeol to support that lupeol may have a potential to be a candidate therapeutic agent for multiple human diseases. Several researchers have reported that systemic administration of lupeol did not exhibit acute and chronic toxicity in animals [4, 32, 70, 87, 96, 103, 119]. For acute toxicity study in rodents, oral administration of lupeol up to 2 g/kg did not cause any adverse effects or mortality after 96 h or seven consecutive days of observation [4, 87]. Lupeol (40 mg/kg, ip) also showed no toxicological sign or mortality in mice [70]. As for subacute toxicity study in rodents, lupeol (50–100 mg/kg/day, po) under various periods (7, 8 or 15 consecutive days) did not cause any systemic toxicity or mortality [32, 96, 119]. In addition, topical treatment of lupeol (2 mg/animal) for 28 weeks (two times/week) did not induce any epidermal hyperplasia, and it did not affect body weight gain and any systemic toxicity effect in mice [103]. We can summarize from thee preclinical toxicological tests that lupeol treatment up to 100 mg/kg under various periods (short-term treatment of 7, 8 or 15 consecutive days) did not exhibit any systemic toxicity in animals, and then, it did not affect skin epidermal histology and gene expression when topical treatment for subacute periods (28 days).

In conclusion, pentacyclic lupane-type triterpene lupeol has a great potential to be a lead candidate compound. Many researchers attempted to synthesize lupeol by various routes such as polyolefin cyclization or enantioselective synthetic pathway [118, 131, 143]. Because the structure of lupeol comprises ten asymmetric centers, it causes the stereochemical challenge and the higher degree of difficulty in synthesis processes. There is a tendency to obtain lupeol from lupeol-rich plants such as *C. nurvala, Mangifera indica* L. and birch barks or from industrial residues of cork processing [1, 100, 116, 147] because this way is less polluting and cheaper.

On the other hand, lupeol is expected to exhibit poor bioavailability by oral route because of high lipophilic and low solubility. Some researchers synthesized lupeol derivatives by esterification, heterocycle or substituted insertion (such as aromatic or nicotinic groups) at C-2 and C-3 positions to increase its solubility, bioavailability and pharmacological activities [29, 30, 33, 91, 119–124, 127, 130]. Further, the inserted substitutions at C-2/C-3 or C-20/C-30 positions of lupeol, the effective doses and the duration of treatment with different human diseases should be taken into account when lupeol will be used as a lead compound to synthesize lupeol derivatives (prodrugs) which possess more potent and bioavailability than lupeol. Preclinical pharmacokinetic data and clinical evidence of lupeol and lupeol derivatives also shall be investigated in the future.

References

1. Agarwal SK, Kumar S (2003) An improved process for the extraction of lupeol, an antiurotithic compound from *Crateva nurvala*. Indian. INXXAPIN 191625 A1 20031206: 11
2. Agra LC, Ferro JN, Barbosa FT, Barreto E (2015) Triterpenes with healing activity: a systematic review. J Dermatol Treat 26:465–470
3. Ahmad SF, Pandey A, Kour K, Bani S (2010) Downregulation of pro-inflammatory cytokines by lupeol measured using cytometric bead array immunoassay. Phytotherapy Res 24:9–13
4. Al-Rehaily AJ, El-Tahir KEH, Mossa JS, Rafatullah S (2001) Pharmacological studies of various extracts and the major constituent, lupeol, obtained from hexane extract of *Teclea nobilis* in Rodents. Nat Prod Sci 7:76–82
5. Akihisa T, Kojima N, Kikuchi T, Yasukawa K, Tokuda H, Masters E, Manosroi A, Manosroi J (2010) Anti-inflammatory and chemopreventive effects of triterpene cinnamates and acetates from shea fat. J Oleo Sci 59:273–280
6. Akihisa T, Yasukawa K, Oinuma H, Kasahara Y, Yamanouchi S, Takido M, Kumaki K, Tamura T (1996) Triterpene alcohols from the flowers of compositae and their anti-inflammatory effects. Phytochemistry 43:1255–1260
7. Alqahtani A, Hamid K, Kam A, Wong KH, Abdelhak Z, Razmovski-Naumovski V, Chan K, Li KM, Groundwater PW, Li GQ (2013) The pentacyclic triterpenoids in herbal medicines and their pharmacological activities in diabetes and diabetic complications. Curr Med Chem 20:908–931
8. Ambasta RK, Jha SK, Kumar D, Sharma R, Jha NK, Kumar P (2015) Comparative study of anti-angiogenic activities of luteolin, lectin and lupeol biomolecules. J Transl Med 13:307
9. Annabi B, Vaillancourt-Jean E, Beliveau R (2013) MT1-MMP expression level status dictates the *in vitro* action of lupeol on inflammatory biomarkers MMP-9 and COX-2 in medulloblastoma cells. Inflammopharmacology 21:91–99
10. Ardiansyah YE, Shirakawa H, Hata K, Hiwatashi K, Ohinata K, Goto T, Komai M (2012) Lupeol supplementation improves blood pressure and lipid metabolism parameters in stroke-prone spontaneously hypertensive rats. Biosci Biotechnol Biochem 76:183–185
11. Asha R, Devi VG, Abraham A (2016) Lupeol, a pentacyclic triterpenoid isolated from *Vernonia cinerea* attenuate selenite induced cataract formation in Sprague Dawley rat pups. Chem Biol Interact 245:20–29
12. Ashalatha K, Venkateswarlu Y, Priya AM, Lalitha P, Krishnaveni M, Jayachandran S (2010) Anti inflammatory potential of *Decalepis hamiltonii* (Wight and Arn) as

evidenced by down regulation of pro inflammatory cytokines-TNF-alpha and IL-2. J Ethnopharmacol 130:167–170
13. Badshah H, Ali T, Rehman SU, Amin FU, Ullah F, Kim TH, Kim MO (2016) Protective effect of lupeol against lipopolysaccharide-induced neuroinflammation via the p38/c-Jun N-terminal kinase pathway in the adult mouse Brain. J Neuroimmune Pharmacol 11:48–60
14. Baliga MS, Thilakchand KR, Rai MP, Rao S, Venkatesh P (2013) *Aegle marmelos* (L.) Correa (Bael) and its phytochemicals in the treatment and prevention of cancer. Integr Cancer Ther 12:187–196
15. Bani S, Kaul A, Khan B, Ahmad SF, Suri KA, Gupta BD, Satti NK, Qazi GN (2006) Suppression of T lymphocyte activity by lupeol isolated from *Crataeva religiosa*. Phytotherapy Res 20:279–287
16. Beveridge TH, Li TS, Drover JC (2002) Phytosterol content in American ginseng seed oil. J Agric Food Chem 50:744–750
17. Bhandari P, Patel NK, Bhutani KK (2014) Synthesis of new heterocyclic lupeol derivatives as nitric oxide and pro-inflammatory cytokine inhibitors. Bioorg Med Chem Lett 24:3596–3599
18. Chappell J (2002) The genetics and molecular genetics of terpene and sterol origami. Curr Opin Plant Biol 5:151–157
19. Chatterjee I, Chakravarty AK, Gomes A (2006) *Daboia russellii* and *Naja kaouthia* venom neutralization by lupeol acetate isolated from the root extract of Indian sarsaparilla *Hemidesmus indicus* R.Br. J Ethnopharmacol 106:38–43
20. Chen YF, Ching C, Wu TS, Wu CR, Hsieh WT, Tsai HY (2012) *Balanophora spicata* and lupeol acetate possess antinociceptive and anti-inflammatory activities in vivo and in vitro. Evid Based Complement Altern Med 2012:371273
21. Connolly JD, Hill RA (2008) Triterpenoids. Nat Prod Rep 25:794–830
22. Correa RS, Coelho CP, dos Santos MH, Ellena J, Doriguetto AC (2009) Lupeol. Acta Crystallogr C 65:O97–O99
23. de Lima FO, Alves V, Barbosa Filho JM, Almeida JR, Rodrigues LC, Soares MB, Villarreal CF (2013) Antinociceptive effect of lupeol: evidence for a role of cytokines inhibition. Phytotherapy Res 27:1557–1563
24. de Miranda AL, Silva JR, Rezende CM, Neves JS, Parrini SC, Pinheiro ML, Cordeiro MC, Tamborini E, Pinto AC (2000) Anti-inflammatory and analgesic activities of the latex containing triterpenes from *Himatanthus sucuuba*. Planta Med 66:284–286
25. Deutschlander MS, Lall N, Van de Venter M, Hussein AA (2011) Hypoglycemic evaluation of a new triterpene and other compounds isolated from *Euclea undulata Thunb*. var. *myrtina* (Ebenaceae) root bark. J Ethnopharmacol 133:1091–1095
26. Duke JA (1992) Handbook of phytochemical constituents of GRAS herbs and other economic plants, vol CRC. Press, Boca Raton
27. Fernandez A, Alvarez A, Garcia MD, Saenz MT (2001a) Anti-inflammatory effect of *Pimenta racemosa* var. *ozua* and isolation of the triterpene lupeol. Farmaco 56:335–338
28. Fernandez MA, de las Heras B, Garcia MD, Saenz MT, Villar A (2001b) New insights into the mechanism of action of the anti-inflammatory triterpene lupeol. J Pharm Pharmacol 53:1533–1539
29. Fotie J, Bohle DS, Leimanis ML, Georges E, Rukunga G, Nkengfack AE (2006) Lupeol long-chain fatty acid esters with antimalarial activity from *Holarrhena floribunda*. J Nat Prod 69:62–67
30. Furukawa S, Takagi N, Ikeda T, Ono M, Nafady AM, Nohara T, Sugimoto H, Doi S, Yamada H (2002) Two novel long-chain alkanoic acid esters of lupeol from alecrim-propolis. Chem Pharm Bull (Tokyo) 50:439–440
31. Gandhi GR, Ignacimuthu S, Paulraj MG (2012) Hypoglycemic and beta-cells regenerative effects of *Aegle marmelos* (L.) Corr. bark extract in streptozotocin-induced diabetic rats. Food Chem Toxicol 50:1667–1674
32. Geetha T, Varalakshmi P (1999) Effect of lupeol and lupeol linoleate on lysosomal enzymes and collagen in adjuvant-induced arthritis in rats. Mol Cell Biochem 201:83–87

33. Geetha T, Varalakshmi P (2001) Anti-inflammatory activity of lupeol and lupeol linoleate in rats. J Ethnopharmacol 76:77–80
34. Geetha T, Varalakshmi P, Latha RM (1998) Effect of triterpenes from *Crataeva nurvala* stem bark on lipid peroxidation in adjuvant induced arthritis in rats. Pharmacol Res 37:191–195
35. Golechha M, Sarangal V, Ojha S, Bhatia J, Arya DS (2014) Anti-inflammatory effect of *Emblica officinalis* in rodent models of acute and chronic inflammation: involvement of possible mechanisms. Int J Inflamm 2014:178408
36. Gupta R, Sharma AK, Sharma MC, Dobhal MP, Gupta RS (2012) Evaluation of antidiabetic and antioxidant potential of lupeol in experimental hyperglycaemia. Nat Prod Res 26:1125–1129
37. Hao J, Pei Y, Ji G, Li W, Feng S, Qiu S (2011) Autophagy is induced by 3β-O-succinyl-lupeol (LD9-4) in A549 cells via up-regulation of Beclin 1 and down-regulation mTOR pathway. Eur J Pharmacol 670:29–38
38. Harish BG, Krishna V, Santosh Kumar HS, Khadeer Ahamed BM, Sharath R, Kumara Swamy HM (2008) Wound healing activity and docking of glycogen-synthase-kinase-3-β-protein with isolated triterpenoid lupeol in rats. Phytomedicine 15:763–767
39. Hata K, Hori K, Takahashi S (2003) Role of p38 MAPK in lupeol-induced B16 2F2 mouse melanoma cell differentiation. J Biochem 134:441–445
40. Hata K, Mukaiyama T, Tsujimura N, Sato Y, Kosaka Y, Sakamoto K, Hori K (2006) Differentiation-inducing activity of lupane triterpenes on a mouse melanoma cell line. Cytotechnology 52:151–158
41. Hata K, Ogihara K, Takahashi S, Tsuka T, Minami S, Okamoto Y (2010) Effects of lupeol on melanoma in vitro and in vivo: fundamental and clinical trials. Anim Cell Technol Basic Appl Aspects 16:339–344
42. He Y, Liu F, Zhang L, Wu Y, Hu B, Zhang Y, Li Y, Liu H (2011) Growth inhibition and apoptosis induced by lupeol, a dietary triterpene, in human hepatocellular carcinoma cells. Biol Pharm Bull 34:517–522
43. Itoh H, Mukaiyama T, Goto T, Hata K, Azuma K, Tsuka T, Osaki T, Imagawa T, Okamoto Y (2014) Non-surgical treatment of canine oral malignant melanoma: a case study of the application of complementary alternative medicine. Oncol Lett 7:1829–1830
44. Jin Y, Lyu Y, Tang X, Zhang Y, Chen J, Zheng D, Liang Y (2015) Lupeol enhances radiosensitivity of human hepatocellular carcinoma cell line SMMC-7721 in vitro and in vivo. Int J Radiat Biol 91:202–208
45. Jyotshna, Srivastava P, Killadi B, Shanker K (2015) Uni-dimensional double development HPTLC-densitometry method for simultaneous analysis of mangiferin and lupeol content in mango (*Mangifera indica*) pulp and peel during storage. Food Chem 176:91–98
46. Kahlos K, Kangas L, Hiltunen R (1989) Ergosterol peroxide, an active compound from *Inonotus radiatus*. Planta Med 55:389–390
47. Kardar MN, Zhang T, Coxon GD, Watson DG, Fearnley J, Seidel V (2014) Characterisation of triterpenes and new phenolic lipids in *Cameroonian propolis*. Phytochemistry 106:156–163
48. Katkar GD, Sharma RD, Vishalakshi GJ, Naveenkumar SK, Madhur G, Thushara RM, Narender T, Girish KS, Kemparaju K (2015) Lupeol derivative mitigates *Echis carinatus* venom-induced tissue destruction by neutralizing venom toxins and protecting collagen and angiogenic receptors on inflammatory cells. Biochim Biophys Acta 1850:2393–2409
49. Katzung BG, Masters SB, Trevor AJ (2012) Nosteroidal anti-inflammatory drugs, disease-modifying antirheumatic drugs, nonopoid analgesics, and drugs used in gout. Basic and clinical pharmacology. McGraw-Hill Medical, pp 635–636
50. Khan MF, Maurya CK, Dev K, Arha D, Rai AK, Tamrakar AK, Maurya R (2014) Design and synthesis of lupeol analogues and their glucose uptake stimulatory effect in L6 skeletal muscle cells. Bioorg Med Chem Lett 24:2674–2679
51. Kim MJ, Bae GS, Choi SB, Jo IJ, Kim DG, Shin JY, Lee SK, Kim MJ, Song HJ, Park SJ (2015) Lupeol protects against cerulein-induced acute pancreatitis in mice. Phytotherapy Res 29:1634–1639

52. Kim SJ, Cho HI, Kim SJ, Kim JS, Kwak JH, Lee DU, Lee SK, Lee SM (2014) Protective effects of lupeol against D-galactosamine and lipopolysaccharide-induced fulminant hepatic failure in mice. J Nat Prod 77:2383–2388
53. Kumar A, Tantry BA, Rahiman S, Gupta U (2011) Comparative study of antimicrobial activity and phytochemical analysis of methanolic and aqueous extracts of the fruit of *Emblica officinalis* against pathogenic bacteria. J Tradit Chin Med 31:246–250
54. Kumari A, Kakkar P (2012) Lupeol prevents acetaminophen-induced in vivo hepatotoxicity by altering the Bax/Bcl-2 and oxidative stress-mediated mitochondrial signaling cascade. Life Sci 90:561–570
55. Kumari A, Kakkar P (2012) Lupeol protects against acetaminophen-induced oxidative stress and cell death in rat primary hepatocytes. Food Chem Toxicol 50:1781–1789
56. Kwon HH, Yoon JY, Park SY, Min S, Kim YI, Park JY, Lee YS, Thiboutot DM, Suh DH (2015) Activity-guided purification identifies lupeol, a pentacyclic triterpene, as a therapeutic agent multiple pathogenic factors of acne. J Invest Dermatol 135:1491–1500
57. Lakshmi V, Gupta P, Tiwari P, Srivastava AK (2006) Antihyperglycemic activity of *Rhizophora apiculata* Bl. in rats. Nat Prod Res 20:1295–1299
58. Lee TK, Castilho A, Cheung VC, Tang KH, Ma S, Ng IO (2011) Lupeol targets liver tumor-initiating cells through phosphatase and tensin homolog modulation. Hepatology 53:160–170
59. Li W, Hao J, Xiao Y (2013) Synthesis and in vitro antitumor activities of lupeol dicarboxylic acid monoester derivatives. Arch Pharm Res 36:1447–1453
60. Lima LM, Perazzo FF, Tavares Carvalho JC, Bastos JK (2007) Anti-inflammatory and analgesic activities of the ethanolic extracts from *Zanthoxylum riedelianum* (Rutaceae) leaves and stem bark. J Pharm Pharmacol 59:1151–1158
61. Lira SR, Rao VS, Carvalho AC, Guedes MM, de Morais TC, de Souza AL, Trevisan MT, Lima AF, Chaves MH, Santos FA (2009) Gastroprotective effect of lupeol on ethanol-induced gastric damage and the underlying mechanism. Inflammopharmacology 17:221–228
62. Liu Y, Bi T, Dai W, Wang G, Qian L, Shen G, Gao Q (2015a) Lupeol induces apoptosis and cell cycle arrest of human osteosarcoma cells through PI3K/AKT/mTOR Pathway. Technol Cancer Res Treat pii: 1533034615609014
63. Liu Y, Bi T, Shen G, Li Z, Wu G, Wang Z, Qian L, Gao Q (2016) Lupeol induces apoptosis and inhibits invasion in gallbladder carcinoma GBC-SD cells by suppression of EGFR/MMP-9 signaling pathway. Cytotechnology 68:123–133
64. Liu Y, Bi T, Wang G, Dai W, Wu G, Qian L, Gao Q, Shen G (2015b) Lupeol inhibits proliferation and induces apoptosis of human pancreatic cancer PCNA-1 cells through AKT/ERK pathways. Naunyn Schmiedebergs Arch Pharmacol 388:295–304
65. Lucetti DL, Lucetti EC, Bandeira MA, Veras HN, Silva AH, Leal LK, Lopes AA, Alves VC, Silva GS, Brito GA, Viana GB (2010) Anti-inflammatory effects and possible mechanism of action of lupeol acetate isolated from *Himatanthus drasticus* (Mart.) Plumel. J Inflamm (Lond) 7:60
66. Malini MM, Lenin M, Varalakshmi P (2000) Protective effect of triterpenes on calcium oxalate crystal-induced peroxidative changes in experimental urolithiasis. Pharmacol Res 41:413–418
67. Manjula K, Rajendran K, Eevera T, Kumaran S (2012) Effect of *Costus igneus* stem extract on calcium oxalate urolithiasis in albino rats. Urol Res 40:499–510
68. Manoharan S, Palanimuthu D, Baskaran N, Silvan S (2012) Modulating effect of lupeol on the expression pattern of apoptotic markers in 7, 12-dimethylbenz(a)anthracene induced oral carcinogenesis. Asian Pac J Cancer Prev 13:5753–5757
69. Martelanc M, Vovk I, Simonovska B (2009) Separation and identification of some common isomeric plant triterpenoids by thin-layer chromatography and high-performance liquid chromatography. J Chromatogr A 1216:6662–6670
70. Murtaza I, Saleem M, Adhami VM, Hafeez BB, Mukhtar H (2009) Suppression of cFLIP by lupeol, a dietary triterpene, is sufficient to overcome resistance to TRAIL-mediated apoptosis in chemoresistant human pancreatic cancer cells. Cancer Res 69:1156–1165

71. Na M, Kim BY, Osada H, Ahn JS (2009) Inhibition of protein tyrosine phosphatase 1B by lupeol and lupenone isolated from *Sorbus commixta*. J Enzyme Inhib Med Chem 24:1056–1059
72. Nagaraj M, Sunitha S, Varalakshmi P (2000) Effect of lupeol, a pentacyclic triterpene, on the lipid peroxidation and antioxidant status in rat kidney after chronic cadmium exposure. J Appl Toxicol 20:413–417
73. Narvaez-Mastache JM, Garduno-Ramirez ML, Alvarez L, Delgado G (2006) Antihyperglycemic activity and chemical constituents of *Eysenhardtia platycarpa*. J Nat Prod 69:1687–1691
74. Nazaruk J, Borzym-Kluczyk M (2015) The role of triterpenes in the management of diabetes mellitus and its complications. Phytochem Rev 14:675–690
75. Nguemfo EL, Dimo T, Dongmo AB, Azebaze AG, Alaoui K, Asongalem AE, Cherrah Y, Kamtchouing P (2009) Anti-oxidative and anti-inflammatory activities of some isolated constituents from the stem bark of *Allanblackia monticola* Staner L.C (Guttiferae). Inflammopharmacology 17:37–41
76. Nigam N, Prasad S, George J, Shukla Y (2009) Lupeol induces p53 and cyclin-B-mediated G2/M arrest and targets apoptosis through activation of caspase in mouse skin. Biochem Biophys Res Commun 381:253–258
77. Nigam N, Prasad S, Shukla Y (2007) Preventive effects of lupeol on DMBA induced DNA alkylation damage in mouse skin. Food Chem Toxicol 45:2331–2335
78. Nikiema JB, Vanhaelen-Fastre R, Vanhaelen M, Fontaine J, De Graef C, Heenen M (2001) Effects of antiinflammatory triterpenes isolated from *Leptadenia hastata* latex on keratinocyte proliferation. Phytotherapy Res 15:131–134
79. Nitta M, Azuma K, Hata K, Takahashi S, Ogiwara K, Tsuka T, Imagawa T, Yokoe I, Osaki T, Minami S, Okamoto Y (2013) Systemic and local injections of lupeol inhibit tumor growth in a melanoma-bearing mouse model. Biomed Rep 1:641–645
80. Nkobole N, Houghton PJ, Hussein A, Lall N (2011) Antidiabetic activity of *Terminalia sericea* constituents. Nat Prod Commun 6:1585–1588
81. Ogihara K, Naya Y, Okamoto Y, Hata K (2014) Differentiation-inducing and anti-proliferative activities of lupeol on canine melanoma cells. Springerplus 3:632
82. Ogiwara K, Hata K (2009) Melanoma cell differentiation induced by lupeol separates into two stages: morphological and functional changes. J Nat Med 63:323–326
83. Omoyeni OA, Hussein A, Meyer M, Green I, Iwuoha E (2015) *Pleiocarpa pycnantha* leaves and its triterpenes induce apoptotic cell death in Caco-2 cells in vitro. BMC Complement Altern Med 15:224
84. Ortiz-Andrade RR, Garcia-Jimenez S, Castillo-Espana P, Ramirez-Avila G, Villalobos-Molina R, Estrada-Soto S (2007) alpha-Glucosidase inhibitory activity of the methanolic extract from *Tournefortia hartwegiana*: an anti-hyperglycemic agent. J Ethnopharmacol 109:48–53
85. Palanimuthu D, Baskaran N, Silvan S, Rajasekaran D, Manoharan S (2012) Lupeol, a bioactive triterpene, prevents tumor formation during 7,12-dimethylbenz(a)anthracene induced oral carcinogenesis. Pathol Oncol Res 18:1029–1037
86. Papi Reddy K, Singh AB, Puri A, Srivastava AK, Narender T (2009) Synthesis of novel triterpenoid (lupeol) derivatives and their in vivo antihyperglycemic and antidyslipidemic activity. Bioorg Med Chem Lett 19:4463–4466
87. Patocka J (2003) Biologically active pentacyclic triterpenes and their current medicine signification. J Appl Biomed 1:7–12
88. Pereira AC, Pereira AB, Moreira CC, Botion LM, Lemos VS, Braga FC, Cortes SF (2015) *Hancornia speciosa* Gomes (Apocynaceae) as a potential anti-diabetic drug. J Ethnopharmacol 161:30–35
89. Phillips DR, Rasbery JM, Bartel B, Matsuda SP (2006) Biosynthetic diversity in plant triterpene cyclization. Curr Opin Plant Biol 9:305–314

90. Piaulino CA, Carvalho FC, Almeida BC, Chaves MH, Almeida FR, Brito SM (2013) The stem bark extracts of *Cenostigma macrophyllum* attenuates tactile allodynia in streptozotocin-induced diabetic rats. Pharm Biol 51:1243–1248
91. Poumale HM, Awoussong KP, Randrianasolo R, Simo CC, Ngadjui BT, Shiono Y (2012) Long-chain alkanoic acid esters of lupeol from *Dorstenia harmsiana* Engl. (Moraceae). Nat Prod Res 26:749–755
92. Prabhu B, Balakrishnan D, Sundaresan S (2015) Antiproliferative and anti-inflammatory properties of diindolylmethane and lupeol against N-butyl-N-(4-hydroxybutyl) nitrosamine induced bladder carcinogenesis in experimental rats. Hum Exp Toxicol (in press)
93. Prasad S, Kalra N, Shukla Y (2007) Hepatoprotective effects of lupeol and mango pulp extract of carcinogen induced alteration in Swiss albino mice. Mol Nutr Food Res 51:352–359
94. Prasad S, Kumar Yadav V, Srivastava S, Shukla Y (2008) Protective effects of lupeol against benzo[a]pyrene induced clastogenicity in mouse bone marrow cells. Mol Nutr Food Res 52:1117–1120
95. Prasad S, Madan E, Nigam N, Roy P, George J, Shukla Y (2009) Induction of apoptosis by lupeol in human epidermoid carcinoma A431 cells through regulation of mitochondrial, Akt/PKB and NFkappaB signaling pathways. Cancer Biol Ther 8:1632–1639
96. Preetha SP, Kanniappan M, Selvakumar E, Nagaraj M, Varalakshmi P (2006) Lupeol ameliorates aflatoxin B1-induced peroxidative hepatic damage in rats. Comp Biochem Physiol C Toxicol Pharmacol 143:333–339
97. Rahman K (2007) Studies on free radicals, antioxidants, and co-factors. Clin Interv Aging 2:219–236
98. Ramirez Apan AA, Perez-Castorena AL, de Vivar AR (2004) Anti-inflammatory constituents of *Mortonia greggii* Gray. Z Naturforsch C 59:237–243
99. Righi AA, Alves TR, Negri G, Marques LM, Breyer H, Salatino A (2011) Brazilian red propolis: unreported substances, antioxidant and antimicrobial activities. J Sci Food Agric 91:2363–2370
100. Ruiz-Montanez G, Ragazzo-Sanchez JA, Calderon-Santoyo M, Velazquez-de la Cruz G, de Leon JA, Navarro-Ocana A (2014) Evaluation of extraction methods for preparative scale obtention of mangiferin and lupeol from mango peels (*Mangifera indica* L.). Food Chem 159:267–272
101. Rutters F, Pilz S, Koopman AD, Rauh SP, Te Velde SJ, Stehouwer CD, Elders PJ, Nijpels G, Dekker JM (2014) The association between psychosocial stress and mortality is mediated by lifestyle and chronic diseases: the Hoorn Study. Soc Sci Med 118:166–172
102. Saleem M (2009) Lupeol, a novel anti-inflammatory and anti-cancer dietary triterpene. Cancer Lett 285:109–115
103. Saleem M, Afaq F, Adhami VM, Mukhtar H (2004) Lupeol modulates NF-kappaB and PI3K/Akt pathways and inhibits skin cancer in CD-1 mice. Oncogene 23:5203–5214
104. Saleem M, Alam A, Arifin S, Shah MS, Ahmed B, Sultana S (2001) Lupeol, a triterpene, inhibits early responses of tumor promotion induced by benzoyl peroxide in murine skin. Pharmacol Res 43:127–134
105. Saleem M, Kaur S, Kweon MH, Adhami VM, Afaq F, Mukhtar H (2005) Lupeol, a fruit and vegetable based triterpene, induces apoptotic death of human pancreatic adenocarcinoma cells via inhibition of Ras signaling pathway. Carcinogenesis 26:1956–1964
106. Saleem M, Kweon MH, Yun JM, Adhami VM, Khan N, Syed DN, Mukhtar H (2005) A novel dietary triterpene lupeol induces fas-mediated apoptotic death of androgen-sensitive prostate cancer cells and inhibits tumor growth in a xenograft model. Cancer Res 65:11203–11213
107. Saleem M, Maddodi N, Abu Zaid M, Khan N, bin Hafeez B, Asim M, Suh Y, Yun JM, Setaluri V, Mukhtar H (2008) Lupeol inhibits growth of highly aggressive human metastatic melanoma cells in vitro and in vivo by inducing apoptosis. Clin Cancer Res 14:2119–2127
108. Saleem M, Murtaza I, Tarapore RS, Suh Y, Adhami VM, Johnson JJ, Siddiqui IA, Khan N, Asim M, Hafeez BB, Shekhani MT, Li B, Mukhtar H (2009) Lupeol inhibits proliferation of human prostate cancer cells by targeting beta-catenin signaling. Carcinogenesis 30:808–817

109. Saleem M, Murtaza I, Witkowsky O, Kohl AM, Maddodi N (2009) Lupeol triterpene, a novel diet-based microtubule targeting agent: disrupts survivin/cFLIP activation in prostate cancer cells. Biochem Biophys Res Commun 388:576–582
110. Santiago LA, Mayor AB (2014) Lupeol: an antioxidant triterpene in *Ficus pseudopalma* Blanco (Moraceae). Asian Pac J Trop Biomed 4:109–118
111. Saratha V, Subramanian SP (2012) Lupeol, a triterpenoid isolated from *Calotropis gigantea* latex ameliorates the primary and secondary complications of FCA induced adjuvant disease in experimental rats. Inflammopharmacology 20:27–37
112. Siddique HR, Mishra SK, Karnes RJ, Saleem M (2011) Lupeol, a novel androgen receptor inhibitor: implications in prostate cancer therapy. Clin Cancer Res 17:5379–5391
113. Siddique HR, Saleem M (2011) Beneficial health effects of lupeol triterpene: a review of preclinical studies. Life Sci 88:285–293
114. Siveen KS, Nguyen AH, Lee JH, Li F, Singh SS, Kumar AP, Low G, Jha S, Tergaonkar V, Ahn KS, Sethi G (2014) Negative regulation of signal transducer and activator of transcription-3 signalling cascade by lupeol inhibits growth and induces apoptosis in hepatocellular carcinoma cells. Br J Cancer 111:1327–1337
115. Slimen IB, Najar T, Ghram A, Dabbebi H, Ben Mrad M, Abdrabbah M (2014) Reactive oxygen species, heat stress and oxidative-induced mitochondrial damage. A review. Int J Hyperth 30:513–523
116. Sousa AF, Pinto PC, Silvestre AJ, Pascoal Neto C (2006) Triterpenic and other lipophilic components from industrial cork byproducts. J Agric Food Chem 54:6888–6893
117. Srivastava S, Sonkar R, Mishra SK, Tiwari A, Balaramnavar VM, Mir S, Bhatia G, Saxena AK, Lakshmi V (2013) Antidyslipidemic and antioxidant effects of novel Lupeol-derived chalcones. Lipids 48:1017–1027
118. Stork G, Uyeo S, Wakamatsu T, Grieco P, Labovitz J (1971) Total synthesis of lupeol. J Am Chem Soc 93:4945–4947
119. Sudhahar V, Ashok Kumar S, Varalakshmi P, Sujatha V (2008) Protective effect of lupeol and lupeol linoleate in hypercholesterolemia associated renal damage. Mol Cell Biochem 317:11–20
120. Sudhahar V, Ashokkumar S, Varalakshmi P (2006) Effect of lupeol and lupeol linoleate on lipemic–hepatocellular aberrations in rats fed a high cholesterol diet. Mol Nutr Food Res 50:1212–1219
121. Sudhahar V, Kumar SA, Sudharsan PT, Varalakshmi P (2007) Protective effect of lupeol and its ester on cardiac abnormalities in experimental hypercholesterolemia. Vascul Pharmacol 46:412–418
122. Sudhahar V, Kumar SA, Varalakshmi P (2006) Role of lupeol and lupeol linoleate on lipemic-oxidative stress in experimental hypercholesterolemia. Life Sci 78:1329–1335
123. Sudhahar V, Kumar SA, Varalakshmi P, Sundarapandiyan R (2007) Mitigating role of lupeol and lupeol linoleate on hepatic lipemic-oxidative injury and lipoprotein peroxidation in experimental hypercholesterolemia. Mol Cell Biochem 295:189–198
124. Sudhahar V, Veena CK, Varalakshmi P (2008) Antiurolithic effect of lupeol and lupeol linoleate in experimental hyperoxaluria. J Nat Prod 71:1509–1512
125. Sudharsan PT, Mythili Y, Selvakumar E, Varalakshmi P (2005) Cardioprotective effect of pentacyclic triterpene, lupeol and its ester on cyclophosphamide-induced oxidative stress. Hum Exp Toxicol 24:313–318
126. Sudharsan PT, Mythili Y, Selvakumar E, Varalakshmi P (2006) Lupeol and its ester ameliorate the cyclophosphamide provoked cardiac lysosomal damage studied in rat. Mol Cell Biochem 282:23–29
127. Sudharsan PT, Mythili Y, Selvakumar E, Varalakshmi P (2006) Lupeol and its ester exhibit protective role against cyclophosphamide-induced cardiac mitochondrial toxicity. J Cardiovasc Pharmacol 47:205–210
128. Sultana N, Saify ZS (2012) Naturally occurring and synthetic agents as potential anti-inflammatory and immunomodulants. Antiinflammatory Antiallergy Agents Med Chem 11:3–19

129. Sultana S, Saleem M, Sharma S, Khan N (2003) Lupeol, a triterpene, prevents free radical mediated macromolecular damage and alleviates benzoyl peroxide induced biochemical alterations in murine skin. Indian J Exp Biol 41:827–831
130. Sunitha S, Nagaraj M, Varalakshmi P (2001) Hepatoprotective effect of lupeol and lupeol linoleate on tissue antioxidant defence system in cadmium-induced hepatotoxicity in rats. Fitoterapia 72:516–523
131. Surendra K, Corey EJ (2009) A short enantioselective total synthesis of the fundamental pentacyclic triterpene lupeol. J Am Chem Soc 131:13928–13929
132. Suzuki M, Ikekawa N (1966) Studies on the sterol of *Bombyx mori*. V. Lupeol in silkworm blood. Chem Pharm Bull (Tokyo) 14:1049–1051
133. Tarapore RS, Siddiqui IA, Adhami VM, Spiegelman VS, Mukhtar H (2013) The dietary terpene lupeol targets colorectal cancer cells with constitutively active Wnt/β-catenin signaling. Mol Nutr Food Res 57:1950–1958
134. Tarapore RS, Siddiqui IA, Saleem M, Adhami VM, Spiegelman VS, Mukhtar H (2010) Specific targeting of Wnt/β-catenin signaling in human melanoma cells by a dietary triterpene lupeol. Carcinogenesis 31:1844–1853
135. Thimmappa R, Geisler K, Louveau T, O'Maille P, Osbourn A (2014) Triterpene biosynthesis in plants. Annu Rev Plant Biol 65:225–257
136. Tomosaka H, Koshino H, Tajika T, Omata S (2001) Lupeol esters from the twig bark of Japanese pear (*Pyrus serotina* Rehd.) cv. Shinko. Biosci Biotechnol Biochem 65:1198–1201
137. Vasconcelos JF, Teixeira MM, Barbosa-Filho JM, Lucio AS, Almeida JR, de Queiroz LP, Ribeiro-Dos-Santos R, Soares MB (2008) The triterpenoid lupeol attenuates allergic airway inflammation in a murine model. Int Immunopharmacol 8:1216–1221
138. Vidya L, Lenin M, Varalakshmi P (2002) Evaluation of the effect of triterpenes on urinary risk factors of stone formation in pyridoxine deficient hyperoxaluric rats. Phytotherapy Res 16:514–518
139. von Ruesten A, Feller S, Bergmann MM, Boeing H (2013) Diet and risk of chronic diseases: results from the first 8 years of follow-up in the EPIC-Potsdam study. Eur J Clin Nutr 67:412–419
140. Wu XT, Liu JQ, Lu XT, Chen FX, Zhou ZH, Wang T, Zhu SP, Fei SJ (2013) The enhanced effect of lupeol on the destruction of gastric cancer cells by NK cells. Int Immunopharmacol 16:332–340
141. Xue Z, Li J, Cheng A, Yu W, Zhang Z, Kou X, Zhou F (2015) Structure identification of triterpene from the mushroom *Pleurotus eryngii* with inhibitory effects against breast cancer. Plant Foods Hum Nutr 70:291–296
142. Yasukawa K, Yu S, Yamanouchi S, Takido M, Akihisa T, Tamura T (1995) Some lupane-type triterpenes inhibit tumor promotion by 12-O-tetradecanoylphorbol-13-acetate in two-stage carcinogenesis in mouse skin. Phytomedicine 1:309–313
143. Yoder RA, Johnston JN (2005) A case study in biomimetic total synthesis: polyolefin carbocyclizations to terpenes and steroids. Chem Rev 105:4730–4756
144. Yokoe I, Azuma K, Hata K, Mukaiyama T, Goto T, Tsuka T, Imagawa T, Itoh N, Murahata Y, Osaki T, Minami S, Okamoto Y (2015) Clinical systemic lupeol administration for canine oral malignant melanoma. Mol Clin Oncol 3:89–92
145. Yokozawa T, Kim HY, Kim HJ, Okubo T, Chu DC, Juneja LR (2007) Amla (*Emblica officinalis* Gaertn.) prevents dyslipidaemia and oxidative stress in the ageing process. Br J Nutr 97:1187–1195
146. Yoon YP, Lee HJ, Lee DU, Lee SK, Hong JH, Lee CJ (2015) Effects of lupenone, lupeol, and taraxerol derived from *Adenophora triphylla* on the gene expression and production of airway MUC5AC mucin. Tuberc Respir Dis (Seoul) 78:210–217
147. Yunusov MS, Komissarova NG, Belenkova NG (2006) Method for preparing betulin and lupeol from white from white-stem brich bark. Russian. RUXXE7 RU 2270202 C1 20060220: 6

148. Zhang L, Tu Y, He W, Peng Y, Qiu Z (2015) A novel mechanism of hepatocellular carcinoma cell apoptosis induced by lupeol via brain-derived neurotrophic factor inhibition and glycogen synthase kinase 3 beta reactivation. Eur J Pharmacol 762:55–62
149. Zhang L, Zhang Y, Zhang L, Yang X, Lv Z (2009) Lupeol, a dietary triterpene, inhibited growth, and induced apoptosis through down-regulation of DR3 in SMMC7721 cells. Cancer Invest 27:163–170

Gingerol and Its Role in Chronic Diseases

Yasmin Anum Mohd Yusof

Abstract Since antiquity, ginger or *Zingiber officinale*, has been used by humans for medicinal purposes and as spice condiments to enhance flavor in cooking. Ginger contains many phenolic compounds such as gingerol, shogaol and paradol that exhibit antioxidant, anti-tumor and anti-inflammatory properties. The role of ginger and its constituents in ameliorating diseases has been the focus of study in the past two decades by many researchers who provide strong scientific evidence of its health benefit. This review discusses research findings and works devoted to gingerols, the major pungent constituent of ginger, in modulating and targeting signaling pathways with subsequent changes that ameliorate, reverse or prevent chronic diseases in human studies and animal models. The physical, chemical and biological properties of gingerols are also described. The use of ginger and especially gingerols as medicinal food derivative appears to be safe in treating or preventing chronic diseases which will benefit the common population, clinicians, patients, researchers, students and industrialists.

Keywords Gingerol · Signaling pathways · Chronic diseases · Physicochemical · Biological properties

1 Introduction

A multitude of research in the last two decades provides strong evidence that many phytochemicals found in medicinal plants, fruits and vegetables either taken alone or in combination may be used to prevent or treat chronic diseases [3, 16]. Most of these phytochemicals such as epigallocatechin-3-gallate [EGCC], curcumin in

Y.A. Mohd Yusof (✉)
Department of Biochemistry, Faculty of Medicine, Universiti Kebangsaan Malaysia, Level 17, Pre-Clinical Building, Jalan Yaacob Latif, Bandar Tun Razak, 56000 Cheras, Kuala Lumpur, Malaysia
e-mail: rahmatyasmin@yahoo.com

S.C. Gupta et al. (eds.), *Drug Discovery from Mother Nature*, Advances in Experimental Medicine and Biology 929,
DOI 10.1007/978-3-319-41342-6_8

turmeric and gingerol in ginger are known to have antioxidant, anti-inflammatory anti-proliferative, anti-invasion and anti-angiogenesis properties.

Zingiber officinale Roscoe Zingiberaceae or commonly known as ginger was first used by the Indians and Chinese to treat illnesses almost 5000 years ago [15]. The plant was initially cultivated in South East Asia before it is widely grown in many parts of tropical Asian countries as well as in western parts of the world [89]. The word ginger comes from the Middle English *gingivere*, while in Arabic it is known as *zanjabil*, in Hindi, *adarakha*, in Chinese, *jiang*, in Malay, *halia,* and in Indonesia, *jahe*. Across all cultures, ginger is known for its medicinal properties and as spice condiments to enhance flavor in cooking. Traditionally, it has been used for the treatment of many ailments including colds and flu, nausea, asthma, arthritis, gastrointestinal disturbances and migraines. Ginger is also used to prevent nausea resulting from chemotherapy, motion sickness and surgery [17, 20]. The medicinal and nutraceutical values of ginger root or rhizome can be attributed to the number of bioactive compounds including gingerols, shogaols, paradols, zerumbones and zingiberene [20, 104]. Gingerols, which are the main constituents of fresh ginger, have been shown to exhibit many biological properties beneficial for human health including cancer prevention or chemoprevention. The term cancer chemoprevention was first introduced by Sporn [106]. It was defined as the utilization of chemically active compounds to "reverse, suppress or prevent progression of disease from pre-invasive cancer to frank malignancy". However, as time progresses with a plethora of studies on chemoprevention, it is now best defined as the use of non-toxic substances, including dietary food substances, to modulate or target molecular processes in signaling pathways of cancer development or carcinogenesis, causing the death of cancer cells.

It is interesting to note that several population-based studies conducted showed that people from South East Asia have a lower risk of acquiring colon, gastrointestinal, prostate, breast and other cancers when compared to their western counterparts. It is highly possible that the constituents in their diet such as soy, ginger, onion, chilies and green tea play an important role in suppressing the early tumorigenesis process, which includes inflammation, hyper-proliferation, transformation and the final stages of carcinogenesis, angiogenesis and metastasis [31].

Similar to other herbal plants, ginger is known to have many health benefits from anecdotal accounts, resulting in a current population who is overly conscious of including herbal supplements as dietary regiments to maintain good health and to prevent from getting chronic diseases. However, it is of great importance to conduct scientific experiments and clinical trials to ensure the safety and efficacy of ginger and its bioactive components for human consumption [112].

There is a great deal of interest among researchers for the past years in the search for the mechanism of chemoprevention and therapeutic role of ginger and its constituents. Excellent work and reviews on the aspect of the physicochemical, pharmacological, medicinal and cancer preventing properties of ginger and its major compounds have been reported [8, 15–17, 20, 29, 41, 56, 94, 104, 105, 109]. This review will discuss scientific evidence from animal and human studies regarding the therapeutic properties of gingerols and how they modulate signaling pathways in preventing the growth of cancer cells and their nutraceutical effects in treating and preventing chronic diseases.

2 Physico–chemical Properties of Gingerol

The odor of ginger is attributed to the volatile oil or oleoresin which comprised of monoterpenoids (e.g., geraniol, curcumene, citral) and sesquiterpenoids (e.g., zerumbone, zingiberene, beta-bisabolene, zingiberol), while the non-volatile pungent component of ginger is primarily due to the presence of gingerols, shogaols and paradols which are vanillyl ketones or phenols (Fig. 1). Jolad et al. [55, 56] found that fresh ginger and commercially processed dry ginger contain over 115 compounds of which major constituents in fresh ginger are gingerol-related compounds with [6]-gingerol being the most abundant constituent. Other gingerols are present in lesser amounts, such as [4]-, [8]-, [10]- and [12]-gingerols and [6]-gingerdione [53]. Shogaols are formed from the corresponding gingerols during thermal processing and drying [122, 131]. Figure 1a shows the chemical structure of gingerol and shogaol isolated from the ginger rhizome.

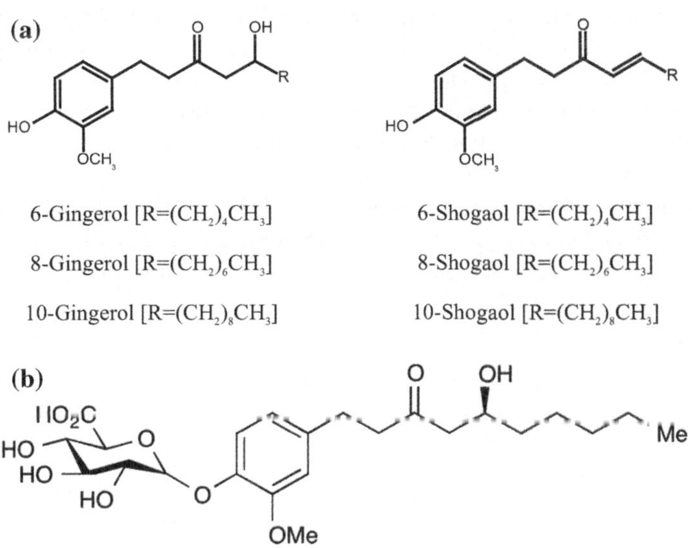

Fig. 1 **a** Chemical structures of the various gingerol and shogaol analogues isolated from ginger rhizome (reproduced with permission from [104]). **b** Chemical structure of (*S*)-6-gingerol-4′-O-β-glucuronide

2.1 Pharmacokinetic of [6]-Gingerol and its Metabolism

It is not clearly understood how [6]-gingerol is metabolized once it gets into the bloodstream. One study reported that it is rapidly cleared from rat plasma following intravenous administration of 3 mg/kg [6]-gingerol with total body clearance of 16.8 ml/min/kg [29]. It was also reported to be enzymatically metabolized to gingerdiol in cell suspensions of rat liver [110]. The pharmacokinetics of [6]-, [8]-, [10]-gingerol and [6]-shogaol were examined in human subjects by Zick et al. [132] who gave them ginger starting from 100 mg to 2 g in escalating manner to different groups. No participant had detectable free [6]-, [8]-, [10]-gingerol or [6]-shogaol in their serum, but instead [6]-, [8]-, [10]-gingerol and [6]-shogaol glucuronides were detected. The metabolic fate of [6]-gingerol was also investigated by Nakazawa and Ohsawa [81] and a primary metabolite, (*S*)-[6]-gingerol-4′-O-β-glucuronide, was detected in the bile of rats given oral administration of [6]-gingerol, suggesting the conjugation and oxidation reactions of its phenolic side chain (Fig. 1b).

In another study, [6]-, [8]-, and [10]-gingerols from natural ginger extract were shown to have higher bioavailability compared to gingerols in a synthetically prepared ginger mix and the gingerols were detected in feces upon intravenous administration confirming hepatobiliary elimination [39]. Bhattarai et al. [13] reported that [6]-shogaol and [6]-gingerol undergo first-order reversible dehydration and hydration reactions under an acidic condition to form [6]-gingerol and [6]-shogaol, respectively, in simulated gastric and intestinal fluids after prolonged incubation. Their study indicates that gingerol and shogaol interconvert between one and another in the intestine. [6]-Gingerol was shown to have greater stability than [6]-shogaol whereby after 21 days of incubation only 30 % of gingerol had degraded compared to 80 % of shogaol.

During drying or thermal processing, gingerols being thermally labile due to the presence of beta hydroxy group in the structure either dehydrate to the corresponding shogaols or are degraded by a retro-aldol reaction to zingerone and the corresponding aldehyde [29].

2.2 Biosynthesis of Gingerols

In the laboratory, gingerols can be synthesized in several ways. The synthesis of [6]-gingerol [(5S)-5-hydroxy-1-(4-hydroxy-3-methoxyphenyl) decan-3-one, MW $C_{17}H_{26}O_4$], begins from the precursor amino acid phenylalanine which is then converted to p-coumaric acid, followed by conversion to dihydroferulic acid and subsequently to 6-gingerdione and finally to [6]-gingerol [27]. An alternative pathway was suggested by Ramirez-Ahumada et al. [98] using the same starting material, phenylalanine. Some key enzymes that are involved include phenylalanine ammonia lyase (PAL), *p*-coumaroyl shikimate transferase (CST), *p*-coumaroyl quinate transferase (CQT), caffeic acid *O*-methyltransferase (COMT) and

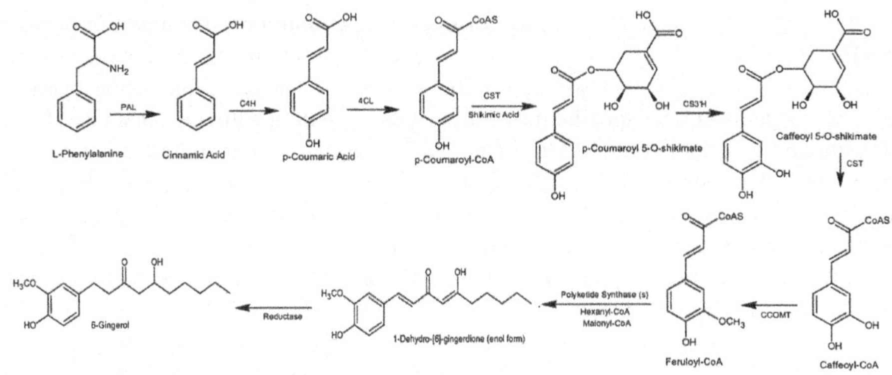

Fig. 2 Biosynthesis of [6]-gingerol as proposed by Ramirez-Ahumada et al. [98]

caffeoyl-CoA-*O*-methyltransferase (CCOMT), and reductase (Fig. 2). Using eugenol as starting material, Kumar et al. [68] synthesized [6]-, [7]- and [9]-gingerols, producing the nitro-derivative of eugenol which then reacts with terminal alkenes to form isoxazolines, which then yields the corresponding gingerols through catalytic hydrogenation with Raney nickel [68]. Ma et al. [76] have developed an enantioselective approach for the synthesis of (+)-(*S*)-[6], [8]- and [10]-gingerols, which included an organo-catalytic enantioselective aldol as a key step for efficient production of the gingerols.

3 Modulation of Cell Signaling Pathways by Gingerol

An accumulating body of research data indicates that many cancers can be prevented by diet mostly attributed to the presence of phytochemicals known to have antioxidant, anti-inflammatory and anticancer properties. Some of these compounds act alone or in combination in modulating the genes and proteins of the signaling pathways. Therefore, identifying the specific signal transduction pathways, protein and gene targets, and mechanisms explaining the properties of various phytochemicals may provide effective therapeutic interventions or methods of disease prevention.

Signal transduction is the process by which information from an extracellular signal is transmitted from the plasma membrane into the cell eliciting an intracellular cascade of signaling molecules to stimulate highly orchestrated cellular and nuclear responses. Interestingly, modulation of cell signaling pathways is not a feature of carcinogens alone but is also shared by chemotherapeutic and chemopreventive agents. Carcinogens direct cells toward uncontrolled proliferation and malignancy with changes seen such as activation of oncogenes, inhibition of tumor suppressor genes, induction of the inflammatory response, induction of angiogenesis and upregulation of genes responsible for the survival of cancer cells, while chemopreventive agents target specific molecules of the signaling pathways that have been deregulated by tumor cells development and consequently inducing death of cancer cells. The chemopreventive mechanism of many dietary compounds is shown to reverse, ameliorate or modulate the damage triggered by carcinogens with subsequent cellular responses including apoptosis and/or cell cycle arrest [3, 14, 88].

Gingerols like other dietary bioactive components were reported to target and modulate multiple cell signaling pathways in the prevention (chemoprevention) and treatment of cancer and other chronic diseases. Molecular targets of gingerols include protein kinases (MAPK, JNK, IKK, AKT, PI3 K), transcription factors (NF-κB, activator protein-1 (AP-1)], apoptosis and anti-apoptosis proteins (Bcl-2, Bcl-XL, caspases,), tumor suppressor gene p53, growth factors (EGF, TGF, PDGF, TNF), metastasis proteins (COX2, iNOS, MMPs, VEGF) and cell cycle proteins (cyclin D1, CDK 1, 2, 4, 6, 7) [3]. A summary of the molecular targets of gingerol in modulating signaling pathways associated with cancer is presented in Table 1.

Table 1 Molecular targets of gingerol in modulating signaling pathways

Signaling proteins/pathways	Effect	References
MAPK, NF-κB, COX2	[6]-Gingerol inhibits TPA-induced COX2 by blocking p38 MAPK/NF-κB pathway and suppressing IκBα degradation and p65 nuclear translocation in mouse skin carcinogenesis	Kim et al. [63]
	[6]-Gingerol inhibits TPA-induced COX-2 expression, by suppressing NF-κB DNA binding in mouse skin carcinogenesis	Kim et al. [64]
	[8]-Gingerol inhibits melanogenesis through downregulation of MAPK and PKA pathways in murine melanoma cells	Huang et al. [45]
MAPK/PI3K/Akt/NF-κB	[6]-Gingerol inhibits Hep3B hepatoma cells invasion via inhibition of MAPK/PI3 K/Akt signaling pathways and inactivation of NF-κB	Weng et al. [120]
NF-κB/COX2/AP-1	[6]-Gingerol inhibits NF-κB, AP-1, COX2, MAPK, pJNK and pERK in pancreatic tumor cells	Park et al. [93]
NF-κB/TNF α	Ginger oleoresin (gingerol as major compound) suppressed NF-κB and TNF α elevation in liver cancer-induced rats	Habib et al. [41]
ERK.NFκB/Snail	[6]-Gingerol strengthens tight junction proteins in invasive human pancreatic cancer cells through inactivation of ERK/NF-κB snail	Kim and Kim [62]
AP-1	[6]-gingerol inhibits EGF-induced cell transformation and AP-1 activation in mouse epidermal cells and human skin keratinocytes	Bode et al. [18]

(continued)

Table 1 (continued)

Signaling proteins/pathways	Effect	References
Cyclin D1, Cyclin A, Cyclin B/β-catenin	[6]-Gingerol suppressed proliferation of HCT116 colon cancer cells via induction of apoptosis, inhibition of cyclin D1 and β-catenin	Lee et al. [73]
	[6]-Gingerol induced G2/M phase arrest, increased expressions of p27Kip1 and p21Cip1, decreased cyclin A, cyclin B1 and CDK1 levels in LoVo colon cancer cells	Lin et al. [75]
Apoptosis/MAPK/ERK/AP-1	[6]-Gingerol induced apoptotic cell death in mutant p53-expressing pancreatic cancer cells but not in wild-type HPAC cells	Park et al. [93]
	[6]-Gingerol inhibits cellular proliferation and induces apoptosis via activation of caspases 3, 7, 8 and 9 and downregulates PMA-induced activation of ERK1/2, JNK, MAPK/AP-1 in SW-48 human colon cancer cell line	Radhakrishnan et al. [97]
	[10]-Gingerol induces mitochondrial apoptosis through activation of MAPK/JNK/P38 and ERK pathway in HCT116 colon cancer cells and increases Bax/Bcl-2, caspases 3 and 9	Ryu and Chung [102]
p53/apoptosis	[6]-Gingerol inhibits growth of A431 epidermoid cancer cells and induces release of cytochrome c and upregulates Apaf-1 protein and caspases	Nigam et al. [83]
	[6]-Gingerol increases p53 and Bax levels in benzo [a]pyrene-induced mouse skin carcinogenesis and increases Apaf-1 and cytochrome c release	Nigam et al. [84]
	[6]-Gingerol decreases expression of anti-apoptotic proteins (survivin, c-FLIP, Bcl-2 and XIAP) and increases pro-apoptotic protein, Bax and truncate Bid in glioblastoma cells	Lee et al. [70]
	[6]-gingerol induces apoptosis of gastric cancer cells by increasing caspase 3/7 activation, inhibiting TRAIL-induced NF-κB activation	Prasad and Tyagi [95]
mTOR/Wnt/β-catenin	Combined ginger extract and Gelam honey inhibits mTOR/Wnt/β-catenin pathway in HT29 colon cancer cells	Wee et al. [116]

3.1 MAPK

The mitogen-activated protein kinases (MAPKs) comprise a family of extracellular signal-regulated protein kinases(ERKs), c-Jun N-terminal kinases/(JNKs) and p38 kinases which mediate a succession of signaling cascades activated by outside stimuli such as tumor promoters, (e.g., tetradecanoyl phorbol-13-acetate, TPA), growth factors such as epidermal growth factor (EGF) and platelet-derived growth factor (PDGF) which controls growth, proliferation, differentiation, migration and apoptosis [24]. Deregulation of MAP kinases and/or their target molecules is observed in a variety of human cancers and experimental animals.

3.2 ERK/RAS/RAF

Activation of RAS-RAF proteins by tyrosine kinases-mediated extracellular signals leads to the phosphorylation and activation of ERK and its nuclear translocation where it phosphorylates a variety of transcription factors that are important in tumor and cancer development. The transcription factors include activator protein-1 (AP-1) and nuclear factor-kappaB (NF-κ B), which then upregulates COX-2, TNF, cyclin D1, MMPs and iNOS gene products known to stimulate proliferation, inflammation, angiogenesis, invasion and inhibition of apoptosis in tumorigenesis [3, 82, 96, 108]. Park et al. [93] investigated the chemopreventive effect of [6]-gingerol on HPAC (wild type) and BxPC-3 (p53 deficient) pancreatic tumor cell lines and found that protein expression analysis of MAPK, pJNK and pERK was inhibited in both cell types after [6]-gingerol treatment, while AKT phosphorylation was increased in HPAC but not in BxPC-3 cells. Interestingly, we have shown that fresh ginger extract which contains gingerols induced death of HT29 colon cancer cells by downregulating KRAS, ERK, AKT and NF-κB (p65) genes [111]. Weng et al. [120] revealed that [6]-gingerol inhibits Hep3B hepatoma cells invasion by blocking of MAPK/PI3 K/Akt signaling pathways. In a separate study by Radhakrishnan et al. [97], [6]-gingerol was shown to downregulate phorbol myristate acetate (PMA)-induced phosphorylation of ERK1/2 and JNK MAP kinases but with very little effect on phosphorylation of p38 MAP kinase in colon cancer cells. Kim and Kim [62] demonstrated that [6]-gingerol regulates and strengthens tight junction-related proteins and suppresses NF-κB/Snail and ERK pathway of human pancreatic duct cell-derived cancer cell line, PANC-1.

3.3 NF-κB/COX2

NF-κB and COX2 are both involved in inflammatory processes, and there is increasing evidence supporting that chronic inflammation may lead to chronic diseases including cancer development of many organs such as skin, stomach, colon, breast, prostate and pancreas [3, 77]. NF-κB is a family of closely related protein dimers of five subunits: p65 (RelA), c-Rel, RelB, p50/NF-κB1 and p52/NF-κB2. NF-κB resides in the cytoplasm bound to specific inhibitory proteins, IκB families. It can be translocated into the nucleus when activated by cytokines, inflammatory stimuli and other oxidative stress molecules. Once in the nucleus, it will bind to a specific region of DNA and induces many genes that promote cellular proliferation, transformation, invasion, metastases and genes which suppress apoptosis, leading to a variety of chronic diseases including cancer. Several dietary agents including gingerols have been shown to be potent inhibitors of NF-κB [3, 77].

Cyclooxygenases (COX) are prostaglandin H synthase, which converts arachidonic acid (AA) into prostaglandins. Two isoforms of COX are COX-1 and

COX-2. The latter has been associated with tumorigenesis and is overexpressed in premalignant and malignant cancers of many organs such as colon, skin, stomach and esophagus [108]. COX-2 has been recognized as a molecular target for many anti-inflammatory as well as chemopreventive agents. Kim et al. [63] found that [6]-gingerol inhibits TPA-induced COX-2 expression in mouse skin by blocking the p38 MAPK-NF-κB signaling pathway with a corresponding inhibition of Iκ Bα degradation, p65 nuclear translocation and its interaction with cAMP response element-binding (CREB) protein, a transcriptional coactivator of NF-κB.

3.4 *AP-1*

Activator protein-1 is a transcription factor composed of homodimers and or heterodimers of Jun, Fos, ATF (activating transcription factor) and MAF (musculoaponeurotic fibrosarcoma) protein families [10]. AP-1 plays a major role in cell transformation and is crucial in tumor promotion, progression and metastasis [30]. It is associated with the regulation of genes involved in apoptosis and proliferation and may promote cell proliferation by activating the cyclin D1 gene and repressing tumor suppressor genes, such as p53, p21cip1/WAF1 and p16 [3].

Bode et al. [18] found that [6]-gingerol inhibited EGF-induced cell transformation and AP-1 activation in mouse epidermal cells and AP-1 activation in human skin keratinocytes, while Radhakrishnan et al. [97] recently showed that [6]-gingerol downregulated phorbol myristate acetate (PMA)-induced activation of AP-1 transcription factor.

3.5 *PI3K/AKT*

Phosphatidylinositol-3 kinases, PI3Ks, constitute a lipid kinase family characterized by their ability to phosphorylate inositol phospholipids to generate the second messenger phosphatidylinositol-3,4,5-trisphosphate (PI3) which will phosphorylate and activate Akt kinase. Akt/PKB is a serine/threonine protein kinase that functions as a critical regulator of cell survival and proliferation. In mammals, there are three known isoforms of the Akt kinase: PKBα/Akt1, PKBβ/Akt2 and PKBγ/Akt3 [107]. Activation of Akt/PKB was evident in various types of cancers [23, 26]. Activated Akt promotes cell survival by activating the NF-κB signaling pathway [87] and by inhibiting apoptosis [21]. Park et al. [93] showed that [6]-gingerol induced mostly apoptotic death in the mutant p53-expressing pancreatic cancer cells, while no signs of early apoptosis were detected in wild-type p53-expressing cells which were related to the increased phosphorylation of AKT.

Treatment of MDA–MB–231 breast cancer cells with [10]-gingerol inhibited cell proliferation through downregulation of cyclin-dependent kinases and cyclins, and G1 phase arrest. In addition, 10-gingerol treatment blocked cell invasion in response to mitogenic stimulation which is mediated through inactivation of Akt and p38 MAPK activity, and suppression of epidermal growth factor receptor expression [57]. Weng et al. [121] demonstrated that [6]-gingerol inhibits Hep3B hepatoma cells invasion via blocking phosphorylation of mitogen-activated protein kinase (MAPK) and PI3K/Akt signaling, inactivation of NF-κB and preventing the translocation of NF-κB and STAT3 into the nucleus.

3.6 β-Catenin/Wnt Pathway

Aberrant Wnt signaling pathway occurs in many types of cancers, predominantly in colorectal cancers [11, 37]. Cytoplasmic β-catenin levels are normally kept low through continuous proteosome-mediated degradation by adenomatous polyposis coli (APC)/glycogen synthase kinase-3β (GSK-3β)/Ax in complex. When Wnt signal is initiated in tumor promotion, the degradation of β-catenin is inhibited and levels of β-catenin build up in the cytoplasm and nucleus, which then interacts with transcription factors for the regulation of genes involved in tumor progression [113]. Lee et al. [73] reported that [6]-gingerol suppressed cellular proliferation and induced apoptosis and G1 cell cycle arrest with subsequent suppression of the *cyclin D1* gene in the human colorectal cell line, HCT116. The latter event is associated with inhibition of translocation of β-catenin into the nucleus and increased proteolysis of cyclin D1 protein.

3.7 Cell Cycle

The loss of the regulation of cell cycle is implicated in many types of cancer. Cyclin D1 is the rate-limiting factor in the progression of cells through the G1 phase of the cell cycle. Overexpression of cyclin D1 and cyclin-dependent kinases is a features of tumorigenesis [28]. [6]-Gingerol has been shown to inhibit progression of the cell cycle of human colon cancer cells by downregulating the expression of cyclin D1 [73]. In addition, Park et al. [93] reported that [6]-gingerol arrested the cell cycle in G1 phase by decreasing cyclin A and Cdk proteins in both wild-type and p53-deficient pancreatic tumor cell lines.

3.8 Apoptosis

Apoptosis is a form of programmed cell death triggered by outside stimuli such as anticancer drugs, various cytokines and natural food components which activate "death receptors" such as Fas ligand receptors and tumor necrosis factor receptors (extrinsic pathway), leading to proteolytic cleavage and activation of initiator caspases (caspases 8, 9, 10). The release of cytochrome c will activate executioner caspases (caspases 3, 6, 7) (mitochondrial or intrinsic pathway), leading to cell death. Phytochemicals known to inhibit NF-κB or AP-1 can suppress cellular proliferation and induce cell toward apoptosis [12, 36]. Deregulated apoptotic mechanisms have been implicated in numerous pathologic diseases including Alzheimer's disease, autoimmunity (lupus, type 1 diabetes, rheumatoid arthritis), infectious diseases, cancer, cardiovascular and osteoporosis. Accumulating evidence indicates that dietary bioactive agents can trigger specific targets of apoptosis pathway of cancer cells causing its death [99]. Radhakrishnan et al. [97] showed that [6]-gingerol inhibited proliferation and induced apoptosis of colon cancer cell line, SW-48, via activation of caspases 3, 7, 8 and 9, while Ryu and Chung [102] reported that [10]-gingerol-treated HCT116 colon cancer cells exhibited an increased ratio of Bax/Bcl-2 (ratio of pro-apoptosis to anti-apoptosis protein), resulting in the activation of caspases 3 and 9 indicating an apoptosis event. In addition, they found that [10]-gingerol induced apoptosis of the colon cancer cells was accompanied by phosphorylation of the mitogen-activated protein kinase (MAPKs) family, c-Jun N-terminal kinase (JNK), p38 MAPK (p38) and extracellular signal-regulated kinase (ERK).

3.9 Tumor Suppressor Gene P53

p53 is a transcription factor, which also plays an important role as a regulator, or SOS gene in signal transduction pathway by removing damaged DNA, thus suppressing the tumor formation. It activates transcription of downstream genes, p21WAF1 and Bax to induce apoptosis of tumor cells [115]. [6]-Gingerol was shown to increase p53 and Bax levels, which were downregulated, by the carcinogen benzo[a]-pyrene in mouse skin carcinogenesis model. [6]-Gingerol treatment also resulted in the release of cytochrome c, caspases activation and increase in apoptotic protease-activating factor-1 (Apaf-1) as mechanism of apoptosis induction [84].

3.10 mTOR

The mammalian target of rapamycin, mTOR, is the key factor in regulating cell growth and proliferation. The pathway is activated in tumorigenesis, due to mutations in certain proteins closely related to mTOR pathway, including amplification of PIK3CA gene, loss or inactivation of phosphatase and tensin homolog (PTEN), mutations of TSC1/2 complex and p53 [38]. mTOR/Wnt/B-catenin pathways share the same Akt upstream target. Akt activation by PI3K mediates the activation and inhibition of several targets which include the three pathways: mTOR, GSK3/Akt and Wnt/Beta catenin, leading to increase in target genes, protein synthesis and inhibition of apoptosis [35]. The search for mTOR inhibitors could be potential therapeutic agents against cancer. There are yet no data specifically showing gingerol as an inhibitor of mTOR. However, [6]-shogaol, the major constituent of dried ginger, was shown to modulate AKT/mTOR pathway by blocking the activation of AKT and downstream targets, mTOR, fork head transcription factors (FKHR) and glycogen synthase kinase-3beta (GSK-3 β) in human non-small cell lung cancer A549 cells. Phosphorylation of mTOR's downstream targets, p70 ribosomal protein S6 kinase (p70S6 kinase) and 4E-BP1, was also diminished. [6]-Shogaol was also shown by the same group to inhibit cell proliferation by inducing autophagic cell death and not by apoptosis [46]. Interestingly, our laboratory has shown that when ginger extract was combined with honey, gene expressions of Akt, mTOR, Raptor, Rictor, β-catenin, Gsk3β, Tcf4 and cyclin D1 were downregulated, while cytochrome C and caspase 3 genes were shown to be upregulated in HT29 colon cancer cells [116].

4 Role of Gingerol in Chronic Diseases

Many diseases have been associated with aberrantly regulated signaling pathways ultimately leading to inflammation, hyper-proliferation or inhibition of apoptosis and propagation of diseases. Chemoprevention by plant-based compounds rich in phytochemicals provides a promising approach in the search for a safe therapeutic mode of treatment. Gingerols have been shown to target many of the pathways described above in combating many diseases such as cancer, cardiovascular disease, diabetes and gastrointestinal disturbances.

4.1 Role of Gingerol in Cancer

An accumulating body of scientific evidence indicates that many cancers are preventable since diet and nutrition are key factors in the modulation of cancer risk. Compelling scientific evidence suggests that the chemopreventive action of ginger and its natural components is attributed to the polyphenolic antioxidants properties. The mechanism of action of ginger and its bioactive components has been associated with inhibiting proliferation and inducing apoptosis [71] inducing cell cycle arrest [2, 73, 111] and suppressing inflammation by inactivating NF-κB activity [41, 93, 111].

4.1.1 Skin Cancer

One of the earlier studies using ginger as an anticancer agent was in mouse model skin carcinogenesis [59]. They reported that [6]-gingerol applied to DMBA initiated skin cancer in SENCAR mice afforded a significant protection against skin cancer with lower tumor burden. Nigam et al. [83] reported that [6]-gingerol inhibited the growth of human epidermoid A431 cells by generating reactive oxygen species (ROS). The increase in ROS led to perturbation of mitochondrial membrane potential with the release of cytochrome c and upregulation of Apaf-1, subsequently leading to caspases cascade induction indicating an apoptotic event. Their study suggests that [6]-gingerol can be effectively used for the treatment of skin cancer.

A similar study by the same researchers on benzo[a]pyrene-induced skin cancer in mice showed that [6]-gingerol given prior and after benzo[a]pyrene treatment for 32 weeks was able to reduce the number of skin tumors and volume, increased the suppressed p53 and Bax levels, while decreasing the expression of Bcl-2 and survivin. [6]-Gingerol treatment also resulted in apoptosis event, with release of cytochrome c, caspases activation and increase in apoptotic protease-activating factor-1 (Apaf-1) [84].

4.1.2 Brain Cancer

Glioblastoma multiforme (GBM) is the most lethal, aggressive and malignant astrocytoma of primary brain tumors in adults. [6]-Gingerol was shown by Lee et al. [72] to induce TRAIL-mediated apoptosis of glioblastoma. The bioactive compound of ginger increased death receptor (DR) 5 levels in a p53-dependent manner and decreased the expression of anti-apoptotic proteins (survivin, c-FLIP, Bcl-2 and XIAP) and increased pro-apoptotic protein, Bax and truncate Bid, by generating reactive oxygen species (ROS). The study suggests the possibility of combination therapy of TRAIL and [6]-gingerol in TRAIL-resistant glioblastoma tumor therapy.

4.1.3 Gastrointestinal Cancer

GI cancer is defined as the cancer of organs of the digestive system including the esophagus, gallbladder, liver, pancreas, stomach, small intestine, large intestine, rectum and anus [95]. In vitro study showed that [6]-gingerol induced apoptosis of gastric cancer cells by increasing caspase-3/7 activation. The induction of apoptosis by [6]-gingerol was mediated through downregulation of cytosolic inhibitor of apoptosis (cIAP)-1 and inhibiting TRAIL-induced NF-κB activation [49, 95].

Mahady et al. [78] tested the effects of [6]-, [8]- and [10]-gingerols on 19 strains of *Helicobacter pylori* (HP) including the most sensitive strain 5 CagA+. *H. pylori* is the first bacterium to be classified as a Group 1 carcinogen which causes gastric cancer in humans by the International Agency for Research on Cancer [47, 103]. Infection from CagA+ HP strains significantly increases the risk of developing severe gastric inflammation, atrophic gastritis and non-cardia gastric adenocarcinoma. Their study demonstrated that [10]-gingerol was the most active in inhibiting the growth of all HP strains with MIC of 6.25 μg/ml (range 0.78–50.0 μg/ml), followed by [6]- and [8]-gingerols with MIC of 12.5 μg/ml (range 3.125–100.0 μg/ml) [78].

4.1.4 Liver Cancer

Yagihashi et al. [124] reported that [6]-gingerol inhibited both proliferation and invasion of rat ascites hepatoma AH109A cells. Cell cycle arrest and apoptosis induction are the main causes of the protective effect of [6]-gingerol in these cancerous cells. Ginger oleoresin was demonstrated by Yusof et al. [129] to have a chemopreventive effect against liver cancer in rats, while Habib et al. [41] elucidated that the chemopreventive mechanism of ginger oleoresin was by ameliorating inflammation with reduction in elevated expressions of NF-κB and TNF-α in liver cancer cells. In human HepG2 hepatoma cells, [6]-gingerol induced apoptosis through release of cathepsin D which preceded ROS generation and cytochrome C release from mitochondria [125].

Anti-invasive activity of [6]-gingerol was seen in HepG2 cells, whereby it inhibited the migratory and invasive abilities of phorbol 12-myristate 13-acetate (PMA) mediated by inhibition of MMP-9, urokinase-type plasminogen activator (uPA) and increased expression of tissue inhibitor metalloproteinase protein-1 (TIMP-1). The mechanism of invasion and metastasis was elucidated via inhibition of MAPK and PI3 k/Akt pathways and NF-κB and STAT3 activities [120].

4.1.5 Pancreatic Cancer

Kim and Kim [62] demonstrated that [6]-gingerol regulates tight junction-related proteins and suppresses invasion and metastasis of pancreatic cancer, PANC-1 cells through ERK/NF-κB/Snail signal transduction pathway. In a separate experiment, Akimoto et al. [5] demonstrated that the ginger extract suppressed cell cycle progression and consequently induced the death of human pancreatic cancer cell lines, including Panc-1 cells. The underlying mechanism entailed autosis, a recently characterized form of cell death, but not apoptosis or necroptosis.

4.1.6 Colon Cancer

Colorectal cancer (CRC) is the third most commonly diagnosed cancer among males after lung and prostate cancer, whereas for female, CRC is the second common cancer after breast [51]. A multistep genetic model of colorectal carcinogenesis involving mutation of the APC gene, Kras, PI3K and Wnt/β-catenin and the cross talk between these pathways has been suggested to play a major role in deregulation of cell cycle progression, evasion of apoptosis, induction of genetic instability and enhanced invasiveness and metastasis [80, 123]. Reduced rates of apoptosis in colonic mucosa are associated with an increased risk of colorectal cancer. Treatment of human colon cancer cell LoVo with [6]-gingerol induced significant G2/M phase arrest with increased negative cell cycle regulators p27Kip1 and p21Cip1 while diminishing the level of cyclin A, cyclin B1 and CDK1 [75].

In our laboratory, we showed that fresh ginger extract which contains gingerols induced cell death of colon cancer cells, HT29, associated with upregulation of caspase 9, the pro-apoptosis gene accompanied by downregulation of Bcl-xL, the anti-apoptotic gene. Interestingly, the observed downregulation of the genes involved in cancer pathways, KRAS, ERK, AKT and NF-κB (p65) genes correlated with concomitant upregulation of the inhibitory gene Iκ Bα [111].

In vivo study showed that [6]-gingerol is an effective inhibitor of azoxymethane (AOM)-induced intestinal carcinogenesis in rats by inhibiting the multiplicity of adenocarcinomas after 20-week administration of AOM [128]. Using a reverse-docking approach, [6]-gingerol was shown to suppress colon cancer growth by targeting and inhibiting the activity leukotriene A4 hydrolase, from the leukotrienes family of the arachidonic acid metabolism [52]. Leukotrienes have been implicated in human cancer and chronic inflammation [40].

4.2 *Coronary Heart Disease*

Besides its major role as cancer preventive agent, many scientific findings indicated the protective role of gingerols in other chronic diseases such as cardiovascular, diabetes and asthma.

In 1987, Kobayashi and colleagues found that [8]-gingerol at low concentrations (0.001–0.03 μM) was able to exert a positive inotropic effect on isolated left atrium of guinea pig, suggesting that it can act as a cardiotonic [66]. A study by Maier et al. [79] attested that [10]-gingerol at 0.1 μM exerts a positive inotropic effect by increasing sarcoplasmic reticulum $Ca2^{+}$ uptake in human myocardial homogenates.

Anti-platelet therapy is an effective approach for preventing coronary heart disease. [8]-Gingerol, [8]-shogaol and [8]-paradol were found to be effective anti-platelet aggregation agents better than aspirin. The mechanism underlying AA-induced platelet aggregation inhibition may be related to attenuation of COX-1/Tx synthase enzymatic activity [85]. Gingerols and related phenylalkanol analogs (gingerols 1–7) were shown to inhibit arachidonic acid (AA)-induced platelet serotonin release and aggregation in vitro comparable to aspirin. The mechanism was suggested to be via an effect on cyclooxygenase (COX) activity in platelets [67].

Kamato et al. [58] found that [6]-gingerol (*S*-enantiomer) exhibited a potent anti-atherosclerotic activity by blocking the incorporation of $[^{35}S]$-Met/Cys into proteoglycans and total proteins and inhibiting TGF-β-stimulated proteoglycan synthesis in human vascular smooth muscle cells.

4.3 Asthma

Asthma is a chronic disease characterized by involvement of inflammation and hypersensitivity of airway smooth muscle cells to different substances that induce spasms. Ginger has been used for centuries in treating respiratory illnesses. Gingerols markedly decreased the recruitment of eosinophils to the lungs in ovalbumin-sensitized mice and also suppressed the Th2 cell-driven response to allergen [4]. In isolated human and guinea pig tracheas, [6]-gingerol, [8]-gingerol and [6]-shogaol induced rapid relaxation of precontracted airway smooth muscle (ASM). In A/J mice, the nebulization of [8]-gingerol (100 μM), 15 min before methacholine challenge, significantly attenuated airway resistance. [114].

4.4 Diabetes

Diabetes is a metabolic disorder, and it is one of the major global health problems worldwide. It is caused by low blood insulin level or insulin resistance of target organs. Ginger and the bioactive compounds have been implicated in controlling complications of diabetes via anti-hyperglycemic effect [7]. The exact mechanism of action of ginger in diabetes control is not fully understood, but a few studies suggest that it might be due to the inhibition of oxidative stress and suppression of anti-inflammatory process, thus reducing the severity of associated complications. Oral administration of ethanolic extract of ginger significantly decreased fasting blood glucose level in STZ-treated type 1 diabetic rat model [86]. However, Abdul Sani et al. [1] showed that ginger oleoresin did not have any hypoglycemic effect on STZ-induced diabetic rats, but instead it ameliorated the oxidative stress by restoring the ratio of reduced glutathione: oxidized glutathione and catalase activity in diabetic rats.

Chakraborty et al. [22] reported that [6]-gingerol was able to reduce blood sugar and oxidative stress in sodium arsenite-induced type 2 diabetes mice. They implicated that the hypoglycemic effect of [6]-gingerol is due to stimulation of superoxide dismutase, catalase, glutathione peroxidase and GSH activities. Treatment with [6]-gingerol also resulted in increased plasma insulin levels in mice by improving impaired insulin signaling.

5 Biological Activities of Gingerol

Although it is widely known for culinary uses, ginger extract and its major bioactive components have been proven to exhibit biological activities that are of medicinal values in animal and human studies.

5.1 *In Vitro Biological Activities of Gingerol*

5.1.1 Antioxidant Activity

Oxidative stress imposed by reactive oxygen species (ROS) is linked to the pathophysiology associated with atherosclerosis, neurodegenerative diseases and cancer. Oxidative stress is a result of an imbalance between the generation of ROS from normal cellular metabolism or from exogenous stimuli and their removal. Endogenous enzyme antioxidants such as glutathione peroxidase (GPx), superoxide dismutase (SOD), catalase and non-enzyme antioxidants such as vitamins, polyphenols, flavonoids and minerals found in food work best to remove the ROS generated. However, an excess of ROS causes an imbalance between ROS generation and the antioxidant capacity to remove them, leading to an electrophilic attack of ROS to proteins, DNA and lipid, resulting in cellular and tissue damage.

Many of the naturally dietary compounds found in fruits and vegetables such as resveratrol in grapes, EGCG in green tea, curcumin in turmeric and lycopene in tomatoes exhibit high antioxidant activities that may potentially be chemoprotective against a variety of cancers and other chronic diseases [3]. The antioxidative properties of ginger and its components have been explored in various in vitro and in vivo test systems. [6]-Gingerol, [8]-gingerol, [10]-gingerol and [6]-shogaol exhibited substantial scavenging activities against 1,1-diphenyl-2-picrylhydrazyl, DPPH radical, superoxide radical and hydroxyl radical. The free radical scavenging activity is dose dependent with the concentration of gingerol [32].

Two separate studies by Park et al. [92] and Huang et al. [44] revealed the antioxidant effect of [6]-gingerol in scavenging ROS in TGF-β1-induced nasal polyp-derived fibroblasts and B16F10 murine melanoma cells, respectively. In a separate study by Ippoushi et al. [48], [6]-gingerol was shown to exhibit dose-dependent inhibition of NO production and significant reduction in iNOS in lipopolysaccharide-stimulated macrophages, thus suggesting the protective effect of gingerol against peroxynitrite-mediated oxidation and nitration reactions. We have shown that [6]-gingerol has higher scavenging activity compared to ethanol extract of ginger against 1,1-diphenyl-2-picrylhydrazyl and DPPH radical at lower concentrations (<100 μg/ml), but both ginger extract and [6]-gingerol exhibited same antioxidant potency at higher doses (100 1000 μg/ml) [12].

Contrary to the above findings, some researchers have shown the pro-oxidant effect of gingerols in preventing the growth of cancer cells [75, 126]. Lin and Tsay [75] indicated in their study that 35 and 50 μM of [6]-gingerol can increase the ROS concentration in LoVo colon cancer cell lines with a corresponding increase in p53 levels. However, the elevated levels of ROS production were inhibited by *N*-acetylcysteine, a potent antioxidant. The above studies show the dual function of ROS, either as an antioxidant or pro-oxidant in blocking tumorigenesis depending on the experimental models and the type of cancer cells.

5.1.2 Anticancer Activity

Many preclinical data have shown the chemopreventive efficacy of ginger and its constituents using human or animal cell lines. Ginger extracts and individual ginger constituents such as [6]-gingerol and [6]-shogaol have exhibited antioxidant, anti-proliferative, anti-inflammatory, anti-mutagenic, anti-angiogenic and proapoptotic effects in a variety of different cancer cell lines such as leukemia [71], skin [18, 83], ovarian [100], gastric [49], pancreas, [130], colon [2, 52, 97], liver [42, 120], breast [72] and brain [70].

Various dietary agents rich in phytochemicals including ginger and its bioactive compounds have been reported to inhibit growth and trigger apoptosis causing the death of cancer cells. Park et al. [93] investigated the chemopreventive effect of [6]-gingerol on HPAC (wild type) and BxPC-3 (p53 deficient) pancreatic tumor cell lines and colon cancer cell lines, HCT116, SW480, HT29 and LoVo. They found that [6]-gingerol at various concentrations (50–800 μM) inhibits the growth of both types of pancreatic cancer cells and in some cases dose dependently. However, they reported that apoptosis was only seen in BxPC-3 cells, suggesting that [6]-gingerol can bypass p53 mutant resistance to apoptosis, but it exerts a cytostatic effect on wild-type p53-expressing cells by inducing temporal growth arrest.

Apoptosis was found to be induced in human hepatocellular carcinoma, HepG2 cells after incubation with 0–200 μM [6]-gingerol for 24 h as indicated by the increased ratio of chromatin condensation and fragmented fluorescent nuclei which were dose dependent [125]. The authors suggested the release of cathepsin D to the cytosol appeared to be an early event that preceded the release of cytochrome c from mitochondria in inducing apoptosis. Inhibition of cathepsin D activity resulted in suppressed release of cytochrome c and subsequent apoptosis. We also investigated the apoptosis effect of ginger on hepatoma cell line, HepG2. Ginger oleoresin and [6]-gingerol at doses ranging from 100 to 1000 μg/mL reduced the viability of HepG2 cells dose dependently with a concomitant increase in the rate of apoptosis when treated with [6]-gingerol. However, the anti-proliferative and apoptosis effect was more potent with the use of ginger oleoresin when compared to [6]-gingerol [42].

Using colorectal cancer cell lines LoVo and HCT116, Lee et al. [73] demonstrated that [6]-gingerol induced significant G2/M, G1 cell cycle arrest and apoptosis with inhibition of cyclin D1, cyclin A and cyclin B1. Abdullah et al. [2] reported a dose-dependent increase in apoptosis with cell cycle arrest at G0/G1 and G2/M phases and a corresponding decrease in S-phase DNA synthesis in HCT116 and HT29 colon cancer cells treated with ginger extract. A subsequent study by Tahir et al. [111] showed that combination of ginger and Gelam honey produced a synergistic increase in the rate of apoptosis of colon cancer cells when compared to ginger or honey alone. Stimulation of early apoptosis (upregulation of caspase 9 and IκB genes) was accompanied by downregulation of KRAS, ERK, AKT, Bcl-xL and NFkB (p65) genes in a synergistic manner, implicating the enhanced anticancer properties of ginger when combined with honey.

Pro-apoptosis effect by [6]-gingerol was also evident in promyelocytic leukemia HL-60 cells associated with increased DNA fragmentation and inhibition of Bcl-2 expressions [117].

5.1.3 Anti-inflammatory Activity

Inflammation involves a cascade of cellular and molecular components collectively referred to as inflammation mediators. It can be classified into arachidonic acid (AA)-dependent and AA-independent pathways [127]. AA-dependent pathway mediators include cyclooxygenase (COX), lipooxygenase (LOX) and phospholipase A2 (PLA2), while AA-independent mediators include nitric oxide synthase (NOS), NF-κ B, peroxisome proliferator-activated receptors (PPAR) and NSAID-activated gene-1 (NAG-1) [50, 127].

The anti-inflammatory property of ginger has been known for centuries, but a good deal of scientific evidence has further confirmed its anti-inflammatory property mostly in animal models of inflammation and to a much lesser extent in humans [119]. The anti-inflammatory properties of gingerols were evidenced by its inhibitory effects on prostaglandins and leukotrienes synthesis in RBL-1 cells [65] and by mimicking dual-acting nonsteroidal anti-inflammatory drugs (NSAIDs) in intact human leukocytes in vitro [34]. Kim et al. [61] showed that 30 μM of [6]-gingerol caused a decrease in UVB-induced intracellular ROS levels, activated caspases 3, 8 9 and Fas expressions, stimulated expression of COX-2 and inhibited the nuclear translocation of NF-κB from the cytosolin HaCaT cells, following the suppression of IκBκ phosphorylation. Gingerols and its derivative [8]-paradol have been reported to be more potent anti-platelet and cyclooxygenase-1 (COX-1) inhibitors than aspirin when tested in vitro [85]. In a separate experiment, Lantz et al. [69] showed that ginger extracts containing either predominantly gingerols or shogaols were highly active at inhibiting LPS-induced PGE_2 production in U937 cells COX-2 expression.

Generation of nitiric oxide, NO, has been implicated in the pathogenesis of inflammatory diseases. Aktan et al. [6] examined the effect of a stable [6]-gingerol metabolite RAC-[6]-dihydroparadol ([6]-DHP) and a closely related gingerol analog [a capsaicin/gingerol (capsarol) analog referred to as ZTX42] on NO production, inducible nitric oxide synthase (iNOS) activity and protein expression levels in a murine macrophage cell line. ZTX42 and [6]-DHP were found to suppress NO production by partially inhibiting iNOS enzymatic activity and reducing iNOS protein production, via attenuation of NF-κB-mediated iNOS gene expression.

5.1.4 Anti-angiogenesis, Anti-invasion and Metastasis Activity

Angiogenesis is a crucial step in tumorigenesis, whereby new blood vessels are formed, supporting the survival and development of metastasized tumors as well as contributing to resistance to chemotherapy and radiation. Vascular endothelial growth factor, VEGF and interleukin-8 (IL-8) are among the important markers of angiogenesis. Matrix metallo-proteinases, MMPs, are proteolytic enzymes that are highly expressed in various malignant tumors. They are important regulators of tumor progression and metastasis. Inhibition of MMPs could be an effective strategy to prevent tumor cell invasion and metastasis.

Accumulating studies have shown the anti-angiogenic property of [6]-gingerol. Kim and colleagues showed that [6]-gingerol inhibited VEGF-induced proliferation of human endothelial cells by causing G1 cell cycle arrest. It also blocked VEGF-induced capillary-like tube formation by endothelial cells and strongly inhibited sprouting of endothelial cells in the rat aorta and formation of a VEGF-induced new blood vessel in the mouse cornea [60]. Weng et al. [120, 121] demonstrated that [6]-gingerol reduced VEGF and IL-8 secretion in Hep3B hepatoma cells. Using HUVEC cells via tube formation assay, they further proved that capillary tube formation can be blocked and its length reduced by [6]-gingerol, suggesting its anti-angiogenic and anti-invasive effects. A separate study by the same group suggested that [6]-gingerol might exert anti-invasive activity against hepatoma cells (HepG2 and Hep3B) through regulation of MMP-9 (matrix metalloproteinase) and TIMP-1 (tissue inhibitor metalloproteinase protein [121]. In addition, Kim et al. [60] reported an anti-angiogenic activity of [6]-gingerol which inhibits both vascular endothelial growth factor (VEGF)- and basic fibroblast growth factor-induced proliferation and capillary-like tube formation in human endothelial cells and ovarian cancer cells.

In a separate study by Lee et al. [72] and Kim and Kim [62], it was shown that [6]-gingerol exhibited anti-invasion activity by inhibiting the activities of MMP-2 and MMP-9 in MDA-MB-231 human breast cancer cells and PANC-1 cells (pancreatic duct-like cancer), respectively.

5.1.5 Anti-microbial and Anti-fungal Activity

[6]-gingerol and [12]-gingerol, isolated from ginger rhizome, demonstrated antibacterial activity against periodontal Gram-negative bacteria, *Porphyromonas gingivalis* ATCC 53978, *Porphyromonas endodontalis* ATCC 35406 and *Prevotella intermedia* ATCC 2561 [91], while [10]-gingerol showed antibacterial activity against of *M. avium* and *M. tuberculosis* [43]. Riaz et al. [101] showed that ginger extract exhibited anti-microbial activity against *Escherichia Coli, Bacillus subtilis, Staphylococcus aureus, Streptococcus faecalis* and anti-fungal activity against *Candida albicans and Aspergillus Niger.*

5.1.6 Neuroprotective Activity

Neuroprotective activity of [6]-gingerol was examined in Aβ(25-35)-induced oxidative stress in neuroblastoma cells, SH-SY5Y. It was found that [6]-gingerol effectively suppressed intracellular accumulation of ROS and restored Aβ(25-35)-depleted endogenous antioxidant glutathione levels and upregulated the mRNA and protein expression of antioxidant enzymes such as γ-glutamylcysteine ligase (GCL) and heme oxygenase-1 (HO-1) mediated by activation of NF-E2-related factor 2 (Nrf2) [74].

5.2 In Vivo Biological Activity of Gingerol: Anticancer Property

Similar to in vitro study, ginger extract or oleoresin and its bioactive compounds have exhibited antioxidant, anticancer and anti-inflammatory effects in animals induced with cancer including mouse skin [63], rat liver [41, 129] and rat colon [128].

5.2.1 Colon Carcinogenesis

In 2005, Kim and colleagues injected C57BL/6 mice intraperitoneally with [6]-gingerol (3 or 5 mg/kg body weight) prior to injection of B16F10 melanoma cells. With a higher dosage of [6]-gingerol (5 mg/kg body weight), they managed to show 100 % suppression of the presence of metastatic colonies seen in the lung after 3 weeks of treatment [60, 64]. Jeong et al. [52] demonstrated the anti-tumor effect of [6]-gingerol given to nude mice prior to injecting human HCT116 colon cancer cells. They found that when [6]-gingerol was injected three times per week, fewer tumor growth of smaller volume was seen 4 weeks after the injection of HCT116 colon cancer cells and the mice lived longer than the untreated mice with measurable tumor size of 1 cm or larger. Using reverse-docking technique, the authors suggested that suppression of tumors was an effect mediated by inhibition of LTA4H activity, the molecular target of [6]-gingerol.

5.2.2 Skin Carcinogenesis

In 1998, Park et al. [90] and collaborators were able to induce two-stage skin carcinogenesis model (initiation and promotion) by single topical application of DMBA and repeated applications of TPA. Topical application of [6]-gingerol on the shaved backs of female ICR mice decreased the incidence of skin papilloma. Kim et al. [64] investigated the anti-tumor effect of [6]-gingerol on TPA-induced skin cancer in mice. They attested that [6]-gingerol inhibited TPA-induced COX-2 expression, an inflammatory marker involved in carcinogenesis, by blocking the p38 MAP kinase NF-kB signaling pathway.

Nigam et al. [84] investigated the anticancer effect of [6]-gingerol in mouse skin carcinogenesis model using benzo[a]pyrene as a carcinogen. Mice treated with benzo[a]pyrene and received [6]-gingerol (2.5 μM/animal) pre- or post-treatment for 32 weeks resulted in a reduced number of tumors by about 55 and 74 %, respectively, and reduced tumor volume by about 51 and 65 %, respectively. Further to their investigation, [6]-gingerol treatment also resulted in the induction of apoptosis as seen by the increasing benzo[a]pyrene-suppressed p53 levels, upregulation of Bax expression, protease-activating factor-1 (Apaf-1), the release of cytochrome c, caspases activation and decreased Bcl-2 expression.

5.2.3 Liver Carcinogenesis

We investigated the effect of ginger oleoresin on rats induced with liver cancer using ethionine as a carcinogen in the drinking water. The tumor burden in rats with liver cancer reduced significantly from 100 to 17 %, with tumor size shrinking from 1 to 0.1 cm when rats were fed with ginger oleoresin. Interestingly, there was a concomitant increase in antioxidant enzyme, SOD and reduction in MDA level in the blood with reduction in tumor burden, suggesting the antioxidant activity of ginger in blocking tumorigenesis [129].

6 Biological Activities of Gingerol in Humans

There are not many human studies or clinical trials to suggest the protective effect of [6]-gingerol on chronic diseases; however, many studies were conducted using ginger extract or its oleoresin.

6.1 Anti-emetic Effect

Earlier clinical studies on ginger were mainly on the anti-emetic effect on pregnant women. Seventy pregnant women with nausea and vomiting in pregnancy consented to take part in the study, and they were given oral ginger 1 g per day, for 4 days. Subjects graded the severity of their nausea using visual analog scales and recorded number of vomiting for the period of ginger treatment. Nausea decreased significantly in the ginger group compared with the placebo group. The number of vomiting episodes also decreased significantly in the ginger group compared with the placebo group. [116]. Based on Medline, EMBASE and the Cochrane Library search (six RCTs, $n = 675$ and one cohort study, $n = 187$) on women suffering from pregnancy-related nausea and vomiting, such as morning sickness and hyperemesis gravidarum, Borrelli et al. [19] concluded that ginger may be a safe and effective option for the treatment of nausea and vomiting in pregnancy, but further research is required to confirm these findings. A systematic review of the evidence from randomized controlled trials for or against the efficacy of ginger for nausea and vomiting reported that ginger favored over placebo especially on postoperative nausea, and it was suggested that ginger was equally effective as metoclopramide, the anti-emetic drug [33].

6.2 Anticancer Effect

A pilot study by Citronberg et al. [25] on individuals with increased risk of colorectal cancer (CRC) has suggested the anti-proliferative and anti-inflammatory properties of ginger. Individuals at high risk of colon cancer were given ginger extract (2 g/day for 28–30 days), and biomarkers of cell proliferation [human telomerase reverse transcriptase (hTERT), MIB-1], differentiation (p21WAF1/cip1) and apoptosis (Bax, Bcl-2) in colonic mucosa from individuals at high risk of colorectal cancer were measured. Results from the trial suggest that ginger may reduce proliferation in the normal-appearing colorectal epithelium (reflecting the pre-malignant stage) and increase apoptosis especially in the differentiation zone of colon crypts.

In a separate study by Jiang et al. [54], 20 individuals at increased risk of CRC were randomized and given 2.0 g/day ginger or placebo for 28 days. Flexible sigmoidoscopy was used to obtain colon biopsies at baseline and end of the study. Ginger significantly lowered COX-1 protein expression, in individuals with increased risk of colon cancer, suggesting the chemopreventive effect of ginger.

Zick et al. [133] tested the effect of ginger on 20 subjects with increased risk of CRC. They were given 2 g/day ginger for 28 days. Decreased arachidonic acid (AA) and increased LTB4 were found in the biopsies of normal-appearing colonic mucosa. Increased AA has been associated with the inflammatory marker in cancer development.

6.3 Lipid-Lowering Effect

Ginger was shown by Alizadeh-Nawaie et al. [9] to have lipid-lowering effect. Ginger capsules (3 g/day) supplemented to 45 patients with hyperlipidemia for 45 days resulted in significant reduction in serum triglyceride, cholesterol, low-density lipoprotein (LDL) and very-low-density lipoprotein (VLDL) compared to placebo group (lactose 3 g/day).

7 Conclusion

Ginger is popularly known for its medicinal benefit rather than as flavor-enhancing agent. Gingerols, the pungent component of ginger, are the major phytochemicals found in fresh ginger rhizome, and [6]-gingerol is the most extensively studied bioactive component along with [6]-shogaol. Although [6]-gingerol is shown to be more therapeutic compared to its natural form, the safety of its consumption in larger doses is uncertain and may not be advisable unless intensive clinical trials in human subjects and its bioavailability were evaluated.

The pharmacokinetic study indicates that gingerols accumulate in the gastrointestinal tract and they can be metabolized in the liver to the glucuronides. Gingerol can be converted to shogaol with prolonged incubation in the intestine. [6]-Gingerol acts as a potent antioxidant and anticancer in vitro and in vivo studies. It also appears to exert an anti-inflammatory effect by suppressing COX-2 with subsequent inhibition of prostaglandin and leukotriene biosynthesis. This review clearly shows that [6]-gingerol is able to modulate cell signaling pathways known to be activated in tumorigenesis, such as MAPK/ERK/NF-κB/AP-1/PI3K, and apoptosis. In some cases, gingerol can even cross talk between the pathways in exerting its chemopreventive effect.

The results of human trials conducted by Citronberg et al. [25], Jiang et al. [54] and Zick et al. [133] so far suggest that ginger extract has only modest effects on biomarkers of cell proliferation, apoptosis and differentiation, as well as on arachidonic acid metabolism, in normal-appearing colonic tissues when administered at a dose of 2 g/day. It warrants perhaps future studies to consider using higher doses of ginger. However, one disadvantage noted in their study is that the normal-appearing colonic epithelium in individuals with high risk of colorectal cancer may not directly mimic the premalignant stage of colorectal cancer.

With convincing evidence that ginger is an effective therapeutic and chemopreventive agent in animal and human studies, it is perhaps advantageous to investigate further the effects of ginger and its constituents directly on premalignant tissues such as rectal polyps in familial APC (adenomatous polyposis coli) patients, or patients with ulcerative colitis and other GIT-related diseases linked to colorectal or on cancer tissues before surgery which may then reveal accurate and useful information.

In summary, ginger and its bioactive components, have been proven to possess many pharmacological and nutraceutical properties. In spite of the lack of intensive clinical trials, and the fact that long-term use of synthetic drugs is often associated with serious side effects, the use of ginger and especially gingerols appears to be safe and the convincing evidence highlighted in this review regarding the medicinal effects of gingerols in treating or preventing chronic diseases will benefit the common population, clinicians, patients, researchers and industrialists.

References

1. Abdul Sani NF, Belani LK, Chong PS et al (2014) Effect of the Combination of Gelam honey and ginger on oxidative stress and metabolic profile in streptozotocin-induced diabetic sprague-dawley rats. Bio Med Res Int. doi:10.1155/2014/160695
2. Abdullah S, Abidin SAZ, Murad NA, Makpol S, Wan Ngah WZ, Mohd Yusof YA (2010) Ginger extract (*Zingiber officinale*) triggers apoptosis and G0/G1 cells arrest in HCT 116 and HT 29 colon cancer cell lines. Afr J Biochem Res 4:134–142

3. Aggarwal BB, Shishodia S (2006) Molecular targets of dietary agents for prevention and therapy of cancer. Biochem Pharmacol 71:1397–1421
4. Ahui ML, Champy P, Ramadan A et al (2008) Ginger prevents Th2-mediated immune responses in a mouse model of airway inflammation. Int Immunopharmacol 8(12):1626–1632
5. Akimoto M, Iizuka M, Kanematsu R et al (2015) Anticancer effect of ginger extract against pancreatic cancer cells mainly through reactive oxygen species-mediated autotic cell death. PLoS ONE 10(5):e0126605. doi:10.1371/journal.pone.0126605
6. Aktan F, Henness S, Tran VH et al (2006) Gingerol metabolite and a synthetic analogue capsarol inhibit macrophage NF-kappa B-mediated iNOS gene expression and enzyme activity. Planta Med 72:27–734
7. Al-Amin ZM, Thomson M, Al-Qattan KK et al (2006) Antidiabetic and hypolipidemic properties of ginger in streptozotocin induced diabetic rats. Br J Nutr 96:660–666
8. Ali BH, Blunden G, Tanira MO et al (2008) Some phytochemical, pharmacological and toxicological properties of ginger (*Zingiber officinale Roscoe*): a review of recent research. Food Chem Toxicol 46(2):409–420
9. Alizadeh-Navaei R, Roozbeh F, Saravi M et al (2008) Investigation of the effect of ginger on the lipid levels. A double blind controlled clinical trial. Saudi Med J 29:1280–1284
10. Angel P, Karin M (1991) The role of Jun, Fos and the AP-1 complex in cell-proliferation and transformation. Biochim Biophys Acta 1072:129–157
11. Behrens J (2005) The role of the Wnt signalling pathway in colorectal tumorigenesis. Biochem Soc Trans 33:672–675
12. Bharti AC, Aggarwal BB (2002) Nuclear factor-kappaB and cancer: its role in prevention and therapy. Biochem Pharmacol 64(5–6):883–888
13. Bhattarai S, Tran VH, Duke CC (2007) Stability of [6]-gingerol and [6]-shogaol in simulated gastric and intestinal fluids. J Pharmaceut Biomed Anal 45:648–653
14. Bode AM (2004) Cancer prevention by food factors through targeting signal transduction pathways. Nutr 20(1):80–94. doi:10.1016/j.nut.2003.09
15. Bode AM, Dong Z (2004) Ginger. In: Packer L, Ong CN, Halliwell B (eds) Herbal and traditional medicine: molecular aspects of health. Marcel Dekker, New York, pp 131–156
16. Bode AM, Dong Z (2008) Modulation of cell signal transduction by tea and ginger. In: Dong Z, Surh YJ (ed) Dietary modulation of cell signaling pathways. CRC Press/Taylor & Francis, Boca Raton (FL), pp 45–74
17. Bode AM, Dong Z (2011) The amazing and mighty ginger. In: Benzie IFF, Wachtel-Galor S (ed) Herbal medicine: biomolecular and clinical aspects, 2nd edn. CRC Press/Taylor & Francis, Boca Raton (FL), pp 129–154
18. Bode AM, Ma WY, Surh YJ et al (2001) Inhibition of epidermal growth factor-induced cell transformation and activator protein 1 activation by [6]-gingerol. Cancer Res 61:850–853
19. Borrelli F, Capasso R, Aviello G et al (2005) Effectiveness and safety of ginger in the treatment of pregnancy induced Nausea and vomiting. Database of abstracts of reviews of effects (DARE): quality assessed reviews [Internet]. Centre for Reviews and Dissemination (UK), York (UK)
20. Butt MS, Sultan MT (2011) Ginger and its health claims: molecular aspects. Crit Rev Food Sci Nutr 51:383–393
21. Cardone MH, Roy N, Stennicke HR et al (1998) Regulation of cell death protease caspase-9 by phosphorylation. Science 282:1318–1321
22. Chakraborty D, Mukherjee A, Sikdar S et al (2012) [6]-gingerol isolated from ginger attenuates sodium arsenite induced oxidative stress and plays a corrective role in improving insulin signaling in mice. Toxicol Lett 210:34–43
23. Chang F, Lee JT, Navolanic PM et al (2003) Involvement of PI3K/Akt pathway in cell cycle progression, apoptosis, and neoplastic transformation: a target for cancer chemotherapy. Leukemia 17(3):590–596
24. Chen Z, Gibson TB, Robinson F et al (2001) MAP kinases. Chem Rev 101:2449–2476

25. Citronberg J, Bostick R, Ahern T et al (2013) Effects of ginger supplementation on cell cycle biomarkers in the normal-appearing colonic mucosa of patients at increased risk for colorectal cancer: results from a pilot, randomized, controlled trial. Cancer Prev Res 6: 271–281
26. Clarke RB (2003) p27KIP1 phosphorylation by PKB/Akt leads to poor breast cancer prognosis. Breast Cancer Res 5(3):162–163
27. Denniff P, Macleod I, Whiting DA (1980) Studies in the biosynthesis of [6]-gingerol, pungent principle of ginger (*Zingiber officinale*). J Chem Soc Perkin Trans 1:2637–2644
28. Diehl JA (2002) Cycling to cancer with cyclin D1. Cancer Biol Ther 1(3):226–231
29. Ding GH, Naora K, Hayashibara M et al (1991) Pharmacokinetics of [6]-gingerol after intravenous administration in rats. Chem Phar Bull (Tokyo) 39:1612–1614
30. Dong Z, Birrer MJ, Watts RG et al (1994) Blocking of tumor promoter-induced AP-1 activity inhibits induced transformation in JB6 mouse epidermal cells. Proc Natl Acad Sci U S A 91:609–613
31. Dorai T, Aggarwal BB (2004) Role of chemopreventive agents in cancer therapy. Cancer Lett 215:129–140
32. Dugasani S, Pichika MR, Nadarajah VD et al (2010) Comparative antioxidant and anti-inflammatory effects of [6]-gingerol, [8]-gingerol, [10] gingerol and [6]-shogaol. J Ethnopharmacol 127:515–520
33. Ernst E, Pittler MH (2000) Efficacy of ginger for nausea and vomiting: a systematic review of randomized clinical trials. Br J Anaesth 84(3):367–371
34. Flynn DL, Rafferty MF, Boctor AM (1968) Inhibition of human neutrophil 5-lipoxygenase activity by gingerdione, shogaol, capsaicin and related pungent compounds. Prostaglandins Leukot Med 24:195–198
35. Fresno-Vara JA, Casado E, Castro J et al (2004) PI3K/Akt signaling pathway and cancer. Cancer Treatment Rev 30:193–204
36. Fulda S, Debatin KM (2006) Extrinsic versus intrinsic apoptosis pathways in anticancer chemotherapy. Oncogene 25(34):4798–4811
37. Giles RH, van Es JH, Clevers H (2003) Caught up in a Wnt storm: Wnt signaling in cancer. Biochim Biophys Acta 1653:1–24
38. Guertin DA, Sabatini DM (2007) Defining the role of mTOR in cancer. Cancer Cell 12:9–22
39. Gundala SR, Mukkavilli R, Yang C et al (2014) Enterohepatic recirculation of bioactive ginger phytochemicals is associated with enhanced tumor growth-inhibitory activity of ginger extract. Carcinogenesis 35(6):1320–1329. doi:10.1093/carcin/bgu011
40. Gunning WT, Kramer PM, Steele VE et al (2002) Chemoprevetion by lipoxygenase and leukotriene pathway inhibitors of vinyl carbamate-induced lung tumours in mice. Cancer Res 62:4199–4201
41. Habib SH, Makpol S, Abdul Hamid NA et al (2008) Ginger extract (*Zingiber officinale*) has anti-cancer and anti-inflammatory effects on ethionine-induced hepatoma rats. Clinics (Sao Paulo) 63(6):807–813
42. Harliyansyah H, Murad NA, Wan Ngah WZ et al (2007) Antiproliferative, antioxidant and apoptosis effects of *Zingiber officinale* and 6-gingerol on HepG2 cells. Asian J Biochem 2 (6):421–426
43. Hiserodt RD, Franzblau SG, Rosen RT (1998) Isolation of 6-, 8-, and 10-gingerol from ginger rhizome by HPLC and preliminary evaluation of inhibition of *Mycobacterium avium* and *Mycobacterium tuberculosis*. Agric Food Chem 46:2504–2508
44. Huang HC, Chiu SH, Chang TM (2011) Inhibitory effect of [6]-gingerol on melanogenesis in B16F10 melanoma cells and a possible mechanism of action. Biosci Biotechnol Biochem 75 (6):1067–1072
45. Huang HC, Chou YC, Wu CY et al (2013) [8]-gingerol inhibits melanogenesis in murine melanoma cells through down-regulation of the MAPK and PKA signal pathways. Biochem Biophys Res Commun 438:375–381

46. Hung JY, Hsu YL, Li CT et al (2009) 6-Shogaol, an active constituent of dietary ginger, induces autophagy by inhibiting the AKT/mTOR pathway in human non-small cell lung cancer A549 cells. J Agric Food Chem 57:9809–9816
47. IARC monographs on the evaluation of carcinogenic risks to humans (1994) Lyon, France: international agency for research on cancer; IARC working group on the evaluation of carcinogenic risks to humans, *schistomsomes*, liver flukes and *Helicobacter pylori.* Infect *Helicobacter pylori* 61:177–201
48. Ippoushi K, Azuma K, Ito H et al (2003) [6]-gingerol inhibits nitric oxide synthesis in activated J774.1 mouse macrophages and prevents peroxynitrite-induced oxidation and nitration reactions. Life Sci 73:3427–3437
49. Ishiguro K, Ando T, Maeda O et al (2007) Ginger ingredients reduce viability of gastric cancer cells via distinct mechanisms. Biochem Biophys Res Commun 362(1):218–223
50. Issa AY, Volate SR, Wargovich MJ (2006) The role of phytochemicals in inhibition of cancer and inflammation: new directions and perspectives. J Food Compost Anal 19: 405–419
51. Jemal A, Bray F, Center M et al (2011) Global cancer statistics. CA: Cancer J Clin 61: 69–90
52. Jeong CH, Bode AM, Pugliese A et al (2009) [6]-gingerol suppresses colon cancer growth by targeting Leukotriene A4 Hydrolase. Cancer Res 69:5584–5591
53. Jiang H, Solyom AM, Timmermann BN et al (2005) Characterization of gingerol-related compounds in ginger rhizome (*Zingiber officinale Rosc.*) by high-performance liquid chromatography/ electrospray ionization mass spectrometry. Rapid Commun Mass Spectrom 19(20):2957–2964
54. Jiang Y, Turgeon DK, Wright BD et al (2013) Effect of ginger root on cyclooxygenase-1 and 15-hydroxyprostaglandin dehydrogenase expression in colonic mucosa of humans at normal and increased risk for colorectal cancer. Europ J Cancer Prevent 22(5):455–460
55. Jolad SD, Lantz RC, Solyon AM et al (2004) Fresh organically grown ginger (*Zingiber officinale*): composition and effects on LPS-induced PGE2 production. Phytochem 65: 1937–1954
56. Jolad SD, Lantz RC, Chen GJ et al (2005) Commercially processed dry ginger (*Zingiber officinale*): composition and effects on LPS-stimulated PGE2 production. Phytochem 66 (13):1614–1635
57. Joo JH, Hong SS, Cho YR et al (2015) [10]-gingerol inhibits proliferation and invasion of MDA-MB-231 breast cancer cells through suppression of Akt and p38MAPK activity. Oncol Reports. doi:10.3892/or.2015.4405
58. Kamato D, Rezaei HB, Getachew R et al (2013) (S)-[6]-Gingerol inhibits TGF-β-stimulated biglycan synthesis but not glycosaminoglycan hyperelongation in human vascular smooth muscle cells. J Pharm Pharmacol 65:1026–1036
59. Katiyar SK, Agarwal R, Mukhtar H (1996) Inhibition of tumor promotion in SENCAR mouse skin by ethanol extract of *Zingiber officinale*rhizome. Cancer Res 56(5):1023–1030
60. Kim EC, Min JK, Kim TY et al (2005) [6]-gingerol, a pungent ingredient of ginger, inhibits angiogenesis in vitro and in vivo. Biochem Biophys Res Commun 335(2):300–308
61. Kim JK, Kim Y, Na KM et al (2007) [6]-Gingerol prevents UVB induced ROS production and COX-2 expression in vitro and in vivo. Free Rad Res 41:603–614
62. Kim SO, Kim MR (2013) [6]-gingerol prevents disassembly of cell junctions and activities of MMPs in invasive human pancreas cancer cells through ERK/NF-κB/snail signal transduction pathway. Evid Based Complement Alternat Med 2013:761852. doi:10.1155/2013/761852
63. Kim SO, Chun KS, Kundu JK et al (2004) Inhibitory effects of [6]-gingerol on PMA-induced COX-2 expression and activation of NF-kB and p38 MAPK in mouse skin. BioFactors 21:27–31
64. Kim SO, Kundu JK, Shin YK et al (2005) [6]-gingerol inhibits COX-2 expression by blocking the activation of p38 MAP kinase and NF-kappa B in phorbol ester-stimulated mouse skin. Oncogene 24(15):2558–2567

65. Kiuchi F, Shibuya M, Sankawa U (1982) Inhibitors of prostaglandin biosynthesis from ginger. Chem Pharm Bull (Tokyo) 30:754–757
66. Kobayashi M, Ishida Y, Shoji N et al (1988) Cardiotonic action of [8]-gingerol, an activator of the Ca2+-pumping adenosine triphosphatase of sarcoplasmic reticulum, in guinea pig atrial muscle. J Pharmacol Exp Ther 246:667–673
67. Koo KL, Ammit AJ, Tran VH et al (2001) Gingerols and related analogues inhibit arachidonic acid-induced human platelet serotonin release and aggregation. Thromb Res 103 (5):387–397
68. Kumar NV, Srinivas P, Bettadaiah BK (2012) New scalable and eco-friendly synthesis of gingerols. Tetrahedron Lett 53:2993–2995
69. Lantz RC, Chen GJ, Sarihan M et al (2007) The effect of extracts from ginger rhizome on inflammatory mediator production. Phytomed 14:123–128
70. Lee DH, Kim DW, Jung CH et al (2014) Gingerol sensitizes TRAIL-induced apoptotic cell death of glioblastoma cells. Toxicol Appl Pharmacol 279(3):253–265. doi:10.1016/j.taap.2014.06.030
71. Lee E, Surh YJ (1998) Induction of apoptosis in HL-60 cells by pungent vanilloids, [6]-gingerol and [6] paradol. Cancer Lett 134:163–168
72. Lee HS, Seo EY, Kang NE, Kim WK (2008) [6]-Gingerol inhibits metastasis of MDS-MB-231 human breast cancer cells. J Nutr Biochem 19:313–319
73. Lee SH, Cekanova M, Baek SJ (2008) Multiple mechanisms are involved in 6-gingerol-induced cell growth arrest and apoptosis in human colorectal cancer cells. Mol Carcinog 47(3):197–208
74. Lee C, Park GH, Kim CY et al (2011) [6]-gingerol attenuates β-amyloid-induced oxidative cell death via fortifying cellular antioxidant defense system. Food ChemToxicol 49: 1261–1269
75. Lin CC, Tsay GJ (2012) 6-gingerol inhibits growth of colon cancer cell LoVo via induction of G2/M arrest. Evid Based Complement Alternat Med. doi:10.1155/2012/326096
76. Ma S, Zhang S, Duan W et al (2009) An enantioselective synthesis of (+)-(*S*)-[*n*]-gingerols via the L-proline-catalyzed aldol reaction. Bioorganic Medic Chem Lett 19:3909–3911
77. Maeda S, Omata M (2008) Inflammation and cancer: role of nuclear factor-kappa B activation. Cancer Sci 99:836–842
78. Mahady GB, Pendland SL, Yun GS et al (2003) Ginger (*Zingiber officinale* Roscoe) and the gingerols inhibit the growth of Cag A+ strains of helicobacter pylori. Anticancer Res 23:3699–3702
79. Maier LS, Schwan C, Schillinger W et al (2000) Gingerol, isoproterenol and ouabain normalize impaired post-rest behavior but not force-frequency relation in failing human myocardium. Cardiovasc Res 45:913–924
80. Moran A, Ortega P, de Juan C et al (2010) Differential colorectal carcinogenesis: molecular basis and clinical relevance. World J Gastrointest Oncol 2:151–158. doi:10.4251/wjgo.v2.i3.151
81. Nakazawa T, Ohsawa K (2002) Metabolism of [6]-gingerol in rats. Life Sci 70:2165–2175
82. Neergheen VS, Bahorun T, Taylor EW et al (2010) Targeting specific cell signaling transduction pathways by dietary and medicinal phytochemicals in cancer chemoprevention. Toxicol 278:229–241
83. Nigam N, Bhui K, Prasad S et al (2009) [6]-gingerol induces reactive oxygen species regulated mitochondrial cell death pathway in human epidermoid carcinoma A431 cells. Chem Biol Interact 181:77–84
84. Nigam N, George J, Srivastava S et al (2010) Induction of apoptosis by [6]-gingerol associated with the modulation of p53 and involvement of mitochondrial signaling pathway in B[a]P-induced mouse skin tumorigenesis. Cancer Chemother Pharmacol 65:687–696
85. Nurtjahja-Tjendraputra E, Ammit AJ, Roufogalis BD et al (2003) Effective anti-platelet and COX-1 enzyme inhibitors from pungent constituents of ginger. Thromb Res 111(4–5):259–265

86. Ojewole JAO (2006) Analgesic, antiinflammatory and hypoglycaemic effects of ethanol extract of *Zingiber officinale* (Roscoe) rhizomes (Zingiberaceae) in mice and rats. Phytother Res 20:764–772
87. Ozes ON, Mayo LD, Gustin JA et al (1999) NF-kappaB activation by tumour necrosis factor requires the Akt serine-threonine kinase. Nature 401(6748):82–85
88. Pana MH, Ho CT (2008) Chemopreventive effects of natural dietary compounds on cancer Development. Chem Soc Rev 37:2558–2574
89. Park EJ, Pezzuto JM (2011) Botanicals in cancer chemoprevention. Cancer Metastasis Rev 21:231–255
90. Park KK, Chun KS, Lee JM et al (1998) Inhibitory effects of [6]-gingerol, a major pungent principle of ginger, on phorbol ester-induced inflammation, epidermal ornithine decarboxylase activity and skin tumor promotion in ICR mice. Cancer Lett 129(2):139–144
91. Park M, Bae J, Lee DS (2008) Antibacterial activity of [10]-gingerol and [12]-gingerol isolated from ginger rhizome against periodontal bacteria. Phytother Res 22:1446–1449
92. Park SA, Park IH, Cho JS et al (2012) Effect of [6]-gingerol on myofibroblast differentiation in transforming growth factor beta 1-induced nasal polyp-derived fibroblasts. Am J Rhinol Allergy 26(2):97–103
93. ParkYJ; Wen J, Bang S et al (2006) [6]-gingerol induces cell cycle arrest and cell death of mutant p 53-expressing pancreatic cancer cells. Yonsei Med J 47(5): 688–697
94. Poltronieri J, Becceneri AB, Fuzer AM et al (2014) [6]-gingerol as a cancer chemopreventive agent: a review of its activity on different steps of the metastatic process. Mini Rev Med Chem 14(4):313–321
95. Prasad S, Tyagi AK (2015) Ginger and its constituents: role in prevention and treatment of gastrointestinal cancer. Gastroenterol Res Practice. doi:10.1155/2015/142979
96. Prescott SM, Fitzpatrick FA (2000) Cyclooxygenase-2 and carcinogenesis. Biochim Biophys Acta 1470:M69–M67
97. Radhakrishnan EK, Bava SV, Narayanan SS et al (2014) [6] gingerol induces caspase-dependent apoptosis and prevents PMA-induced proliferation in colon cancer cells by inhibiting MAPK/AP-1 signaling. PLoS ONE, 26:9(8):e104401. doi:10.1371/journal.pone.0104401
98. Ramirez-Ahumada MC, Timmermann BN, Gang DR (2006) Biosynthesis of curcuminoids and gingerols in turmeric (*Curcuma longa*) and ginger (*Zingiber officinale*): identification of curcuminoid synthase and hydroxycinnamoyl-CoA thioesterases. Phytochem 67:2017–2029
99. Reed J (2001) Apoptosis-regulating proteins as targets for drug discovery. Trends Mol Med 7:314–319
100. Rhode J, Fogoros S, Zick S et al (2007) Ginger inhibits cell growth and modulates angiogenic factors in ovarian cancer cells. BMC Complement Alternat Med 7:44
101. Riaz H, Begum A, Raza SA et al (2015) Antimicrobial property and phytochemical study of ginger found in local area of Punjab, Pakistan. Internat Curr Pharmaceut J 4(7):405–409
102. Ryu MJ, Chung HS (2015) [10]-gingerol induces mitochondrial apoptosis through activation of MAPK pathway in HCT116 human colon cancer cells. Vitro Cell Dev Biol Anim 51 (1):92–101. doi:10.1007/s11626-014-9806-6
103. Scheiman JM, Cutler AF (1999) Helicobacter pylori and gastric cancer. Am J Med 106:222–226
104. Semwal RB, Semwal DK, Combrinck S et al (2015) Gingerols and shogaols: important nutraceutical principles from ginger. Phytochem 117:554–568
105. Shukla Y, Singh M (2007) Cancer preventive properties of ginger: a brief review. Food Chem Toxicol 45(5):683–690
106. Sporn MB, Dunlop NM, Newton DL et al (1976) Prevention of chemical carcinogenesis by vitamin A and its synthetic analogs (retinoids). Fed Proc 35:1332–1338
107. Song G, Quyang G, Bao S (2005) The activation of Akt/PKB signaling pathway and cell survival. J Cell Mol Med 9(1):59–71

108. Subbaramaiah K, Dannenberg AJ (2003) Cyclooxygenase 2: a molecular target for cancer prevention and treatment. Trends Pharmacol Sci 24:96–102
109. Surh YJ, Lee E, Lee JM (1998) Chemoprotective properties of some pungent ingredients present in red pepper and ginger. Mutat Res 402(1–2):259–267
110. Surh YJ, Lee SS(1994) Enzymic reduction of gingerol, a major pungent principle of ginger, in the cell-free preparation of rat liver. Life Sci 54:PL321–PL326
111. Tahir AA, Abdul Sani NF, Morad NA et al (2015) Combined ginger extract and gelam honey modulate Ras/ERK and P13/AKT pathway genes in colon cancer HT29 cells, Nutr J 13:31
112. Talalay P (2001) The importance of using scientific principles in the development of medicinal agents from plants. Acad Med 76(3):238–247
113. Tarapore RS, Siddiqui IA, Mukhtar H (2012) Modulation of Wnt/β-catenin signaling pathway by bioactive food components. Carcinogenesis 33(3):483–491. doi:10.1093/carcin/bgr305
114. Townsend EA, Siviski ME, Zhang Y et al (2013) Effects of ginger and its constituents on airway smooth muscle relaxation and calcium regulation. Am J Respir Cell Mol Biol 48 (2):157–163. doi:10.1165/rcmb.2012-0231OC
115. Vogelstein B, Kinzler KW (1992) p53 function and dysfunction. Cell 70(4):523–526
116. Vutyavanich T, Kraisin T, Ruangsri R (2001) Ginger for nausea and vomiting in pregnancy: randomized, double-masked, placebo-controlled trial. Obstet Gynecol 97(4):577–582
117. Wang CC, Chen LG, Lee LT et al (2003) Effects of 6-gingerol, an antioxidant from ginger, on inducing apoptosis in human leukemic HL-60 cells. In Vivo 17:641–645
118. Wee LH, Morad NA, Aan GJ et al (2015) Mechanism of chemoprevention against colon cancer cells using combined Gelam honey and ginger extract via mTOR and Wnt/β-catenin pathways. Asian Pac J Cancer Prev 16:6549–6556
119. Wei QY, Ma JP, Cai YJ et al (2005) Cytotoxic and apoptotic activities of diarylheptanoids and gingerol-related compounds from the rhizome of Chinese ginger. J Ethnopharmacol 102:177–184
120. Weng CJ, Wu CF, Huang HW et al (2010) Anti-invasion effects of 6-shogaol and 6-gingerol, two active components in ginger, on human hepatocarcinoma cells. Mol Nutr Food Res 54 (11):1618–1627
121. Weng CJ, Chou CP, Ho CT et al (2012) Molecular mechanism inhibiting human hepatocarcinoma cell invasion by 6-shogaol and 6-gingerol. Mol Nutr Food Res 56(8): 1304–1314
122. Wohlmuth H, Leach DN, Smith MK et al (2005) Gingerol content of diploid and tetraploid clones of ginger (*Zingiber officinale Roscoe*). J Agric Food Chem 53:5772–5778
123. Wu KK, Wang XJ, Cheng AS et al (2013) Dysregulation and crosstalk of cellular signaling pathways in colon carcinogenesis. Crit Rev Oncol/Hemato l86: 251–277
124. Yagihashi S, Miura Y, Yagasaki K (2008) Inhibitory effect of gingerol on the proliferation and invasion of hepatoma cells in culture. Cytotechnology 57:129–136
125. Yang G, Wang S, Zhong L et al (2012) [6]-gingerol induces apoptosis through lysosomal-mitochondrial axis in human hepatoma G2 cells. Phytother Res 26(11):1667–1673
126. Yang G, Zhong L, Jiang L et al (2010) Genotoxic effect of 6-gingerol on human hepatoma G2 cells. Chem Biol Interact 185(1):12–17
127. Yoon JH, Baek SJ (2005) Molecular targets of dietary polyphenols with anti-inflammatory properties. Yonsei Med J 46(5):585–596. doi:10.3349/ymj.2005.46.5.585
128. Yoshimi N, Wang A, Morishita Y et al (1992) Modifying effects of fungal and herb metabolites on azoxymethane-induced intestinal carcinogenesis in rats. Jpn J Cancer Res 83 (12):1273–1278
129. Yusof YAM, Ahmad N, Das S et al (2009) Chemopreventive efficacy of ginger (*Zingiber officinale*) in ethionine induced rat hepatocarcinogenesis. Afr J Tradit Complem Altern Med 6:87–93

130. Zhang S, Liu Q, Liu Y et al (2012) Zerumbone, a Southeast Asian ginger sesquiterpene, induced apoptosis of pancreatic carcinoma cells through p53 signaling pathway. Evid Based Complement Alternat Med. doi:10.1155/2012/936030
131. Zhang YX, Li JS, Chen LH et al (2012) Simultaneous determination of five gingerols in raw and processed ginger by HPLC. Chinese Pharm J 47:471–474
132. Zick SM, Djuric Z, Ruffin MT et al (2008) Pharmacokinetics of 6-, 8-, 10-gingerols and 6-shogaol and conjugate metabolites in healthy human subjects. Cancer Epidemiol Biomarkers Prev 17(8):1930–1936. doi:10.1158/1055-9965.EPI-07-2934
133. Zick SM, Turgeon DK, Ren J et al (2015) Pilot clinical study of the effects of ginger root extract on eicosanoids in colonic mucosa of subjects at increased risk for colorectal cancer. Mol Carcinog 54(9):908–915. doi:10.1002/mc.22163

Potential Use of Flavopiridol in Treatment of Chronic Diseases

Thejal Srikumar and Jaya Padmanabhan

Abstract This chapter describes the potential use of flavopiridol, a CDK inhibitor with anti-inflammatory and anti-proliferative activities, in the treatment of various chronic diseases. Flavopiridol arrests cell cycle progression in the G1 or G2 phase by inhibiting the kinase activities of CDK1, CDK2, CDK4/6, and CDK7. Additionally, it binds tightly to CDK9, a component of the P-TEFb complex (CDK9/cyclin T), and interferes with RNA polymerase II activation and associated transcription. This in turn inhibits expression of several pro-survival and anti-apoptotic genes, and enhances cytotoxicity in transformed cells or differentiation in growth-arrested cells. Recent studies indicate that flavopiridol elicits anti-inflammatory activity via CDK9 and NFκB-dependent signaling. Overall, these effects of flavopiridol potentiate its ability to overcome aberrant cell cycle activation and/or inflammatory stimuli, which are mediators of various chronic diseases.

Keywords Flavopiridol · Hematologic malignancies · Solid tumors · Neurodegenerative diseases · Coronary heart disease · Infectious disease · CDKs · Inflammation

T. Srikumar
Morsani College of Medicine, University of South Florida, Tampa, FL 33612, USA

J. Padmanabhan (✉)
Department of Molecular Medicine, Morsani College of Medicine,
University of South Florida, Tampa, FL 33612, USA
e-mail: jpadmana@health.usf.edu

J. Padmanabhan
USF Health Byrd Alzheimer's Institute, University of South Florida,
4001 E. Fletcher Ave., Tampa, FL 33613, USA

S.C. Gupta et al. (eds.), *Drug Discovery from Mother Nature*,
Advances in Experimental Medicine and Biology 929,
DOI 10.1007/978-3-319-41342-6_9

1 Introduction

Several studies have shown that natural food sources and ingredients have protective properties against low-level inflammation [1–4]. This chapter focuses on the potential use of one such compound, namely flavopiridol, as a nutritional pharmaceutical ('nutraceutical'). Flavopiridol (alvocidib, HMR-1275, L868275) is a semi-synthetic flavonoid derived from Rohitukine, a chromone alkaloid extracted from the Indian plant *Dysoxylum binectariferum*. In addition to flavopiridol, other agents from the flavonoid class are being investigated for their therapeutic potential as nutraceuticals, including catechins, genistein, and quercetin [5]. Flavopiridol was originally identified as an anti-cancer agent in an empirical study performed in 1992, where it was found to inhibit cyclin-dependent kinases CDK1, CDK2 and CDK4 [6]. In 1994, it was shown that in vitro concentrations at which flavopiridol inhibits CDKs could be safely achieved in vivo in humans. Hence, it entered clinical trials, mainly for its role in hematologic malignancy [7]. Here, we will discuss the properties, pathways, and roles of the anti-inflammatory nutraceutical flavopiridol in a wide spectrum of chronic diseases, with a focus on its role in treatment of malignancy and neurodegenerative diseases.

2 Physio-chemical Properties of Flavopiridol

Flavopiridol (IUPAC name 2-(2-chlorophenyl)-5,7-dihydroxy-8-[(3S,4R)-3-hydroxy-1-methylpiperidin-4-yl]chromen-4-one) is a free base form of synthetic *N*-methylpiperidinyl chlorophenyl flavone that is derived from the *D. binectariferum* plant. The molecular formula is $C_{21}H_{20}ClNO_5$ and has a molecular weight of 401.8402 g/mol. It has 3 hydrogen bond donors and 6 hydrogen bond acceptors, in addition to 2 rotatable bonds, and a heavy atom count of 28. It has no formal charge and is soluble in organic solvents such as ethanol, DMSO, dimethyl formamide (DMF), with limited solubility in aqueous buffers [8].

A recent study has shown that flavopiridol directly interacts with DNA, leading to structural, conformational, and thermodynamic changes [9]. Using surface-enhanced Raman Spectroscopy (SERS) and attenuated total reflectance Fourier Transform Infrared Spectroscopy (ATR-FTIR), it was shown that flavopiridol binds with the DNA nitrogenous bases guanine and thymine via a groove-directed intercalation. This interaction is of moderate strength, with an association constant of $K_a = 1.18 \times 10^4\ M^{-1}$.

3 Modulation of Cell Signaling Pathways by Flavopiridol

Flavopiridol (Alvocidib) has been shown to induce differentiation, inhibit proliferation, and enhance cytotoxicity in cells via several mechanisms , a summary of which can be seen in Fig. 1. Initially, it was shown to inhibit cyclin-dependent kinases

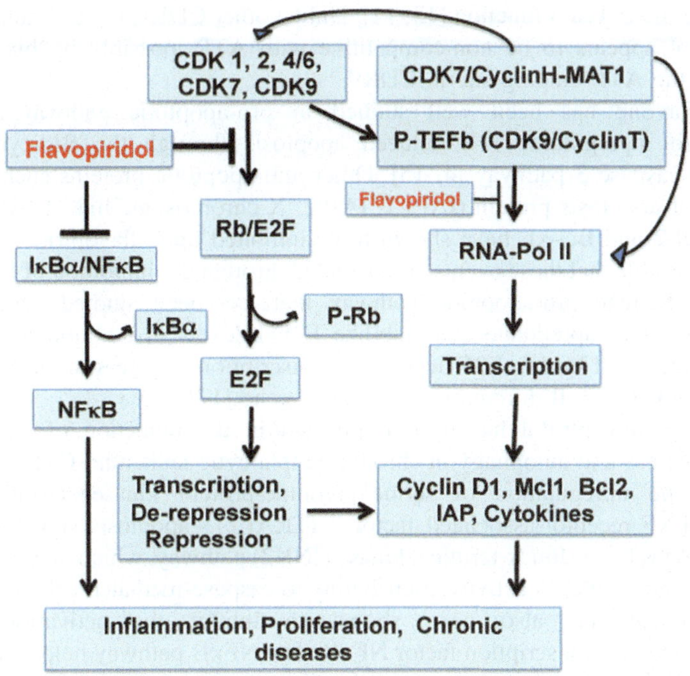

Fig. 1 Schematic summarizing the signaling mechanisms affected by flavopiridol: Flavopiridol prevents cell cycle progression in G1 or G2 phases of cell cycle by competitively binding to the ATP binding sites in CDK1, CDK2, or CDK4/6. This interferes with Rb-E2F-signaling and cell cycle progression. Flavopiridol is also known to inhibit CDK7, which associates with cyclin H and induces activation of CDKs, in addition to phosphorylation and activation of RNA Polymerase II. Further, it is known to bind tightly to the ATP binding site of CDK9 in a non-competitive manner and inhibit the P-TEFb-mediated phosphorylation and activation of RNA polymerase II, thereby affecting the RNA Pol II-dependent transcription. Flavopiridol also interferes with phosphorylation and degradation of IκBα, therefore preventing NFκB nuclear translocation and associated gene transcription, inflammatory signaling and/or cell proliferation, which are important players in induction of chronic diseases

CDK1, CDK2, CDK4, and CDK7 in a concentration-dependent manner, thereby inducing cell cycle arrest in G1 and G2 phases [7, 10, 11]. Structure-based studies have shown that flavopiridol binds to the ATP binding site of CDKs, thereby competitively inhibiting the kinase [12]. Since flavopiridol potently inhibits cell cycle activation and transcription by inhibiting CDKs, it is expected that the diseases that show activation of these kinases and unwarranted cell cycle entry would benefit from flavopiridol treatment.

Although initially developed as a CDK inhibitor, flavopiridol has been shown to inhibit RNA Pol II-dependent transcription by inactivating the positive transcription elongation factor P-TEFb, which is a complex of CDK9 and cyclin T1. P-TEFb phosphorylates the C-terminal domain of RNA Pol II, leading to its activation. Flavopiridol appears to specifically inhibit the elongation phase of transcription by interfering the P-TEFb function [13, 14]. Unlike other CDKs, P-TEFb inhibition by flavopiridol appears to be non-competitive with ATP, possibly by binding very tightly to the ATP binding site in CDK9.

This flavone has been well studied in pro-apoptotic pathways as well. Flavopiridol upregulates TNF-induced apoptosis through the Bid-cytochrome-caspase 9-caspase 3 pathway [4, 15]. Other anti-apoptotic proteins such as AKT, inhibitor of apoptosis protein (IAP)-1, IAP-2, X-chromosome-linked IAP (XIAP), Mcl-1, Bcl-2 and Bcl-xL have shown to be inhibited upon flavopiridol treatment, and it is possible that these events are mediated through the inhibition of P-TEFb [4, 16]. An alternate pro-apoptotic pathway that has been studied suggests that flavopiridol may upregulate and stabilize E2F-1 levels in addition to inhibiting CDK2, which will lead to E2F-dependent transcriptional repression of the induced myeloid leukemia cell differentiation (Mcl-1) gene [17].

Recently, flavopiridol has been implicated in the induction of endoplasmic reticulum stress and autophagy in chronic lymphocytic leukemia (CLL) cells. This involved the upregulation of serine/threonine-protein kinase/endoribonuclease (IRE1)—TNF receptor-associated factor 2 (TRAF2)—apoptosis signal-regulating kinase 1 (ASK1)—c-Jun N-terminal kinase (JNK2) pathway, which in turn increased caspase 4 and caspase 8 activity contributing to caspase-mediated cell death [18].

Flavopiridol has also been shown to inhibit the activation of the pro-inflammatory transcription factor NFκB. The NFκB pathway helps regulate the expression of genes involved in several cell functions, including transformation, survival, proliferation, invasion, and angiogenesis, and has been studied extensively for its role in cancer development and metastasis [4]. Flavopiridol inhibits NFκB by preventing IκBα kinase phosphorylation, ubiquitination, and degradation, and thus abrogating the nuclear translocation of the p65 subunit of NFκB. This in turn leads to an inhibition of COX-2, cyclin-D1, and matrix-metalloproteinase-9 synthesis, which are known to play a role in oncogenic transformation and metastasis [19]. IκB-NFκB-dependent signaling has been implicated in multiple hematopoietic malignancies such as multiple myeloma and acute myeloid leukemia (AML), both of which will be discussed further later in the chapter.

Although the pathways listed all have associations with inflammation, flavopiridol directly influences the levels of pro-inflammatory syndrome markers as well, such as interleukins. Treatment with flavopiridol has been shown to inhibit expression of IL-6-inducible acute phase proteins by interfering with CDK9-STAT3 complex formation. This suggests that CDK9 plays an important role in induction of inflammation-associated transcription and translation, and flavopiridol brings about its effects by interfering with the P-TEFb function [20].

Finally, flavopiridol has been shown to play a role in tumor angiogenesis as well. Flavopiridol inhibits hypoxia-mediated HIF-1α expression, VEGF secretion, and tumor cell migration in glioma cell lines, thereby interfering with tumor growth. Flavopiridol was also tested in murine models of glioma, and monotherapy showed inhibition of glioma tumor growth. In vitro analysis of the intracranial gliomas showed reduced vascularity of the samples treated with flavopiridol, further supporting a role for flavopiridol in pathways related to angiogenesis [21].

4 Role of Flavopiridol in Chronic Diseases

Due to the wide array of pathways that are modulated by flavopiridol, this compound has been studied in the treatment of a large variety of chronic diseases. Here, we will review the studies on flavopiridol in hematologic malignancies, solid tumors, neurological disorders, cardiovascular disease, and infectious diseases.

4.1 *Flavopiridol and Hematologic Malignancies*

4.1.1 Chronic Lymphocytic Leukemia

CLL, the most prevalent leukemia in the elderly, is characterized by an accumulation of immature, non-actively proliferating B cells that express high levels of the anti-apoptotic protein B cell lymphoma (Bcl2), which offers resistance against chemotherapeutic agents. CLL shows high heterogeneity and varies from asymptomatic progression-free survival for decades to rapidly progressive disease [22]. Deletion of 17p13.1 (del17p3) and 11q22.3 (del11q22.3) is considered to be a poor prognostic factors associated with accelerated progression and reduced survival in CLL patients [23, 24]. It has been shown that the increased expression of Bcl2 delays apoptosis and promotes drug resistance in the B cells [25, 26].

In vitro cell culture studies and clinical trials in patients with advanced disease have shown potent, p53-independent, anti-cancer effects of flavopiridol [27]. Studies in the CLL cells showed that flavopiridol treatment reduces expression of the anti-apoptotic Bcl2, Mcl-1 (myeloid cell leukemia 1), and XIAP proteins, which are known to play an important role in the survival of CLL cells. The effect on these pro-survival genes could be mediated through inhibition of P-TEFb and transcription elongation phase [27]. Studies in CLL cells have also shown that flavopiridol induces apoptosis through activation of caspase 3 [15]. These data therefore imply that flavopiridol interferes with not only cell cycle progression but also transcription and pro-survival signaling to inhibit cancer progression.

Studies by Mahoney and colleagues show that cells from CLL patient cells treated with flavopiridol show an induction of autophagy [18]. Although a moderate amount of endoplasmic reticulum (ER) stress has shown protective effects against CLL cell death, flavopiridol potentiates an excessive amount of ER stress, thereby activating apoptosis signal-regulated kinase 1 (ASK1) and caspase 4. As a result, flavopiridol induced enhanced cell death in otherwise resistant cells.

In addition to studies investigating flavopiridol as a single-agent drug, several studies have looked at flavopiridol in combination with other known agents for the development of novel chemotherapeutic regimens in CLL [28]. Flavopiridol has been shown to potentiate other chemotherapeutic agents such as paclitaxel, docetaxel, gemcitabine, and doxorubicin [29–33]. One such novel combinatorial therapy involves the use of flavopiridol and lenalidomide, the former acting as a direct cytotoxic agent and the latter as an immunomodulatory agent [34]. Lenalidomide is known to activate T cells and natural killer cells and downregulate pro-survival cytokines, thereby modifying the microenvironment. Phase I and phase II trials have shown that flavopiridol and lenalodomide can act individually to downregulate Mcl-1 and enhance immune cell function [35, 36]. A phase I trial was carried out with flavopiridol administered as a single agent in cycle 1 to reduce the number of tumor cells, followed by administration of both flavopiridol and lenalidomide concomitantly (in increasing doses) in the following cycles 2–8. This mode of treatment did not show any additional increase in toxicities associated with single-agent use of flavopiridol, including tumor lysis syndrome (TLS), tumor flare, or opportunistic infection. TLS is characterized by a set of metabolic complications that arise from the treatment, namely hyperkalemia, hyperphosphatemia, hypocalcemia, and hyperuricemia, due to the fact that a large number of newly generated cells are killed. This trial showed significant response rate (51 %) in relapsed and heavily pre-treated patients. The response rate was also significant in patients with poor prognostic cytogenetic features (del17p13.1 and del11q22.3) as well. This study also showed that patients pre-treated with flavopiridol were able to tolerate higher doses of lenalidomide [23].

Fludarabine, a purine analogue that inhibits DNA synthesis, has been widely used in the clinical setting to treat patients with CLL. Patients who are resistant to fludarabine are known to have a dismal prognosis, with an estimated survival of 10 months. There are inadequate treatment options for such patients, and a multicenter, international phase II study tested the efficacy of flavopiridol on such patients [37]. A total of 165 patients were enrolled in this study and 159 were treated. A treatment strategy of 30-min intravenous bolus (IVB) of flavopiridol followed by 4-h continuous intravenous infusion (CIVI) was used, as this was shown to be a more efficacious dosing regimen of flavopiridol than 24–72 h of CIVI in a phase I trial [38, 39]. This mode of administration showed significant activity of flavopiridol in relapsed, fludarabine-treated, refractory CLL, with the overall response rate in these patients at 25 %, with mostly partial responses [37]. These results imply that flavopiridol could serve as a potent therapeutic agent alone or in combination with other therapies as described to treat high-risk CLL or other hematologic malignancies that are fludarabine refractory.

Though patients with refractory CLL have shown significant response with flavopiridol, the main dose-limiting side effect of this drug is TLS, especially in people with leukocyte count of 200×10^9/L. To help overcome the limiting factor of development of TLS, a novel combinatorial drug treatment strategy was studied to determine whether inclusion of cyclophosphamide and rituximab together with flavopiridol helps to prevent severe toxicity from TLS [40]. This combinatorial treatment is referred to as CAR (cyclophosphamide, alvocidib, rituximab, a chimeric CD20 antibody) therapy. A phase I trial used the CAR regimen with delayed introduction of flavopiridol, only introducing it on cycle 1 day 8. Using this delayed strategy, severe grade 3 and 4 TLS was avoided in these patients [40]. This study proved CAR to be efficacious in high-risk CLL patients and protected against TLS, thereby suggesting that this combinatorial therapy could be of potential benefit to the high-risk group patients.

4.1.2 Other Hematologic Neoplasms

Proteasomal inhibitors have been a mainstay of treatment in several hematologic malignancies [41–44]. Studies are being done to develop novel treatment strategies to combine the use of flavopiridol with proteasome inhibitors due to similarities in pathway and may therefore possibly have a synergistic effect. The proteasome inhibitor bortezomib has been shown to inhibit NFκB signaling by interfering with the degradation of NFκB-inhibitory IκBα [45]. Since flavopiridol is known to induce apoptosis and inhibit NFκB signaling, studies have been undertaken to test whether combining flavopiridol with the proteasome inhibitor bortezomib shows any additive or synergistic effects on resistant, relapsed, or refractory tumors. A phase I clinical trial was carried out in 16 patients with recurrent or refractory B cell neoplasms including 9 Non-Hodgkin's Lymphoma patients (6 of which were mantle cell lymphoma), 6 multiple myeloma patients, and 1 Extra-Medullary Plasmacytoma patient [46]. Flavopiridol (30 mg/m^2) and bortezomib (1.3 mg/m^2), both administered as 30-min bolus and 4-h infusion, showed an overall response rate of 44 % in these patients. Again, one of the side effects noticed with this therapy regimen was hyperacute TLS. Another study with the combinatorial treatment of bortezomib and flavopiridol showed synergistic effect on enhanced lysis of leukemia cells, which was associated with downregulation of Mcl-1 and XIAP [47]. These cells also showed activation of JNK and inactivation of the NFκB signaling, contributing to the reduced survival. This combination induced apoptosis in imatinib-resistant CML cell lines, raising the possibility that combinatorial therapies using the proteasome inhibitor and flavopiridol may effectively prevent multiple hematologic malignancies [48].

Flavopiridol has also been studied as a single agent and in combinatorial chemotherapies for AML, which is a malignancy distinguished by clonal proliferation and transformation of immature myeloid precursor cells [49]. A phase 1 trial was undertaken in 2003 by Karp et al. which looked at flavopiridol as an initial cytoreductive agent, followed by cytarabine and mitoxantrone in a sequential manner (also known as FLAM therapy) [50]. Response to therapy was higher in AML (overall response rate 31 %) in comparison with acute lymphoblastic leukemia and chronic myeloid leukemia patients, again with significant side effects of TLS, diarrhea, and oral mucositis. A phase II trial was conducted with FLAM therapy for patients with refractory, relapsed, and high-risk AML. Flavopiridol in the context of FLAM therapy was found to induce anti-leukemic cytotoxicity in 44 % of the patients enrolled in the trial, as measured by >50 % decrease in peripheral blood blast counts [51]. Several other phase I and phase II trials have followed these initial studies, corroborating their findings.

Multiple myeloma is a plasma cell neoplasm for which several novel therapies, including bortezomib, immune modulators, thalidomide, and lenalidomide, have greatly increased the length of survival for patients who suffer from this disease [52–54]. This is thought to be accomplished by interferon regulatory factor-4 inhibition and caspase-mediated apoptosis. A phase I trial was recently undertaken to look at the role of flavopiridol in patients with relapsed multiple myeloma [55]. In this trial, 15 patients with relapsed myeloma were treated with a bolus of flavopiridol at 3 dose levels, followed by a continuous infusion for 4 weeks out of a 5-week cycle. It was found that flavopiridol achieved only marginal responses in myeloma and that patients incurred significant side effects including cytopenias, diarrhea, and transaminase elevation. However, as mentioned above, studies are still being undertaken to evaluate for the combinatorial use of flavopiridol with proteasome inhibitors in multiple myeloma patients.

4.2 Flavopiridol and Its Role in Solid Tumors

Flavopiridol is known to inhibit CDKs by binding to the ATP binding sites, and inhibits cyclin D1 and VEGF by interfering with transcriptional and post-transcriptional mechanisms [56]. Any tumors that show activation of the CDK1, CDK2, CDK4/6, CDK7, or CDK9 are expected to show some response to treatment with flavopiridol. Although the most convincing data on clinical efficacy of flavopiridol are evident from research done on hematologic malignancies such as CLL, studies have been conducted to assess how flavopiridol affects solid tumors as well. A phase I study looked at flavopiridol in pancreatic, breast, esophageal, colon, melanoma, lung, ovarian, sarcoma, carcinoid, and gastric cancer patients, and identified flavopiridol as a safe and tolerable regimen. Promising clinical activity was seen, especially among refractory germ cell, pancreatic, gastric, and sweat gland tumors [57]. Here, we will provide a brief review of the role of flavopiridol specifically in breast cancer, sarcoma, colon cancer, and pancreatic cancer.

4.2.1 Sarcoma

Sarcomas are a group of heterogeneous malignancies that are mesenchymal in origin. Treatment options for advanced sarcomas are limited and patients often have poor prognoses. The main treatment options currently available for advanced sarcomas, especially those that are metastatic or unresectable, are systemic use of chemotherapy including doxorubicin, gemcitabine, docetaxel, ifosfamide, and dacarbazine. Studies in Rb-null osteosarcoma have shown that flavopiridol potentiates the anti-tumor activity of doxorubicin [58]. In a study done by Luke et al. in 2012, the authors determined whether flavopiridol elicits similar effects on well-differentiated and de-differentiated soft tissue sarcomas [59]. In addition to amplification of the MDM2 proto-oncogene, the majority of soft tissue sarcomas show amplification of CDK4. Since flavopiridol is a potent inhibitor of CDK4, co-treatment with doxorubicin and flavopiridol was expected to elicit synergistic effect [60]. LS141 and MPNST cell lines derived from a patient with high-grade retroperitoneal de-differentiated liposarcoma or high-grade peripheral nerve sheath tumor of the thigh were used for in vitro cell culture and in vivo tumor xenograft studies. Results showed that combinatorial treatment with doxorubicin and flavopiridol shows significant inhibition of cell growth compared to single-agent treatment [60]. Following this, a phase I dose escalation clinical trial was completed in patients with advanced sarcoma to determine maximum tolerable dose and activity of flavopiridol in combination with doxorubicin [59]. This study showed that combinatorial therapy with doxorubicin and flavopiridol had tolerable adverse effects and provided significant disease control. The progression-free survival at 12 weeks was calculated at 57 % and at 24 weeks at 32 %, which suggests that combinatorial therapy with flavopiridol and doxorubicin would be beneficial in treatment of well-differentiated and de-differentiated soft tissue sarcomas.

4.2.2 Breast Cancer

Breast cancer is the second leading cause of cancer-related death in women, despite huge strides in early detection of malignancy [61]. Studies using directed therapies such as trastuzumab (antibody therapy) and lapatinib (receptor tyrosine kinase inhibitor, RTK) have shown efficacy toward breast cancer but is overshadowed by tumor heterogeneity, drug resistance, and off-target effects. It is known that the overexpression of the RTKs such as epidermal growth factor receptor (EGFR) and HER-2 contributes significantly to the cancer pathogenesis by signaling via the Ras-Raf-MEK-ERK and PI3K-Akt signaling pathways [62]. In addition to these pathways, the cancer cells also show activation of CDKs and Rb-E2F signaling. Knockdown of cyclin D1 and CDK4/6 has been shown to increase or inhibit cell migration in estrogen receptor (ER)-positive or negative tumors, respectively [63]. Treatment with flavopiridol could reproduce similar effects, implying the potential use of this drug for treatment of ER-negative tumors. Recently, it was shown that sorafenib (a tyrosine kinase inhibitor, TKI) together with flavopiridol provides greater cytotoxicity at lower doses compared to combination of sorafenib with RTK inhibitors, in both EGFR/HER-2 overexpressing and K-Ras-B-Raf-mutation associated breast tumor cells. This suggests a potential use of flavopiridol in combination with sorafenib for treatment of breast cancer patients [62]. Flavopiridol appears to interact with lapatinib and reduce expression of Mcl-1. Additionally, inclusion of Mcl-1 inhibitor obatoclax appeared to enhance the lethality of both lapatinib and flavopiridol by promoting BAX-BAK-dependent mitochondrial dysfunction and cellular apoptosis in vitro [64].

4.2.3 Colon Cancer

Colorectal cancer is the second leading cause of cancer-related deaths among both men and women in the USA [61]. Studies in colon cancer cells that are positive or negative for p53 have shown that sequential treatment with CPT-11 (irinotecan, topoisomerase inhibitor) and flavopiridol shows more beneficial effects in the p53-positive tumors and the effect was mediated through p53-dependent suppression of Rad51 and promotion of apoptosis [65]. Further, studies in colon cancer cells have also shown that sequential treatment with γ-irradiation followed by flavopiridol significantly inhibits tumor growth and this was associated with a loss of p21 [66]. HCT-116 colon cancer cells that lacked p21 responded to γ-irradiation and flavopiridol treatment much more effectively, implying that loss of p21 expression potentiates the efficacy of the co-treatment. In vitro and in vivo studies have shown that sequential treatment with docetaxel for 1 h, followed by flavopiridol 24 h, followed by 5-fluorouracil (a thymidylate synthase inhibitor) 24 h, showed significant inhibition of HCT116 colon cancer cell proliferation, colony formation on soft agar, as well as reduced tumor growth and increased survival in xenograft models [67]. Flavopiridol together with irinotecan has shown significant tumor growth inhibition in xenograft models. To test the efficacy of flavopiridol in patients with advanced CRC, a pre-clinical study was carried out with irinotecan followed by flavopiridol. Results were promising and patients who were wild type (WT) for p53 appeared to respond by interfering with p21 and Drg1 (differentiation-associated gene 1) expression [68]. Similarly, a phase I trial with FOLFIRI and flavopiridol appeared to have potent anti-tumor activity in solid tumors. Once again, the effectiveness correlated with the presence of WT p53 expression, and the addition of flavopiridol stabilized the disease in patients with irinotecan-refractory colorectal tumor [69].

4.2.4 Pancreatic Cancer

Despite its low prevalence, pancreatic cancer is the fourth leading cause of cancer-related death in the USA due to the lack of effective screening tools, vague symptoms, and aggressive nature of the disease [61]. Current therapies directed toward pancreatic cancer show marginal effects and combinatorial therapies with gemcitabine show promising results [70–72]. Treatment with gemcitabine has been shown to enhance expression of ribonucleotide reductase M2 subunit and flavopiridol appears to inhibit its expression and enhance cytotoxic effects of gemcitabine [30]. A phase II study was undertaken to evaluate flavopiridol in 10 pancreatic adenocarcinoma patients with gemcitabine refractory tumors. Docetaxel was followed by flavopiridol, and the combination showed only minimal effect with high toxicity, thereby raising potential problems in this treatment strategy to overcome pancreatic adenocarcinoma [73].

4.3 *Flavopiridol in Neurological Disorders*

4.3.1 Neurodegenerative Diseases

While apoptosis is important for the sculpting of the developing brain, apoptosis in terminally differentiated neurons has been associated with the development of neuropathology [74]. Studies in patients with Alzheimer's disease or other neurodegenerative diseases have shown evidence for enhanced expression and activation of cell cycle regulatory proteins in terminally differentiated neurons [75–84]. Treatment of the neurons with CDK inhibitors such as flavopiridol, roscovitine, or olomoucine showed protection against apoptosis induced by specific insults such as activity withdrawal, DNA-damaging agent exposure, and growth factor deprivation, confirming that aberrant neuronal cell cycle entry promotes neurodegeneration and apoptosis in mature neurons [85–92]. Furthermore, studies conducted with organotypic cultures of cerebellar sections have shown that axotomy-induced apoptosis can be prevented by treatment with flavopiridol, olomoucine, or roscovitine [93].

Studies in neurons have shown that transcription and translation are upregulated under apoptotic conditions [94, 95]. Earlier studies from our laboratory have shown that flavopiridol inhibits the activity of cyclin D1/CDK, Cycin E/CDK complexes, and Rb phosphorylation while protecting cerebellar neurons from death induced by KCl withdrawal [85]. We recently showed that this KCl withdrawal-induced apoptosis is associated with upregulation of RNA Pol II phosphorylation and transcription [96]. Treatment with flavopiridol, as well as DRB (5,6-dichloro-1-beta-D-ribobenzimidazole), a more specific inhibitor of RNA Pol II, protected the neurons against apoptosis, which was associated with inhibition of Pol II phosphorylation and activation. Upon removal of these drugs, the neurons showed enhanced phosphorylation of Pol II and increased apoptosis. In addition to transcriptional inhibition, the neurons also showed reduced incorporation of ^{35}S-Methionine, indicative of reduced translation. This correlated with inhibition of P70S6 kinase phosphorylation and activation. It is possible that flavopiridol brings about the protective effect on the neurons by inhibiting RNA Pol II and P70S6 kinase-mediated transcription and translation, respectively, of specific 5′-Terminal oligopyrimidine (TOP) tract mRNAs that play an essential role in neuronal apoptosis. Identification of these specific mRNAs will help in the development of more targeted inhibitors to prevent neuronal apoptosis in chronic neurodegenerative diseases.

4.3.2 Stroke

Stroke is the fourth leading cause of death in the USA, and it is estimated that by 2030 greater than 3 million people will be suffering from this debilitating degenerative disease. Stroke can be categorized as ischemic (not enough blood flow to the brain) and hemorrhagic (where the blood vessels in the brain rupture). Studies in rat models of ischemia-induced stroke have shown that one of the underlying mechanisms of neurodegeneration is deregulation of cell cycle machinery that causes aberrant cell cycle entry of the differentiated neurons. Neurons in these models showed activation of CDK4, cyclin D1, Rb phosphorylation and E2F1 induction [97]. In vivo intracerebroventricular administration of flavopiridol via implanted cannula connected to an osmotic pump showed significant reduction in neuronal death, indicative of aberrant CDK activation in promotion of ischemia-induced cell death. Furthermore, the rats treated with flavopiridol also showed signs of increased spatial learning behavior and functional recovery [98]. This suggests that flavopiridol may have therapeutic potential toward prevention of irreversible neuronal damage in ischemia-induced stroke.

4.3.3 Traumatic Brain Injury

Traumatic brain injury (TBI) is associated with neuronal death, activation of microglia, inflammation, and astrogliosis [99–102]. Such a reaction can lead to permanent tissue loss and glial scar formation. Thus, long-term sequelae of traumatic brain injuries can occur, creating a picture of neurodegenerative disease. Flavopiridol was studied in etoposide-treated primary cortical neurons and was found to decrease the number of apoptotic cells via several proposed mechanisms, including downregulation of caspase 3, regulation of cell cycle via downregulation of cyclin D1, and upregulation of CDK inhibitor p27. In rat brain astrocyte culture, flavopiridol addition was able to decrease cell proliferation in a dose-dependent manner [103]. Flavopiridol was also studied in rats that underwent TBI and was found to decrease microglial proliferation and invasion, which was associated with decrease in lesion volume and increase in functional recovery in these models [99].

Evidence suggests that inflammatory modulators induce neuronal cell cycle entry and inhibition of cell cycle prior to induction of inflammation protects against neurodegeneration [104]. In this regard, the finding that flavopiridol acts as an anti-inflammatory agent is of significant importance and suggests that this CDK inhibitor might be beneficial in protecting against neuroinflammation through inhibition of CDK9, and this could be one of the mechanisms by which flavopiridol brings about the neuroprotection observed in stroke and TBI animal models [105].

4.4 Flavopiridol in Cardiovascular Disease

Coronary artery disease (CAD) is by far the leading cause of morbidity and mortality in developed nations worldwide. It is characterized by atherosclerosis, which is the build up of plaque that is composed of lipids and fibrous elements, in the coronary arteries. Recently, CDK9 levels were found to be very high in plaque samples, serum, and monocytes in patients with atherosclerotic disease [106]. The infiltration of inflammatory cells such as monocytes and macrophages within the plaque was found to be associated with CDK9 expression, suggesting that CDK9 could potentially be a marker of atherosclerosis [106]. Furthermore, flavopiridol has been shown to inhibit leukocyte adhesion to the endothelium by inhibiting the expression of adhesion molecules, which was brought about by inhibition of CDK9 [105]. As such, due to the potent inhibitory activity of flavopiridol on CDK9, this nutraceutical could potentially show major benefit in patients with CAD and atherosclerosis. However, no studies to this end have been completed as of yet.

Flavopiridol has also been utilized in the drug-eluting stents within atherosclerotic arteries. A common complication of stent placement is the possibility of re-stenosis of the vasculature due to proliferation of coronary smooth muscle cells into the lumen. Jaschke et al. [107] showed that, in addition to p53, flavopiridol potently inhibits the proliferation and migration of coronary smooth muscle cells in vitro via cell cycle inhibition and increase in CDK inhibitors p21 and p27. Flavopiridol also decreased Rb hyperphosphorylation in these cells, thereby preventing G1/S progression. When the flavopiridol drug-eluting stents were placed in the carotid arteries of rats, a reduction in neointima injury formation could be observed in comparison with control [107]. These studies imply that inclusion of flavopiridol in stents used for atherosclerotic vessels could increase the patency of these vessels by preventing the formation of re-stenosis.

4.5 *Flavopiridol in Infectious Disease*

4.5.1 Human Immunodeficiency Virus-1 (HIV-1)

Human immunodeficiency virus-1 (HIV-1) and its development into acquired immunodeficiency syndrome (AIDS) has caused a huge worldwide burden of disease. HIV-1 is a retrovirus that is dependent on cell cycle machinery to replicate and proliferate. Specifically, the CDK9/cyclin T (P-TEFb) complex activates the transcription of the HIV-1 long-terminal repeat promoter, making P-TEFb both essential and a limiting factor in HIV-1 replication [108]. As discussed earlier, flavopiridol is a potent P-TEFb inhibitor and has been shown to block HIV-1 Tat transactivation and viral replication [13, 109]. Flavopiridol has been shown to significantly inhibit the replication of HIV-1 in HeLa cell models as well [110].

Studies have also been done to evaluate the role of flavopiridol in HIV-induced nephropathy. Nelson et al. [111] found that in in vitro models, flavopiridol inhibited HIV transcription in infected podocytes without significant toxic effects. In 2003, the same group created an HIV-1 NL4-3 transgenic mouse model of HIV-associated nephropathy (HIVAN) [112]. Flavopiridol administration for a 20-day course was utilized, and the results showed that HIV-1 proviral expression had decreased significantly throughout the kidney. Furthermore, the nephrotic changes visualized in histologic and transcriptional activity of the endogenous mouse renal cells had been reversed with flavopiridol administration up to 82 %.

Although no clinical trials have yet been conducted, research into synthetic analogues of flavopiridol is being studied to help minimize toxicity.

4.5.2 Human Herpes Simplex Virus 1 (HSV-1)

Herpes simplex virus 1 (HSV-1) is a double-stranded DNA virus of the *Herpesviridae* family. Similar to HIV-1, HSV-1 is dependent upon human cell cycle machinery for viral transcription. In a 2013 study, it was shown that serine-2 phosphorylated RNA Polymerase II was required for HSV-1 transcription [113]. Inhibition of the RNA Polymerase II via CDK9 inhibition with flavopiridol decreased the level of late viral proteins, led to poor formation of viral transcription compartments, and decreased RNA synthesis in vitro. To date, no studies of the role of flavopiridol in HSV-1 treatment have been conducted in animal or human models.

5 Conclusions

Flavopiridol has shown potential efficacy in a wide array of disorders. Several clinical trials with flavopiridol as a single agent or in combination with other chemotherapeutic agents have shown significant benefits in treating chronic diseases, especially hematologic malignancies such as CLL. Additionally, studies in solid tumors also have shown promising results with this CDK inhibitor as a sole treatment or in combination with other chemotherapy regimens. The toxicities associated with flavopiridol treatment, primarily TLS, are manageable and other combinatorial therapies such as the CAR treatment, which shows activity against hyperacute TLS. Bolus treatment with flavopiridol for 30 min followed by 4-h infusion appears to provide maximum activity for extended period of time. Studies performed with various disease-relevant cell culture or animal models, as well as human clinical trials, imply that flavopiridol as a single agent or in combination with other agents would also prove to be beneficial in treatment of neurodegenerative diseases, stroke, TBI, atherosclerosis, HIV, and HSV infection. Results from future studies will enable us to determine whether inclusion of flavopiridol would be beneficial in treatment of other chronic diseases that are resistant to the current treatment strategies. Since flavopiridol shows potent inhibitory effect toward CDK9, additional flavopiridol mimetics are being developed to determine whether more selective inhibitors with reduced toxicity can be used to achieve similar efficacy. In this regard, the CDK9 inhibitor FIT-03, which has shown promising results with drug-resistant HSVs and other DNA viruses, or fluoroflavopiridol, with 40-fold more selectivity toward P-TEFb function, might prove to cause lower levels of toxicity [114, 115]. Regardless, due to the ubiquitous role of flavopiridol in several critical cell cycle and inflammatory pathways, there is no doubt that this nutraceutical has boundless potential in the management of disease states.

Acknowledgments The work in JP's laboratory is supported by funds from Anna Valentine Moffitt/USF Collaborative Grant and Small Grant Program from USF Health Byrd Alzheimer's Institute.

References

1. Rafi MM, Yadav PN, Maeng I-K (2003) Targeting inflammation using nutraceuticals. In Ho C-T, Lin J-K, Zheng QY (Eds.), Oriental Food and Herbs: Chemistry and Health Benefits (ACS Symposium Series) (48–63). United States of America: Oxford University Press.
2. Rajasekaran A, Sivagnanam G, Xavier R (2008) Nutraceuticals as therapeutic agents: a review. Res J Pharm Tech 1(4):328–340
3. Das L et al (2012) Role of nutraceuticals in human health. J Food Sci Technol 49(2):173–183
4. Gupta SC et al (2010) Regulation of survival, proliferation, invasion, angiogenesis, and metastasis of tumor cells through modulation of inflammatory pathways by nutraceuticals. Cancer Metastasis Rev 29(3):405–434
5. Wang HK (2000) The therapeutic potential of flavonoids. Expert Opin Investig Drugs 9 (9):2103–2119
6. Losiewicz MD et al (1994) Potent inhibition of CDC2 kinase activity by the flavonoid L86-8275. Biochem Biophys Res Commun 201(2):589–595
7. Senderowicz AM (1999) Flavopiridol: the first cyclin-dependent kinase inhibitor in human clinical trials. Invest New Drugs 17(3):313–320
8. CID = 5287969 (2015) National Center for Biotechnology Information
9. Ray B et al (2015) Structural, conformational and thermodynamic aspects of groove-directed-intercalation of flavopiridol into DNA. J Biomol Struct Dyn, 1–47
10. Senderowicz AM, Sausville EA (2000) Preclinical and clinical development of cyclin-dependent kinase modulators. J Natl Cancer Inst 92(5):376–387
11. Sedlacek H et al (1996) Flavopiridol (L86 8275; NSC 649890), a new kinase inhibitor for tumor therapy. Int J Oncol 9(6):1143–1168
12. De Azevedo WF Jr et al (1996) Structural basis for specificity and potency of a flavonoid inhibitor of human CDK2, a cell cycle kinase. Proc Natl Acad Sci U S A 93(7):2735–2740
13. Chao SH et al (2000) Flavopiridol inhibits P-TEFb and blocks HIV-1 replication. J Biol Chem 275(37):28345–28348
14. Aleem E, Arceci RJ (2015) Targeting cell cycle regulators in hematologic malignancies. Front Cell Dev Biol 3:16
15. Byrd JC et al (1998) Flavopiridol induces apoptosis in chronic lymphocytic leukemia cells via activation of caspase-3 without evidence of bcl-2 modulation or dependence on functional p53. Blood 92(10):3804–3816
16. Takada Y et al (2008) Flavopiridol suppresses tumor necrosis factor-induced activation of activator protein-1, c-Jun N-terminal kinase, p38 mitogen-activated protein kinase (MAPK), p44/p42 MAPK, and Akt, inhibits expression of antiapoptotic gene products, and enhances apoptosis through cytochrome c release and caspase activation in human myeloid cells. Mol Pharmacol 73(5):1549–1557
17. Ma Y, Cress WD, Haura EB (2003) Flavopiridol-induced apoptosis is mediated through up-regulation of E2F1 and repression of Mcl-1. Mol Cancer Ther 2(1):73–81
18. Mahoney E et al (2012) ER stress and autophagy: new discoveries in the mechanism of action and drug resistance of the cyclin-dependent kinase inhibitor flavopiridol. Blood 120 (6):1262–1273
19. Takada Y, Aggarwal BB (2004) Flavopiridol inhibits NF-κB activation induced by various carcinogens and inflammatory agents through inhibition of IκBα kinase and p65 phosphorylation: abrogation of cyclin D1, cyclooxygenase-2, and matrix metalloprotease-9. J Biol Chem 279(6):4750–4759

20. Hou T, Ray S, Brasier AR (2007) The functional role of an interleukin 6-inducible CDK9. STAT3 complex in human gamma-fibrinogen gene expression. J Biol Chem 282(51): 37091–37102
21. Newcomb EW et al (2005) Flavopiridol downregulates hypoxia-mediated hypoxia-inducible factor-1alpha expression in human glioma cells by a proteasome-independent pathway: implications for in vivo therapy. Neuro Oncol 7(3):225–235
22. Chen R et al (2005) Transcription inhibition by flavopiridol: mechanism of chronic lymphocytic leukemia cell death. Blood 106(7):2513–2519
23. Maddocks K et al (2015) Reduced occurrence of tumor flare with flavopiridol followed by combined flavopiridol and lenalidomide in patients with relapsed chronic lymphocytic leukemia (CLL). Am J Hematol 90(4):327–333
24. Dighiero G et al (1991) B-cell chronic lymphocytic leukemia: present status and future directions. French cooperative group on CLL. Blood 78(8):1901–1914
25. Robertson LE et al (1996) Bcl-2 expression in chronic lymphocytic leukemia and its correlation with the induction of apoptosis and clinical outcome. Leukemia 10(3):456–459
26. Adachi M et al (1990) Preferential linkage of bcl-2 to immunoglobulin light chain gene in chronic lymphocytic leukemia. J Exp Med 171(2):559–564
27. Kitada S et al (2000) Protein kinase inhibitors flavopiridol and 7-hydroxy-staurosporine down-regulate antiapoptosis proteins in B-cell chronic lymphocytic leukemia. Blood 96 (2):393–397
28. Desai AV, El-Bakkar H, Abdul-Hay M (2015) Novel agents in the treatment of chronic lymphocytic leukemia: a review about the future. Clin Lymphoma Myeloma Leuk 15 (6):314–322
29. Motwani M et al (2001) Augmentation of apoptosis and tumor regression by flavopiridol in the presence of CPT-11 in Hct116 colon cancer monolayers and xenografts. Clin Cancer Res 7(12):4209–4219
30. Jung CP, Motwani MV, Schwartz GK (2001) Flavopiridol increases sensitization to gemcitabine in human gastrointestinal cancer cell lines and correlates with down-regulation of ribonucleotide reductase M2 subunit. Clin Cancer Res 7(8):2527–2536
31. Motwani M, Delohery TM, Schwartz GK (1999) Sequential dependent enhancement of caspase activation and apoptosis by flavopiridol on paclitaxel-treated human gastric and breast cancer cells. Clin Cancer Res 5(7):1876–1883
32. Wall NR et al (2003) Suppression of survivin phosphorylation on Thr34 by flavopiridol enhances tumor cell apoptosis. Cancer Res 63(1):230–235
33. Bible KC, Kaufmann SH (1997) Cytotoxic synergy between flavopiridol (NSC 649890, L86-8275) and various antineoplastic agents: the importance of sequence of administration. Cancer Res 57(16):3375–3380
34. Crane E, List A (2005) Lenalidomide: an immunomodulatory drug. Future Oncol 1(5): 575–583
35. Byrd JC et al (2007) Flavopiridol administered using a pharmacologically derived schedule is associated with marked clinical efficacy in refractory, genetically high-risk chronic lymphocytic leukemia. Blood 109(2):399–404
36. Chanan-Khan A et al (2006) Clinical efficacy of lenalidomide in patients with relapsed or refractory chronic lymphocytic leukemia: results of a phase II study. J Clin Oncol 24 (34):5343–5349
37. Lanasa MC et al (2015) Final results of EFC6663: a multicenter, international, phase 2 study of alvocidib for patients with fludarabine-refractory chronic lymphocytic leukemia. Leuk Res 39(5):495–500
38. Schwartz GK et al (2002) Phase I study of the cyclin-dependent kinase inhibitor flavopiridol in combination with paclitaxel in patients with advanced solid tumors. J Clin Oncol 20 (8):2157–2170
39. Lin TS et al (2002) Seventy-two hour continuous infusion flavopiridol in relapsed and refractory mantle cell lymphoma. Leuk Lymphoma 43(4):793–797

40. Stephens DM et al (2013) Cyclophosphamide, alvocidib (flavopiridol), and rituximab, a novel feasible chemoimmunotherapy regimen for patients with high-risk chronic lymphocytic leukemia. Leuk Res 37(10):1195–1199
41. Esparis-Ogando A et al (2005) Bortezomib is an efficient agent in plasma cell leukemias. Int J Cancer 114(4):665–667
42. Adams J (2002) Proteasome inhibition: a novel approach to cancer therapy. Trends Mol Med 8(4 Suppl):S49–S54
43. Landis-Piwowar KR et al (2006) The proteasome as a potential target for novel anticancer drugs and chemosensitizers. Drug Resist Updates 9(6):263–273
44. Mitsiades CS et al (2006) Proteasome inhibition as a new therapeutic principle in hematological malignancies. Curr Drug Targets 7(10):1341–1347
45. Sunwoo JB et al (2001) Novel proteasome inhibitor PS-341 inhibits activation of nuclear factor-κB, cell survival, tumor growth, and angiogenesis in squamous cell carcinoma. Clin Cancer Res 7(5):1419–1428
46. Holkova B et al (2011) Phase I trial of bortezomib (PS-341; NSC 681239) and alvocidib (flavopiridol; NSC 649890) in patients with recurrent or refractory B-cell neoplasms. Clin Cancer Res 17(10):3388–3397
47. Holkova B, Grant S (2011) Combining proteasome with cell cycle inhibitors: a dual attack potentially applicable to multiple hematopoietic malignancies. Expert Rev Hematol 4 (5):483–486
48. Dai Y et al (2004) Bortezomib and flavopiridol interact synergistically to induce apoptosis in chronic myeloid leukemia cells resistant to imatinib mesylate through both Bcr/Abl-dependent and -independent mechanisms. Blood 104(2):509–518
49. Zeidner JF, Karp JE (2015) Clinical activity of alvocidib (flavopiridol) in acute myeloid leukemia. Leuk Res 39(12):1312–1318
50. Karp JE et al (2005) Phase I and pharmacokinetic study of flavopiridol followed by 1-β-D-arabinofuranosylcytosine and mitoxantrone in relapsed and refractory adult acute leukemias. Clin Cancer Res 11(23):8403–8412
51. Zeidner JF et al (2015) Randomized multicenter phase II study of flavopiridol (alvocidib), cytarabine, and mitoxantrone (FLAM) versus cytarabine/daunorubicin (7 + 3) in newly diagnosed acute myeloid leukemia. Haematologica 100(9):1172–1179
52. Zhu YX, Kortuem KM, Stewart AK (2013) Molecular mechanism of action of immune-modulatory drugs thalidomide, lenalidomide and pomalidomide in multiple myeloma. Leuk Lymphoma 54(4):683–687
53. San Miguel JF et al (2008) Bortezomib plus melphalan and prednisone for initial treatment of multiple myeloma. N Engl J Med 359(9):906–917
54. Richardson PG et al (2005) Bortezomib or high-dose dexamethasone for relapsed multiple myeloma. N Engl J Med 352(24):2487–2498
55. Hofmeister CC et al (2014) A phase I trial of flavopiridol in relapsed multiple myeloma. Cancer Chemother Pharmacol 73(2):249–257
56. Senderowicz AM (2003) Novel direct and indirect cyclin-dependent kinase modulators for the prevention and treatment of human neoplasms. Cancer Chemother Pharmacol 52 (Suppl 1):S61–S73
57. Rathkopf D et al (2009) Phase I study of flavopiridol with oxaliplatin and fluorouracil/leucovorin in advanced solid tumors. Clin Cancer Res 15(23):7405–7411
58. Li W, Fan J, Bertino JR (2001) Selective sensitization of retinoblastoma protein-deficient sarcoma cells to doxorubicin by flavopiridol-mediated inhibition of cyclin-dependent kinase 2 kinase activity. Cancer Res 61(6):2579–2582
59. Luke JJ et al (2012) The cyclin-dependent kinase inhibitor flavopiridol potentiates doxorubicin efficacy in advanced sarcomas: preclinical investigations and results of a phase I dose-escalation clinical trial. Clin Cancer Res 18(9):2638–2647
60. Dei Tos AP et al (2000) Coordinated expression and amplification of the MDM2, CDK4, and HMGI-C genes in atypical lipomatous tumours. J Pathol 190(5):531–536
61. Siegel RL, Miller KD, Jemal A (2015) Cancer statistics, 2015. CA Cancer J Clin 65(1):5–29

62. Nagaria TS et al (2013) Flavopiridol synergizes with sorafenib to induce cytotoxicity and potentiate antitumorigenic activity in EGFR/HER-2 and mutant RAS/RAF breast cancer model systems. Neoplasia 15(8):939–951
63. Lamb R et al (2013) Cell cycle regulators cyclin D1 and CDK4/6 have estrogen receptor-dependent divergent functions in breast cancer migration and stem cell-like activity. Cell Cycle 12(15):2384–2394
64. Mitchell C et al (2010) Inhibition of MCL-1 in breast cancer cells promotes cell death in vitro and in vivo. Cancer Biol Ther 10(9):903–917
65. Ambrosini G et al (2008) The cyclin-dependent kinase inhibitor flavopiridol potentiates the effects of topoisomerase I poisons by suppressing Rad51 expression in a p53-dependent manner. Cancer Res 68(7):2312–2320
66. Jung C et al (2003) The cyclin-dependent kinase inhibitor flavopiridol potentiates gamma-irradiation-induced apoptosis in colon and gastric cancer cells. Clin Cancer Res 9 (16 Pt 1):6052–6061
67. Guo J et al (2006) Efficacy of sequential treatment of HCT116 colon cancer monolayers and xenografts with docetaxel, flavopiridol, and 5-fluorouracil. Acta Pharmacol Sin 27(10): 1375–1381
68. Shah MA et al (2005) A phase I clinical trial of the sequential combination of irinotecan followed by flavopiridol. Clin Cancer Res 11(10):3836–3845
69. Dickson MA et al (2010) A phase I clinical trial of FOLFIRI in combination with the pan-cyclin-dependent kinase (CDK) inhibitor flavopiridol. Cancer Chemother Pharmacol 66 (6):1113–1121
70. Schaal C, Padmanabhan J, Chellappan S (2015) The role of nAChR and calcium signaling in pancreatic cancer initiation and progression. Cancers (Basel) 7(3):1447–1471
71. Woods NK, Padmanabhan J (2013) Inhibition of amyloid precursor protein processing enhances gemcitabine-mediated cytotoxicity in pancreatic cancer cells. J Biol Chem 288 (42):30114–30124
72. Marks E, Saif MW, Jia Y (2014) Updates on first-line therapy for metastatic pancreatic adenocarcinoma. JOP 15(2):99–102
73. Carvajal RD et al (2009) A phase II study of flavopiridol (Alvocidib) in combination with docetaxel in refractory, metastatic pancreatic cancer. Pancreatology 9(4):404–409
74. Pallas M et al (2005) Flavopiridol: an antitumor drug with potential application in the treatment of neurodegenerative diseases. Med Hypotheses 64(1):120–123
75. Vincent I, Pae CI, Hallows JL (2003) The cell cycle and human neurodegenerative disease. Prog Cell Cycle Res 5:31–41
76. Vincent I et al (2001) Constitutive Cdc25B tyrosine phosphatase activity in adult brain neurons with M phase-type alterations in Alzheimer's disease. Neuroscience 105(3):639–650
77. Stone JG et al (2011) The cell cycle regulator phosphorylated retinoblastoma protein is associated with tau pathology in several tauopathies. J Neuropathol Exp Neurol 70(7): 578–587
78. Alquezar C et al (2015) Targeting cyclin D3/CDK6 activity for treatment of Parkinson's disease. J Neurochem 133(6):886–897
79. Hoglinger GU et al (2007) The pRb/E2F cell-cycle pathway mediates cell death in Parkinson's disease. Proc Natl Acad Sci U S A 104(9):3585–3590
80. Seward ME et al (2013) Amyloid-beta signals through tau to drive ectopic neuronal cell cycle re-entry in Alzheimer's disease. J Cell Sci 126(Pt 5):1278–1286
81. Arendt T et al (1996) Expression of the cyclin-dependent kinase inhibitor p16 in Alzheimer's disease. NeuroReport 7(18):3047–3049
82. Arendt T (2000) Alzheimer's disease as a loss of differentiation control in a subset of neurons that retain immature features in the adult brain. Neurobiol Aging 21(6):783–796
83. Arendt T (2002) Dysregulation of neuronal differentiation and cell cycle control in Alzheimer's disease. J Neural Transm Suppl 62:77–85
84. Herrup K, Arendt T (2002) Re-expression of cell cycle proteins induces neuronal cell death during Alzheimer's disease. J Alzheimers Dis 4(3):243–247

85. Padmanabhan J et al (1999) Role of cell cycle regulatory proteins in cerebellar granule neuron apoptosis. J Neurosci 19(20):8747–8756
86. Park DS et al (2000) Involvement of retinoblastoma family members and E2F/DP complexes in the death of neurons evoked by DNA damage. J Neurosci 20(9):3104–3114
87. Park DS et al (1998) Cyclin-dependent kinases participate in death of neurons evoked by DNA-damaging agents. J Cell Biol 143(2):457–467
88. Verdaguer E et al (2005) Inhibition of multiple pathways accounts for the antiapoptotic effects of flavopiridol on potassium withdrawal-induced apoptosis in neurons. J Mol Neurosci 26(1):71–84
89. Kruman II et al (2004) Cell cycle activation linked to neuronal cell death initiated by DNA damage. Neuron 41(4):549–561
90. Kim AH, Bonni A (2008) Cdk1-FOXO1: a mitotic signal takes center stage in post-mitotic neurons. Cell Cycle 7(24):3819–3822
91. Folch J et al (2012) Role of cell cycle re-entry in neurons: a common apoptotic mechanism of neuronal cell death. Neurotox Res 22(3):195–207
92. Copani A et al (2001) Activation of cell-cycle-associated proteins in neuronal death: a mandatory or dispensable path? Trends Neurosci 24(1):25–31
93. Padmanabhan J, Brown K, Shelanski ML (2007) Cell cycle inhibition and retinoblastoma protein overexpression prevent Purkinje cell death in organotypic slice cultures. Dev Neurobiol 67(6):818–826
94. Freeman RS, Estus S, Johnson EM Jr (1994) Analysis of cell cycle-related gene expression in postmitotic neurons: selective induction of Cyclin D1 during programmed cell death. Neuron 12(2):343–355
95. Iwasaki K et al (1996) Changes in gene transcription during a beta-mediated cell death. Mol Psychiatry 1(1):65–71
96. Padmanabhan J et al (2015) Functional role of RNA polymerase II and P70 S6 kinase in KCl withdrawal induced cerebellar granule neuron apoptosis. J Biol Chem 290(9):5267–5279
97. Osuga H et al (2000) Cyclin-dependent kinases as a therapeutic target for stroke. Proc Natl Acad Sci U S A 97(18):10254–10259
98. Wang F et al (2002) Inhibition of cyclin-dependent kinases improves CA1 neuronal survival and behavioral performance after global ischemia in the rat. J Cereb Blood Flow Metab 22 (2):171–182
99. Di Giovanni S et al (2005) Cell cycle inhibition provides neuroprotection and reduces glial proliferation and scar formation after traumatic brain injury. Proc Natl Acad Sci U S A 102 (23):8333–8338
100. Otori T et al (2004) Traumatic brain injury elevates glycogen and induces tolerance to ischemia in rat brain. J Neurotrauma 21(6):707–718
101. Raghupathi R (2004) Cell death mechanisms following traumatic brain injury. Brain Pathol 14(2):215–222
102. McGraw J, Hiebert GW, Steeves JD (2001) Modulating astrogliosis after neurotrauma. J Neurosci Res 63(2):109–115
103. Cernak I et al (2005) Role of the cell cycle in the pathobiology of central nervous system trauma. Cell Cycle 4(9):1286–1293
104. Varvel NH et al (2009) NSAIDs prevent, but do not reverse, neuronal cell cycle reentry in a mouse model of Alzheimer disease. J Clin Invest 119(12):3692–3702
105. Schmerwitz UK et al (2011) Flavopiridol protects against inflammation by attenuating leukocyte-endothelial interaction via inhibition of cyclin-dependent kinase 9. Arterioscler Thromb Vasc Biol 31(2):280–288
106. Han Y et al (2016) Serum cyclin-dependent kinase 9 is a potential biomarker of atherosclerotic inflammation. Oncotarget 7(2):1854–1862
107. Jaschke B et al (2004) Local cyclin-dependent kinase inhibition by flavopiridol inhibits coronary artery smooth muscle cell proliferation and migration: Implications for the applicability on drug-eluting stents to prevent neointima formation following vascular injury. FASEB J 18(11):1285–1287

108. Bieniasz PD et al (1999) Recruitment of cyclin T1/P-TEFb to an HIV type 1 long terminal repeat promoter proximal RNA target is both necessary and sufficient for full activation of transcription. Proc Natl Acad Sci U S A 96(14):7791–7796
109. Chao SH, Price DH (2001) Flavopiridol inactivates P-TEFb and blocks most RNA polymerase II transcription in vivo. J Biol Chem 276(34):31793–31799
110. Pumfery A et al (2006) Potential use of pharmacological cyclin-dependent kinase inhibitors as anti-HIV therapeutics. Curr Pharm Des 12(16):1949–1961
111. Nelson PJ, Gelman IH, Klotman PE (2001) Suppression of HIV-1 expression by inhibitors of cyclin-dependent kinases promotes differentiation of infected podocytes. J Am Soc Nephrol 12(12):2827–2831
112. Nelson PJ et al (2003) Amelioration of nephropathy in mice expressing HIV-1 genes by the cyclin-dependent kinase inhibitor flavopiridol. J Antimicrob Chemother 51(4):921–929
113. Ou M, Sandri-Goldin RM (2013) Inhibition of cdk9 during herpes simplex virus 1 infection impedes viral transcription. PLoS ONE 8(10):e79007
114. Yamamoto M et al (2014) CDK9 inhibitor FIT-039 prevents replication of multiple DNA viruses. J Clin Invest 124(8):3479–3488
115. Ali A et al (2009) Identification of flavopiridol analogues that selectively inhibit positive transcription elongation factor (P-TEFb) and block HIV-1 replication. ChemBioChem 10 (12):2072–2080

Plumbagin and Its Role in Chronic Diseases

Pharkphoom Panichayupakaranant and Md Iftekhar Ahmad

Abstract Plumbagin (5-hydroxy-2-methyl-1,4-naphthoquinone) is a plant-derived naphthoquinones obtained mainly from three families, including Plumbaginaceae, Droseraceae, and Ebenaceae. Plumbagin has exhibited its potential therapeutic benefits on numerous chronic diseases, i.e., breast cancer, non-small cell lung cancer, melanoma, ovarian, squamous cell carcinomas, pancreatic cancer, and prostate cancer. In addition, its anti-inflammatory and antimicrobial activities as well as control of diabetes and cardiovascular diseases have been reported. Thus, plumbagin is a promising agent for development as a new drug for the treatment or control of chronic diseases. Studies on controlled drug release or drug delivery systems have been involved for improvement of its therapeutic efficacy as well as for the reduction of its toxicity. However, most of the recent research information is from in vitro and in vivo studies. Further clinical studies are therefore required for its developments and applications as a novel drug used to treat chronic diseases.

Keywords Plumbagin · Chronic diseases · Anticancer · Antimicrobial · Anti-inflammation · Antidiabetic · Cardiovascular · Toxicity

P. Panichayupakaranant (✉)
Department of Pharmacognosy and Pharmaceutical Botany, Faculty of Pharmaceutical Sciences, Prince of Songkla University, Hat-Yai, Songkhla 90112, Thailand
e-mail: pharkphoom.p@psu.ac.th

P. Panichayupakaranant · M.I. Ahmad
Excellent Research Laboratory, Phytomedicine and Pharmaceutical Biotechnology Excellence Center, Faculty of Pharmaceutical Sciences, Prince of Songkla University, Hat-Yai, Songkhla 90112, Thailand

S.C. Gupta et al. (eds.), *Drug Discovery from Mother Nature*,
Advances in Experimental Medicine and Biology 929,
DOI 10.1007/978-3-319-41342-6_10

1 Introduction

Chronic diseases are long-lasting conditions that can be controlled but can rarely be cured with vaccines or medication. Chronic diseases tend to become more common with age. The leading chronic diseases in developed countries include cancer, cardiovascular diseases, AIDS, diabetes, depression, and other pain syndromes. These chronic diseases inflicted on humans are treated by different medications that often cause serious side effects to the human body. Medicines obtained from plants often play important roles in the primary healthcare needs of humans as well as animals from time immemorial. Many plants exhibit various properties like antimicrobial, antiviral, anti-inflammatory, antioxidant, and anticancer activities due to the presence of secondary metabolites, e.g., essential oils, alkaloid, glycosides, terpenoids, flavonoids, quinones, coumarins, and other phenolic compounds [1]. Secondary plant metabolites have interesting biological properties, which make them desirable for optimizing any pharmacological activities to develop new drugs [2]. Thus, it is very important to look for drugs obtained from natural sources to optimize their activities and yield new drugs and development processes.

Naphthoquinones constitute the largest and diverse groups of plant secondary metabolites many of which have biological activities, including antimicrobial, antifeedant, and allelopathic activities, all of which can contribute toward plant defenses against disease [3–7]. Naphthoquinones commonly occur in the reduced and glycosidic forms and may be found as monomers as well as dimers or trimers in some plant species (e.g., Diospyros, Ebenaceae). They are biosynthesized via a variety of pathways including the acetate and malonate pathways (plumbagin), shikimate/succinyl CoA combined pathway (lawsone), and shikimate/mevalonate pathway (alkannin) [8]. Naphthoquinones also possess pharmacological activities, such as anticancer [9], antifertility, antihyperlipidemic [10], antiestrogenic [11], malignant furunculous scabies [12], antiplasmodial [13], antimicrobial [14], antifungal [15], anti-inflammatory [16], antibacterial [17], antidiabetic [18], and hypolipidemic activities [19]. The therapeutic activities of naphthoquinones are mainly due to their abilities to act as potent inhibitors of electron transport, as uncouplers of oxidative phosphorylation, as intercalating agents in the DNA double helix, as bioreductive alkylating agents of biomolecules, and as producers of reactive oxygen radicals by redox cycling in aerobic conditions.

Plumbagin (Fig. 1) is one of the simplest secondary plant naphthoquinones of three major phylogenic families, including Plumbaginaceae, Droseraceae, and Ebenaceae. Plumbagin is produced by members of the Plumbaginaceae and is accumulated mostly in the plant root [20]. Plumbagin is mainly isolated from *Plumbago zeylanica* [21]. The other main sources of plumbagin are *Drosophyllum lusitanicum*, *Drosera natalensis* [22], *D. capensis* [23], and *D. gigantea* [24]. Plumbagin is also found in *Juglans regia* (English walnut), *Juglans cinerea* (butternut and white walnut), and *Juglans nigra* (blacknut) [25]. Plumbagin has shown its potential therapeutic benefits on numerous chronic diseases like breast cancer, non-small cell lung cancer, melanoma, ovarian, squamous cell carcinomas,

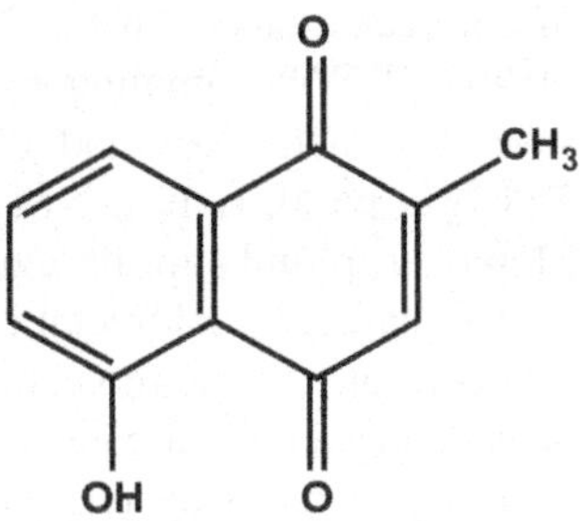

Fig. 1 Chemical structure of plumbagin

pancreatic cancer, and prostate cancer [26]. It has also been investigated for any anti-inflammatory action, antibacterial, antifungal, control of diabetes, and hypolipidemia. This chapter is focused on the role of plumbagin on the treatment of chronic diseases.

2 Physicochemical Properties of Plumbagin

Plumbagin or 5-hydroxy-2-methyl-1,4-naphthoquinone or 5-hydroxy-2-methyl-1, 4-naphthalenedione (Fig. 1) is a naphthoquinone compound with the molecular formula of $C_{11}H_8O_3$ and the molecular weight of 188.17 g/mol, isolated from the plant species of *Plumbago*, *Drosera,* and *Diospyros.* The name 'plumbagin' is derived from the plant genus Plumbago, from which it was first isolated [27]. The yellow needles of plumbagin that are crystallized from alcohol have a melting point of 78–79 °C. It has an irritating odor and can be sublimated or volatilized with steam. It is slightly soluble in hot water and soluble in alcohol, acetone, chloroform, benzene, and acetic acid [28].

3 Modulation of Cell Signaling Pathways by Plumbagin

Quinones are a group of compounds that are highly reactive organic chemical species. They may interact with biological systems to promote inflammatory, anti-inflammatory, and anticancer actions as well as sometimes inducing toxicity. Recently, targeting programmed cell death and other important pathways has become a promising approach to treat cancer through regulating cancer cell apoptosis and autophagy. Plumbagin induces cell death in cancer cells by affecting various signaling pathways, such as the Wnt, p53, Ras, and epithelial–mesenchymal transition (EMT) signaling pathways.

Wnt signaling is important in the early stages of cell development [29]. It is also essential for maintaining homeostasis by assisting in the self-renewal of intestinal epithelial cells [30]. Deregulation in the Wnt signaling pathway can cause cancer [31]. Wnt signaling plays an important role in pathogenesis and in the progression of colorectal cancer. It has been demonstrated that plumbagin-mediated downregulation of Wnt signaling is p53 independent. It also inhibited the expression of several co-activators and downstream targets of Wnt signaling, i.e., β-catenin, TCF7L2, p300, Bcl9 l, c-Myc, vimentin, and cyclin D1 in colorectal cancer cells. Moreover, plumbagin upregulated the expression of HBP1, a negative regulator of Wnt signaling in colorectal cancer cells. Downregulation of Wnt signaling could be therefore one of the molecular mechanisms for the inhibitory effects of plumbagin on human colorectal cancer cells [32].

The p53 pathway responds to stresses that can disrupt the accuracy of DNA replication and cell division. A stress signal is transmitted to the p53 protein by post-translational modifications. This results in the activation of the p53 protein as a transcription factor that initiates a program of cell cycle arrest, cellular senescence, or apoptosis. Thus, the p53 pathway plays a significant role in modulating the cell cycle and by inducing apoptosis when DNA is damaged or as a cell response to stress in human cells [33]. The p53-induced cell cycle arrest and apoptosis require transactivation of p21 and other cell cycle-related elements, such as cyclin B1 and cyclin D1. In addition, the murine double minute 2 (MDM2) plays a key role in negatively moderating the p53 activity. It has been reported that the p53 gene was activated by inhibiting the expression of MDM2 [34]. Inhibition of the expression of MDM2 induces apoptosis in tumors that retain wild-type p53 [35]. Plumbagin significantly inhibited the growth of osteosarcoma cells by upregulating the expression of p53 and p21 in the osteosarcoma cell lines causing cell cycle arrest by decreasing the expression of MDM2/cyclin B1 and cyclin D1. Moreover, plumbagin altered the ratio of Bax/Bcl-2 and may have triggered the mitochondrial apoptotic pathway that resulted in activation of caspase-3 and caspase-9. Plumbagin also induced the generation of reactive oxygen species (ROS) in osteosarcoma cell lines. Thus, plumbagin exerts its anticancer activity against osteosarcoma cells by inducing the p53 signaling pathway and by modulating the intracellular ROS that causes induction of apoptosis [36].

Angiogenesis, the growth of new blood vessels from pre-existing ones, is a marker of tumor development and metastatic progression. Inhibition of angiogenesis is therefore a promising strategy for the development of anticancer drugs. A major proangiogenic cytokine is vascular endothelial growth factor (VEGF) that comprises several isotypes, including VEGF-A, vascular permeability factor, VEGF-B, VEGF-C, and VEGF-D. The VEGF-A and VEGF-B promote vascular angiogenesis primarily through activation of two receptors, VEGFR1 and VEGFR2 [37]. In the VEGF/VEGFR2-mediated intracellular signaling pathways, the small guanine nucleotide-bound protein Ras (21 kDa) plays various roles in angiogenesis and the growth of tumors [38]. After stimulation by VEGF, GDP-bound inactive Ras is transformed to the GTP-bound active Ras [39], and this activates a number of angiogenic signaling pathways such as the Rac and MEK pathways [40] that ultimately control the critical processes of angiogenesis [39, 41]. Increased Ras activity is frequently detected in human cancers due to genetic mutations and amplifications [42]. Ras signaling pathways are therefore believed to be important targets for anticancer therapies [43].

Antiangiogenic drugs that target VEGF pathway were found to decrease the disease progression in patients with cancer. Plumbagin inhibited tumor angiogenesis and tumor growth by the VEGF receptor (VEGFR)2-mediated Ras signaling pathway in endothelial cells [44]. Moreover, plumbagin inhibited angiogenesis and growth in human colon carcinoma and prostate cancer mouse models. At a molecular level, plumbagin blocked the Ras/Rac/cofilin and Ras/MEK signaling pathways mediated by VEGFR2 in the human umbilical vein endothelial cells (HUVECs). It has been reported that both cisplatin-sensitive, *BRCA2*-deficient and cisplatin-resistant, *BRCA2*-proficient ovarian cancer cells are sensitive to plumbagin irrespective of the *BRCA2* status in both normoxia and hypoxia. Plumbagin effectively inhibits VEGF-A and GLUT1 in cisplatin-sensitive, *BRCA2*-deficient and cisplatin-resistant, *BRCA2*-proficient ovarian cancer cells. Plumbagin also restricts the VEGF-induced proangiogenic signaling in HUVECs and subsequently the proliferation of endothelial cell. In addition, plumbagin may significantly inhibit Ki67 and vWF expressions, which then had an effect on tumor regression in OVCAR-5 (human ovarian cancer cells) tumor-bearing mice. Plumbagin also significantly reduced expression of CD31. These findings indicated that plumbagin exhibited its anticancer activity against ovarian cancer cells through inhibition of proliferation and angiogenesis [45].

Epithelial–mesenchymal transition (EMT) is a process involving the transdifferentiation of epithelial cells into motile mesenchymal cells. EMT has been involved in the regulation of cancer stem cell properties, cancer regression as well as immune suppression. Metastatic dissemination of cancer cells from the primary tumor is believed to be initiated by the reactivation of an embryonic development program referred to as EMT, whereby epithelial cells lose apicobasal polarity and cell–cell contacts and gain mesenchymal phenotypes with increased migratory and invasive capabilities. There is evidence that indicates that the EMT process is activated during prostate cancer development, growth, progression, and metastasis [46, 47]. The EMT process is selected by prostate cancer cells during their metastatic dissemination from a primary organ to secondary sites [48]. Intervention of the EMT signaling pathways may therefore represent a novel strategy to prevent prostate cancer metastasis. It has been reported that plumbagin significantly modulated the expression of critical proteins that regulate the cell cycle, apoptosis, and the EMT signaling pathways in human prostate cancer PC-3 cells but not in human prostate cancer DU145 cells [49]. However, Western blotting analysis has confirmed the modulating effects of plumbagin on important proteins that regulate cell cycle, apoptosis, autophagy, and EMT in PC-3 and DU145 cells. The data from the Western blot analysis did not display significant differences between PC-3 and DU145 cells. This indicated that plumbagin stimulated different proteomic responses in the PC-3 and DU145 cells and involved proteins and pathways that regulate the cell cycle, apoptosis, autophagy, production of reactive oxygen species, and antioxidation/oxidation homeostasis. Inhibition of nuclear factor erythroid 2-related factor 2 (Nrf-2) can partly explain the inhibitory effect of plumbagin against EMT. Plumbagin suppressed the translocation of Nrf2 from cytosol to nucleus, resulting in an inhibition in the expression of downstream targets.

Plumbagin may be therefore considered as a promising anticancer compound via inhibiting Nrf2-mediated oxidative stress signaling pathway [50]. Moreover, Nrf-2 blockade by plumbagin may lead to protection against osteoporosis [51].

Plumbagin has been reported to be a potent inhibitor of the NF-kappaB activation pathway that leads to the suppression of NF-kappaB-regulated gene products. Activation of the transcription factor NF-kappaB therefore regulated the modulation of the cellular proliferation, anticarcinogenic, and radio resistance activities of plumbagin [52].

4 Role of Plumbagin in Chronic Diseases

Chronic disease is long-lasting condition that can be controlled but cannot be prevented by vaccines or cured by medications. Chronic diseases tend to become more common with age. The root of *Plumbago zeylanica*, a major source of plumbagin, has been traditionally used in Ayurvedic medicines as a cardiotronic, hepatoprotective, neuroprotective, and antiatherogenic agent [53]. Recently, plumbagin has been shown to possess a broad range of pharmacological activities, such as anticarcinogenic, antimicrobial, antiatherosclerotic, and antidiabetic activities. It is therefore considered to be a natural agent with the potential for controlling chronic diseases.

4.1 Cancer Diseases

Plumbagin has been recently evaluated for its anticancer activities against different cancer cells. There have been several studies on its anticancer activity that have indicated a potential role for plumbagin in the prevention and/or treatment of cancer diseases. Some preclinical studies for the anticancer effects of plumbagin and its mechanisms of action are described as follows.

Breast cancer is currently the major cause of cancer-related deaths in women. It has been reported that plumbagin significantly inhibited the growth of breast cancer cells with no effect on normal breast epithelial cells [54]. In addition, plumbagin induced apoptosis with a concomitant inactivation of Bcl-2 and the DNA binding activity of NF-kappaB. The inhibition of cell growth and induction of apoptosis by plumbagin are in part due to its inactivation of the NF-kappaB/Bcl-2 pathway. It has been reported that approximately 30 % of breast cancers overexpress the Her2 oncogene and plumbagin has been shown to induce apoptosis in Her2-overexpressing breast cancers through a mitochondrial-mediated pathway [55]. In addition, encapsulation using poly(D,L-lactide)-*co*-glycolide (PLGA) was carried out to reduce toxicity as well as increase stability and estrogen receptor specificity of plumbagin [56].

Plumbagin also induced apoptosis of ovarian cancer cells by binding to the active site of the estrogen receptor (ER) alpha. Moreover, plumbagin may have chemotherapeutic potential in BRCA1-mutant/defective ER-positive cancers [57].

Prostate cancer is one of the major causes of cancer-related deaths in men. Hormone-refractory invasive prostate cancer is the end stage leading to the majority of prostate cancer patient deaths. Plumbagin inhibited prostate cancer cell invasion and selectively induced apoptosis in prostate cancer cells and had no effect on normal prostate epithelial RWPE-1 cells. Plumbagin inhibited the growth and invasion of PCa, both in vitro and in vivo preclinical models. Moreover, plumbagin inhibited multiple molecular targets including PKC epsilon, a predictive biomarker of prostate cancer aggressiveness. Plumbagin may be considered to be a potential agent for the control of hormone-refractory prostate cancer [58]. Plumbagin also inhibited the growth of human prostate cancer cells (PC-3, LNCaP, and C4-2) by mediating a decrease in cell viability that was correlated with the induction of apoptosis, and was accompanied by the generation of reactive oxygen species (ROS) and the depletion of intracellular glutathione levels. Plumbagin also altered the expression of genes responsible for the metabolism of ROS, i.e., superoxide dismutase 2. This indicated that ROS played an important role in plumbagin-induced apoptosis in human prostate cancer cells [59]. Recently, a nanoformulation of plumbagin nanoparticles was explored as a potential natural drug against prostate cancer [60]. Plumbagin nanoparticles exhibited higher cytocompatibility with normal cells when compared to plumbagin crude extract. In addition, the nanoformulation had a dose-dependent toxicity to prostate cells.

Pancreatic cancer is another of the most resistant malignancies. Plumbagin inhibited the growth of pancreatic cancer cell lines, i.e., PANC-1 and BxPC-3 cells. Plumbagin induced apoptosis in human pancreatic cancer cells primarily through the mitochondrial-related pathway followed by both caspase-dependent and caspase-independent cascades [61]. Plumbagin also possessed a potent anticancer effect against pancreatic cancer by inducing cell cycle arrest in human pancreatic cancer (PANC-1 and BxPC-3) cells *via* the modulation of cell cycle regulators, i.e., CDK1/CDC2, cyclin B1, cyclin D1, p21 Waf1/Cip1, p27 Kip1, and p53. It promoted cell cycle arrest and autophagy but inhibited the epithelial to mesenchymal transition phenotype in pancreatic cancer cells that involved the PI3K/protein kinase B/mammalian target of rapamycin and p38 MAPK-mediated pathways [62]. This indicated that plumbagin can be potentially developed as a therapeutic agent for treating pancreatic cancer.

Lung cancer is one of the major causes of cancer-related deaths in the USA. Plumbagin significantly inhibited the growth of non-small cell lung cancer, including H460 and A549 cell lines, by modulating the prosurvival and proapoptotic signaling that caused induction of apoptosis [63–65]. It upregulated the expression of the p53 and p21 (CIP1/WAF1) causing cell cycle arrest in the G2/M phase by downregulating the G2/M regulatory proteins (cyclin B1 and CDC25B) in H460 cells. Moreover, it activated the JNK/p38 signaling that led to caspase-3 activation and resulted in the induction of apoptosis.

Radiotherapy is the primary line for the treatment of cervical cancer. However, radiotherapy is limited by the total given dose that causes no normal tissue damage. It has been reported that a combination of plumbagin and radiation increased the inhibition of cell growth compared to a treatment by a single higher radiation dose. This has clearly indicated that plumbagin may be used to potentiate the induction of apoptosis by acting as a radiosensitizer [66]. Additionally, plumbagin–silver nanoparticle complex enhanced the cellular uptake as well as its antiproliferative, antimitotic, and apoptotic activities of plumbagin [67].

Plumbagin also showed great potential in controlling brain cancer, especially the brain cancer cells that are sensitive to radiation [68]. Plumbagin treatment on brain cancer cells, including human glioblastoma multiforme cells (KNS60, A172, and U251MG) and medulloblastoma cells (ONS76), resulted in the induction of DNA damage, cell cycle arrest, and apoptosis, followed by the suppression of their colony-forming ability. These effects were proven by the upregulation of TNFRSF1A and downregulation of E2F1 genes, together with a decrease in MDM2, cyclin B1, survivin, and BCL2 protein expression as well as an induced increased level of caspase-3/7 activity. Plumbagin also upregulated PTEN gene, a negative regulator of the AKT cell survival pathway [68].

Since plumbagin is a natural compound, it may have advantages over other synthetic chemotherapeutic agents due to its specific action on the cancer cells and also due to its slightly effect on normal tissue. However, further studies are essential to confirm its therapeutic effect and safety.

Moreover, several studies on novel delivery/formulation systems of plumbagin have been recently performed in order to develop new anticancer drugs. One possible strategy is to synthesize a metal complex derived from plumbagin, i.e., Cu(II) compounds derived from plumbagin. Folic acid–human serum albumin (FA-HSA) has been used as a carrier for copper–plumbagin complexes. Anticancer activities and targeting of the Cu(II) compound are improved when bound to FA-HSA [69].

4.2 *Cardiovascular Diseases*

The structure of plumbagin is similar to that of vitamin K. Thus, it might have an effect on blood coagulation. It has been reported that at a low dosage level (2 mg/kg body weight), a *Plumbagin zeylanica* extract as well as its naphthoquinone component given to individual animal groups prolonged the bleeding time by altering platelet adhesiveness and coagulation [70]. This anticoagulation property might be used to help to control some cardiovascular diseases.

4.3 *Diabetes Mellitus*

Recently, there has been a report on the antidiabetic activity of plumbagin [71]. Sunil et al. [18] carried out a study to evaluate the antidiabetic effects of plumbagin on streptozotocin-induced diabetic rats. Plumbagin significantly reduced the blood glucose level as well as altering all other investigated biochemical parameters that included body weight, plasma insulin, total protein, urea, creatinine, liver glycogen, plasma enzymes (SGOT, SGPT, and ALP), and the carbohydrate metabolism enzymes (glucose-6-phosphatase, fructose-1,6-bisphosphatase, and hexokinase) to almost normal levels. Plumbagin also increased hexokinase activity, but decreased glucose-6-phosphatase and fructose-1,6-bisphosphatase activities in the treated diabetic rats. It also enhanced GLUT4 mRNA and protein expression that contributed to glucose homeostasis. Plumbagin therefore has been targeted as a potential source of drug for controlling diabetes.

4.4 *Infectious Diseases*

Plumbagin might be considered to be a potential source of new antimicrobial drugs. There are several studies that have confirmed its antimicrobial activities against Gram-positive and Gram-negative bacteria, antibiotic-resistant bacteria as well as fungi and yeasts [72]. Plumbagin exhibited antibacterial activity against *Staphylococcus aureus* with a minimum inhibitory concentration (MIC) of 1.56 μg/mL and minimum bactericidal concentration (MBC) of 25.0 μg/mL as well as anti-*Candida albicans* with an MIC of 0.78 μg/mL and minimum fungicidal concentration (MFC) of 1.56 μg/mL [73]. Plumbagin exhibited antibacterial activity against the human intestinal pathogen, *Helicobacter pylori* that causes peptic ulcer with an MIC of 0.97 μg/mL [74]. Plumbagin and its derivatives, 3,3′-biplumbagin and ellipticine, also possessed antibacterial activity against bacteria involved with acne. Among these, plumbagin exhibited the strongest antibacterial activity against *Propionibacterium acnes*, *Stapylococcus aureus*, and *S.epidermidis* with MICs of 12.5, 3.1, 0.02 μg/mL and MBCs of 50, 12.5, 3.1 μg/mL, respectively [75, 76]. The method for the preparation of plumbagin-derivative-rich *Plumbago indica* root extract and its antibacterial activity compared to its constituted three naphthoquinones was also described [76]. Moreover, plumbagin possessed antibacterial activity against methicillin- and multidrug-resistant *S. aureus* with MICs between 4.0 and 10.7 μg/mL. In addition, a combination of plumbagin (2.0 μg/mL) and oxacillin exhibited a synergistic effect against two epidemic methicillin-resistant *S. aureus* strains, EMRSA15 and MRSA1 [77]. It is therefore a promising antimicrobial agent for controlling a number of infectious diseases.

5 Other Pharmacological Activity of Plumbagin

Several studies on other pharmacological activities have been published as summarized in Table 1. These pharmacological activities may be a guide for further study for the development of plumbagin to be a novel drug for controlling chronic

Table 1 Other pharmacological activities of plumbagin

Pharmacological activity	Assay method	Effect/potency	Reference
Antimutagenicity	Ames test and RNA polymerase B (rpoB)-based rifampicin resistance assay	Strong antimutagenic (against ultraviolet and ethyl methanesulfonate)	[78]
Antioxidant	Radical scavenging assays and reducing power measurement	Very low (percent scavenging of hydroxyl and superoxide radicals was 26 and 27 %, respectively, at $\geq$120 μM; ferric reducing power 5–9 %, at 160 μM)	[78]
Protection of cells and DNA	Survival analysis and gel electrophoresis profiling	Reduction of cell death (exposed to gamma radiation at 250 Gy) by ~14 % at 25 μM of plumbagin	[78]
Antimalarial	In vitro assay against K1 (chloroquine-resistant) and 3D7 (chloroquine-sensitive) *Plasmodium falciparum*: SYBR green I-based assay	IC_{50} against 3D7 and K1 *P. falciparum* of 580 and 370 nM, respectively	[79]
	In vitro assay: inhibit isoforms of human cytochrome P450 (CYP), including CYP1A2, CYP2C19, and CYP3A4 using human liver microsomes	IC_{50} for CYP2C19, CYP1A2, and CYP3A4 was 0.78, 1.39, and 2.37 μM, respectively	[80]
	In vivo assay: *Plasmodium berghei*-infected mouse model (a 4-day suppressive test)	Plumbagin (25 mg/kg body weight given for 4 days) was safe, but exhibited weak antimalarial activity	[79]
Anti-inflammatory and analgesic	In vivo assay: oral administration 5–20 mg/kg body weight in rats	– Suppressed the paw edema of rats induced by carrageenan – Reduced the number of writhings of mice induced by the intra-peritoneal injection of acetic acid – Suppressed proinflammatory mediators, i.e., histamine, serotonin, bradykinin, prostaglandin E2 – Decreased production of the proinflammatory cytokines interleukin-1, interleukin-6, and tumor necrosis factor – Inhibited the expression of the proinflammatory mediators: inducible nitric oxide synthase and cyclooxygenase 2 – inhibited phosphorylation of the p65 subunit of NF-κB	[81]

(continued)

Table 1 (continued)

Pharmacological activity	Assay method	Effect/potency	Reference
Cytoprotective (protection against osteoporosis)	In vitro assay: glucocorticoid-induced cell damage in osteoblastic cells (MC3T3-E1)	– 10 μM plumbagin treatment effectively ameliorated dexamethasone (DEX)-induced cell death by increasing the cell viability to 92 % – Reversed the levels of oxidative stress and apoptotic markers and protected against DEX-induced cell damage – Improved the expression of osteogenic markers compared to DEX treatment	[51]
Antidepressant	In vivo assay: tail suspension test and sucrose preference test (oral administration 4, 8, and 16 mg/kg body weight for 3 successive weeks in mice)	Highest dose (16 mg/kg) of plumbagin: – Decreased immobility period of unstressed and stressed mice – Restored the reduced sucrose preference (%) in stressed mice – Inhibited brain MAO-A activity – Decreased plasma nitrite, brain malondialdehyde, and catalase levels – Increased reduced glutathione levels – Reversed stress-induced increase in plasma corticosterone levels	[82]
Hepatoprotective	In vivo assay: CCl_4-induced liver fibrosis in rat models (4 and 8 mg/kg plumbagin plus a 5 % CCl_4 mixed peanut oil solution (0.5 ml/100 g), gavaged 3 times a week for 8 weeks)	– Decreased the serum concentrations of liver functional enzymes, ALT, AST, ALB, TBIL – Reduced the levels of inflammatory cytokine, IL-6, TNF-α – Decreased collagen markers, HA, LN, PCIII, and CIV – Improved hepatocellular impairments – downregulating NF-κB and TLR-4 mRNA – Reduced levels of α-SMA and TNF-α immunoreactive cells in liver tissue	[83]

diseases, especially its anti-inflammatory activity, because inflammation has been described to be the root of almost all chronic diseases, such as cancer, cardiovascular diseases, and autoimmune diseases.

6 Toxicity Assessment of Plumbagin

Although plumbagin has been used in traditional medicine, there has been concern about its safety due to reports on its vesicant and abortifacient properties. However, there have been no epidemiological studies or case reports to indicate that exposure to plumbagin can be a cancer risk for humans, although some toxic side effects, including diarrhea, skin rashes, increases in white blood cells, and neutrophil counts, increased serum phosphatase and acid phosphatase levels, and hepatic toxicity have been reported [84]. Plumbagin has been studied using several standard assays for its mutagenicity, chromosomal aberrations, and DNA damage. Several studies have reported that plumbagin was not mutagenic in stationary phase cells but was moderately mutagenic in exponential-phase cells based on assays with *Escherichia coli* AQ634 cells and by measuring the Trp-ø Trp1 reversion frequency. Plumbagin at lower concentrations behaved like a spindle poison by inhibiting entry of cells into mitosis, but at higher concentrations, it also exhibited radiomimetic nucleotoxic and cytotoxic effects [85]. Plumbagin showed exceptional antimutagenicity, when tested for its antimutagenic potency with respect to mutagenicities induced by 2-nitrofluorene (2NF), 3-nitrofluoranthene (3-NFA), and 1-nitropyrene (1-NP) in *Salmonella typhimurium* TA98 [86].

There is some evidence to indicate that plumbagin exhibited cytotoxic effects on cancer cells but not to normal cells. For examples, plumbagin inhibited the cell growth of MDA-MB-231 and MCF-7 cells with an effective induction of apoptosis, but had no effect on MCF-10A cells, the non-tumorigenic 'normal' breast epithelial cells [54]. Plumbagin also exhibited an efficient induction of apoptosis on prostate cancer cells (DU145, CWR22rv1, and LNCaP) but had no significant effect on non-tumorigenic immortalized prostate epithelial RWPE-1 cells [62]. These are very encouraging results; however, further preclinical animal studies are warranted.

Toxicity and mutagenicity of plumbagin and the induction of a possible new DNA repair pathway have been determined using *E. coli*. Actively growing *E. coli* exposed to plumbagin were mutagenized or killed. The toxicity of plumbagin was not found to be mediated by membrane damage. The bacteria pretreated with plumbagin could partially reactivate lambda phage damaged by exposure to riboflavin plus light, a treatment that produced active oxygen species. The result indicated the induction of a DNA repair response. It is proposed that *E. coli* has an inducible DNA repair response specific for the type of oxidative damage generated during incubation with plumbagin [87].

Mutagenicity of plumbagin has been assessed using the in vivo micronucleus assay and glutathione *S*-transferase (GST) activity determination in Swiss albino mice. Plumbagin was found to induce micronuclei at all the doses studied (4, 8, 16 mg/kg body weight), and it was toxic to bone marrow cells of Swiss albino mice. In addition, there was no significant change in GST activity observed with a plumbagin dose of 4 mg/kg body weight, whereas the GST activity was significantly inhibited by higher doses of plumbagin (8 mg and 16 mg/kg body weight) and also cyclophosphamide used a positive control [88].

Acute and subacute toxicity assessments in a mouse model indicated that plumbagin had relatively low toxicity at doses of up to 100 mg/kg body weight (single oral administration) and 25 mg/kg body weight (daily oral administrations for 14 days) for acute and subacute toxicity, respectively [79].

It has been reported that niosomal plumbagin prepared using a lipid layer hydration method reduced toxicity of plumbagin and improved its anticancer and antifertility activities [89, 90]. Niosome-encapsulated plumbagin was less toxic than free plumbagin. The antitumor activity of plumbagin against a solid tumor (sarcoma-180) and Ehrlich ascites model was also better after encapsulation. A poly (lactic-co-glycolic) acid injectable gel implant for the delivery of plumbagin has also been formulated to reduce its toxicity and improve antitumor efficacy. The toxicity of plumbagin was reduced in mice after subcutaneous injection of a gel containing plumbagin compared to free plumbagin. The volume doubling time was significantly higher for the gel compared to free plumbagin. The gel implant could be therefore an effective drug delivery system for reducing toxicity and enhancing the antitumor therapeutic efficacy of plumbagin [91]. Plumbagin has been also encapsulated either as a conventional or as a long circulating liposomal formulation to enhance its biological half-life and antitumor efficacy [92]. The liposomes were prepared by a thin-film hydration method and were assayed for their pharmacokinetic and pharmacodynamic efficacy against mice bearing the B16F1 melanoma as well as by an evaluation of its in vivo toxicity. The optimized formulations of plumbagin exhibited better antitumor efficacy in vivo with no signs of normal tissue toxicity.

7 Conclusions

Plumbagin is a simple naturally occurring naphthoquinone that is obtained from the roots of the plants in the family Plumbaginaceae. Plumbagin possesses several pharmacological activities associated with the treatment of chronic diseases, especially cancers and infectious diseases. Thus, it is a promising agent for development as a new drug for the treatment or control of chronic diseases. Studies on controlled drug release or drug delivery systems are essential for improvement of its therapeutic efficacy as well as for the reduction of its toxicity. However, most of the recent research information is from in vitro and in vivo studies. Further clinical studies are therefore required for its developments and applications as a novel drug used to treat chronic diseases.

References

1. Sandhy B, Thomas S, Isabel W, Shenbagavathai R (2006) Ethno medicinal plants used by the valaiyan community of Piranmalai hills (Reserved forest), Tamil Nadu, India. A pilot study. Afr J Tradit Complements Altern Med 3:101–114
2. Gu XD, Sun MY, Zhang L, Fu HW, Cui L, Chen RZ, Zhang DW, Tian JK (2010) UV-B induced changes in the secondary metabolites of *Morusalba* L. Leaves Mol 15:2980–2993
3. Babula P, Mikelova R, Adam V, Kizek R, Havel L, Sladky Z (2006) Naphthoquinones-biosynthesis, occurrence and metabolism in plants. CeskaSlov Farm 55:151–159
4. Babula P, Adam V, Havel L, Kizek R (2007) Naphthoquinones and their pharmacological properties. CeskaSlov Farm 56:114–120
5. Krolicka A, Szpitter A, Maciag M, Biskup E, Gilgenast E, Romanik G, Kaminski M, Wegrzyn G, Lojkowska E (2009) Antibacterial and antioxidant activity of the secondary metabolites from in vitro cultures of *Droseraaliciae*. Biotechnol Appl Biochem 53:175–184
6. Weissenberg M, Meisner J, Klein M, Schaeffler I, Eliyahu M, Schmutterer H, Ascher KRS (1997) Effect of substituent and ring changes in naturally occurring naphthoquinones on the feeding response of larvae of the Mexican bean beetle. Epilachnavarivestis. J Chem Ecol 23:3–18
7. Duroux L, Delmotte FM, Lancelin JM, Keravis G, Jay-Allemand C (1998) Insight into naphthoquinone metabolism: beta-glucosidase-catalysed hydrolysis of hydrojuglone beta-D-glucopyranoside. Biochem J 333:275–283
8. Babula P, Adam V, Havel L, Kizek R (2009) Note worthy secondary metabolites naphthoquinones-their occurrence, pharmacological properties and analysis. Curr Pharm Anal 5:47–68
9. Moammir HA, Nancy E, Dreckschmidt, Ajit K (2008) Plumbagin, a medicinal plant-derived naphthoquinone, is a novel inhibitor of the growth and invasion of hormone-refractory prostate cancer. Cancer Res 68:9024–9032
10. Dutta S, Vankatesh D, Souza R, Shenoy BD, Udupi RH, Udupa N (2002) Niosomal delivery of plumbagin ester for better antifertility activity. Indian Drugs 39:163–165
11. Pendurkar, Sudha R, Mengi, Sushma A (2009) Antihyperlipidemic effect of aqueous extract of *Plumbago zeylanica* roots in diet induced hyperlipidemic rat. Pharm Biol 47:1004–1010
12. Jiangsu New Medical College, Zhongyao Dictionary (Encyclopedia of Chinese MateriaMedica). Scientific & Technological Press, Shanghai, 1979; 711–712
13. Simonsen HT, Nordskjold JB, Smitt UW, Nyman U, Palpu P, Joshi P, Varughese G (2001) In vitro screening of Indian medicinal plants for antiplasmodial activity. J Ethnopharmacol 74:195–204
14. Ahmad I, Mehmood Z, Mohammad F, Ahmad S (2000) Antimicrobial potency and synergistic activity of five traditionally used Indian medicinal plants. J Med Aromatic Plant Sci 23:173–176
15. Mehmood Z, Ahmad I, Mohammad F, Ahmad S (1999) Indian medicinal plants: a potential source of anticandidal drugs. Pharm Biol 37:237–242
16. Oyedapo OO (1996) Studies on the bioactivity of the extract of *Plumbago zeylanica*. Phytotherapy Res 13:346–348
17. Jeyachandran R, Mahesh A, Cindrella L, Sudhakar S, Pazhanichamy K (2009) Antibacterial activity of plumbagin and root extracts of *Plumbago zeylanica* L. Acta Biologica Cracoviensia Series Botanica 51:17–22
18. Sunil C, Duraipandiyan V, Agastian P, Ignacimuthu S (2012) Antidiabetic effect of plumbagin isolated from *Plumbago zeylanica* L. root and its effect on GLUT4 translocation in streptozotocin-induced diabetic rats. Food Chem Toxicol 50:4356–4363
19. Kanchana N, Sadiq AM (2011) Hepatoprotective effect of *Plumbago zeylanica* on paracetamol induced liver toxicity in rats. Int J Pharm Pharm Sci 3:151–154
20. Sharma I, Gusain D, Dixit VP (1991) Hypolipidaemic and ant atherosclerotic effects of plumbagin in rabbits. Indian J Physiol Pharmacol 35:10–14

21. Van-der VLM (1974) Distribution of plumbagin in the Plumbaginaceae. Phytochemistry 11:3247–3248
22. Nahalka J, Blanarik P, Gemeiner P, Matusova E, Partlova I (1996) Production of plumbagin by cell suspension cultures of *Drosophyllum lusitanicum*. J Biotechnol 49:153–161
23. Crouch IJ, Finnie JF, Staden JV (1990) Studies on the isolation of plumbagin from in vitro and *in vivo* grown *Drosera* species. Plant Cell Tissue Organ Cult 21:79–82
24. Budzianowski J (2000) Naphthoquinone glucosides of *Droseragigantea* from in vitro cultures. Planta Medica 66:667–669
25. Sung B, Oyajobi B, Aggarwal BB (2012) Plumbagin inhibits osteoclastogenesis and reduces human breast cancer-induced osteolytic bone metastasis in mice through suppression of RANKL signaling. Mol Cancer Ther 11(2):350–359
26. Hafeeza BB, Zhongb W, Fischera JW, Mustafaa A, Shic X, Meskea L, Hongd H, Caid W, Havighurste T, Kime KM, Ajit K, Verma AK (2013) Plumbagin, a medicinal plant (*Plumbago zeylanica*)-derived 1, 4-naphthoquinone, inhibits growth and metastasis of human prostate cancer PC-3 M-luciferase cells in an orthotopic xenograft mouse model. Mol Oncol 7:428–439
27. van der Vijver LM (1972) Distribution of plumbagin in the Plumbaginaceae. Phytochemistry 11:3247–3248
28. Windholz M (ed) (1983) The merck index, 10th edn. Merck & Co Inc, N.J.
29. Cadigan KM, Nusse R (1997) Wnt signaling: a common theme in animal development. Genes Dev 11:3286–3305
30. Gregorieff A, Clevers H (2005) Wnt signaling in the intestinal epithelium: from endoderm to cancer. Genes Dev 19:877–890
31. Reya T, Clevers H (2005) Wnt signalling in stem cells and cancer. Nature 434:843–850
32. Raghu D, Karunagaran D (2014) Plumbagin down regulates Wnt signaling independent of p53 in human colorectal cancer cells. J Nat Prod 77:1130–1134
33. Harris SL, Levine AJ (2005) The p53 pathway: positive and negative feedback loops. Oncogene 24:2899–2908
34. Zhang Y, Wolf GW, Bhat K (2003) Ribosomal protein L11 negatively regulates oncoprotein MDM2 and mediates a p53-dependent ribosomal-stress checkpoint pathway. Mol Cell Biol 23:8902–8912
35. Dickens MP, Fitzgerald R, Fischer PM (2010) Small-molecule inhibitors of MDM2 as new anticancer therapeutics. Semin Cancer Biol 20:10–18
36. Tian L, Yin D, Ren Y (2012) Plumbagin induces apoptosis via the p53 pathway and generation of reactive oxygen species in human osteosarcoma cells. Molecular Medicine Reports 5:126–132
37. Huang Y, Chen X, Dikov MM (2007) Distinct roles of VEGFR-1 and VEGFR-2 in the aberrant hematopoiesis associated with elevated levels of VEGF. Blood 110:624–631
38. Rak J, Kerbel RS (2001) Ras regulation of vascular endothelial growth factor and angiogenesis. Methods Enzymol 333:267–283
39. Meadows KN, Bryant P, Pumiglia K (2001) Vascular endothelial growth factor induction of the angiogenic phenotype requires as activation. J Biol Chem 276:49289–49298
40. Dancey JE (2002) Agents targeting Ras signaling pathway. Curr Pharm Des 8:2259–2267
41. Meadows KN, Bryant P, Vincent PA (2004) Activated Ras induces a proangiogenic phenotype in primary endothelial cells. Oncogene 23:192–200
42. Hoa M, Davis SL, Ames SJ (2002) Amplification of wild-type K-ras promotes growth of head and neck squamous cell carcinoma. Cancer Res 62:7154–7156
43. Morgan MA, Ganser A, Reuter CW (2007) Targeting the RAS signaling pathway in malignant hematologic diseases. Curr Drug Targets 8:217–235
44. Lai L, Liu J, Zhai D (2012) Plumbagin inhibits tumor angiogenesis and tumor growth through VEGFR2-mediated Ras signaling pathway. Br J Pharmacol 165:1084–1096
45. Sinha S, Pal K, Elkhanany A (2013) Plumbagin inhibits tumorigenesis and angiogenesis of ovarian cancer cells in vivo. Int J Cancer 132:1201–1212
46. Zheng H, Kang Y (2014) Multilayer control of the EMT master regulators. Oncogene 33:1755–1763

47. Lamouille S, Xu J, Derynck R (2014) Molecular mechanisms of epithelial-mesenchymal transition. Nat Rev Mol Cell Biol 15:178–196
48. Nauseef JT, Henry MD (2011) Epithelial-to-mesenchymal transition in prostate cancer: paradigm or puzzle? Nat Rev Urol 8:428–439
49. Qui JX, Zhou ZW, He ZX (2015) Plumbagin elicits differential proteomic responses mainly involving cell cycle, apoptosis, autophagy, and epithelial-to-mesenchymal transition pathways in human prostate cancer PC-3 and DU145 cells. Drug Design Develop Ther 9:349–417
50. Pan S-T, Qin Y, Zhou Z-W, He Z-X, Zhang X, Yang T, Yang Y-X, Wang D, Zhou S-F, Qiu J-X (2015) Plumbagin suppresses epithelial to mesenchymal transition and stemless via inhibiting Nrf2-mediated signaling pathway in human tongue squamous cell carcinoma cells. Drug Design Develop Ther 9:5511–5551
51. Zhang S, Li D, Yang J-Y, Yan T-B (2015) Plumbagin protects against glucocorticoid-induced osteoporosis through Nrf-2 pathway. Cell Stress Chaperones 20:621–629
52. Sandur SK, Ichikawa H, Sethi G, Ahn KS, Aggarwal BB (2006) Plumbagin (5-hydroxy-2-methyl-1,4-naphthoquinone) suppresses NF-kappaB activation and NF-kappaB-regulated gene products through modulation of p65 and IkappaBalpha kinase activation, leading to potentiation of apoptosis induced by cytokine and chemotherapeutic agents. J Biol Chem 281:17023–17033
53. Shyur L, Lau ASY (2012) Advances in botanical research: recent trends in medicinal plants research, vol 62. Academic Press, London
54. Ahmad A, Banerjee S, Wang Z, Kong D, Sarkar FH (2008) Plumbagin-induced apoptosis of human breast cancer cells is mediated by inactivation of NF-kappaB and Bcl-2. J Cell Biochem 105:1461–1471
55. Kawiak A, Zawacka-Pankau J, Lojkowska E (2012) Plumbagin induces apoptosis in Her2-overexpressing breast cancer cells through the mitochondrial-mediated pathway. J Nat Prod 75:747–751
56. Kilcar AY, Tekin V, Muftuler FZB, Medine EI (2015) 99mTc labeled plumbagin: estrogen receptor dependent examination against breast cancer cells and comparison with PLGA encapsulated form. J Radio Anal Nuclear Chem. doi:10.1007/s10967-015-4284-1
57. Thasnil KA, Rakesh S, Rojini GG, Ratheeshkumar T, Srinivas G, Priya S (2008) Estrogen-dependent cell signaling and apoptosis in BRCA1-blocked BG1 ovarian cancer cells in response to plumbagin and other chemotherapeutic agents. Ann Oncol 19:696–705
58. Wang F, Wang Q, Zhou Z-W, Yu S-N, Pan S-T, He Z-X, Zhang X, Wang D, Yang Y-X, Yang T, Sun T, Li M, Qiu J-X, Zhou S-F (2015) Plumbagin induces cell cycle arrest and autophagy and suppresses epithelial to mesenchymal transition involving PI3K/Akt/mTOR-mediated pathway in human pancreatic cancer cells. Drug Design Develop Ther 9 537–560
59. Powolny AA, Singh SV (2008) Plumbagin-induced apoptosis in human prostate cancer cells is associated with modulation of cellular redox status and generation of reactive oxygen species. Pharm Res 25:2171–2180
60. Nair HA, Snima KS, Kamath RC, Nair SV, Lakshmanan V-K (2015) Plumbagin nanoparticles induce dose and pH dependent toxicity on prostate cancer cells. Curr Drug Deliv 12:709–716
61. Chen CA, Chang HH, Kao CY, Tsai TH, Chen YJ (2009) Plumbagin, isolated from *Plumbago zeylanica,* induces cell death through apoptosis in human pancreatic cancer cells. Pancreatology 9:797–809
62. Aziz MH, Dreckschmidt NE, Verma AK (2008) Plumbagin, a medicinal plant-derived naphthoquinone, is a novel inhibitor of the growth and invasion of hormone-refractory prostate cancer. Cancer Res 68:9024–9032
63. Hsu YL, Cho CY, Kuo PL, Huang YT, Lin CC (2006) Plumbagin (5-hydroxy-2-methyl-1,4-naphthoquinone) induces apoptosis and cell cycle arrest in A549 cells through p53 accumulation via c-Jun NH2-terminal kinase-mediated phosphorylation at serine 15 in vitro and in vivo. J Pharm Exp Ther 318:484–494
64. Gomathinayagam R, Sowmyalakshmi S, Mardhatillah F, Kumar R (2008) AkbarshaMA, Damodaran C. Anticancer mechanism of plumbagin, a natural compound, on non-small cell lung cancer cells. Anticancer Res 28:785–792

65. Acharya BR, Bhattacharyya B, Chakrabarti G (2008) The natural naphthoquinone plumbagin exhibits ant proliferative activity and disrupts the microtubule network through tubulin binding. Biochemistry 47:7838–7845
66. Nair S, Nair RR, Srinivas P, Srinivas G, Pillai MR (2008) Radiosensitizing effects of plumbagin in cervical cancer cells is through modulation of apoptotic pathway. Mol Carcinog 47:22–33
67. Appadurai P, Rathinasamy K (2015) Plumbagin-silver nanoparticle formulations enhance the cellular uptake of plumbagin and its antiproliferative activities. IET Nanobiotechnol 9:264–272
68. Khaw AK, Sameni S, Venkatesan S, Kalthur G, Hande MP (2015) Plumbagin alters telomere dynamics, induces DNA damage and cell death in human brain tumour cells. Mutation Res/Genetic Toxicol Environ Mutagen 793:86–95
69. Gou Y, Zhang Z, Qi J, Liang S, Zhou Z, Yang F, Liang H (2015) Folate-functionalized human serum albumin carrier for anticancer copper(II) complexes derived from natural plumbagin. J Inorg Biochem 153:13–22
70. Vijayakumar R, Senthilvelan M, Ravindran R (2006) Sheela Devi R. *Plumbago zeylanica* action on blood coagulation profile with and without blood volume reduction. Vascul Pharmacol 45:86–90
71. Sunil C, Duraipandiyan V, Agastian P, Ignacimuthu S (2012) Antidiabetic effect of plumbagin isolated from *Plumbago zeylanica* L. root and its effect on GLUT4 translocation in streptozotocin-induced diabetic rats. Food Chem Toxicol 50:4356–4363
72. Lajubutu BA, Pinney RJ, Roberts MF, Odelola HA, Oso BA (1995) Antibacterial activity of diosquinone and plumbagin from the root of *Diospyrosmespiliformis* (Hostch) (Ebenaceae). Phytother Res 9:346–350
73. de Paiva SR, Figueiredo MR, Aragão TV, Kaplan MA (2003) Antimicrobial activity in vitro of plumbagin isolated from *Plumbago* species. Memórias do Instituto Oswaldo Cruz 98:959–961
74. Renuga G, Babuthandapani A (2013) Evaluation on antimicrobial potential of root extracts *Plumbago zeylanica* L against human intestinal microflora. Int J Pharm Biol Res 4: 146–158
75. Kaewbumrung S, Panichayupakaranant P (2012) Isolation of three antibacterial naphthoquinones from *Plumbago indica* roots and development of a validated quantitative HPLC analytical method. Nat Prod Res 26:2020–2023
76. Kaewbumrung S, Panichayupakaranant P (2014) Antibacterial activity of plumbagin derivative-rich *Plumbago indica* root extracts and chemical stability. Nat Prod Res 28:835–837
77. Rondevaldova J, Novy P, Kokoska L (2015) *In vitro* combinatory antimicrobial effect of plumbagin with oxacillin and tetracycline against *Staphylococcus aureus*. Phytother Res 29:144–147
78. Kumar S1, Gautam S, Sharma A (2013) Antimutagenic and antioxidant properties of plumbagin and other naphthoquinones. Mutatation Res 755:30–41
79. Sumsakul W, Plengsuriyakarn T, Chaijaroenkul W, Viyanant V, Karbwang J, Na-Bangchang K (2014) Antimalarial activity of plumbagin *in vitro* and in animal models. BMC Complement Altern Med 14:1–6. http://bmccomplementalternmed.biomedcentral.com/articles/10.1186/1472-6882-14-15
80. Sumsakul W, Chaijaroenkul W, Na-Bangchang K (2015) In vitro inhibitory effects of plumbagin, the promising antimalarial candidate, on human cytochrome P450 enzymes. Asian Pac J Trop Med 8:914–918
81. Luo P, Wong YF, Ge L, Zhang ZF, Liu Y, Liu L, Zhou H (2010) Anti-inflammatory and analgesic effect of plumbagin through inhibition of nuclear factor-κB activation. J Pharmacol Exp Ther 335:735–742
82. Dhingra D, Bansal S (2015) Antidepressant-like activity of plumbagin in unstressed and stressed mice. Pharmacol Rep 67:1024–1032
83. Wei Y, Huang M, Liu X, Yuan Z, Peng Y, Huang Z, Duan X, Zhao T (2015) Anti-fibrotic effect of plumbagin on CCl4-Lesioned rats. Cell Physiol Biochem 35:1599–1608
84. Singh UV, Udupa N (1997) Reduced toxicity and enhanced antitumor efficacy of betacyclodextrin plumbagin inclusion complex in mice bearing Ehrlich ascites carcinoma. Indian J Physiol Pharmacol 41:171–175

85. Santhakumari G, Saralamma PG, Radhakrishnan N (1980) Effect of plumbagin on cell growth and mitosis. Indian J Exp Biol 18:215–218
86. Edenharder R, Tang X (1997) Inhibition of the mutagenicity of 2-nitrofluorene, 3-nitrofluoranthene and 1-nitropyrene by flavonoids, coumarins, quinones and other phenolic compounds. Food Chem Toxicol 35:357–372
87. Farr SB, Natvig DO, Kogoma T (1985) Toxicity and mutagenicity of plumbagin and the induction of a possible new DNA repair pathway in *Escherichia coli*. J Bacteriol 164:1309–1316
88. SivaKumar V, Prakash R, Murali MR, Devaraj H, NiranjaliDevaraj S (2005) In vivo micronucleus assay and GST activity in assessing genotoxicity of plumbagin in Swiss albino mice. Drug Chem Toxicol 28:499–507
89. Raja Naresh RA, Udupa N, Uma Devi P (1996) Niosomal plumbagin with reduced toxicity and improved anticancer activity in BALB/C mice. J Pharm Pharmacol 48:1128–1132
90. Kini DP, Pandey S, Shenoy BD, Singh UV, Udupa N, Umadevi P, Kamath R (1997) Nagarajkumari, Ramanarayan K. Antitumor, and antifertility activities of plumbagin controlled release formulations. Indian J Exp Biol 35:374–379
91. Singh UV, Bisht KS, Rao S, Uma Devi P, Udupa N (1997) Reduced toxicity, and enhanced antitumor efficacy of plumbagin using poly (Lactic-co-glycolic) biodegradable injectable implant. Indian J Pharmacol 29:168–172
92. Kumar MR, Aithal BK, Udupa N, Reddy MS, Raakesh V, Murthy RS, Raju DP, Rao BS (2011) Formulation of plumbagin loaded long circulating pegylated liposomes: in vivo evaluation in C57BL/6J mice bearing B16F1 melanoma. Drug Deliv 18:511–522

Anethole and Its Role in Chronic Diseases

Ana Clara Aprotosoaie, Irina-Iuliana Costache and Anca Miron

Abstract Anethole is the main fragrance and bioactive compound of anise, fennel, and star anise spices and more than other 20 plant species. It is widely used as flavor agent in food industry and other industries, in cosmetics, perfumery, and pharmaceuticals. In the last few years, various studies have revealed multiple beneficial effects of anethole for human health, such as anti-inflammatory, anti-carcinogenic and chemopreventive, antidiabetic, immunomodulatory, neuroprotective, or antithrombotic, that are mediated by the modulation of several cell signaling pathways, mainly NF-kB and TNF-α signaling, and various ion channels. This chapter aims to review the scientific data and attempts to provide an insight into pharmacological activity of anethole and its therapeutic potential in human chronic diseases.

Keywords Anethole · Anti-inflammatory · Anticarcinogenic · NF-kB · TNF-α · MAPK · STAT · AP-1 signaling pathways

1 Introduction

Anethole (1-methoxy-4-propenyl-benzene, isoestragole) is an alkoxy-propenylbenzene derivative and an important flavoring component of essential oils of more than 20 plant species [1]. Essential oils from seeds of anise (*Pimpinella*

A.C. Aprotosoaie (✉) · A. Miron
Department of Pharmacognosy, Faculty of Pharmacy, University of Medicine and Pharmacy "Grigore T. Popa", Iasi, Romania
e-mail: anaclara70@yahoo.com; ana.aprotosoaie@umfiasi.ro

A. Miron
e-mail: ancamiron@umfiasi.ro

I.-I. Costache
Department of Internal Medicine, Faculty of Medicine, "Sf. Spiridon" University Hospital Iasi, University of Medicine and Pharmacy "Grigore T. Popa", Iasi, Romania
e-mail: irinaiulianacostache@yahoo.com

S.C. Gupta et al. (eds.), *Drug Discovery from Mother Nature*,
Advances in Experimental Medicine and Biology 929,
DOI 10.1007/978-3-319-41342-6_11

Table 1 Botanical sources of anethole

Essential oil	Plant sources	Anethole content (%)	References
Anise	Seeds of *Pimpinella anisum* L., Apiaceae	77–94	[68–70]
Star anise	Seeds, leaves and branches of *Illicium verum* Hook.f., Magnoliaceae	72–92	[68, 70]
Sweet fennel	Seeds of *Foeniculum vulgare* var.*dulce*, Apiaceae	81.63–95	[71]
Maggot killer	Leaves of *Clausena anisata* (Willd.) Hook f.ex. Benth., Rutaceae	85–100	[72, 73]
Anise myrtle	Leaves of *Syzygium anisatum* (Vickery) Craven and Biffen, Myrtaceae	93–95	[74]
Croton zehntneri	Leaves, branches of *Croton zehntneri* Pax et Hoffm, Euphorbiaceae	42–86.8	[49, 60, 75]
Cicely	Different parts of *Myrrhis odorata* (L.) Scop, Apiaceae	85.48	[76]
Amberoot	Roots of *Osmorhiza longistylis* (Torr.) DC, Apiaceae	95.43	[76]
Cake bush	Leaves of *Piper marginatum* Jacq. sin. *Piper anisatum* Kunth, Piperaceae	80.47	[76]
Bitter fennel	Seeds of *Foeniculum vulgare* Mill. var. *vulgare*, Apiaceae	55–75	[77]
Florence fennel	Leaves of *Foeniculum vulgare* Mill. ssp. *vulgare* var.*azoricum*	60–66.3	[78]

anisum L.), star anise (*Illicium verum* Hook.f), and sweet fennel (*Foeniculum vulgare* Mill. var. *dulce*) are the main sources used for the isolation of anethole (Table 1). Two isomers of anethole occur in nature: E- or *trans*-anethole and Z-or *cis*-anethole (Fig. 1). About 90 % of natural anethole is *trans*-isomer [2]. Besides separation from natural essential oils, anethole is obtained using the rectification of crude sulfate turpentine and/or the organic synthesis starting from methylchavicol or anisole and propionic anhydride [3]. Compared to natural compound, synthetic *trans*-anethole is impurified with higher amounts of *cis*-isomer [4].

Worldwide, traditional uses of plants that contain anethole include mainly gastro-intestinal and nervous disturbances, cutaneous inflammatory conditions, or catarrh of the respiratory tract. Besides, many of them are spices (anise, star anise, fennel) or are used as sweeteners (*Croton zehntneri* Pax et Hoffm) [5] or for mouth fresheners (fennel) [6]. Only *trans*-anethole is considered as food grade. It is used as flavor agent in food and confectionary products (baked goods, seasonings, ice-creams, candy), alcoholic beverages, such as anise-flavored liqueurs (Pernaud, Sambuco, Ouzo, Raki, Anisette), as well as in perfumery and pharmaceuticals [3, 7]. Generally, aniseed drinks contain between 0.125 and 4.04 g/L *trans*-anethole [2]. In perfumery, it adds fresh and fruity-anisic nuances to fragrances [8]. *Trans*-anethole can cover unpleasant odors, mainly acid, rancid, sulfurous malodors, so it is widely used as masking agent in cosmetics, soaps, and oral hygiene products

Fig. 1 Chemical structures of anethole isomers

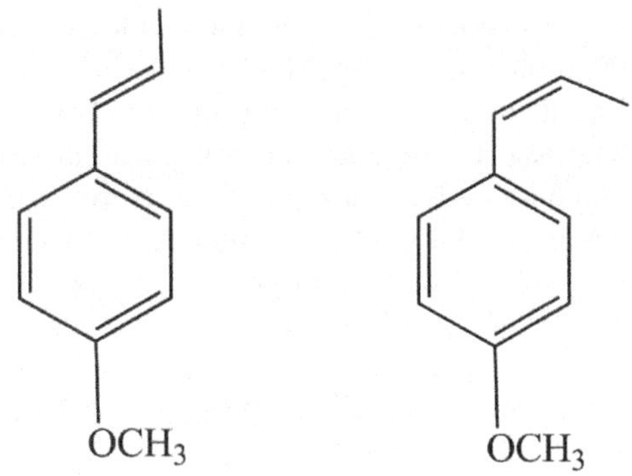

Trans-anethole *Cis*-anethole

(toothpaste, mouthwash) [3, 7]. Also, *trans*-anethole is used in food preservation, industrial products, feed additives, synthetic flavors, and pesticides [3].

Trans-anethole is considered non-genotoxic, non-carcinogenic, being generally recognized as safe agent (GRAS) by the *Expert Panel of the Flavour and Extract Manufacturers Association* (FEMA) and *Food and Drug Administration* (FDA) [1, 3]. *The International Joint FAO/WHO Expert Committee on Food Additives* (JECFA) established an acceptable daily intake (ADI) of 0–2 mg/kg bw [9].

2 Physicochemical Properties of Anethole

Pure anethole is a colorless to faintly yellow liquid at above 23 °C [10]. It is poorly soluble in water, is highly soluble in alcohol, and is miscible with ether and chloroform. The two isomers of anethole have different aroma profile and toxicity. *Trans*-anethole has a sweet herbaceous smooth odor profile [7] and a sweet taste, being more than 10 times sweeter than common sugar [11]. It is perceived as being pleasant to the taste even at higher concentrations [12]. *Cis*-anethole has an acid pungent, camphoraceous, and unpleasant odor [3, 13]. The main physicochemical constants of anethole are presented in Table 2.

Table 2 Physicochemical properties of anethole [3]

Molecular formula	$C_{10}H_{12}O$
Relative density (20 °C)	0.986–0.991
Refractive index (20 °C)	1.5570–1.5620
Boiling point (°C)	234–237
Optical rotation $[\alpha]_D^{25}$	−0.15 to +0.15 °C
Vapor pressure (kPa)	5.45
Flash point (°C)	90

Ultraviolet (UV) light and visible (VIS) light, temperature, atmospheric oxygen, the prolonged storage significantly influence the chemical stability of anethole. The degradation of anethole through oxidation, isomerization, and cyclization reactions may lead to some sensory, physical, and toxicological alterations [14]. Under the influence of light or high temperatures, *trans*-anethole is converted into *cis*-isomer that is about 15–38 times more toxic to animals than *trans*-form [15]. As a result of long-term storage (more of 2 months) of sweet fennel essential oil, *trans*-anethole is completely oxidized to anisaldehyde or isomerized to *cis*-anethole. Sunlight or UV-irradiation may induce the formation of a photoanethole (4,4′-dimethoxystilbene) through photocycloaddition between anethole and anisaldehyde (Fig. 2). The formation of inclusion complex between anethole and β-cyclodextrin could be an efficient way to improve its aqueous solubility and physicochemical stability. Besides, the complex can maintain the fragrance of anethole for a long time and its release behavior can be controlled [16].

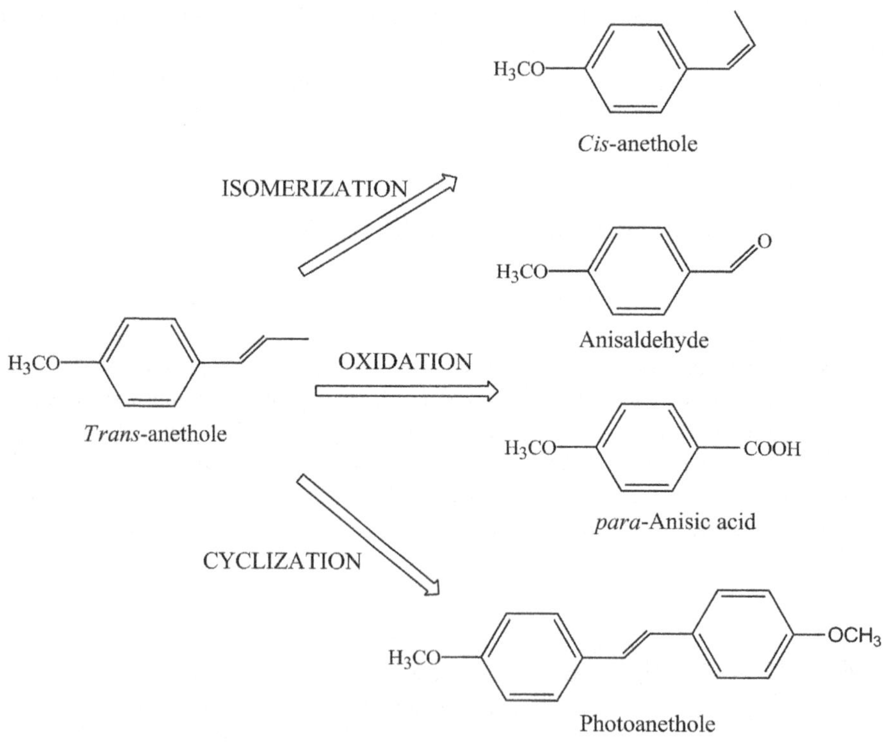

Fig. 2 Degradation products of anethole

3 Pharmacokinetic Profile of Anethole

Anethole satisfies Lipinski's rule of five (molecular weight <500; octanol/water partition coefficient, log $P < 5$; hydrogen bond donors <5; hydrogen bond acceptors <10) (Table 3), and ADMET (absorption, distribution, excretion, metabolism, toxicology) properties [17]. It is able to show drug likeliness, being orally bioavailable [18]. Experimental studies on rats and mice showed that the anethole is completely absorbed but slowly after oral administration. The major metabolic pathways involve *O*-demethylation, oxidation of the C3-side chain [19], and conjugation with glucuronic acid, glycine, sulfate, and glutathione [20]. The main metabolites of anethole are 4-methoxy-hippuric acid, 4-methoxy-benzoic acid, 4-hydroxypropenylbenzene, 2-hydroxy-1-methylthio-1-(4′-methoxyphenyl)-propane, 4-methoxy derivatives of acetophenone, cinnamic alcohol, and cinnamic acid. The elimination of anethole occurs within 48–72 h, and the major routes are renal, pulmonary, and fecal excretion [19]. The metabolism and excretion of anethole are dose-dependent in animals. Low doses of anethole are mainly metabolized via *O*-demethylation and eliminated via exhalation as CO_2. With increasing doses, the metabolism of anethole involves side-chain oxidation and epoxidation, and the renal excretion predominates. In humans, anethole is mainly metabolized to anisic acid, *p*-hydroxybenzoic acid, and 4-methoxy-hippuric acid. Anethole metabolites are eliminated within 8 h after anethole administration, and the major routes include renal excretion (54–69 %) and exhalation (13–17 %) [19].

4 Modulation of Cell Signaling Pathways by Anethole

Various studies provide evidence that anethole may interfere several important signaling pathways such as NF-kB (nuclear factor k-light-chain enhancer of activated B cells), MAPK (mitogen-activated protein kinase), STAT (signal transducer and activator of transcription) and AP-1 (activator protein-1), as well as cytokine signaling [TNF-α (tumor necrosis factor), interferon (IFN)-γ], or matrix metalloproteinase (MMPs) activities (Fig. 3).

Table 3 Lipinski properties of anethole [79]

Molecular weight	148.2 g/mol
Hydrogen bond donors	0
Hydrogen bond acceptors	1
Rotatable bonds	2
Topological polar surface area	9.2 angstrom squared
Log *P*	2.91
Molar refractivity	48.99
Dipole	1.409
% of human oral absorption	100

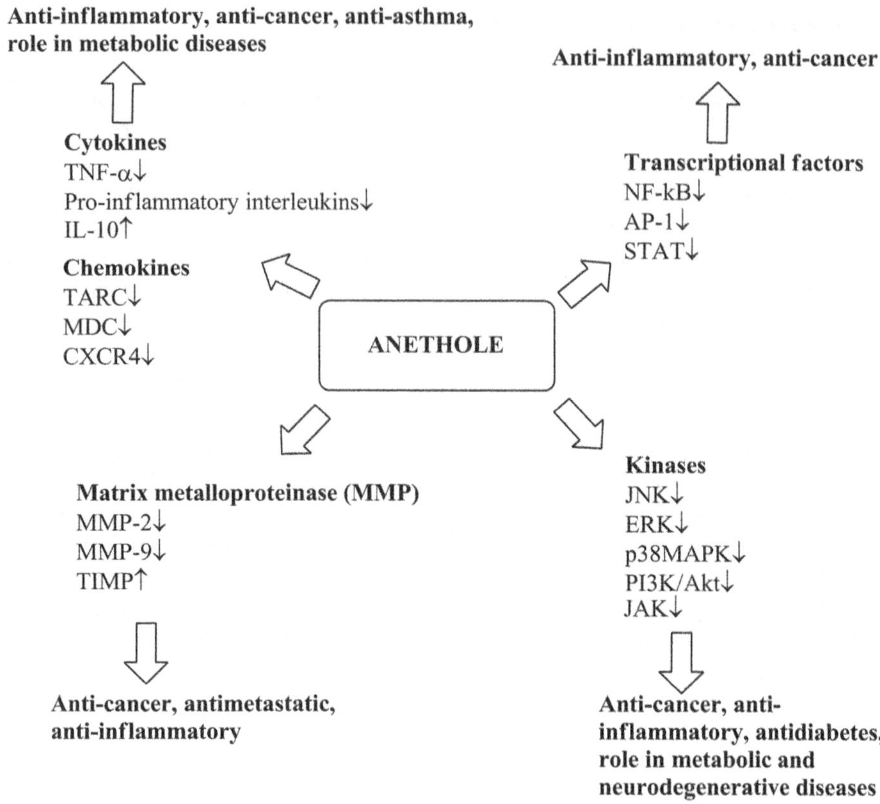

Fig. 3 Molecular targets of anethole. *NF-kB* nuclear factor B; *AP-1* activator protein 1; *STAT* signal transducer and activator of transcripition; *JNK* c-Jun N-terminal kinase; *ERK* extracellular receptor kinase; *p38MAPK* p38 mitogen-activated protein kinase; *PI3K/Akt* phosphoinositide-3-kinase-protein kinase B; *JAK* janus kinase; *TNF-α* tumor necrosis factor α; *IL-10* interleukin-10; *TARC* thymus and activation-regulated chemokine; *MDC* macrophage-derived chemokine; *CXCR4* chemokine receptor type 4; *TIMP* tisssue inhibitor of metalloproteinase gene expression

Chainy et al. [21] reported that anethole blocked both early and late cellular responses transduced by TNF-α, having an effect on NF-kB, AP-1, JNK (c-Jun N-terminal kinases), MAPK pathways, and apoptosis. It is a potent inhibitor of NF-kB signaling pathway *via* the blockade of IkBα (inhibitor of NF-kB) degradation and phosphorylation. Compared to some anti-inflammatory drugs such as sodium salicylate that suppresses NF-kB activation at suprapharmacological concentrations (>5 mM), anethole is active at low concentrations (1 mM). Thus, the incubation of ML1a cells with anethole (1 mM) effectively inhibits TNF-induced NF-kB activation. The inhibitory effect of anethole seems to be not cell type specific since the compound suppresses NF-kB activation in other cells such as myeloid (U-397) and epithelial (HeLa) cells. It completely inhibits NF-kB activation induced by phorbol ester, LPS, okadaic acid, and ceramide, acting at a step common to all these agents in the signal-transduction NF-kB pathway. Also, anethole may suppress H_2O_2-induced NF-kB activation, but in this case, for the complete inhibition, a higher concentration than 1 mM is required [21].

An ethanolic extract of star anise containing *trans*-anethole as major component has showed a repressive effect on NF-kB pathway. The extract inhibited NF-kB translocation into the nucleus and dose-dependently inhibited TNF-α/IFN-γ-induced nuclear localization of NF-kB p65 as well as phosphorylation and degradation of IkBα in human keratinocyte HaCaT cell line [22, 23]. The treatment of human breast cancer cells (MCF-7, MDA-MB-231) with anethole at concentrations of 10^{-6}–10^{-3} M causes a significant decrease of NF-kB transcriptional activity independent of estrogen receptor status [24]. Besides, anethole (50, 100 μM) inhibits NF-kB activation in highly metastatic human fibrosarcoma cell line (HT-1080) [25]. Different mechanisms contribute to the suppressant effect of anethole on TNF-α-induced NF-kB activation, such as inhibition of free oxygen radical generation and lipid peroxidation, increase of cellular GSH levels, inhibition of mitogen-activated protein kinase kinase (MEK) activity [21].

Anethole treatment (1 mM) suppresses TNF-α-induced activation of AP-1 in ML1a cells [21], and it down-regulates AP-1 in phorbol 12-myristate 13-acetate (PMA) or ionomycin-stimulated EL 4 mouse T cells [26]. The effect of anethole on AP-1 may result from the inhibition of NF-kB reporter activity of adaptor molecule TRAF 2 as well as the abolition of MEK activation [21]. Also, anethole (1 mM) abolishes TNFα-induced JNK activation in ML1a cells. The effect is gradual; at concentrations below 1 mM, anethole only partially inhibits JNK activation. The potent inhibition of MEK activation by anethole supports its suppressive effect on JNK pathway [21].

Anethole can modulate not only JNK module of MAPK pathways as it has already shown, but also ERK and p38 cascades. At concentration of 1 mM, anethole inhibits TNF-induced MAPK kinase activation in ML1a cells [21]. It suppresses, in a dose-dependent manner, ERK and p38 MAPK signaling pathways in HT-1080 human fibrosarcoma cells [25]. Besides, an ethanolic extract from *I. verum* containing *trans*-anethole as main component has been shown to inhibit TNF-α/interferon (IFN)-γ-induced activation of ERK and p38 MAPK pathways in HaCaT human keratinocytes [22, 23]. The inhibitory effects of anethole on leukocyte chemotaxis stimulated by chemotactic agents such as formyl-methionyl-leucyl-phenylalanine (fMLP) and leukotriene B4 (LTB_4) may be explained, at least partially, by its suppressive activity on MAPK signaling [27].

Sung et al. [28] have reported that the ethanolic extract of *I. verum* (100 μg/mL) containing anethole as main component suppresses IFN-γ-induced JAK/STAT activation and ICAM-1 (intracellular adhesion molecule-1) expression in HaCaT keratinocytes. The extract inhibits IFN-γ expression and further STAT 1 phosphorylation and activation. Also, it up-regulates SOCS1 (suppressor of cytokine signaling 1). SOCS1 belongs to a protein family that negatively regulates STAT pathway. In addition, anethole up-regulates the expression of PTEN (phosphatase and tensin homologue) and suppresses CXCR4 chemokine expression in DU145 and LNCaP prostate cancer cells [29]. PEN negatively regulates STAT signaling.

Since CXCR4/CXCL12 axis stimulates JAK/STAT signaling, antagonist effect of anethole on CXCR4 may be associated with a suppression of this signal-transduction pathway. Rhee et al. [29] have found that anethole (25, 50, 100 μM) reduces the phosphorylation of Akt (protein kinase B) and PI3K (phosphoinositide-3-kinase) via PTEN activation in DU145 prostate cell cancer. In addition, anethole suppresses the phosphorylation of Akt in HT-1080 human fibrosarcoma cells [25]. Also, treatment with a star anise ethanolic extract containing *trans*-anethole as main compound inhibits TNFα/IFNγ-induced phosphorylation of Akt and down-regulates the expression of some pro-inflammatory cytokines (IL-1, IL-6) and chemokines [thymus and activation-regulated chemokine (TARC), macrophage-derived chemokine (MDC)] in HaCaT human keratinocytes line [22, 23].

Besides the effect on cellular events transduced by TNF-α, anethole directly affects the production of this pleiotropic cytokine. Oral treatment with anethole inhibits production or release of TNF-α induced by intraplantar carrageenan and Complete Freund's adjuvant (CFA) in mice and it decreases the carrageenan-induced pleural level of TNF-α in rats [30]. At concentrations of 50 mg/kg (i.p), anethole suppresses TNF-α production in a rat model of lipopolysaccharide (LPS)-induced periodontitis [31]. However, Domiciano et al. [32] did not identify a decrease of TNF-α pleural level in same model of a carrageenan-induced pleurisy in rats, after anethole treatment. These contradictory findings can be attributed to the fact that Domiciano et al. have tested star anise essential oil and not pure anethole, and its administration was performed as single dose. It seems that the prolonged treatment with anethole produces more evident inhibitory effects on TNF-α levels [30]. Anethole suppresses the release of some interleukins that mediate a broad spectrum of inflammatory and hyper nociceptive signaling responses (IL-1β, IL-2, IL-3, IL-4, IL-5, IL-6, IL-13, and IL-17) (Table 4). Also, it may increase IL-10 levels [33], an anti-inflammatory cytokine with protective role in allergic diseases, asthma, autoimmune diseases, and diabetes mellitus [34].

Table 4 Main functions of anethole-suppressed interleukins [22, 34, 80, 81]

Interleukin	Function	Related diseases
IL-1β	Proliferation, differentiation of specific immunocompetent cells and nonadaptive cells; synthesis of chemokines; vascular permeability; induction of COX2, iNOS; activation of acute-phase proteins in the liver	Autoimmune disease, rheumatoid arthritis, atherosclerosis, inflammatory bowel diseases, allergic diseases, cancer
IL-2	Growth factor for T cells, proliferation, activation, stimulus for antibody cells	Psoriasis
IL-3	Hematopoietic growth factor, differentiation and growth of different cell lineages	Neurodegenerative diseases, allergic diseases, cancer

(continued)

Table 4 (continued)

Interleukin	Function	Related diseases
IL-4	Proliferation of B and cytotoxic T cells, differentiation of antigen-stimulated naive T cells, IgE and IgG production	Allergic diseases
IL-5	Growth, mobilization, differentiation, survival of eosinophils, chemotaxis of eosinophils, Ig A and IgM production	Allergic asthma
IL-6	Hematopoiesis, maturation of B cells into antibody-producing plasma cells, T-cell activation, recruitment of neutrophils and mononuclear cells	Autoimmune diseases, allergic diseases, chronic inflammatory proliferative diseases, B-cell malignancy, diabetes mellitus, psoriasis
IL-13	Eosinophils and mast cell activation, fibrosis, tissue remodeling	Allergic diseases, asthma
IL-17	Recruitment and activation of neutrophils, induction of colony-stimulating factors (GM-CSF), metalloproteases	Rheumatoid arthritis, inflammatory bowel diseases, asthma, psoriasis

5 Role of Anethole in Chronic Diseases

The animal and cell-line data suggest that anethole may have beneficial effects in many chronic diseases linked with inflammation, such as inflammatory conditions, cancer, diabetes, neurological diseases, since it targets many of the key players in the inflammation to cancer sequence or in the inflammation to metabolism sequence.

5.1 Anethole and Inflammatory Process

The inflammation is a biological response to noxious stimuli (pathogens, physical injury, damaged cells) and a crucial process for tissue's homeostasis. Acute inflammation is considered as a protective reaction to stimuli and the chronic inflammation is a dys-regulated, maladaptive response that results in cellular and tissue malfunction. The prolonged inflammation is involved in the onset and maintenance of a large number of chronic human disorders, including cancer, arthritis, asthma, atherosclerosis, type 2 diabetes, obesity, neurodegenerative diseases, and atopic dermatitis [35–37]. Anethole alleviates the cellular and vascular events associated with inflammation and it also has an important antinociceptive activity. It may be effective in controlling some nonimmune inflammation-related diseases [32], in inflammatory pain [30] and periodontitis [31]. Oral treatment with anethole even for a prolonged time seems to be devoid of specific side effects of non-steroidal anti-inflammatory drugs such as hepatotoxicity, nephrotoxicity, and ulcerogenicity.

In addition, *trans*-anethole suppresses airway inflammation and exerts favorable effects in asthma through up-regulation of regulatory T cells [33]. Therefore, anethole may be a useful therapeutic candidate for inflammatory skin diseases such as atopic dermatitis [22, 23]. Oxidative stress-related skin diseases may be another area of application. Pretreatment with anethole (5, 10 μM) prevents the collagen metabolism alteration triggered by H_2O_2 in human skin fibroblasts. It increases collagen synthesis and inhibits the activity of major collagen-degrading enzymes MMP-2 and MMP-9 [38].

Anethole exerts anti-inflammatory activity via multiple mechanisms: negative modulation of NF-kB, TNF-α, Ap-1, MAPK kinase, JAK-STAT signaling pathways, inhibition of the pro-inflammatory cytokines production/release (TNF-α, IL-1β, IL-6, NO, PGE2), and inhibition of MMP-2 and MMP-9 matrix metalloproteinases [21, 39]. Also, anethole may modulate the cellular activities of inflammation-related cells reducing the chemotaxis of neutrophils by inhibiting myeloperoxidase activity and reducing oxidative stress [27, 35]. Modulation of voltage-gated L-type Ca^{2+} channel and KCa^{2+} channels could be another potential anti-inflammatory mechanism since LPS-induced inflammatory mediators production has been shown to be inhibited by the blockade of this type of ionic channels [31].

5.2 Anethole and Cancer

As potential antitumor agent, anethole interferes cancer cell biology by its pro-apoptotic, anti-metastatic and anti-inflammatory effects. Anethole and its synthetic analogues exhibit chemopreventive activity by suppressing the incidence and multiplicity of both invasive and non-invasive adenocarcinomas [29, 40]. Anethole induces apoptosis in human breast cells [24, 41], including triple-negative breast cancer subtype [42] and cervical carcinoma [43], and inhibits cell migration and invasion in human fibrosarcoma [25] and prostate cancer cells [29]. In addition, anethole enhances activity of some anticancer drugs such as cyclophosphamide [44], tamoxifen [41], and reduces chemotherapy toxicity [45, 46].

Anticancer properties of anethole are mediated by modulation of multiple cell pathways: induction of caspase activation pathway (caspase 8, 9), suppression of NF-kB, JNK, Akt and MAPK signaling pathways, and down-regulation of matrix metalloproteinase MMP-2 and MMP-9 expression. The suppression of ERK/p38 MAPK/Akt/NF-kB signaling pathways, down-regulation of MMP-2 and MMP-9, and urokinase plasminogen activator mRNA expressions as well as up-regulation of tissue inhibitor of metalloproteinase gene expression (TIMP) are involved in anti-metastatic effects of anethole [25].

5.3 Anethole and Diabetes

Anethole may serve as a promising candidate in the development of therapeutic agents against type 2 diabetes and control of secondary complications in diabetes. Diabetes mellitus is one of the most prevalent metabolic diseases characterized by chronic hyperglycemia resulting from either insulin dysfunction or insulin insufficiency [47]. Type 2 diabetes is the most common; it represents 90 % of the cases of diabetes worldwide. The beneficial effects of anethole in diabetes are mediated by the improvement of glycemic control mechanisms, amelioration of pancreatic β-cell function, and the stimulation of insulin secretion from existing β-cells [48]. Besides, it has noncompetitive to mixed aldose reductase inhibitory properties and potential anticataract effects. Aldose reductase is a key enzyme in polyol pathway that plays a significant role in the progression of diabetic complications, including cataract [6]. The wound-healing potential of anethole may be useful in the development of effective drugs to treat wound complications from diabetes and venous ulcers [49].

5.4 Anethole and Neurological Diseases

Neuroprotective properties of anethole may be useful in the amelioration of ischemic brain damage and some neurodegenerative symptomatology. Anethole (10 μM) significantly reduces neuronal cell death induced by oxygen-glucose deprivation/reoxygenation and mechanisms involve antioxidant and anti-excitotoxic effects as well as mitochondrial protection [50]. Beneficial effects in neurodegenerative diseases such as Alzheimer's and Parkinson's diseases can arise through cholinesterase inhibitory properties. Anethole is more active on acetylcholinesterase (IC_{50} = 39.89 μg/mL) than butyrylcholinesterase (IC_{50} = 75.35 μg/mL) [51]. Inhibition of acetylcholinesterase plays an important role in the prevention of cognitive impairment associated with cholinergic deficit. Anethole dithiolethione (Fig. 4), a synthetic analogue of anethole, has an attractive potential in the development of neuroprotective agents in Parkinson's disease due to its multifaceted antioxidant activity coupled with inhibition of monoamine oxidase (MAO)-B activity in clinically relevant dose range

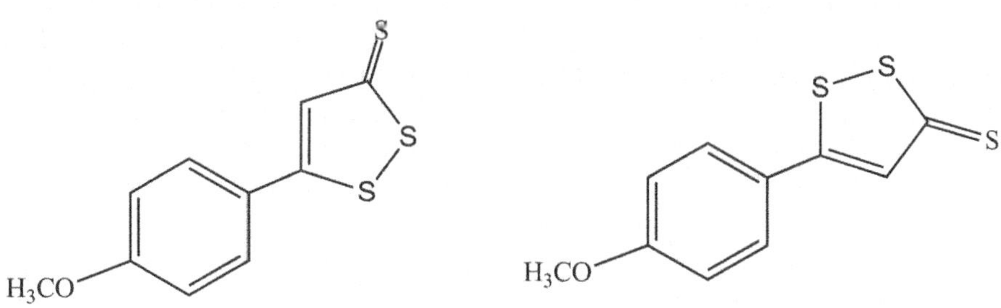

Anethole dithiolethione Anethole trithione

Fig. 4 Synthetic analogues of anethole

(0.03–30 μM). The MAO-catalyzed oxidation of dopamine generates oxidative stress that is involved in the degeneration of dopaminergic neurons in the substantia nigra, a relevant phenomenon in Parkinson's disease pathogenesis [52].

6 Biological Activities of Anethole in Animal Models

6.1 Anti-inflammatory and Antihypernociceptive Activities

Anethole showed anti-inflammatory effects in different experimental models of acute inflammation and/or chronic inflammation. It acts mainly anti-oedematously, inhibits leukocyte chemotaxis and vascular permeability, and attenuates tissue damage associated with inflammation. Oral administration of anethole (3, 10, and 30 mg/kg) inhibits the paw edema elicited by carrageenan and some pro-inflammatory mediators (substance P, bradykinine, TNF-α, serotonin, histamine) in Swiss mice [53]. Pretreatment with anethole (250 and 500 mg/kg, oral) reduces acute inflammatory responses such as carrageenan-induced pleurisy and migration of leukocytes in rats or ear-edema induced by croton-oil in mice. In the latter case, the effects of anethole were similarly to indomethacin (10 mg/kg, oral), a well-known non-steroidal anti-inflammatory drug, and only oral administration was effective; topical application of anethole had no inflammatory effects [32] suggesting that either anethole has an unfavorable pharmacokinetic profile for this way of administration, either it behaves as prodrug. Thus, anethole metabolites generated by its hepatic biotransformation are responsible for the anti-inflammatory effects [32]. In fact, Freire et al. [54] have showed that some hydroxylated derivatives of anethole display a greater anti-inflammatory activity than anethole itself. These derivatives (30, 300 mg/kg, oral) inhibit the increase of vascular permeability induced by acetic acid in mice, being as active as the control drug, indomethacin (10 mg/kg, oral). The introduction of hydroxyl groups at double bound from propenyl moiety of anethole enhances the anti-inflammatory activity [54].

Prolonged administration of *trans*-anethole (10, 50 mg/kg/day, i.p, 10 days) has a potent inhibitory activity on *Escherichia coli* LPS-induced periodontitis in rats. In this experimental model, anethole exerts an anti-inflammatory effect that was almost similar to ketoprofen, a non-steroidal anti-inflammatory drug (10 mg/kg, i.p) [31]. Also, anethole prevents LPS-induced lung inflammation in mice [55]. Co-administration of anethole with ibuprofen, both at low doses, produces a synergic anti-inflammatory effect compared to the corresponding monotherapy (anethole or ibuprofen alone) in carrageenan-induced pleurisy and paw edema in rats [56]. In ovalbumin-sensitized BALB/c mice, prolonged treatment with anethole inhibits eosinophilia, and infiltration of lymphocytes in lung tissues, reducing airway hyperresponsiveness [33].

Single oral administration of anethole (250, 500 mg/kg) reduces carrageenan-induced acute inflammatory pain in mice. Also, daily pretreatment with anethole (250 mg/kg, oral) for 7 days causes a significant reduction of CFA-induced mechanical hypernociception in mice. In these models, the antihypernociceptive effects of anethole were similar to indomethacin (2.5 mg/kg). Oral treatment with anethole (62.5, 125, and 250 mg/kg) significantly reduces the nociceptive responses induced by glutamate in mice. In contrast, anethole does not affect the neurogenic pain which occurs in the first phase of formalin test and has no effect on thermal nociception in hot-plate test. An important feature of anethole activity is that its antinociceptive doses do not cause alterations in motor coordination or sedation as observed in the open-field test [57].

6.2 Immunomodulatory Activity

In immunocompetent mice, high doses of *trans*-anethole (250, 500 mg/kg, oral, once a day) cause a significant decrease of delayed-type hypersensitivity response induced by sheep red blood cells and increase of antibody production as well as the leukocyte count in peripheral blood. Also, in immunosuppressed mice with cyclophosphamide (50 mg/kg, ip), treatment with *trans*-anethole (500 mg/kg, oral) improves the humoral response. It produces an increase of white blood cell count and antibody levels close to normal values compared to the non-immunosuppressed control group. The immune effect of anethole may be related not only to an increase of IL-10 production, a cytokine involved in the suppression of T helper cell response, but also to a reduction of T_H1-type cytokines (IL-2) levels. The immunomodulatory profile of anethole may offer promising alternative therapy to counteract the effects of cytotoxic chemotherapeutic agents [46].

6.3 Antitumor Activity

Al-Harbi et al. [44] provided evidence for the anticarcinogenic and cytotoxic effects of anethole in Ehrlich ascites tumor in mice. The compound increases the survival time and reduces tumor weight and volume. In mice with Sarcoma-180 solid tumor, anethole (10, 20, 40 mg/kg, *per os*) reduces tumor load through apoptotic effects. The combinatorial use of anethole with cyclophosphamide, a classic anticancer drug, exhibits more tumoricidal activity. Also, it protects against side effects induced by cyclophosphamide without influencing drug anticancer activity [45]. Anethole trithione (Fig. 4), a dithiolthione analogue, inhibits aflatoxin B1-induced hepatic tumorigenicity [58] and azoxymethane-induced colon carcinogenesis in rats [59]. Dietary exposure to anethole trithione (200, 400 ppm) decreases dimethylbenzanthracene-induced mammary cancer multiplicity in female Sprague-Dawley rats. Its chemopreventive properties may be related to the induction of phase II drug metabolizing enzymes [40].

6.4 Cardiovascular Activity

In normotensive conscious rats, intravenous (iv) injections of anethole (1–10 mg/kg) as well as the essential oil of *Croton zehntneri* (1–20 mg/kg) induce biphasic changes in blood pressure and bradycardia. Initial cardiovascular response includes a pronounced arterial hypotension and a rapid bradycardia (phase I). The subsequent response (phase II) consists in an increase of blood pressure and a second period of more lasting bradycardia. The hypotensive effect of anethole is mediated mainly by a cholinergic mechanism, and the pressor response could occur *via* an indirect vasoconstriction through inhibition of endothelial production [60]. In anaesthetized rats, iv injection of anethole (10 mg/kg) elicits hypotension and bradycardia responses. Therefore, iv administration of *Croton zehntneri* essential oil evokes a capsaicin-like bradycardia and depressor reflex that appear to be mediated by the activation of vanilloid TPRV1 receptors located on sensory vagal nerves [5].

6.5 Antithrombotic Activity

Anethole as well as fennel essential oil exhibit antithrombotic properties which are linked to a broad spectrum antiplatelet activity, clot destabilizing effect, spasmolytic, and vasorelaxant abilities. Subacute treatment with anethole or fennel essential oil (30 mg/kg/day for 5 days, oral) prevents pulmonary microembolism and subsequent paralysis events induced by collagen-epinephrine injection in mice (83 and 70 % protection, respectively) being more active than aspirin (100 mg/kg/day, 35 % protection). In vitro findings strongly support the antiplatelet effects of anethole. In guinea pig plasma, anethole inhibits platelet aggregation stimulated by arachidonic acid, collagen, ADP, or U46619, a thromboxane A2 agonist. Moreover, it is able to destabilize clot retraction triggered by thrombin in rat platelet-rich plasma. At antiplatelet concentration, anethole displays NO- and PG-independent vasorelaxant properties, reducing phenylephrine or KCl-induced contractions of rat isolated aorta irrespective of the endothelium presence [61]. Soares et al. [62] have showed that anethole has a complex pharmacological profile of activity on vascular smooth muscle contractility. At low concentrations (10^{-6}–10^{-4} M), it causes the contraction of rat isolated aortic rings precontracted with phenylephrine, and at high concentrations (10^{-3}–10^{-2} M), anethole elicits a complete retraction. It seems that the contractile effects of anethole are mediated by the modulation of voltage-dependent Ca^{2+} channels while the relaxant effects involve multiple mechanisms, including actions on various ion channels. In contrast with many antithrombotic synthetic agents, anethole is devoid of prohemorragic and gastrolesive undesired effects [61].

6.6 Antidiabetic Activity

Trans-anethole exhibits a hypoglycemic activity that is almost similar to glibenclamide, a standard antidiabetic drug. Oral administration of *trans*-anethole (80 mg/kg/day for 45 days) in streptozotocin-induced type 2 diabetic rats prevents the rise of plasma glucose and glycosylated hemoglobin levels, and the decrease of glycogen content in liver and muscle tissues. In addition, it increases the level of insulin and restores the altered activities of key enzymes involved in carbohydrate metabolism (hexokinase, glucose-6-phosphate dehydrogenase, glucose-6-phosphatase, fructose-1,6-bisphosphatase) to near normal levels. Moreover, anethole ameliorates histopathological changes of pancreatic β-cells in diabetic rats [48]. Pari et al. [63] reported that *trans*-anethole restores the altered glycoprotein components in plasma, liver, and kidney of diabetic rats to near normal values. Besides, *trans*-anethole displays anticataract activity through the inhibition of lens aldose reductase (IC_{50} = 3.8 μg/mL) and antioxidant activity. It increases SOD and catalase activities and restores GSH levels in the sugar induced lens opacification [6].

6.7 Gastroprotector Activity

Trans-anethole (30, 300 mg/kg, oral) protects against ethanol-induced gastric lesions in male Swiss mice. Its gastroprotective properties may be related to the stimulation of mucus gastric secretion. The conjugated double bond of propenyl moiety of anethole significantly contributes to this effect [54].

6.8 Local Anesthetic Activity

In the conjunctival reflex assay in rabbit, the administration of *trans*-anethole (10–100 μg/mL) increases the number of stimuli required to evoke reflex in a concentration-dependent manner. Also, in vitro, *trans*-anethole (0.001–1 μg/mL) reduces the electrically evoked contractions of the isolated rat phrenic nerve hemidiaphragm. *Trans*-anethole exhibits a profile of activity similar to the local anesthetic drug, procaine [64].

6.9 Anxiolytic Activity

Inhalation of *trans*-anethole (1 μL/L air) for 90 mins produces an anxiolytic-like effect in male ICR mice. The methoxyl group and 1-propenyl substituent in the *para* position of the benzene ring are required for the anxiolytic properties [65].

6.10 *Wound-Healing Activity*

In an excision wound model in mice, administration of pharmaceutical formulation with 20 % anethole twice daily for 15 days accelerates wound closure of injured tissue, enhances the number of fibroblasts and collagen fibers. Anethole acts in the inflammatory and remodeling phases of the wound-healing process promoting mainly extracellular matrix remodeling. Also, the antioxidant and antimicrobial properties of anethole significantly contribute to the improvement of cutaneous wound condition [49].

7 Biological Activities of Anethole in Humans

To the best of our knowledge, there are no clinical trials with anethole. Only a single clinical study has been performed with synthetic anethole dithiolethione in lung cancer. Anethole dithiolethione [5-p(methoxyphenyl)-3H-1,2-dithiole-3-thione) (Fig. 4) is a sulfur-containing compound that belongs to the dithiolethiones class. It is an approved drug in Canada and Europe for the treatment of xerostomia, including drug- and radiation-induced hyposalivation. In a randomized, double-blind, placebo-controlled, phase IIb clinical trial in smokers with bronchial dysplasia, Lam et al. [66] have reported that anethole dithiolethione at 25 mg orally thrice daily for 6 months prevents the development and progression of pre-existing dysplastic lesions. Cancer chemoprevention activity of anethole dithiolethione may be related to the increase of intracellular glutathione, up-regulation of phase II detoxification enzymes such as glutathione-S-transferase, and inhibition of NF-kB signaling activation [67].

8 Conclusions

Evidence indicate that anethole is a natural bioactive compound with multiple beneficial effects in human health such as anti-inflammatory, anticancer, chemopreventive, neuroprotective, spasmolytic, hypotensive, antithrombotic, immunomodulatory, and antidiabetic. It may offer a safe approach in treatment of several chronic diseases, particularly in skin and lung inflammatory disorders, cancer, type 2 diabetes, neurological diseases. The underlying mechanisms for anethole efficacy seem to be the modulation of several signaling pathways, especially, NF-kB, TNF-α, MAPK pathways. Long-term clinical studies are needed to validate its usefulness.

References

1. Newberne P, Smith RL, Doull J, Goodman JI, Munro IC, Portoghese PS, Wagner BM, Weil CS, Woods LA, Adams TB, Lucas CD, Ford RA (1999) The FEMA GRAS assessment of trans-anethole used as flavouring substance. Food Chem Toxicol 37:789–811
2. Jurado JM, Alcázar A, Pablos F, Martín MJ (2006) LC determination of anethole in aniseed drinks. Chromatographia 64:223–226
3. Zongliang H (2012) Anethole development trends. In: Conference proceedings of IFEAT international conference "Essential Asia", Singapore, 4–8 Nov 2012
4. Özgüven M (2012) Aniseed. In: Peter KW (ed) Handbook of herbs and spices, 2nd edn. Woodhead Publishing Limited, Cambridge, pp 139–150
5. Siqueira RJB, Leal-Cardoso JH, Couture R, Lahlou S (2006a) Role of capsaicin-sensitive sensory nerves in mediation of the cardiovascular effects of the essential oil of *Croton zehntneri* leaves in anaesthetized rats. Clin Exp Pharmacol Physiol 33:238–247
6. Dongare V, Kulkarni C, Kondawar M, Magdum C, Haldavnekar V, Arvindekar A (2012) Inhibition of aldose reductase and anti-cataract action of trans-anethole isolated from *Foeniculum vulgare* Mill. fruits. Food Chem 132:385–390
7. De Rovira Sr D (2008) Dictionary of flavors, 2nd edn. Wiley-Blackwell, Hoboken
8. Milne GWA (ed) (2005) Gardner's commercially important chemicals. Synonyms, trade names, and properties. Wiley, Hoboken
9. Carratù B, Federici E, Gallo FR, Geraci A, Guidotti M, Multari G, Palazzino G, Sanzini E (2010) Plants and parts of plants used in food supplements: an approach to their safety assessment. Ann Ist Super Sanità 46:370–388
10. Food Chemical Codex (2010) The United States pharmacopeial convention. United Book Press Inc, Baltimore
11. Cabral PHB, de Morais Campos R, Fonteles MC, Santos CF, Cardoso JHL, do Nascimento NRF (2014) Effects of the essential oil of *Croton zehntneri* and its major components, anethole and estragole, on the rat corpora cavernosa. Life Sci 112:74–81
12. Panda H (2010) Perfumes and flavours technology handbook. Asia Pacific Business Press Inc, Delhi
13. Singhal RS, Kulkarni PR, Rege DV (1997) Handbook of indices of food quality and authenticity. Woodhead Publishing Limited, Cambridge
14. Turek C, Stintzing FC (2013) Stability of essential oils: a review. Compr Food Sci Food 12:40–53
15. Andallu B, Rajeshwari CU (2011) Aniseeds (*Pimpinella anisum* L.) in health and disease. In: Preedy VR, Ross Watson R, Patel VB (eds) Nuts & seeds in health and disease prevention, 1st edn. Elsevier, Amsterdam, pp 175–181
16. Zhang W, Liu X, Yu T, Yuan L, Rao G, Li D, Mu C (2015) Preparation, physicochemical characterization and release behavior of the inclusion complex of trans-anethole and β-cyclodextrin. Food Res Int 74:55–62
17. Pitchai D, Manikkam R, Sukamaran S, Kandhasamy S, Periyasamy V (2011) In-silico docking studies on anticancerous polyphenolic phytocompounds targeting the BH3 domain of Bcl-XL receptor in apoptotic pathway. J Pharm Res 4:1626–1631
18. Kadam RU, Roy N (2007) Recent trends in drug-likeness prediction: a comprehensive review of in silico methods. Indian J Pharm Sci 69:609–615
19. Committee of Experts on Cosmetic Products (2008) Active ingredients used in cosmetics: safety survey. Partial Agreement Division in the Social and Public Health Field, Council of Europe Publishing, Strasbourg
20. Bounds SV, Caldwell J (1996) Pathways of metabolism of [1′-14C]-trans-anethole in the rat and mouse. Drug Metab Dispos 24:717–724
21. Chainy GBN, Manna SK, Chaturvedi MM, Aggarwal BB (2000) Anethole blocks both early and late cellular responses transduced by tumor necrosis: effect on NF-kB, AP-1, JNK, MAPKK and apoptosis. Carcinogenesis 19:2943–2950

22. Sung B, Prasad Y, Yadav VR, Aggarwal BB (2012a) Cancer cell signaling pathways targeted by spice-derived nutraceuticals. Nutr Cancer 64:173–194
23. Sung Y-Y, Kim YS, Kim HK (2012b) *Illicium verum* extract inhibits TNF-α and IFN-γ-induced expression of chemokines and cytokines in human keratinocytes. J Ethnopharmacol 144:182–189
24. Chen CH, de Graffenried LA (2012) Anethole suppressed cell survival and induced apoptosis in human breast cancer cells independent of estrogen receptor status. Phytomedicine 19:763–767
25. Choo EJ, Rhee Y-H, Jeong S-J, Lee H-J, Kim HS, Ko HS, Kim J-H, Kwon T-R, Jung JH, Kim JH, Lee H-J, Lee E-O, Kim DK, Chen C-Y, Kim S-H (2011) Anethole exerts antimetastatic activity via inhibition of matrix metalloproteinase 2/9 and AKT/mitogen-activated kinase/nuclear factor kappa B signaling pathways. Biol Pharm Bull 34:41–46
26. Yea SS, Jeong HS, Choi CY, Park KR, Oh S, Shin JG, Yun CH (2006) Inhibitory effect of anethole on T-lymphocyte proliferation and interleukin-2 production through down-regulation of the NF-AT and AP-1. Toxicol In Vitro 20:1098–1105
27. Estevão-Silva CF, Kummer R, Fachini-Queiroz FC, Grespan R, de Melo GAN, Baroni S, Cuman RKN, Bersani-Amado CA (2014) Anethole and eugenol reduce in vitro and in vivo leukocyte migration induced by fMLP, LTB_4, and carrageenan. J Nat Med 68:567–575
28. Sung Y-Y, Kim HK (2013) *Illicium verum* extract suppresses IFN-γ-induced ICAM-1 expression via blockade of JAK/STAT pathway in HaCaT human keratinocytes. J Ethnopharmacol 149:626–632
29. Rhee Y-H, Chung P-S, Kim S-H, Ahn JC (2014) CXCR4 and PTEN are involved in the anti-metastatic regulation of anethole in DU145 prostate cancer cells. Biochem Biophys Res Commun 447:557–562
30. Ritter AMV, Domiciano TP, WaldiceuVerri A Jr, Zarpelon AC, da Silva LG, Barbosa CP, Natali MRM, Cuman RKN, Bersani-Amado CA (2013) Antihypernociceptive activity of anethole in experimental inflammatory pain. Inflammopharmacology 21:187–197
31. Moradi J, Abbasipour F, Zaringhalam J, Maleki B, Ziaee N, Khodadoustan A, Janahmadi M (2014) Anethole, a medicinal plant compound, decreases the production of pro-inflammatory TNF-α and IL-1β in a rat model of LPS-induced periodontitis. Iran J Pharm Res 13:1319–1325
32. Domiciano TP, de Oliveira Dalalio MD, Silva EL, Ritter AMV, Estevão-Silva C, Ramos FS, Caparroz-Assef SM, Cuman RKN, Bersani-Amado CA (2013) Inhibitory effect of anethole in nonimmune acute inflammation. Naunyn-Schmiedeberg's Arch Pharmacol 386:331–338
33. Kim S-H, Dong-Seon K, Yoon-Young S, Kyoung KH (2015) Suppression of airway inflammation by *Illicium verum* and trans-anethole. Paper presented at the 10th international congress on complementary medicine research in 2015 (ICCMR 2015), Jeju, 13–15 May 2015
34. Akdis M, Burgler S, Crameri R, Eiwegger T, Fujita H, Gomez E, Klunker S, Meyer N, O'Mahony L, Palomares O, Rhyner C, Quaked N, Schaffartzik A, Van de Veen W, Zeller S, Zimmermann M, Akdis CA (2011) Interleukins, from 1 to 37, and interferon-γ: receptors, functions, and roles in diseases. J Allergy Clin Immunol 127:701–721e54
35. Bellik Y, Boukraâ L, Alzahrani HA, Bakhotmah BA, Abdellah F, Hammoudi SM, Iguer-Ouada M (2013) Molecular mechanisms underlying anti-inflammatory and anti-allergic activities of phytochemicals: an update. Molecules 18:322–353
36. De las Heras B, Hortelano S (2009) Molecular basis of the anti-inflammatory effects of terpenoids. Inflamm Allergy Drug Targets 8:28–39
37. Fürst R, Zündorf I (2014) Plant-derived anti-inflammatory compounds: hope and disappointments regarding the translation of preclinical knowledge into clinical progress. Mediators Inflamm. doi:10.1155/2014/146832
38. Galicka A, Krętowski R, Nazaruk J, Cechowska-Pasko M (2014) Anethole prevents hydrogen peroxide-induced apoptosis and collagen metabolism alterations in human skin fibroblasts. Mol Cell Biochem 394(217):224
39. Aggarwal BA, Shishodia S (2006) Molecular targets of dietary agents for prevention and therapy of cancer. Biochem Pharmacol 71:1397–1421

40. Lubet RA, Steele VE, Eto I, Juliana MM, Kelloff GJ, Grubbs CJ (1997) Chemopreventive efficacy of anetholetrithione, N-acetyl-L-cysteine, miconazole and phenethylisothiocyanate in the DMBA-induced rat mammary cancer model. Int J Cancer 72:95–101
41. Chen C, De Gasperi M, Salcedo R, Cavazos D, de Graffenried L (2009) Evaluation of the phytochemical anethole as an anti-tumor agent in MCF-7 cells. Cancer Res 69:abstract nr.3100
42. Muthukumari D, Padma PR, Sumathi S (2013) In vitro analysis of anethole as an anticancerous agent for triple negative breast cancer. Int J Pharm Sci Rev Res 23:314–318
43. Carvalho AA, Andrade LN, de Sousa EBV, de Sousa DP (2015) Antitumor phenylpropanoids found in essential oils. Biomed Res Int. doi:10.1155/392674
44. Al-Harbi MM, Qureshi S, Raza M, Ahmed MM, Giangreco AB, Shah AH (1995) Influence of anethole treatment on the tumour induced by Ehrlich ascites carcinoma cells in paw of Swiss albino mice. Eur J Cancer Prev 4:307–318
45. Jana S, Patra K, Mukherjee G, Bhattacharjee S, Mandal PD (2015) Antitumor potential of anethole single and in combination with cyclophosphamide in murine Sarcoma-180 transplantable tumor model. RSC Adv 5:56549–56559
46. Wiirzler LAM, de Souza Silva-Comar FM, Silva-Filho SE, de Oliveira MJA, Bersani-Amado CA, Cuman RKN (2015) Evaluation of immunomodulatory activity of trans-anethole and estragole, and protective effect against cyclophosphamide-induced suppression of immunity in Swiss albino mice. Int J Appl Res Nat Prod 8:26–33
47. Tiwari AK, Rao JM (2002) Diabetes mellitus and multiple therapeutic approaches of phytochemicals: present status and future prospects. Curr Sci 83:30–38
48. Sheikh BA, Pari L, Rathinam A, Chandramohan R (2015) Trans-anethole, a terpenoid ameliorates hyperglycemia by regulating key enzymes of carbohydrate metabolism in streptozotocin induced diabetic rats. Biochimie 112:57–65
49. Cavalcanti JM, Leal-Cardoso JH, Diniz LRL, Portella VG, Costa CO, Linard CFBM, Alves K, de Paula Rocha MVA, Lima CC, Cecatto VM, Coelho-de-Souza AN (2012) The essential oil of *Croton zehntneri* and trans-anethole improves cutaneous wound-healing. J Ethnopharmacol 144:240–247
50. Ryu S, Seol GH, Park H, Choi I-Y (2014) Trans-anethole protects cortical neuronal cells against oxygen-glucose deprivation/reoxygenation. Neurol Sci 35:1541–1547
51. Bhadra S, Mukherjee PK, Kumar NS, Bandyopadhyay A (2011) Anticholinesterase activity of standardized extract of *Illicium verum* Hook.f.fruits. Fitoterapia 82:342–346
52. Drukarch B, Flier J, Jongenelen CAM, Andringa G, Schoffelmeer ANM (2006) The antioxidant anetholedithiolethione inhibits monoamine oxidase-B but not monoamine oxidase A activity in extracts of cultures astrocytes. J Neural Transm 113:593–598
53. Ponte EL, Sousa PL, Rocha MVAP, Soares PMG, Coelho-de-Souza AN, Leal-Cardoso JHL, Assreuy AMS (2012) Comparative study of the anti-edematogenic effects of anethole and estragole. Pharmacol Rep 64:984–990
54. Freire RS, Morais SM, Catunda-Junior FEA, Pinheiro DCSN (2005) Synthesis and antioxidant, anti-inflammatory and gastroprotector activities of anethole and related compounds. Bioorg Med Chem 13:4353–4358
55. Kang P, Kim KY, Lee HS, Min SS, Seol GH (2013) Anti-inflammatory effects of anethole in lipopolysaccharide-induced acute lung injury in mice. Life Sci 93:955–961
56. Wisniewski-Rebecca ES, Rocha BA, Wiirzler LAM, Cuman RKN, Velazquez-Martinez CA, Bersani-Amado C (2015) Synergistic effects of anethole and ibuprofen in acute inflammatory response. Chem Biol Interact 242:247–253
57. Ritter AMV, Ames FQ, Otani F, de Oliveira RMW, Cuman RKN, Bersani-Amado CA (2014) Effects of anethole in nociception in experimental models. Evid Based Complement Altern Med. doi:10.1155/2014/345829
58. Kensler TW, Egner PA, Dolan PM, Groopman JD, Roebuck BD (1987) Mechanism of protection against aflatoxin tumorigenicity in rats fed 5-(2-pyrazinyl)-4-methyl-1,2-dithiol-3-thione (Oltipraz) and related 1,2-dithiol-3-thiones. Cancer Res 47:4217–4277
59. Reddy BS, Rao VC, Rivenson A, Kellof G (1993) Chemoprevention of colon carcinogenesis by organosulfur compounds. Cancer Res 53:3493–3498

60. Siqueira RJB, Magalhães PJC, Leal-Cardoso JH, Pinto Duarte G, Lahlou S (2006b) Cardiovascular effects of the essential oil of *Croton zehntneri* leaves and its main constituents, anethole and estragole, in normotensive conscious rats. Life Sci 78:2365–2372
61. Tognolini M, Ballabeni V, Bertoni S, Bruni R, Impicciatore M, Barocelli E (2007) Protective effect of *Foeniculum vulgare* essential oil and anethole in an experimental model of thrombosis. Pharmacol Res 56:254–260
62. Soares PMG, Lima RF, de Freitas Pires A, Souza EP, Assreuy AMS, Criddle DN (2007) Effects of anethole and structural analogues on the contractility of rat isolated aorta: involvement of voltage-dependent Ca^{2+}-channels. Life Sci 81:1085–1093
63. Pari L, Sheikh BA (2015) Antihyperglycemic effect of trans-anethole in streptozotocin induced diabetic rats with special reference to glycoprotein components. Int J Adv Res Biol Sci 2:28–34
64. Ghelardini C, Galeotti N, Mazzanti G (2001) Local anaesthetic activity of monoterpenes and phenylpropanes of essential oils. Planta Med 67:564–566
65. Miyagawa M, Satou T, Yukimune C, Ishibashi A, Seimiya H, Yamada H, Hasegawa T, Koike K (2014) Anxiolytic-like effect of *Illicium verum* fruit oil, trans-anethole and related compounds in mice. Phytotherapy Res 28:1710–1712
66. Lam S, MacAulay C, Le Riche JC, Dyachkova Y, Coldman A, Guillaud M, Hawk E, Christen M-O, Gazdar AF (2002) A randomized phase IIb trial of anetholedithiolethione in smokers with bronchial dysplasia. J Natl Cancer Inst 94:1001–1009
67. Switzer CH, Cheng RY-S, Ridrou L, Murray MC, Tazzari V, Sparatore A, Del Soldato P, Hines HB, Glynn SA, Ambs S, Wink DA (2012) Dithiolethiones inhibit NF-kB activity via covalent modification in human estrogen receptor-negative breast cancer. Cancer Res 72:2394–2404
68. Acimovic M, Tesevic V, Todosijevic M, Djisalov J, Oljaca S (2015) Compositional characteristics of the essential oil of *Pimpinella anisum* and *Foeniculum vulgare* grown in Serbia. Bot Serb 39:9–14
69. Arslan N, Gürbüz B, Sarihan O, Bayrak A, Gümüşçü A (2004) Variation in essential oil content and composition in Turkish anise. Turk J Agric For 28:173–177
70. Dzamic A, Sokovic M, Ristic MS, Grijic-Jovanovic S, Vukojevic J, Marin PD (2009) Chemical composition and antifungal activity of *Illicium verum* and *Eugenia caryophyllata* essential oils. Chem Nat Compd 45:259–261
71. Miraldi E (1999) Comparison of the essential oils from ten *Foeniculum vulgare* Miller samples of fruits of different origin. Flavour Fragrance J 14:379–382
72. Addae-Mensaha I, Asomaninga WA, Oteng-Yeboaha A, Garneaub F-X, Gagnonb H, Jeanb F-I, Moudachirouc M, Koumaglod KH (1996) (E)-anethole as a major essential oil constituent of *Clausena anisata*. J Essent Oil Res 8:513–516
73. Osei-Safo D, Addae-Mensaha I, Garneaub F-X, Koumagloc HK (2010) A comparative study of the antimicrobial activity of the leaf essential oils of chemo-varieties of *Clausena anisata* (Willd.) Hook.f.exBenth. Ind Crops Prod 32:634–638
74. Sultanbawa Y (2016) Anise myrtle (*Syzygium anisatum*) oils. In: Preedy V (ed) Essential oils in food preservation, flavors and safety. Elsevier, Amsterdam, pp 215–218
75. Sousa EMBD, Martínez J, Chiavone-Filho O, Rosa PTV, Domingos T, Meireles MAA (2005) Extraction of volatile oil from *Croton zehntneri* Pax et Hoff with pressurized CO_2: solubility, composition and kinetics. J Food Eng 69:325–333
76. Hussain RA, Poveda LJ, Pezzuto JM, Soejarto DD, Kinghorn AD (1998) Sweeting agents of plant origin: phenylpropanoid constituents of sweet-tasting plants. Econ Bot 44:174–182
77. Pauli A, Schilcher H (2016) In vitro antimicrobial activities of essential oils monographed in the European pharmacopoeia, 8th edn. In: HüsnüBaşer K, Buchbauer G (eds) Handbook of essential oils. Science, technology, and applications, 2nd edn. CRC Press, Boca Raton, pp 433–619
78. Senatore F, Oliviero F, Scandolera E, Taglialatela-Scafati O, Roscigno G, Zaccardelli M, de Falco E (2013) Chemical composition, antimicrobial and antioxidant activities of anethole-rich

oil from leaves of selected varieties of fennel [*Foeniculum vulgare* Mill. ssp. vulgare var. azoricum (Mill.) Thell]. Fitoterapia 90:214–219
79. Prathyusha W, Thanuja VS, Reddy KS, Rohith G, Kar K, Sethi A, Archana D, Vasavi S, Maheswari P, Niranjini P, Vimalacharitha L, Damodar AG, Prashanta Kumar BR (2013) Quantitative measurement of some physico-chemical parameters for the medicinally useful natural products. IAJPR 3:9138–9171
80. Paul WE (2008) Fundamental immunology, 6th edn. Wolters Kluwer/Lippincott Williams & Wilkins, Philadelphia
81. Turner MD, Nedjai B, Hurst, Pennington D (2014) Cytokines and chemokines: at the cross roads of cell signaling and inflammatory disease. Biochim Biophys Acta 1843:2563–2582

The Role of Indirubins in Inflammation and Associated Tumorigenesis

Xinlai Cheng and Karl-Heinz Merz

Abstract Indirubin is the major active component of an herbal recipe '*Dangui Luhui Wan*' (当归芦荟丸) in traditional Chinese medicine (TCM). It is widely used in China for the treatment of inflammation, cancer, and other chronic diseases and is known for good efficiency and very low side effects. Primary studies on the mechanism of action revealed that indirubin and derivatives are potent ATP-competitive inhibitors of CDKs and GSK3ß achieving IC_{50} values down to the low nanomolar range. However, the clinical application of indirubins is limited by the extremely poor water solubility (<1 mg/L in general) and consequently the insufficient bioavailability originating from strong binding forces in the crystal lattice. In the last few decades, a lot of efforts had been put into the structure optimization of indirubin derivatives binding selectively to specific kinases. Thus, a number of new indirubins have been developed bearing substituents mainly in the 5- and 3′-position suitable for improved solubility and inhibition against CDKs and GSK3ß, referred to as canonical indirubins. Interestingly, several noncanonical 7- and 7′-indirubin derivatives have been reported, showing a distinct binding model in the ATP-binding pocket and targeting a very different spectrum of protein kinases as seen from kinase profiling. In this chapter, we will review the field of indirubin research from its discovery, synthesis, chemical modification, structure-activity relationship, and mechanism of action to molecular targets comprising recent advantages and new findings in the context of inflammation-associated signaling pathways, in particular in tumorigenesis, including NF-κB, STAT3, TGF-ß, and AhR.

Keywords Indirubin · Inflammation · Cancer · Structure-activity relationship · TGF-ß · STAT3 · NF-κB · AhR

X. Cheng (✉)
Institute of Pharmacy and Molecular Biotechnology, Pharmaceutical Biology, Heidelberg University, Im Neuenheimer Feld 364, 69120 Heidelberg, Germany
e-mail: x.cheng@uni-heidelberg.de

K.-H. Merz
Department of Chemistry, Division of Food Chemistry and Toxicology, University of Kaiserslautern, Erwin-Schrödinger-Str. 52, 67663 Kaiserslautern, Germany

S.C. Gupta et al. (eds.), *Drug Discovery from Mother Nature*,
Advances in Experimental Medicine and Biology 929,
DOI 10.1007/978-3-319-41342-6_12

1 Introduction

Traditional Chinese medicine (TCM) is a pool of useful medical sources comprising animals, plants, acupuncture, and other practical recipes on the basis of the empirical evidence collected over the period of thousands of years in China [37, 53]. In general, TCM is lack of the systematical clinical evaluation and scrupulous scientific proof, but with the strength to elicit synergistic effects from various medical combinations and minimize side effect in particular in long-term treatment. Therefore, TCM provides a promising pharmacopoeia for the modern drug development [21, 37]. A good exemplar is the antimalarial drug 'artemisinin,' also known as Qinghaosu (青蒿素), which was identified by Youyou Tu and her coworkers from more than 500 recipes and herbal extracts [81, 113]. In 2015, Tu became the first Chinese Nobel Laureate in physiology or medicine jointly with William C. Campbell and Satoshi Omura for her significant breakthrough to save millions of people by using artemisinin and its synthetical analogues [33, 81].

Dangui Luhui Wan (当归芦荟丸) is a mixture of 11 medicinal herbs, namely *Angelica sinensis* (Oliv) Diels, *Aloe vera* L., *Gennana scaber* L., *Saussurea lappa* Clarke, *Scutellaria baicalensis* Georgi, *Phillodendron chinensis* Schneid, *Coptis chinensis* Franch, *Gardenia jasminoides* Ellis, *Rheum palmarus* L., *Indigofera tinctoria* L., *and Moschus moschiferus* L [124], and is used for the treatment of a number of chronic diseases in China, including cancer and inflammation. The first recorded history of *Dangui Luhui Wan* can be found in 'Medicine Vol. I–VI' (医学六书) edited by Hejian Liu (刘河间, 1120–1200). In the middle of 20th century, a clinical trial on 22 patients had been performed in China to test the effect of *Dangui Luhui Wan* on chronic myelogenous leukemia (CML). Hematological complete remissions were observed in 4 cases (18 %) and partial remission in 5 cases (23 %) with remarkable low side effects [124]. In following series of clinical trials over 10 years, researchers systematically identified that *I. tinctoria* L. (青黛, indigo naturalis), a cosmetic historically used in Asia, is the active component, in which indirubin is the major active agent of indigo naturalis [13, 32, 39–41, 57, 58, 79, 116, 122–124, 129, 133].

2 Chemical Synthesis and Structure-Activity Relationship

2.1 Chemical Structure and Synthesis of Indirubin

Indirubin is a 3,2′-bisindole (Fig. 1). Like its 2,2′-isomer 'indigo' (Fig. 1), one of the most successful nature pigments, indirubin can be found in diverse natural sources from plants to animals [53]. Moreover, 1-methylisoindigo, a 3,3′-isomer, also known as meisoindigo (Fig. 1), is a synthetic bisindole derivative successfully used in China for the treatment of CML, too [125]. Very recent results

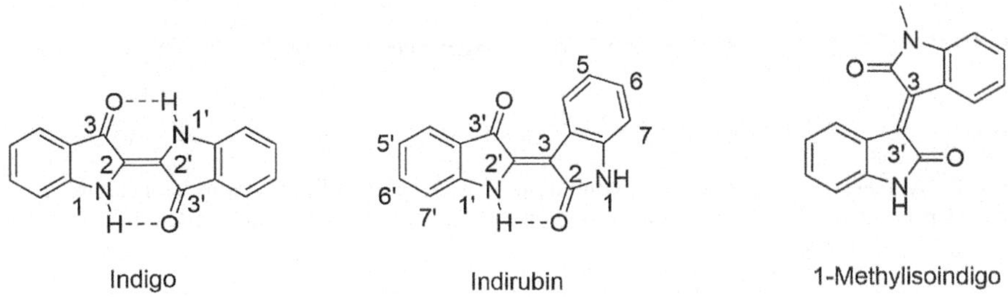

Fig. 1 Structures of indigo (2,2′-bisindole), indirubin (3,2′-bisindole), and 1-methylisoindigo (3, 3′-bisindole). Intramolecular H-bridges were indicated by *dashed lines*

demonstrated that meisoindigo preferentially targets CD133+ pancreatic cancer stem cells by interfering with cellular metabolic signaling pathways [26].

The crystal structure of indirubin had been reported by Pandraud in [91], in which one intramolecular hydrogen bond between 1′-NH and 2-CO groups and another intermolecular hydrogen bond between 1-NH and 2-CO groups were observed, which contributes to a well-organized hydrogen-bonding framework [91], resulting in special physical and chemical properties, such as very planar structure with only 4° deviation, high melting point, and extremely low solubility in most solvents [79]. Since the configuration of indirubin is described as trans-isomer in Pubchem (https://pubchem.ncbi.nlm.nih.gov/compound/Indirubin), it is worth to be mentioned that we never detect this configuration for indirubin or its derivatives in our past researches [27, 28, 53, 76, 80]. Indeed, the formation of intramolecular hydrogen bridge (Fig. 1, dashed lines) induces a significant shift of proton at 1′-position to downfield (between 9 and 11 ppm) in the ^{1}H-NMR spectrum [27, 28, 53], which probably dedicates to the planar cis-configuration of indirubins according to Cahn-Ingold-Prelog priority rules that 1′-NH has a higher priority of 3′-CO. Furthermore, the proximity of the C4-hydrogen atom to the 3′-oxygen atom causes a strong downfield shift of the H4 signal [79].

The nearly flat structure is a double-edged sword, which confers indirubin advanced properties in the application as coloring and medical material, but also makes indirubins insoluble in most solvents and thereby unsatisfying bioavailability, being one of the most critical handicaps for successful trial in clinic. A lot of efforts have been put to improve the aqueous solubility of indirubins by either chemical modification [11, 27, 28, 30, 42, 49, 69, 72, 78, 84, 92–94, 99, 105, 115] or pharmaceutical formation [50–52]. In general, indirubin and its derivatives can be synthesized by coupling isatins with indoxyl derivatives in a good yield (Fig. 2). The first synthesis of indirubin as planned product was achieved by Baeyer in [9] under basic condition in alcoholic solvents [9]. Almost hundred years later, Russell and Kaupp modified this method by replacing semistable indoxyl with stable indoxyl acetate [98]. Alternatively, acetic acid with 10 % concentrated HCl can be used in certain scenarios [56, 77], where reaction participants are sensitive even to mildly basic conditions, like the synthesis of 7,7′-diazaindirubins [27].

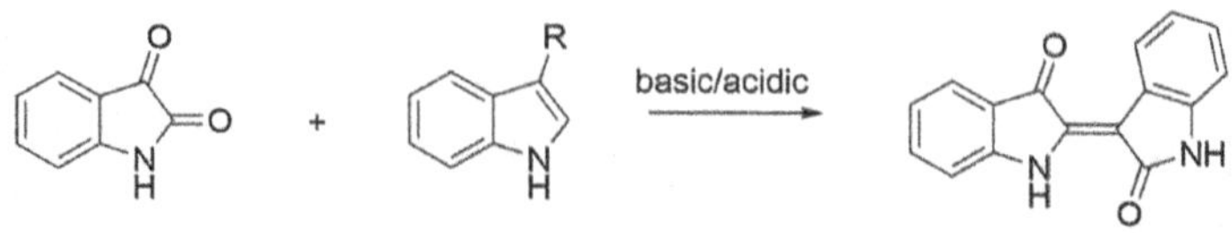

Fig. 2 Synthesis of indirubin. Basic condition: Na_2CO_3, MeOH/EtOH, room temperature, 24 h, R=OH [9] and R=OAc [98]. Acidic condition: acetic acid and 10 % conc. HCl, 100 °C, 24 h, R=OH [77] and R=OAc [56]

2.2 *Structure-Activity Relationship and Chemical Modification*

At the end of 20th century, a number of new indirubin derivatives with improved pharmaceutical properties were synthesized by G. Eisenbrand and his coworkers in Kaiserslautern (Germany), including the widely used indirubin-3′-oxime (IO) and water-soluble indirubin-5-sulfonate (Table 1), which greatly facilitated the investigation of target molecules and mechanism of action of indirubins. In cooperation with L. Meijer and J.A. Endicott, they identified that indirubin and its derivatives are ATP-competitive inhibitors of CDKs [34, 53]. Studying the cocrystal structure of indirubin-5-sulfonate and indirubin-3′-oxime in phospho-CDK2/cyclin A revealed two major hydrogen bonds, NH_{Leu83}–2-C=O_{indi}–NH_{Leu83} (r = 2.7 Å) and C=O_{Leu81}–1-NH_{indi} (r = 3.0 Å). In addition, a minor bond between the backbone oxygen of Glu-83 and the 1′-NH with r = 3.1 Å (Fig. 3, left) is also described, whose contribution to binding affinity, however, might be negligible due to the connection with an unfavorable angle of 94° [34, 53]. More importantly, the lipophilic and aromatic interaction between the apolar, planar ring system of indirubin and hydrophobic and aromatic residues of amino acids in the ATP-binding pocket plays a dominant role [34, 53]. In summary, these results provided the fundamental information for investigating cellular targets of indirubins and pinpointed the available positions for further improving pharmaceutical properties by chemical modification (Fig. 3, right): 5- and 3′-positions bearing to ribose and triphosphate canal, 5′-position, which opens to the solvent [28, 34, 53, 56], and 6-position to enhance the binding affinity to GSK3ß [78, 94].

Under guidance of these criteria, we and other researchers rapidly established new chemical approaches to develop novel indirubins with enhanced water solubility and inhibitory activity [11, 27, 28, 30, 36, 56, 65–67, 69, 72, 78, 80, 84–87, 92–94, 99, 115]. The trivial, but widely used and most effective approach to obtain more soluble indirubins is the modification at 3′-position. Briefly, heating with hydroxylamine hydrochloride in pyridine can convert indirubins to corresponding 3′-oximes, which are more reactive and may serve as nucleophile in ethanol using TMG as base (Fig. 4). With α,ω-dibromoalkanes, this reaction is useful to insert spacers for further nucleophilic substitution reactions (Fig. 4a, c, d).

There are more challenges for chemical optimization at 5- and 6-position, which directly locates in the aromatic ring system. A practical approach has been reported

Table 1 Structures of selected indirubin derivatives

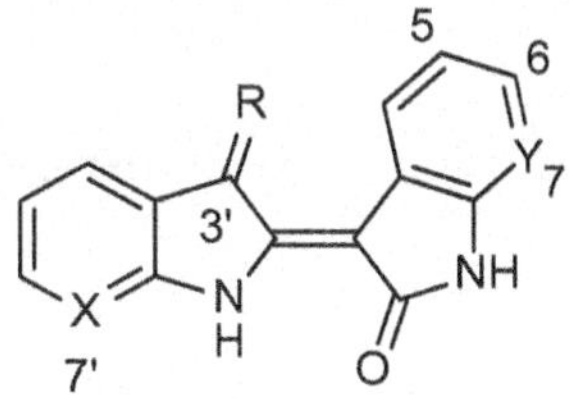

	X	Y	3′	7′	5	6	7
Indirubin-5-sulfonate	C	C	O	–H	$-SO_3^-$	–H	–H
Indirubin-3′-oxime (IO)	C	C	N–OH	–H	–H	–H	–H
Pentafluorophenyl indirubin-5-carboxylate	C	C	O	–H	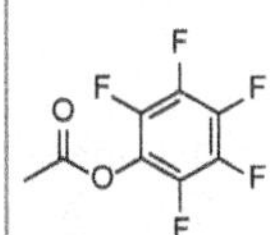	–H	–H
5-Bromoindirubin-3′-oxime (5BIO)	C	C	N–OH	–H	–Br	–H	–H
6-Bromoindirubin-3′-oxime (6BIO)	C	C	N–OH	–H	–H	–Br	–H
7-Bromoindirubin-3′-oxime (7BIO)	C	C	N–OH	–H	–H	–H	–Br
Indirubin-3′-(2,3-dihydroxypropyl)-oxime ether (E804)	C	C	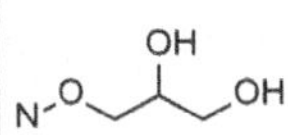	–H	–H	–H	–H
5-Methoxy-indirubin-3′-(2,3-dihydroxypropyl)-oxime ether (E738)	C	C	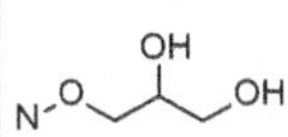	–H	–OMe	–H	–H
5-Methyl-indirubin	C	C	O	–H	–Me	–H	–H
6-Hydroxy-5-methyl-indirubin	C	C	O	–H	–Me	–OH	–H
6,7′-Dihydroxy-5-methyl-indirubin	C	C	O	–OH	–Me	–OH	–H
7-Azaindirubin	C	N	O	–H	–H	–H	–
7′-Azaindirubin	N	C	O	–	–H	–H	–H
7,7′-Diazaindirubin	N	N	O	–	–H	–H	–

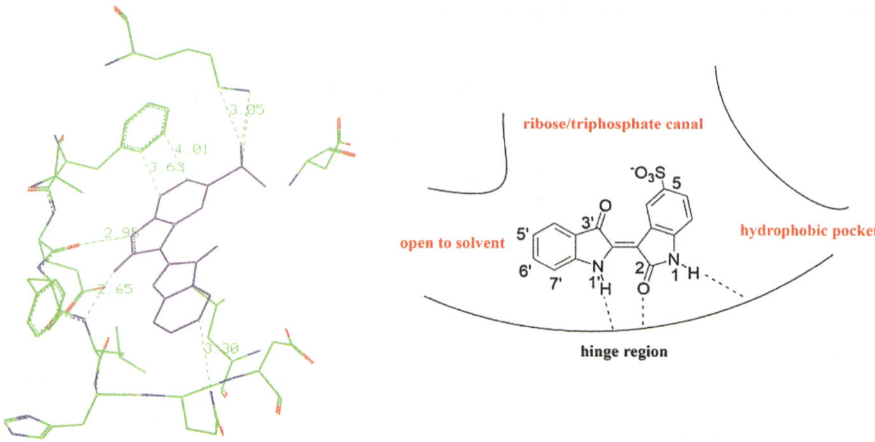

Fig. 3 *Left* Cocrystal structure (PDB: 1E9H) of indirubin-5-sulfonate (purple) in the ATP-binding pocket of CDK2 [53]. The program 'Discovery' was used to represent the binding model of indirubin-5-sulfonate with CDK2. Hydrogen bonds and aromatic and hydrophobic interactions are depicted as *green dashed lines*; distances are given in Å. *Right* Schematic representation of binding mode. Key regions for modification are highlighted (modified from [28])

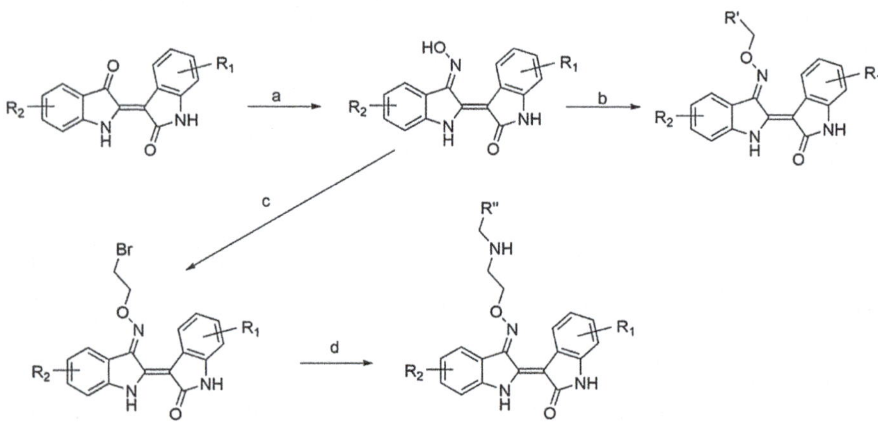

Fig. 4 Synthesis of indirubin-3′-oximes and indirubin-3′-oxime ethers. Reactants and conditions: *a* $NH_2OH{\cdot}HCl$, pyridine, ΔT; *b* functionalized alkyl halides, 1,1,3,3-tetramethylguanidine (TMG), EtOH, ΔT; *c* 1,2-dibromoethane, TMG, EtOH, ΔT; *d* primary or secondary amine, DMF

to modify at 5-position by Eisenbrand's group on the basis of a core active and stable intermediate pentafluorophenyl indirubin-5-carboxylate (Table 1). The reaction is started with the synthesis of 5-carboxyisatin from *p*-aminobenzoic acid in a 5-step reaction. The detailed protocol can be found in the original article and previous review [28, 79]. The resulting indirubin-5-carboxamides carrying hydrophilic amino groups can be easily ionized to their quaternary alkyl ammonium salts or hydrochlorides, which exhibited improved pharmaceutical properties, good

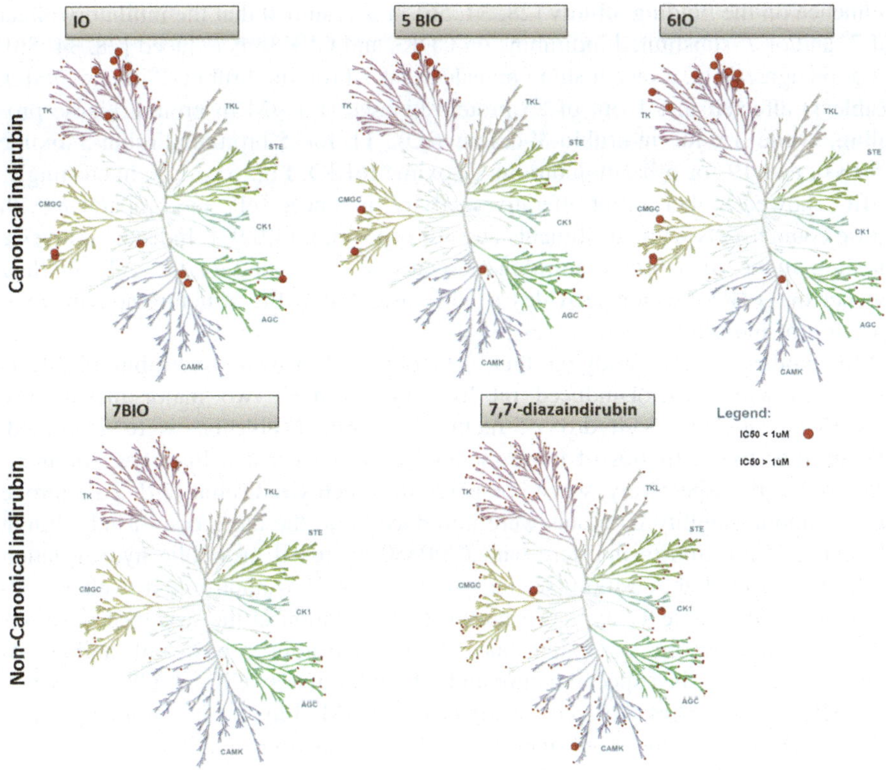

Fig. 5 Protein kinase profiling of canonical and noncanonical indirubins. The kinase profiling of IO, 5BIO, 6BIO, and 7BIO was measured in a panel of 85 protein kinases [97], while 7,7′-diazaindirubin was from 220 kinases [27]

solubility, and enhanced inhibitor effect [28]. Introduction of hydrophilic alkylamino side chains in 3′-oxime position brought about the enhancement of water solubility of 6-bromo-substituted indirubins, designed as GSK3ß inhibitors [94].

Since the ATP-binding pocket of protein kinases is highly conserved in mammals, indirubin derivatives with substituent in 5- and/or 3′-position, like most ATP-competitive kinase inhibitors, target not only CDKs and GSK3ß, but also a wide spectrum of protein kinases [97]. Hence, we refer to as canonical indirubins (Fig. 5) to differ from highly selective noncanonical 7- and/or 7′-indirubin derivatives.

3 Noncanonical Indirubins

According to the binding model in the ATP-binding pocket of CDK2 (Fig. 3), 7- and 7′-positions are close to the hinge region [34, 53]. Additional substituents at those positions may interrupt the formation of H-bridges and thus negatively influence on the binding affinity [28, 34, 56]. It is assumed that the inhibitory effect of 7- and/or 7′-substituted indirubins on CDKs and GSK3ß is reduced [28, 34, 56]. In good agreement, a recent study revealed that 7-bromoindirubin-3′-oxime (7BIO, Table 1) affected just 1 out of 85 protein kinases at 1 μM in protein kinase profiling, while 15 for indirubin-3′-oxime (IO), 11 for 5-bromoindirubin-3′-oxime (5BIO), and 19 for 6-bromoindirubin-3′-oxime (6BIO, Fig. 5). More interestingly, 7BIO showed higher antiproliferative activity in cancer cells in comparison with those counterparts with substituents at 5- or 6-position [42, 97]. Indeed, an inverse binding mode of 7-bromoindirubin derivatives was found in the ATP-binding pocket of DYRK, which provides a new insight into the structure-activity relationship of indirubin-7-derivatives [85].

In another aspect, studying the metabolism of 5-methylindirubin (Table 1) incubated with Aroclor-induced rat liver microsomes, two major metabolites, 6-hydroxy- and 6-7′-dihydroxy-5-methyl-indirubin (Table 1), were identified. Antiproliferative activities of those metabolites in cancer cell lines were dramatically reduced, respectively, when compared to 5-methylindirubin [79]. To improve the metabolic stability, N-atoms were introduced into the backbone of indirubin at 7- and/or 7′-position to interfere with CYP450-mediated metabolic hydroxylation [27]. As expected, the resulting azaindirubins 7- and 7′-azaindirubin as well as 7,7′-diazaindirubin (Table 1) were resistant to hydroxylation at the designed positions [27, 38]. Furthermore, we found that 7,7′-diazaindirubin, a powerful inhibitor of tumor cell growth, is a special compound inhibiting merely CK1c3, CK2a, CK2a2, and SIK in a panel of 220 protein kinases at 1 μM (Fig. 5). Its inhibitory effect against CK2 was further confirmed in cell-based experiments [27].

Those indirubins with the lack of activity toward CDKs and GSK3ß are referred to as noncanonical indirubins to discern from the canonical indirubins, which are potent CDK and GSK3ß inhibitors.

4 Modulation of Signaling Pathways by Indirubins in Inflammation-Associated Cancer

The origin of relationship between inflammation and cancer can be traced back to the observation of leukocytes in neoplasia from a German pathologist, Rudolf Virchow, in the nineteenth century [10]. In the past decades, mounting clinical and experimental evidences were given to confirm his hypothesis that inflammatory places of tissues are more susceptible to the malignant transformation. The concept that an inflammatory microenvironment is of importance in tumorigenesis is now generally accepted. Epidemiological studies showed that less than 10 % of all cancers are caused by germline mutations, while 90 % are related to inflammation associated with unhealthy personal lifestyle and pollution environmental issues [4, 8, 48, 75].

Phosphorylation and dephosphorylation of protein kinases is a fundamental regulator mechanism in cellular post-translational modification and involved in a number

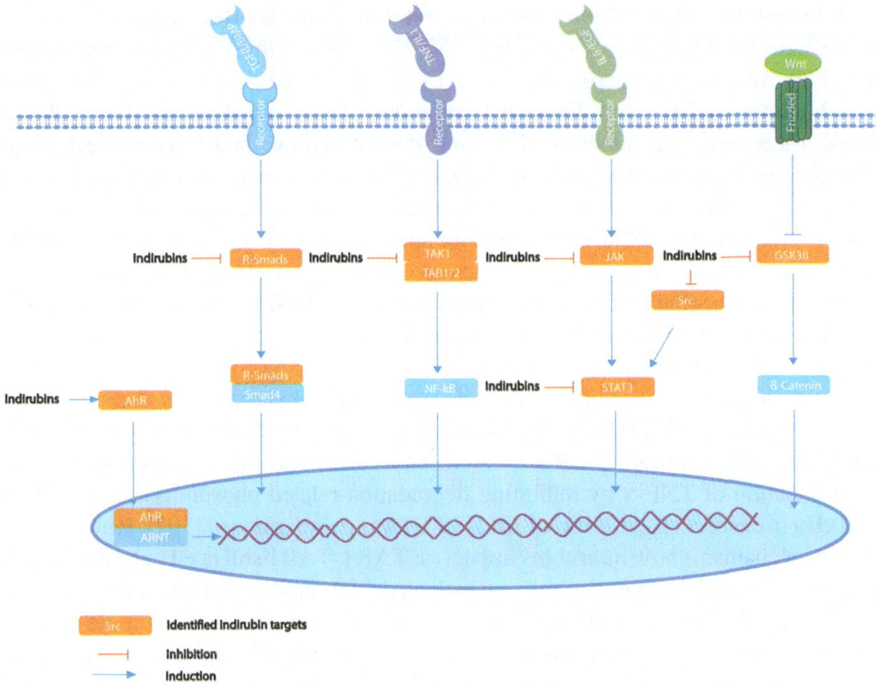

Fig. 6 Molecular targets of indirubins in inflammation and associated tumorigenesis

of biological events. The ATP-binding pocket locates at the catalytic domain of protein kinases between C- and N-terminal lobes, which is highly conserved in all 518 human protein kinases, but with considerable differences in surrounding pockets, which are often exploited for chemical modification toward target selectivity [90]. The high binding affinity to the backbone of the ATP-binding pocket makes indirubin and its derivatives attractive inhibitors against multiple protein kinases involved in a number of signaling pathways [2, 5, 14–17, 22, 42, 45, 54, 55, 59, 68, 70, 71, 74, 76, 82, 83, 86–89, 95–97, 102–104, 106, 111, 114, 117, 118, 121, 130–132]. In this chapter, we will focus on the effect of indirubins on signaling pathways that are involved in inflammation and associated tumorigenesis (Fig. 6).

5 Nuclear Factor-κB

Nuclear factor-κB (NF-κB) is a pro-inflammatory nuclear transcription factor, which was first identified in 1986 and plays an essential role in both inflammation-associated pro- and anticarcinogenesis [10, 48]. In vertebrate, NF-κB is a homo- or heterodimer consisting of proteins with a Rel homology domain, including NF-κB1 (p105 and p50), NF-κB2 (p100 and p52), c-Rel, RelB, and/or

RelA [3, 60, 61]. In nonstimulated cells, inhibitors of κBs (IκBs) directly bind to and restrain NF-κB in the cytoplasm [3, 60, 61]. Upon stimuli of pro-inflammatory cytokines, like tumor necrosis factor-α (TNF-α), interleukin-1 (IL-1), epidermal growth factor (EGF), and lipopolysaccharides (LPS), as well as chemical and physical stresses, like infection, UV, and chemotherapy, IκB kinases (IKKs) are activated by its upstream, such as TAK1 (TGF-ß-activated protein kinase 1). In turn, IκBs are phosphorylated at certain serine residues, leading to IκB degradation in an ubiquitin proteasomal-dependent manner [3, 60, 61]. The released active NF-κB translocates into the nucleus and consequently binds to its DNA target sites, where it promotes the expression of target genes involved in lots of cellular events, including inflammation (TNF-α, IL-6), proliferation (cyclin D), and angiogenesis (VEGF, FGF, and PDGF) [3, 60, 61].

The evidence that indirubins can interfere with NF-κB signaling has been given by Aggarwal and coworkers [102]. As shown in Fig. 6, they found that indirubin-3′-oxime (Table 1) could suppress NF-κB activation and its downstream genes expression under the stimulation of TNF-α by inhibiting degradation-related phosphorylation of IKKs and IκBα in cancer cells, in which TAK1-TAB1was overexpressed [102]. However, the precise mechanisms how indirubins impact on TAK1-TAB1 still need to be elucidated. In good agreement, Kim et al. investigated the application of indirubins on TNF-α-related atherosclerosis and detected that indirubins at low micromole concentrations sufficiently repressed nuclear translocation of NF-κB and activation of JNK [62]. They observed the reduction in the expressions of atherosclerosis-related chemoattractants and adhesion molecules, which might contribute to constrain the attachment of monocytes and macrophages onto endothelium cells [62]. In support, studies on the LPS and DNCB (1-chloro-2,4-dinitrobenzene)-mediated inflammation demonstrated that indirubin-3′-oxime (Table 1) blocked not only the expression of a body of inflammatory mediators and cytokines, but also the alternation of surface markers, suggesting that inflammatory responses upon the stimulation of LPS and DNCB might be generally targeted by indirubin and derivatives in vitro and in animal model [12, 63, 64].

6 Signal Transducer and Activator of Transcription 3

Signal transducer and activator of transcription 3 (STAT3) is one of the seven members of STAT protein family consisting of STAT1, STAT2, STAT3, STAT4, STAT5A, STAT5B, and STAT6 sharing five domains, namely an amino-terminal domain, a transactivation domain, a DNA-binding domain, a SH2 domain, and a carboxy-terminal transactivation domain [128]. As one of the major signaling pathways in response to inflammation, the essential role of STAT3 in embryonic development had been established that the abnormality and consequent lethality could be observed during the development from day 6.0–8.5 in STAT3-deficient mouse embryos [110]. Because of the close relationship between inflammation and tumorigenesis, it is not surprising that aberrantly active STAT3 can be found in lots of inflammation-related tumor cells and tissues originated from breast, AML, CML, melanoma, prostate, pancreatic to brain tumors [126–128].

In general, the activation of STAT3 starts with phosphorylation at Tyr-705 induced by various receptors under stimuli of cytokines (such as IL-6 and LIF), growth factors, and oncogenes (Src) as well as in response to infection, oxidative stress, and chemicals [127]. The phosphorylation leads to form a docking site and subsequently dimerize with STAT3 or other member of STAT via conserved SH2 domain [20, 126]. The active dimer translocates from cytoplasm into the nucleus, binds to DNA, and induces the expression of its target genes, like cyclin D1 and members of BCL-2 family. In addition, the maximal activity of STAT3 can be achieved by additional phosphorylation at Ser-727 [18, 120]. Intriguingly, the latter phosphorylation can endow STAT3 access to mitochondria, where STAT3 interacts with the electron transport chain complexes I and II and participates in the cellular metabolism. As a result, mitochondrial STAT3 facilitates the Ras-induced cell transformation independent of its transcriptional function [47, 119].

The inhibition of indirubins against STAT3 was discovered by screening a panel of indirubin derivatives [87]. Among them, indirubin-3′-(2,3-dihydroxypropyl)-oxime ether, also known as E804 (Table 1), showed the highest activity in DNA-binding affinity assay measured by electrophoretic mobility shift assay (EMSA). Further investigation unveiled that E804 selectively inhibited Src in vitro with an IC_{50} value of 430 nM, but not another upstream kinase, Jak (IC_{50}: 10,000 nM). In a cell-based assay, the compound sufficiently reduced the activity of Src and its related malignant transformation, as well as induced cellular apoptosis indicated with the cleavage of PARP [87, 88]. Remarkably, study on the structure-activity relationship disclosed that indirubins with smart and freely rotatable substituents at 3′-position are more potent than those with bulky substituents, while indirubins carrying methoxy group in 5-position had improved activities. Inspired by this result, a new indirubin derivative with a methoxy substituent at 5-position and 2,3-dihydroxypropyl oxime substituent at 3′-position (Table 1, E738) was synthesized, showing an enhanced water solubility (50 mg/mL). Its inhibitory effect on a panel of STAT3-related protein kinases was evaluated. In comparison with E804, E738 inhibits not only Src with higher efficiency (IC_{50}: 10.7 nM), but also Jak1, Jak2, Jak3, Lyn, and Hck with IC_{50} value of 10.4, 74.1, 0.7, 29.8, and 263.9 nM, respectively (Fig. 6). Moreover, E738 exhibited robust antiproliferative effect on various pancreatic cancer cells in a p53-independent manner [89], one of the most incurable cancer types [25].

7 Transforming Growth Factor-ß

The epithelial-to-mesenchymal transition (EMT) is a fundamental process in the development of adult tissues and functional organs [112] under the restrictive control of TGF-ß (transforming growth factor) superfamily, which can be secreted by various types of immune cells in response to innate and adaptive immunoresponses, including macrophages, dendritic cells, and T cells [44, 46]. In tumor, TGF-ß promotes the dissemination of cancer cells from their original place and in turn reattachment in other places, termed as metastasis, the major cause of mortality in patients [19, 73]. Till now, more than 30 members of TGF-ß have been discovered in mammalian, for instance TGF-ß1/2/3, activinA/B/C, NODAL, bone morphogenetic proteins 2–9 (BMPs), growth and differentiation factors (GDFs), and anti-Müllerian hormone (AMH). Generally, the secreted active intercellular ligand binds to type II receptor on the membrane and in turn phosphorylates type I receptor, which leads to form a binding site to cooperate with regulatory Smads (R-Smads), namely Smad1/5/8 for BMPs/GDFs and Smad2/3 for TGF-ß/activins/NODAL. In cytoplasm, a common Smad (Smad4) is recruited to form a heteromeric Smad complex together with phosphorylated R-Smads, inducing a translocation and accumulation in the nucleus, where it binds to DNA and activates the expressions of its downstream genes [7, 19, 44]. Phosphorylations in the linker region of R-Smad mediated by MAPKs, GSK3ß, and CDKs have been described and play an important role in TGF-ß-mediated cellular events [6, 43, 100]. These cross-activations can be regulated by EGF, Wnt, and cell cycle, via stabilization and prolongation of active R-Smad [6, 23, 43, 100].

6-Bromoindirubin-3′-oxime (6BIO, Table 1) is a well-known GSK3ß inhibitor [78], has been widely used in stem cell research, and showed unique benefits in the maintenance of pluripotency [101] and generation of epiblast stem cells [31]. These results implicate the existence of unveiled target(s) except for its GSK3ß inhibition, which is playing an important role in pluripotency-associated signaling. Therefore, the study of influence of indirubins on TGF-ß signaling was performed by investigating the activity of R-Smad (Fig. 6), which led to identify certain indirubins, e.g., E738, E804, and 6BIO, as potent inhibitors against TGF-ß in a wide spectrum of cell lines [23]. Indeed, the regulation of TGF-ß signaling by indirubins is very complicated [23]. As GSK3ß and CDK inhibitor, indirubins can stabilize phosphorylated R-Smads, whereas nonphosphorylated total R-Smads are ubiquitinated by blocking the activity of two R-Smad-specific deubiquitinases, USP9x and USP34, resulting in the enhancement of TGF-ß activity in short-term treatment due to the accumulation of active R-Smads, but reduction in long-term range as a result of constantly decreased total R-Smads [23]. Interestingly, active noncanonical TGF-ß was observed probably because of the elevation of active receptor but less available R-Smads for signal transmission of canonical TGF-ß pathway [23]. Given the importance of Wnt and TGF-ß signaling pathways in development, E738 can transiently reprogram human primary fibroblasts into ALP-positive cells in a combination with chemical inducers of pluripotency-associated genes [24, 29].

8 Aryl Hydrocarbon Receptor

The aryl hydrocarbon receptor (AhR) is a cytosolic ligand-active helix-loop-helix transcription factor and plays an important role in homeostasis and xenobiotic metabolism, whose ligands include polycyclic aromatic hydrocarbons (PAH), halogenated aromatic hydrocarbon (HAH), and the number of other planar small molecules. The prototypical and most potent AhR ligand is 2,3,7,8-tetrachlorodibenzo-p-dioxin (TCDD). Following exposure to TCDD, AhR is released from a complex comprising two HSP90 (heat shock protein 90), the HSP90-interacting protein p23 and the X-associated protein (XAP2). The active AhR-TCDD complex translocates into the nucleus, where it interacts with the AhR nuclear translocator (ARNT). The resulting heterodimer binds to its specific DNA recognition sites, called dioxin-response elements (DREs), which locate at the promoter region of target genes and thereby activate their expressions. To prevent constitutive activation, AhR is rapidly exported from nucleus after binding to chromosome region maintenance 1 (CRM1) and degraded in ubiquitin proteasomal-dependent manner [35, 108].

The evidence was given that aberrant activation of AhR is associated with tumorigenesis, which, however, occurred in the presence of ligands resistant to cellular metabolism, since the induced negative effects could be observed only after a long-term exposure [35]. Indeed, xenobiotic metabolism and detoxification is one of the major tasks of AhR through overexpression of AhR target genes, encoding cytochrome P450 (CYP) 1A1, CYP1A2, and CYP1B1 for phase I and UGT1A6 and others for phase II metabolism. Moreover, a number of immune responses are activated, including expression of $p27^{Kip1}$ and phosphorylation of Rb for regulating cell cycle and proliferation, activation of NF-κB signaling for inflammation and erythroid 2-related factor 2 (NRF2)-related antioxidant pathway [108].

The relationship between indirubin and AhR was first studied by Adachi and his coworkers (Fig. 6). They identified indirubin as a potent natural AhR agonist by using human urine treated with H_2SO_4 in the yeast reporter assay, showing 50 times higher activity than TCDD [2]. In the competitive binding assay, the binding affinity of indirubin to mouse hepatic AhR is similar to that of TCDF, an analogue of TCDD [49]. In mammalian cells and animal models, indirubins and derivatives can activate the AhR, but with less potency [1, 35, 49, 109]. In MCF7 cells, indirubin-mediated induction of CYP1B1 measured in luciferase reporter assay was comparable to that treated with TCDD after 12-h incubation, but undetectable after 24 h, which could be rescued by adding ellipticine, a CYP1 inhibitor, implicating that indirubin and derivatives are CYP1 inducers and substrates [107]. Thus, the observed antiproliferative effect of indirubins is at least partially caused by activating AhR signaling pathway in kinase inhibition-independent fashion [1, 2, 49, 66].

9 Conclusion

Indirubin is the most active agent of *Dangui Luhui Wan*, a mixture of a medicinal herbal recipe, which was used for the treatment of various chronic diseases in China, including inflammation and cancer. In general, indirubin and its derivatives act as potent inhibitors of CDKs and GSK3ß evidenced by cocrystal structures in the ATP-binding pocket. Under the guideline of a binding model, a number of new canonical indirubin derivatives bearing substituents in 3′- and/or 5-position have been synthesized, which showed an enhanced activity against CDKs, GSK3ß, and other protein kinases with improved pharmaceutical properties. Interestingly, the modification of the 7- and/or 7′- position led to the discovery of noncanonical indirubins, which were more specific in protein kinase profiling and possessed the distinct binding model in comparison with that of canonical indirubins. Mechanistically, the multitarget characteristic confers indirubins' ability to directly regulate numerous inflammation-associated signaling in both protein kinase-dependent and independent manner, including NF-κB, STAT3, TGF-ß, and AhR, therefore showing great benefits in clinical application against inflammation and its related cancer.

Competing Interests
The authors declare that they have no competing interests.

Acknowledgments We thank Gerhard Eisenbrand and Stefan Wölfl for their great supporting. This work is supported by the BMBF grant programs SysToxChip 031A202E. We apologize that we were unable to cite all related primary research papers and excellent reviews due to space limitations.

References

1. Adachi J, Mori Y, Matsui S, Matsuda T (2004) Comparison of gene expression patterns between 2,3,7,8-tetrachlorodibenzo-p-dioxin and a natural arylhydrocarbon receptor ligand, indirubin. Toxicol Sci 80(1):161–169. doi:10.1093/toxsci/kfh129
2. Adachi J, Mori Y, Matsui S, Takigami H, Fujino J, Kitagawa H, Miller CA 3rd, Kato T, Saeki K, Matsuda T (2001) Indirubin and indigo are potent aryl hydrocarbon receptor ligands present in human urine. J Biol Chem 276(34):31475–31478. doi:10.1074/jbc.C100238200
3. Aggarwal BB (2004) Nuclear factor-kappaB: the enemy within. Cancer Cell 6(3):203–208. doi:10.1016/j.ccr.2004.09.003
4. Aggarwal BB, Vijayalekshmi RV, Sung B (2009) Targeting inflammatory pathways for prevention and therapy of cancer: short-term friend, long-term foe. Clin Cancer Res 15 (2):425–430. doi:10.1158/1078-0432.CCR-08-0149
5. Ahn MY, Kim TH, Kwon SM, Yoon HE, Kim HS, Kim JI, Kim YC, Kang KW, Ahn SG, Yoon JH (2015) 5-nitro-5′-hydroxy-indirubin-3′-oxime (AGM130), an indirubin-3′-oxime derivative, inhibits tumor growth by inducing apoptosis against non-small cell lung cancer in vitro and in vivo. Eur J Pharm Sci 79:122–131. doi:10.1016/j.ejps.2015.08.015

6. Alarcon C, Zaromytidou AI, Xi Q, Gao S, Yu J, Fujisawa S, Barlas A, Miller AN, Manova-Todorova K, Macias MJ, Sapkota G, Pan D, Massague J (2009) Nuclear CDKs drive Smad transcriptional activation and turnover in BMP and TGF-beta pathways. Cell 139 (4):757–769. doi:10.1016/j.cell.2009.09.035
7. Alborzinia H, Schmidt-Glenewinkel H, Ilkavets I, Breitkopf-Heinlein K, Cheng X, Hortschansky P, Dooley S, Wolfl S (2013) Quantitative kinetics analysis of BMP2 uptake into cells and its modulation by BMP antagonists. J Cell Sci 126(Pt 1):117–127. doi:10.1242/jcs.109777
8. Anand P, Kunnumakkara AB, Sundaram C, Harikumar KB, Tharakan ST, Lai OS, Sung B, Aggarwal BB (2008) Cancer is a preventable disease that requires major lifestyle changes. Pharm Res 25(9):2097–2116. doi:10.1007/s11095-008-9661-9
9. Baeyer A (1881) Ueber die Verbindungen der Indigogruppe. Chem Ber 14:1741–1750
10. Balkwill F, Mantovani A (2001) Inflammation and cancer: back to Virchow? Lancet 357 (9255):539–545. doi:10.1016/S0140-6736(00)04046-0
11. Beauchard A, Ferandin Y, Frere S, Lozach O, Blairvacq M, Meijer L, Thiery V, Besson T (2006) Synthesis of novel 5-substituted indirubins as protein kinases inhibitors. Bioorg Med Chem 14(18):6434–6443. doi:10.1016/j.bmc.2006.05.036
12. Benson JM, Shepherd DM (2011) Dietary ligands of the aryl hydrocarbon receptor induce anti-inflammatory and immunoregulatory effects on murine dendritic cells. Toxicol Sci 124 (2):327–338. doi:10.1093/toxsci/kfr249
13. Blanz J, Ehninger G, Zeller KP (1989) The isolation and identification of indigo and indirubin from urine of a patient with leukemia. Res Commun Chem Pathol Pharmacol 64 (1):145–156
14. Blazevic T, Heiss EH, Atanasov AG, Breuss JM, Dirsch VM, Uhrin P (2015) Indirubin and indirubin derivatives for counteracting proliferative diseases. Evid Based Complement Alternat Med 2015:654098. doi:10.1155/2015/654098
15. Blazevic T, Schaible AM, Weinhaupl K, Schachner D, Nikels F, Weinigel C, Barz D, Atanasov AG, Pergola C, Werz O, Dirsch VM, Heiss EH (2014) Indirubin-3′-monoxime exerts a dual mode of inhibition towards leukotriene-mediated vascular smooth muscle cell migration. Cardiovasc Res 101(3):522–532. doi:10.1093/cvr/cvt339
16. Braig S, Kressirer CA, Liebl J, Bischoff F, Zahler S, Meijer L, Vollmar AM (2013) Indirubin derivative 6BIO suppresses metastasis. Cancer Res 73(19):6004–6012. doi:10.1158/0008-5472.CAN-12-4358
17. Broecker-Preuss M, Becher-Boveleth N, Gall S, Rehmann K, Schenke S, Mann K (2015) Induction of atypical cell death in thyroid carcinoma cells by the indirubin derivative 7-bromoindirubin-3′-oxime (7BIO). Cancer Cell Int 15:97. doi:10.1186/s12935-015-0251-8
18. Bromberg JF, Wrzeszczynska MH, Devgan G, Zhao YX, Pestell RG, Albanese C, Darnell JE (1999) Stat3 as an oncogene. Cell 98(3):295–303. doi:10.1016/s0092-8674(00)81959-5
19. Calon A, Espinet E, Palomo-Ponce S, Tauriello DV, Iglesias M, Cespedes MV, Sevillano M, Nadal C, Jung P, Zhang XH, Byrom D, Riera A, Rossell D, Mangues R, Massague J, Sancho E, Batlle E (2012) Dependency of colorectal cancer on a TGF-beta-driven program in stromal cells for metastasis initiation. Cancer Cell 22(5):571–584. doi:10.1016/j.ccr.2012.08.013
20. Catlett-Falcone R, Landowski TH, Oshiro MM, Turkson J, Levitzki A, Savino R, Ciliberto G, Moscinski L, Fernandez-Luna JL, Nunez G, Dalton WS, Jove R (1999) Constitutive activation of Stat3 signaling confers resistance to apoptosis in human U266 myeloma cells. Immunity 10(1):105–115. doi:10.1016/s1074-7613(00)80011-4
21. Chan E, Tan M, Xin J, Sudarsanam S, Johnson DE (2010) Interactions between traditional Chinese medicines and Western therapeutics. Curr Opin Drug Discov Devel 13(1):50–65
22. Chan YK, Kwok HH, Chan LS, Leung KS, Shi J, Mak NK, Wong RN, Yue PY (2012) An indirubin derivative, E804, exhibits potent angiosuppressive activity. Biochem Pharmacol 83 (5):598–607. doi:10.1016/j.bcp.2011.12.003
23. Cheng X, Alborzinia H, Merz KH, Steinbeisser H, Mrowka R, Scholl C, Kitanovic I, Eisenbrand G, Wolfl S (2012) Indirubin derivatives modulate TGFbeta/BMP signaling at

different levels and trigger ubiquitin-mediated depletion of nonactivated R-Smads. Chem Biol 19(11):1423–1436. doi:10.1016/j.chembiol.2012.09.008

24. Cheng X, Dimou E, Alborzinia H, Wenke F, Gohring A, Reuter S, Mah N, Fuchs H, Andrade-Navarro MA, Adjaye J, Gul S, Harms C, Utikal J, Klipp E, Mrowka R, Wolfl S (2015) Identification of 2-[4-[(4-methoxyphenyl)methoxy]-phenyl]acetonitrile and derivatives as potent Oct3/4 inducers. J Med Chem 58(12):4976–4983. doi:10.1021/acs.jmedchem.5b00144
25. Cheng X, Holenya P, Can S, Alborzinia H, Rubbiani R, Ott I, Wolfl S (2014) A TrxR inhibiting gold(I) NHC complex induces apoptosis through ASK1-p38-MAPK signaling in pancreatic cancer cells. Mol Cancer 13(1):221. doi:10.1186/1476-4598-13-221
26. Cheng X, Kim JY, Ghafoory S, Duvaci T, Rafiee R, Theobald J, Alborzinia H, Holenya P, Fredebohm J, Merz K-H, Mehrabi A, Hafezi M, Saffari A, Eisenbrand G, Hoheisel JD, Wölfl S (2016) Methylisoindigo preferentially kills cancer stem cells by interfering cell metabolism via inhibition of LKB1 and activation of AMPK in PDACs. Mol Oncol. doi:10.1016/j.molonc.2016.01.008
27. Cheng X, Merz KH, Vatter S, Christ J, Wolfl S, Eisenbrand G (2014) 7,7′-diazaindirubin—a small molecule inhibitor of casein kinase 2 in vitro and in cells. Bioorg Med Chem 22 (1):247–255. doi:10.1016/j.bmc.2013.11.031
28. Cheng X, Rasque P, Vatter S, Merz KH, Eisenbrand G (2010) Synthesis and cytotoxicity of novel indirubin-5-carboxamides. Bioorg Med Chem 18(12):4509–4515. doi:10.1016/j.bmc.2010.04.066
29. Cheng X, Yoshida H, Raoofi D, Saleh S, Alborzinia H, Wenke F, Gohring A, Reuter S, Mah N, Fuchs H, Andrade-Navarro MA, Adjaye J, Gul S, Utikal J, Mrowka R, Wolfl S (2015) Ethyl 2-((4-Chlorophenyl)amino)thiazole-4-carboxylate and derivatives are potent inducers of Oct3/4. J Med Chem 58(15):5742–5750. doi:10.1021/acs.jmedchem.5b00226
30. Choi SJ, Lee JE, Jeong SY, Im I, Lee SD, Lee EJ, Lee SK, Kwon SM, Ahn SG, Yoon JH, Han SY, Kim JI, Kim YC (2010) 5,5′-substituted indirubin-3′-oxime derivatives as potent cyclin-dependent kinase inhibitors with anticancer activity. J Med Chem 53(9):3696–3706. doi:10.1021/jm100080z
31. Chou YF, Chen HH, Eijpe M, Yabuuchi A, Chenoweth JG, Tesar P, Lu J, McKay RD, Geijsen N (2008) The growth factor environment defines distinct pluripotent ground states in novel blastocyst-derived stem cells. Cell 135(3):449–461. doi:10.1016/j.cell.2008.08.035
32. Clinical and experimental studies in the treatment of chronic granulocytic leukemia with indirubin (author's transl) (1979). Zhonghua Nei Ke Za Zhi 18(2):83–88
33. Davey S (2015) 2015 Nobel Prize in physiology or medicine: punishing parasites. Nat Chem 7(12):949. doi:10.1038/nchem.2411
34. Davies TG, Tunnah P, Meijer L, Marko D, Eisenbrand G, Endicott JA, Noble ME (2001) Inhibitor binding to active and inactive CDK2: the crystal structure of CDK2-cyclin A/indirubin-5-sulphonate. Structure 9(5):389–397
35. Denison MS, Nagy SR (2003) Activation of the aryl hydrocarbon receptor by structurally diverse exogenous and endogenous chemicals. Annu Rev Pharmacol Toxicol 43:309–334. doi:10.1146/annurev.pharmtox.43.100901.135828
36. Duensing S, Duensing A, Lee DC, Edwards KM, Piboonniyom SO, Manuel E, Skaltsounis L, Meijer L, Munger K (2004) Cyclin-dependent kinase inhibitor indirubin-3′-oxime selectively inhibits human papillomavirus type 16 E7-induced numerical centrosome anomalies. Oncogene 23(50):8206–8215. doi:10.1038/sj.onc.1208012
37. Efferth T, Li PC, Konkimalla VS, Kaina B (2007) From traditional Chinese medicine to rational cancer therapy. Trends Mol Med 13(8):353–361. doi:10.1016/j.molmed.2007.07.001
38. Eisenbrand G, Cheng X, Zeller J, Merz K-H (2010) Impact of structural modifications on bioactivity and metabolic stability of indirubins. In: Proceedings of the American Association for cancer research annual meeting 51, pp 647–647
39. Eisenbrand G, Hippe F, Jakobs S, Muehlbeyer S (2004) Molecular mechanisms of indirubin and its derivatives: novel anticancer molecules with their origin in traditional Chinese phytomedicine. J Cancer Res Clin Oncol 130(11):627–635. doi:10.1007/s00432-004-0579-2

40. Feng BZ (1984) [Sister chromatid exchange frequency of bone marrow cells and its response to indirubin in chronic myeloid leukemia]. Zhonghua Zhong Liu Za Zhi 6(5):357–360
41. Feng BZ, Zhang YH, Qian LS, Chu YL (1984) [Effect of indirubin on SCE frequencies of BM cells in chronic myeloid leukemia]. Zhongguo Yi Xue Ke Xue Yuan Xue Bao 6(4):308–310
42. Ferandin Y, Bettayeb K, Kritsanida M, Lozach O, Polychronopoulos P, Magiatis P, Skaltsounis AL, Meijer L (2006) 3′-Substituted 7-halogenoindirubins, a new class of cell death inducing agents. J Med Chem 49(15):4638–4649. doi:10.1021/jm060314i
43. Fuentealba LC, Eivers E, Ikeda A, Hurtado C, Kuroda H, Pera EM, De Robertis EM (2007) Integrating patterning signals: Wnt/GSK3 regulates the duration of the BMP/Smad1 signal. Cell 131(5):980–993. doi:10.1016/j.cell.2007.09.027
44. Fuxe J, Karlsson MC (2012) TGF-beta-induced epithelial-mesenchymal transition: a link between cancer and inflammation. Semin Cancer Biol 22(5–6):455–461. doi:10.1016/j.semcancer.2012.05.004
45. Gao X, Zhou Y, Wu KX, Ding YH, Fan DM, Yang M, Zhang YZ, Zhang YJ, Xiong DS (2015) Inhibitory effects of indirubin derivative PHII-7 on invasion and migration in metastatic cancer. Neoplasma 62(2):209–229. doi:10.4149/neo_2015_026
46. Ghafoory S, Mehrabi A, Hafezi M, Cheng X, Breitkopf-Heinlein K, Hick M, Huichalaf M, Herbel V, Saffari A, Wolfl S (2015) Nuclear accumulation of CDH1 mRNA in hepatocellular carcinoma cells. Oncogenesis 4:e152. doi:10.1038/oncsis.2015.11
47. Gough DJ, Corlett A, Schlessinger K, Wegrzyn J, Larner AC, Levy DE (2009) Mitochondrial STAT3 supports Ras-dependent oncogenic transformation. Science 324 (5935):1713–1716. doi:10.1126/science.1171721
48. Grivennikov SI, Greten FR, Karin M (2010) Immunity, inflammation, and cancer. Cell 140 (6):883–899. doi:10.1016/j.cell.2010.01.025
49. Guengerich FP, Sorrells JL, Schmitt S, Krauser JA, Aryal P, Meijer L (2004) Generation of new protein kinase inhibitors utilizing cytochrome p450 mutant enzymes for indigoid synthesis. J Med Chem 47(12):3236–3241. doi:10.1021/jm030561b
50. Heshmati N, Cheng X, Dapat E, Sassene P, Eisenbrand G, Fricker G, Mullertz A (2014) In vitro and in vivo evaluations of the performance of an indirubin derivative, formulated in four different self-emulsifying drug delivery systems. J Pharm Pharmacol 66(11):1567–1575. doi:10.1111/jphp.12286
51. Heshmati N, Cheng X, Eisenbrand G, Fricker G (2013) Enhancement of oral bioavailability of E804 by self-nanoemulsifying drug delivery system (SNEDDS) in rats. J Pharm Sci 102 (10):3792–3799. doi:10.1002/jps.23696
52. Heshmati N, Wagner B, Cheng X, Scholz T, Kansy M, Eisenbrand G, Fricker G (2013) Physicochemical characterization and in vitro permeation of an indirubin derivative. Eur J Pharm Sci 50(3–4):467–475. doi:10.1016/j.ejps.2013.08.021
53. Hoessel R, Leclerc S, Endicott JA, Nobel ME, Lawrie A, Tunnah P, Leost M, Damiens E, Marie D, Marko D, Niederberger E, Tang W, Eisenbrand G, Meijer L (1999) Indirubin, the active constituent of a Chinese antileukaemia medicine, inhibits cyclin dependent kinases. Nat Cell Biol 1(1):60–67. doi:10.1038/9035
54. Hu S, Cui W, Zhang Z, Mak S, Xu D, Li G, Hu Y, Wang Y, Lee M, Tsim KW, Han Y (2015) Indirubin-3-oxime effectively prevents 6OHDA-induced neurotoxicity in PC12 cells via activating MEF2D through the inhibition of GSK3beta. J Mol Neurosci 57(4):561–570. doi:10.1007/s12031-015-0638-y
55. Huang M, Lin HS, Lee YS, Ho PC (2014) Evaluation of meisoindigo, an indirubin derivative: in vitro antileukemic activity and in vivo pharmacokinetics. Int J Oncol 45 (4):1724–1734. doi:10.3892/ijo.2014.2548
56. Jautelat R, Brumby T, Schafer M, Briem H, Eisenbrand G, Schwahn S, Kruger M, Lucking U, Prien O, Siemeister G (2005) From the insoluble dye indirubin towards highly active, soluble CDK2-inhibitors. ChemBioChem 6(3):531–540. doi:10.1002/cbic.200400108
57. Ji XJ, Zhang FR (1985) [Studies on antineoplastic action of indirubin derivatives and analogs and their structure-activity relationships]. Yao Xue Xue Bao 20(2):137–139

58. Ji XJ, Zhang FR, Lei JL, Xu YT (1981) [Studies on the antineoplastic action and toxicity of synthetic indirubin (author's transl)]. Yao Xue Xue Bao 16(2):146–148
59. Jung DW, Hong YJ, Kim SY, Kim WH, Seo S, Lee JE, Shen H, Kim YC, Williams DR (2014) 5-Nitro-5′hydroxy-indirubin-3′oxime is a novel inducer of somatic cell transdifferentiation. Arch Pharm (Weinheim) 347(11):806–818. doi:10.1002/ardp.201400223
60. Karin M (2006) Nuclear factor-kappaB in cancer development and progression. Nature 441 (7092):431–436. doi:10.1038/nature04870
61. Karin M, Greten FR (2005) NF-kappaB: linking inflammation and immunity to cancer development and progression. Nat Rev Immunol 5(10):749–759. doi:10.1038/nri1703
62. Kim EJ, Park WH, Ahn SG, Yoon JH, Kim SW, Kim SA (2010) 5′-nitro-indirubinoxime inhibits inflammatory response in TNF-alpha stimulated human umbilical vein endothelial cells. Atherosclerosis 211(1):77–83. doi:10.1016/j.atherosclerosis.2010.01.040
63. Kim JK, Park GM (2012) Indirubin-3-monoxime exhibits anti-inflammatory properties by down-regulating NF-kappaB and JNK signaling pathways in lipopolysaccharide-treated RAW264.7 cells. Inflamm Res Off J Eur Histamine Res Soc 61(4):319–325. doi:10.1007/s00011-011-0413-7
64. Kim MH, Choi YY, Yang G, Cho IH, Nam D, Yang WM (2013) Indirubin, a purple 3,2-bisindole, inhibited allergic contact dermatitis via regulating T helper (Th)-mediated immune system in DNCB-induced model. J Ethnopharmacol 145(1):214–219. doi:10.1016/j.jep.2012.10.055
65. Kim SH, Kim SW, Choi SJ, Kim YC, Kim TS (2006) Enhancing effect of indirubin derivatives on 1,25-dihydroxyvitamin D3- and all-trans retinoic acid-induced differentiation of HL-60 leukemia cells. Bioorg Med Chem 14(19):6752–6758. doi:10.1016/j.bmc.2006.05.044
66. Knockaert M, Blondel M, Bach S, Leost M, Elbi C, Hager GL, Nagy SR, Han D, Denison M, Ffrench M, Ryan XP, Magiatis P, Polychronopoulos P, Greengard P, Skaltsounis L, Meijer L (2004) Independent actions on cyclin-dependent kinases and aryl hydrocarbon receptor mediate the antiproliferative effects of indirubins. Oncogene 23(25):4400–4412. doi:10.1038/sj.onc.1207535
67. Kritsanida M, Magiatis P, Skaltsounis AL, Peng Y, Li P, Wennogle LP (2009) Synthesis and antiproliferative activity of 7-azaindirubin-3′-oxime, a 7-aza isostere of the natural indirubin pharmacophore. J Nat Prod 72(12):2199–2202. doi:10.1021/np9003905
68. Leclerc S, Garnier M, Hoessel R, Marko D, Bibb JA, Snyder GL, Greengard P, Biernat J, Wu YZ, Mandelkow EM, Eisenbrand G, Meijer L (2001) Indirubins inhibit glycogen synthase kinase-3 beta and CDK5/p25, two protein kinases involved in abnormal tau phosphorylation in Alzheimer's disease. A property common to most cyclin-dependent kinase inhibitors? J Biol Chem 276(1):251–260. doi:10.1074/jbc.M002466200
69. Lee JW, Moon MJ, Min HY, Chung HJ, Park EJ, Park HJ, Hong JY, Kim YC, Lee SK (2005) Induction of apoptosis by a novel indirubin-5-nitro-3′-monoxime, a CDK inhibitor, in human lung cancer cells. Bioorg Med Chem Lett 15(17):3948–3952. doi:10.1016/j.bmcl.2005.05.105
70. Lee MY, Liu YW, Chen MH, Wu JY, Ho HY, Wang QF, Chuang JJ (2013) Indirubin-3′-monoxime promotes autophagic and apoptotic death in JM1 human acute lymphoblastic leukemia cells and K562 human chronic myelogenous leukemia cells. Oncol Rep 29 (5):2072–2078. doi:10.3892/or.2013.2334
71. Liao XM, Leung KN (2013) Indirubin-3′-oxime induces mitochondrial dysfunction and triggers growth inhibition and cell cycle arrest in human neuroblastoma cells. Oncol Rep 29 (1):371–379. doi:10.3892/or.2012.2094
72. Libnow S, Methling K, Hein M, Michalik D, Harms M, Wende K, Flemming A, Kockerling M, Reinke H, Bednarski PJ, Lalk M, Langer P (2008) Synthesis of indirubin-N′-glycosides and their anti-proliferative activity against human cancer cell lines. Bioorg Med Chem 16(10):5570–5583. doi:10.1016/j.bmc.2008.04.003

73. Liu XP, Sun H, Qi J, Wang LL, He SW, Liu J, Feng CQ, Chen CL, Li W, Guo YQ, Qin DJ, Pan GJ, Chen JK, Pei DQ, Zheng H (2013) Sequential introduction of reprogramming factors reveals a time-sensitive requirement for individual factors and a sequential EMT-MET mechanism for optimal reprogramming. Nat Cell Biol 15(7):829–838. doi:10.1038/Ncb2765
74. Lo WY, Chang NW (2013) An indirubin derivative, indirubin-3′-monoxime suppresses oral cancer tumorigenesis through the downregulation of survivin. PLoS ONE 8(8):e70198. doi:10.1371/journal.pone.0070198
75. Mantovani A, Allavena P, Sica A, Balkwill F (2008) Cancer-related inflammation. Nature 454(7203):436–444. doi:10.1038/nature07205
76. Marko D, Schatzle S, Friedel A, Genzlinger A, Zankl H, Meijer L, Eisenbrand G (2001) Inhibition of cyclin-dependent kinase 1 (CDK1) by indirubin derivatives in human tumour cells. Br J Cancer 84(2):283–289. doi:10.1054/bjoc.2000.1546
77. Martinet J, Dornier O (1921) On the new sulfonated derivatives of oxindol and of isatin. Cr Hebd Acad Sci 172:1415–1417
78. Meijer L, Skaltsounis AL, Magiatis P, Polychronopoulos P, Knockaert M, Leost M, Ryan XP, Vonica CA, Brivanlou A, Dajani R, Crovace C, Tarricone C, Musacchio A, Roe SM, Pearl L, Greengard P (2003) GSK-3-selective inhibitors derived from Tyrian purple indirubins. Chem Biol 10(12):1255–1266
79. Merz K-H, Eisenbrand G (2006) Chemistry and structure-activity of indirubins. In: Meijer L, Guyard N, Skaltsounis L, Eisenbrand G (eds) Indirubin, the red shade of indigo. Editions 'Life in progress', Roscoff, pp 203–208
80. Merz KH, Schwahn S, Hippe F, Muhlbeyer S, Jakobs S, Eisenbrand G (2004) Novel indirubin derivatives, promising anti-tumor agents inhibiting cyclin-dependent kinases. Int J Clin Pharmacol Ther 42(11):656–658
81. Miller LH, Su X (2011) Artemisinin: discovery from the Chinese herbal garden. Cell 146 (6):855–858. doi:10.1016/j.cell.2011.08.024
82. Miyoshi K, Takaishi M, Digiovanni J, Sano S (2012) Attenuation of psoriasis-like skin lesion in a mouse model by topical treatment with indirubin and its derivative E804. J Dermatol Sci 65(1):70–72. doi:10.1016/j.jdermsci.2011.10.001
83. Mok CK, Kang SS, Chan RW, Yue PY, Mak NK, Poon LL, Wong RN, Peiris JS, Chan MC (2014) Anti-inflammatory and antiviral effects of indirubin derivatives in influenza A (H5N1) virus infected primary human peripheral blood-derived macrophages and alveolar epithelial cells. Antiviral Res 106:95–104. doi:10.1016/j.antiviral.2014.03.019
84. Moon MJ, Lee SK, Lee JW, Song WK, Kim SW, Kim JI, Cho C, Choi SJ, Kim YC (2006) Synthesis and structure-activity relationships of novel indirubin derivatives as potent anti-proliferative agents with CDK2 inhibitory activities. Bioorg Med Chem 14(1):237–246. doi:10.1016/j.bmc.2005.08.008
85. Myrianthopoulos V, Kritsanida M, Gaboriaud-Kolar N, Magiatis P, Ferandin Y, Durieu E, Lozach O, Cappel D, Soundararajan M, Filippakopoulos P, Sherman W, Knapp S, Meijer L, Mikros E, Skaltsounis AL (2013) Novel inverse binding mode of indirubin derivatives yields improved selectivity for DYRK kinases. ACS Med Chem Lett 4(1):22–26. doi:10.1021/ml300207a
86. Myrianthopoulos V, Magiatis P, Ferandin Y, Skaltsounis AL, Meijer L, Mikros E (2007) An integrated computational approach to the phenomenon of potent and selective inhibition of aurora kinases B and C by a series of 7-substituted indirubins. J Med Chem 50(17):4027–4037. doi:10.1021/jm070077z
87. Nam S, Buettner R, Turkson J, Kim D, Cheng JQ, Muehlbeyer S, Hippe F, Vatter S, Merz KH, Eisenbrand G, Jove R (2005) Indirubin derivatives inhibit Stat3 signaling and induce apoptosis in human cancer cells. Proc Natl Acad Sci USA 102(17):5998–6003. doi:10.1073/pnas.0409467102
88. Nam S, Scuto A, Yang F, Chen W, Park S, Yoo HS, Konig H, Bhatia R, Cheng X, Merz KH, Eisenbrand G, Jove R (2012) Indirubin derivatives induce apoptosis of chronic myelogenous leukemia cells involving inhibition of Stat5 signaling. Mol Oncol 6(3):276–283. doi:10.1016/j.molonc.2012.02.002

89. Nam S, Wen W, Schroeder A, Herrmann A, Yu H, Cheng X, Merz KH, Eisenbrand G, Li H, Yuan YC, Jove R (2013) Dual inhibition of Janus and Src family kinases by novel indirubin derivative blocks constitutively-activated Stat3 signaling associated with apoptosis of human pancreatic cancer cells. Mol Oncol 7(3):369–378. doi:10.1016/j.molonc.2012.10.013
90. Noble ME, Endicott JA, Johnson LN (2004) Protein kinase inhibitors: insights into drug design from structure. Science 303(5665):1800–1805. doi:10.1126/science.1095920
91. Pandraud H (1961) Structure Cristalline De Lindirubine. Acta Crystallogr 14(9):901. doi:10.1107/S0365110x61002667
92. Park EJ, Choi SJ, Kim YC, Lee SH, Park SW, Lee SK (2009) Novel small molecule activators of beta-catenin-mediated signaling pathway: structure-activity relationships of indirubins. Bioorg Med Chem Lett 19(8):2282–2284. doi:10.1016/j.bmcl.2009.02.083
93. Pergola C, Gaboriaud-Kolar N, Jestadt N, Konig S, Kritsanida M, Schaible AM, Li H, Garscha U, Weinigel C, Barz D, Albring KF, Huber O, Skaltsounis AL, Werz O (2014) Indirubin core structure of glycogen synthase kinase-3 inhibitors as novel chemotype for intervention with 5-lipoxygenase. J Med Chem 57(9):3715–3723. doi:10.1021/jm401740w
94. Polychronopoulos P, Magiatis P, Skaltsounis AL, Myrianthopoulos V, Mikros E, Tarricone A, Musacchio A, Roe SM, Pearl L, Leost M, Greengard P, Meijer L (2004) Structural basis for the synthesis of indirubins as potent and selective inhibitors of glycogen synthase kinase-3 and cyclin-dependent kinases. J Med Chem 47(4):935–946. doi:10.1021/jm031016d
95. Prochazkova J, Kozubik A, Machala M, Vondracek J (2011) Differential effects of indirubin and 2,3,7,8-tetrachlorodibenzo-p-dioxin on the aryl hydrocarbon receptor (AhR) signalling in liver progenitor cells. Toxicology 279(1–3):146–154. doi:10.1016/j.tox.2010.10.003
96. Rahman SH, Bobis-Wozowicz S, Chatterjee D, Gellhaus K, Pars K, Heilbronn R, Jacobs R, Cathomen T (2013) The nontoxic cell cycle modulator indirubin augments transduction of adeno-associated viral vectors and zinc-finger nuclease-mediated gene targeting. Hum Gene Ther 24(1):67–77. doi:10.1089/hum.2012.168
97. Ribas J, Bettayeb K, Ferandin Y, Knockaert M, Garrofe-Ochoa X, Totzke F, Schachtele C, Mester J, Polychronopoulos P, Magiatis P, Skaltsounis AL, Boix J, Meijer L (2006) 7-Bromoindirubin-3′-oxime induces caspase-independent cell death. Oncogene 25(47):6304–6318. doi:10.1038/sj.onc.1209648
98. Russell GA, Kaupp G (1969) Oxidation of carbanions. 4. Oxidation of indoxyl to indigo in basic solution. J A Chem Soc 91(14):3851. doi:10.1021/ja01042a028
99. Saito H, Tabata K, Hanada S, Kanda Y, Suzuki T, Miyairi S (2011) Synthesis of methoxy- and bromo-substituted indirubins and their activities on apoptosis induction in human neuroblastoma cells. Bioorg Med Chem Lett 21(18):5370–5373. doi:10.1016/j.bmcl.2011.07.011
100. Sapkota G, Alarcon C, Spagnoli FM, Brivanlou AH, Massague J (2007) Balancing BMP signaling through integrated inputs into the Smad1 linker. Mol Cell 25(3):441–454. doi:10.1016/j.molcel.2007.01.006
101. Sato N, Meijer L, Skaltsounis L, Greengard P, Brivanlou AH (2004) Maintenance of pluripotency in human and mouse embryonic stem cells through activation of Wnt signaling by a pharmacological GSK-3-specific inhibitor. Nat Med 10(1):55–63. doi:10.1038/nm979
102. Sethi G, Ahn KS, Sandur SK, Lin X, Chaturvedi MM, Aggarwal BB (2006) Indirubin enhances tumor necrosis factor-induced apoptosis through modulation of nuclear factor-kappa B signaling pathway. J Biol Chem 281(33):23425–23435. doi:10.1074/jbc.M602627200
103. Sharma S, Taliyan R (2014) Neuroprotective role of Indirubin-3′-monoxime, a GSKbeta inhibitor in high fat diet induced cognitive impairment in mice. Biochem Biophys Res Commun 452(4):1009–1015. doi:10.1016/j.bbrc.2014.09.034
104. Shin EK, Kim JK (2012) Indirubin derivative E804 inhibits angiogenesis. BMC Cancer 12:164. doi:10.1186/1471-2407-12-164

105. Smyth LA, Matthews TP, Collins I (2011) Design and evaluation of 3-aminopyrazolopyridinone kinase inhibitors inspired by the natural product indirubin. Bioorg Med Chem 19(11):3569–3578. doi:10.1016/j.bmc.2011.03.069
106. Song JH, Lee JE, Cho KM, Park SH, Kim HJ, Kim YC, Kim TS (2015) 5-diphenylacetamido-indirubin-3′-oxime as a novel mitochondria-targeting agent with anti-leukemic activities. Mol Carcinog. doi:10.1002/mc.22307
107. Spink BC, Hussain MM, Katz BH, Eisele L, Spink DC (2003) Transient induction of cytochromes P450 1A1 and 1B1 in MCF-7 human breast cancer cells by indirubin. Biochem Pharmacol 66(12):2313–2321
108. Stockinger B, Di Meglio P, Gialitakis M, Duarte JH (2014) The aryl hydrocarbon receptor: multitasking in the immune system. Annu Rev Immunol 32:403–432. doi:10.1146/annurev-immunol-032713-120245
109. Sugihara K, Kitamura S, Yamada T, Okayama T, Ohta S, Yamashita K, Yasuda M, Fujii-Kuriyama Y, Saeki K, Matsui S, Matsuda T (2004) Aryl hydrocarbon receptor-mediated induction of microsomal drug-metabolizing enzyme activity by indirubin and indigo. Biochem Biophys Res Commun 318(2):571–578. doi:10.1016/j.bbrc.2004.04.066
110. Takeda K, Noguchi K, Shi W, Tanaka T, Matsumoto M, Yoshida N, Kishimoto T, Akira S (1997) Targeted disruption of the mouse Stat3 gene leads to early embryonic lethality. P Natl Acad Sci USA 94(8):3801–3804. doi:10.1073/pnas.94.8.3801
111. Tanaka T, Ohashi S, Saito H, Higuchi T, Tabata K, Kosuge Y, Suzuki T, Miyairi S, Kobayashi S (2014) Indirubin derivatives alter DNA binding activity of the transcription factor NF-Y and inhibit MDR1 gene promoter. Eur J Pharmacol 741:83–89. doi:10.1016/j.ejphar.2014.07.035
112. Thiery JP, Acloque H, Huang RY, Nieto MA (2009) Epithelial-mesenchymal transitions in development and disease. Cell 139(5):871–890. doi:10.1016/j.cell.2009.11.007
113. Tu Y (2011) The discovery of artemisinin (qinghaosu) and gifts from Chinese medicine. Nat Med 17(10):1217–1220. doi:10.1038/nm.2471
114. Udumula MP, Medapi B, Dhar I, Bhat A, Desai K, Sriram D, Dhar A (2015) The small molecule indirubin-3′-oxime inhibits protein kinase R: antiapoptotic and antioxidant effect in rat cardiac myocytes. Pharmacology 97(1–2):25–30. doi:10.1159/000441727
115. Vougogiannopoulou K, Ferandin Y, Bettayeb K, Myrianthopoulos V, Lozach O, Fan Y, Johnson CH, Magiatis P, Skaltsounis AL, Mikros E, Meijer L (2008) Soluble 3′,6-substituted indirubins with enhanced selectivity toward glycogen synthase kinase-3 alter circadian period. J Med Chem 51(20):6421–6431. doi:10.1021/jm800648y
116. Wan JH, You YC, Mi JX, Ying HG (1981) [Effect of indirubin on hemopoietic cell production (author's transl)]. Zhongguo Yao Li Xue Bao 2(4):241–244
117. Wang L, Li X, Liu X, Lu K, Chen NA, Li P, Lv X, Wang X (2015) Enhancing effects of indirubin on the arsenic disulfide-induced apoptosis of human diffuse large B-cell lymphoma cells. Oncol Lett 9(4):1940–1946. doi:10.3892/ol.2015.2941
118. Wang Y, Hoi PM, Chan JY, Lee SM (2014) New perspective on the dual functions of indirubins in cancer therapy and neuroprotection. Anticancer Agents Med Chem 14(9):1213–1219
119. Wegrzyn J, Potla R, Chwae YJ, Sepuri NB, Zhang Q, Koeck T, Derecka M, Szczepanek K, Szelag M, Gornicka A, Moh A, Moghaddas S, Chen Q, Bobbili S, Cichy J, Dulak J, Baker DP, Wolfman A, Stuehr D, Hassan MO, Fu XY, Avadhani N, Drake JI, Fawcett P, Lesnefsky EJ, Larner AC (2009) Function of mitochondrial Stat3 in cellular respiration. Science 323(5915):793–797. doi:10.1126/science.1164551
120. Wen Z, Zhong Z, Darnell JE Jr (1995) Maximal activation of transcription by Stat1 and Stat3 requires both tyrosine and serine phosphorylation. Cell 82(2):241–250
121. Wongsaroj L, Sallabhan R, Dubbs JM, Mongkolsuk S, Loprasert S (2015) Cloning of toluene 4-monooxygenase genes and application of two-phase system to the production of the anticancer agent, indirubin. Mol Biotechnol 57(8):720–726. doi:10.1007/s12033-015-9863-4

122. Wu GY, Fang FD (1980) [Studies on the mechanism of indirubin action in the treatment of chronic granulocytic leukemia. II. Effects of indirubin on nucleic acid and protein synthesis in animal transplantable tumor cells and normal proliferating cells in vitro (author's transl)]. Zhongguo Yi Xue Ke Xue Yuan Xue Bao 2(2):83–87
123. Wu GY, Liu JZ, Fang FD, Zuo J (1982) Studies on the mechanism of indirubin action in the treatment of chronic granulocytic leukemia. V. Binding between indirubin and DNA and identification of the type of binding. Sci Sin B 25(10):1071–1079
124. Xiao Z, Hao Y (2006) From Danggui Longhui Wang to meisoindigo: experience in the treatment of chronic myelogenous leukemia in China. In: Meijer L, Guyard N, Skaltsounis L, Eisenbrand, G (eds) Indirubin, the red shade of indigo. Editions 'Life in progress', Roscoff, pp 203–208
125. Xiao Z, Hao Y, Liu B, Qian L (2002) Indirubin and meisoindigo in the treatment of chronic myelogenous leukemia in China. Leukemia Lymphoma 43(9):1763–1768. doi:10.1080/1042819021000006295
126. Yu CL, Meyer DJ, Campbell GS, Larner AC, Cartersu C, Schwartz J, Jove R (1995) Enhanced DNA-binding activity of a STAT3-related protein in cells transformed by the SRC oncoprotein. Science 269(5220):81–83. doi:10.1126/science.7541555
127. Yu H, Lee H, Herrmann A, Buettner R, Jove R (2014) Revisiting STAT3 signalling in cancer: new and unexpected biological functions. Nat Rev Cancer 14(11):736–746. doi:10.1038/nrc3818
128. Yu H, Pardoll D, Jove R (2009) STATs in cancer inflammation and immunity: a leading role for STAT3. Nat Rev Cancer 9(11):798–809. doi:10.1038/nrc2734 (nrc2734 [pii])
129. Yuan ZZ, Sun DT (1987) [Clinical and ultrastructural study on psoriasis treated by indirubin]. Zhonghua Yi Xue Za Zhi 67(1):7–8
130. Zahoor M, Cha PH, Choi KY (2014) Indirubin-3′-oxime, an activator of Wnt/beta-catenin signaling, enhances osteogenic commitment of ST2 cells and restores bone loss in high-fat diet-induced obese male mice. Bone 65:60–68. doi:10.1016/j.bone.2014.05.003
131. Zahoor M, Cha PH, Min do S, Choi KY (2014b) Indirubin-3′-oxime reverses bone loss in ovariectomized and hindlimb-unloaded mice via activation of the Wnt/beta-catenin signaling. J Bone Miner Res 29 (5):1196–1205. doi:10.1002/jbmr.2147
132. Zhang X, Song Y, Wu Y, Dong Y, Lai L, Zhang J, Lu B, Dai F, He L, Liu M, Yi Z (2011) Indirubin inhibits tumor growth by antitumor angiogenesis via blocking VEGFR2-mediated JAK/STAT3 signaling in endothelial cell. Int J Cancer 129(10):2502–2511. doi:10.1002/ijc.25909
133. Zhao PP (1981) [Determination of indirubin by dual wavelength TLC scanner (author's transl)]. Zhong Yao Tong Bao 6(4):28–30

CDDO and Its Role in Chronic Diseases

Bryan J. Mathis and Taixing Cui

Abstract There has been a continued interest in translational research focused on both natural products and manipulation of functional groups on these compounds to create novel derivatives with higher desired activities. Oleanolic acid, a component of traditional Chinese medicine used in hepatitis therapy, was modified by chemical processes to form 2-cyano-3,12-dioxoolean-1,9-dien-28-oic acid (CDDO). This modification increased anti-inflammatory activity significantly and additional functional groups on the CDDO backbone have shown promise in treating conditions ranging from kidney disease to obesity to diabetes. CDDO's therapeutic effect is due to its upregulation of the master antioxidant transcription factor Nuclear factor erythroid 2-related factor 2 (Nrf2) through conformational change of Nrf2-repressing, Kelch-like erythroid cell-derived protein with CNC homology-associated protein 1 (Keap1) and multiple animal and human studies have verified subsequent activation of Nrf2-controlled antioxidant genes via upstream Antioxidant Response Element (ARE) regions. At the present time, positive results have been obtained in the laboratory and clinical trials with CDDO derivatives treating conditions such as lung injury, inflammation and chronic kidney disease. However, clinical trials for cancer and cardiovascular disease have not shown equally positive results and further exploration of CDDO and its derivatives is needed to put these shortcomings into context for the purpose of future therapeutic modalities.

Keywords CDDO · dh404 · TFEA · Nrf2 · Bardoxolone · CDDO-Me · CDDO-Im · Vascular · Hepatotoxic · Cardiorenal · Apoptosis · Keap1

B.J. Mathis
Department of Cell Biology and Anatomy, University of South Carolina School of Medicine, Columbia, SC 29208, USA

T. Cui (✉)
Department of Cell Biology and Anatomy, University of South Carolina School of Medicine, 6439 Garners Ferry Rd., Columbia, SC 29209, USA
e-mail: Taixing.Cui@uscmed.sc.edu

S.C. Gupta et al. (eds.), *Drug Discovery from Mother Nature*,
Advances in Experimental Medicine and Biology 929,
DOI 10.1007/978-3-319-41342-6_13

Definitions

CDDO	2-cyano-3,12-dioxoolean-1,9-dien-28-oic acid
CDDO-Im	CDDO imidazolide
CDDO-Me	CDDO-methyl ester
CDDO-dhTFEA	CDDO-dihydrotrifluoroamide

1 Introduction

Triterpenoids are natural saponin compounds (such as cholesterol and phytosterols) with a multi-carbon skeleton that can be manipulated synthetically, adding various chemical groups for functionality. CDDO, or 2-cyano-3,12-dioxoolean-1,9-dien-28-oic acid, is a synthetic triterpenoid derived from oleanolic acid that was purposely constructed for anti-inflammatory purposes in macrophages and has, over time, been modified with methyl, amine, and imidazolide groups to further affect various signaling pathways such as FLIP/TRAIL, caspase, SMAD, and mTOR. However, the primary target of CDDO and its related compounds is the Kelch-like erythroid cell-derived protein with CNC homology-associated protein 1 (Keap1) that regulates nuclear factor erythroid 2-related factor 2 (Nrf2) that, in turn, acts as a master transcription factor for upregulation of antioxidant response genes such as heme oxygenase-1 (HO-1) and NAD(P)H:quinone oxidoreductase (NQO1). Modulation of Nrf2 by CDDO and related compounds has been repeatedly shown in the literature to positively affect a multitude of disease states in animal models, including amyotrophic lateral sclerosis (ALS), various cancers (breast, prostate, etc.), inflammatory shock, and cardiovascular damage. Phases I and II trials with CDDO in chronic kidney disease have shown much promise. However, well-controlled Phase I cancer trials in humans have not shown dramatic improvements in the disease outcomes. The reasons for these variable results are not well understood, and much work remains to be done in determining the minute details of CDDO-affected signaling pathways in humans. This review will explore a wide range of the literature to provide a framework of understanding about CDDO's chemical properties, its signaling targets, and therapeutic efficacy in animal models. Although CDDO compounds may not yet be the "silver bullet" for some diseases, the clear effect of CDDO treatment on crucial cellular pathways in multiple disease models makes it useful in the laboratory and more work may yet find a derivative compound that proves efficacious in treating human disease.

2 Chemical Properties and Pharmacokinetics

2.1 Chemical Synthesis and Characteristics

Oleanolic acid has been used in China as a therapy for hepatitis and serves as the backbone of CDDO [1]. CDDO was first reported in a series of papers by Honda et al. that stepwise-converted oleanolic and ursolic acids into a compound capable of both inhibiting inducible nitric oxide synthase (iNOS) and cyclooxygenase-2 (COX-2) production in mouse macrophages and growth in an NRP.152 prostate cell line [2–4]. CDDO was originally synthesized from modification of the A and C rings of the saponin compounds with 1-en-3-one functionality, but the C-2 position was found to be critical for activity of the compound [3]. Further studies revealed that α,β-unsaturated carbonyl moieties boost the effect of the compound by several fold [5]. Briefly, oleanolic acid was formylated in the presence of sodium methoxide, with tetrahydrofuran (THF) added. After an isoxazole intermediate was formed via methoxide cleavage and alkali hydrolysis, the nitrile intermediate. A nitrile intermediate was reacted in dimethylfuran (DMF) with lithium iodide in a halogenolysis reaction to form CDDO [3]. A later report from Fu and Gribble [6] introduced a scalable and much more efficient synthesis protocol for CDDO-Me that could prove useful in clinical studies. The polar structure of CDDO lends well to solubility in DMSO for the laboratory while human trials used microcrystalline preparations in gelatin capsules [7]. Functional groups can be added to CDDO, such as a C28 methyl ester, imidazolide, and various amides (ethyl, diethyl, and trifluoroethyl amides) [8, 9]. Each of these compounds has specific kinetics and, taken as a whole group, offer an arsenal of compounds to test in the laboratory.

2.2 Pharmacokinetics of CDDO

CDDO, as synthesized by Honda and Suh [3], has an IC50 of just 0.0004 μM in mouse macrophages, over a thousand times stronger than its parent compound oleanolic acid. Derivatives such as CDDO-Me and CDDO-Im have induced strong NQO1 activity at single doses of as little as 10 μmol/kg in mice while other reports have seen 5–130 nM inhibitory effects in tumor cell lines with CDDO amides [8, 9].

A study undertaken by Noker et al. [10] in rats and dogs found that CDDO is eliminated from plasma in 2 stages, with a mean half-life of 0.06 h for α-phase and 1.95 h for β-phase in rats with total clearance being roughly 9 $L/m^2/h$. Dogs showed a much faster clearance with an α-phase of 0.02 h and a β-phase of 0.65 h with a total clearance of 44.6 $L/m^2/h$ [10] Total results indicated linear pharmacokinetics with side effects (diarrhea, piloerection) but no toxicity even at doses of 50 $mg/m^2/h$ with total maximum tolerated dosages of 2160 mg/m^2 in rats and 6000 mg/m^2 in dogs [10]. This low toxicity with lack of catastrophic side effects makes CDDO an ideal compound for in vivo animal studies. Further studies on

Table 1 Animal studies involving CDDO

Drug	Animal model	Studies and references
CDDO-Me	Murine	Lung injury [125], tumor vaccination [106], colon cancer [93, 126], breast cancer [101, 102], lung cancer [99, 127, 128], pancreatic cancer [129], prostate cancer [35, 94, 103], Leukemia [87], immunosuppression [130], kidneys [41, 80], nephritis [77], gene profiling [8, 26, 78, 109, 131]
CDDO-Im	Murine	Obesity [65], gene profiling [52], chondrogenesis [62], kidneys [76], lung cancer [99, 127], colitis [132], liver damage/hepatotoxicity [98, 133–135], immune neoplasms [46], retinal death [89, 91], neural ischemia [136], diabetes [137]
CDDO-TFEA/CDDO-EA	Murine	Retinal injury [59], ALS [138], lung cancer [99], Liver injury [133, 139]

methodology for bioanalytical methods for in vivo studies with CDDO found that its electrophilic nature caused it to react with glutathione (GSH) and nucleophilic groups in proteins as well as *N*-acetylcysteine, forming covalently adducted metabolites that can be measured with protein precipitation, Edman degradation, and ammonium hydroxide [11]. Clearly, CDDO's main mode of chemical action is for the functional electrophilic groups to attack sulfhydryl and cysteine moieties on target proteins. A clinical trial in humans by Hong et al. [7] explored the more complex pharmacokinetics in chronic kidney disease patients treated with CDDO-Me, finding a maximum tolerated dosage to be 900 mg/day and a maximum peak plasma time of 4 h with a mean half-life of about 39 ± 20 h. Hong et al. concluded that 900 mg/day was the appropriate dosage for any further Phase II trials. Clinical testing has been done in human volunteers with an amorphous spray-dried dispersion (SDD) microcrystalline version of CDDO-Me to increase bioavailability and this was found to be superior in bioavailability to the microcrystalline version used in the Hong trial [12] (Table 1).

3 Signaling Pathways Affected by CDDO

3.1 Antioxidant Response and Nrf2 Regulation

Although CDDO compounds may directly interact with proteins in multiple signaling pathways, the primary mode of CDDO action is the upregulation of Nrf2. Nrf2 is in the Cap "n" Collar (CNC) family of basic leucine zipper (bZip) transcription factors constitutively expressed in the cell and resident in the cytoplasm [13, 14]. The forked Keap1, a substrate adaptor of the E3 ubiquitin ligase Cullin3 complex, contains two large spheres (β-propeller regions) that repress Nrf2 constitutively and represents the most popular target of treatments to modulate Nrf2 activity [15–17]. Upon ubiquitination, Nrf2 is rapidly degraded by the proteasome, but CDDO (and some other small electrophilic molecules) can bind to a key cysteine residue in the Broad complex, Tramtrack, and Bric-a-Brac (BTB) domain of Keap1 to inhibit ubiquitination and proteasomal degradation of Nrf2 [15, 18–20]. Other signaling pathways of Keap1 regulation have been reported, specifically that $p21^{Cip1/WAF1}$ can compete with Nrf2 for Keap1 binding, increasing levels of free Nrf2 to localize to the nucleus and that p62 directly binds to Keap1 on three specific arginine residues to inhibit Keap-1-mediated Nrf2 ubiquitination (linking Nrf2 and autophagy) [21, 22]. Whether or not these alternate pathways may be affected by CDDO is still unclear. If Keap1 is active, the half-life of Nrf2 is very short, on the order of about 20 min [23]. Although this may make probing for nominal levels of Nrf2 difficult, the rapid turnover allows for rapid response. Once translocated to the nucleus, Nrf2 binds with the adaptor protein Maf and binds to antioxidant response elements (ARE) which attracts CREB and p300 to form a complex that can attract RNA polymerases to transcribe antioxidant genes such as superoxide dismutase (SOD), glutathione peroxidase (GPx), gamma-glutamylcysteine synthetase (γ-GCS), HO-1, and NQO1 [13, 24–27]. The Keap1-Nrf2 axis in antioxidant response has been extensively reviewed and, as CDDO has a potent ability to effect a conformational change in Keap1 to reduces its ability to catalyze Nrf2 for K48 ubiquitination, this axis serves as the basis for CDDO's use in disease therapy models [13, 16, 24–26, 28]. Therefore, it is safe to say that any use of CDDO will involve Nrf2 as an upstream modulator of genes of interest, made possible by Nrf2's master ability to affect downstream pathways by ARE activity. Note that natural compounds such as α-lipoic acid and polyphenols like quercetin have also been extensively shown to increase Nrf2 activity by upstream pathways such as PI3 K/Akt, especially in liver and cardiovascular studies [29–33] (Fig. 1).

4 Reactive Oxygen Species and Cell Death: The Primary Target of CDDO

4.1 Apoptosis and Necrosis: CDDO Affects Cell Death via Nrf2

The two known types of cell death are apoptosis and necrosis. Cellular damage from reactive oxygen species (ROS) or nitrogen species (NOS) can affect mitochondria, membranes, and cell nuclei, triggering checkpoint genes such as p53 to induce apoptosis or system wide damage, resulting in necrosis [34]. In apoptosis, death occurs in an "implosive" style with programmed and sequential events shutting down the cell to avoid damage to surrounding cells. Necrosis, on the other hand, can be considered "explosive," where cellular debris (especially highly reactive mitochondrial cytochrome c) and cytokine release cause inflammation and

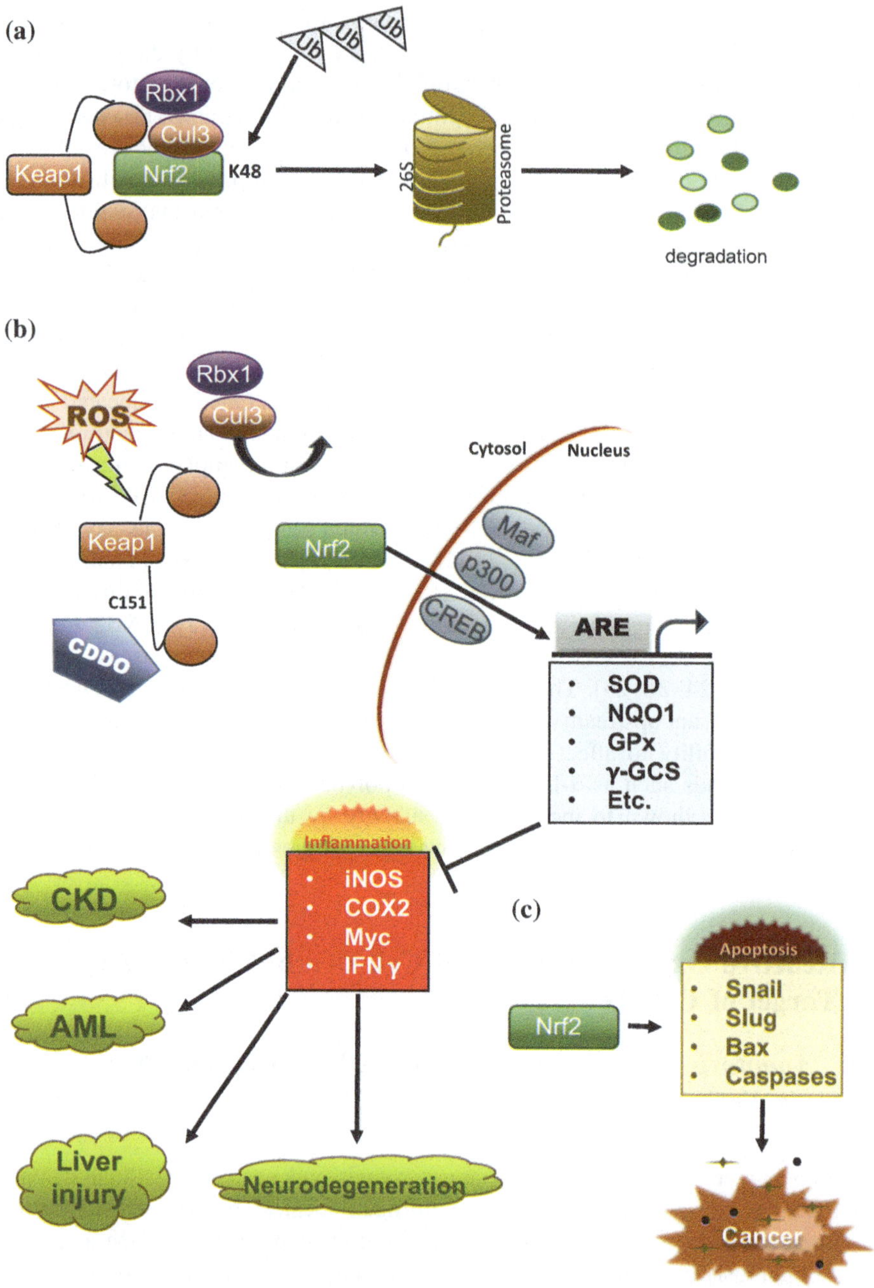

Fig. 1 **a** The Keap1-Nrf2 regulatory pathway features Cul3-mediated K48-linked polyubiquitination of Nrf2, causing subsequent degradation in the proteasome. **b** Damage by ROS or interaction with CDDO on Cysteine 151 of Keap1 releases Nrf2 to the nucleus, where it upregulates antioxidant protective factors that can counter inflammation and related disease states. **c** Nrf2 regulates many apoptotic factors in cancer cells that it does not in healthy cells. This may be due to defects in cellular metabolism that render cancer cells uniquely vulnerable to Nrf2-mediated apoptosis

damage to cascade into surrounding tissue [35]. Nrf2 is directly involved in reducing necrotic cell death by upregulation of antioxidant factors such as HO-1, super oxide dismutase (SOD), and NQO1, but can actually cause apoptosis in cancer cells by affecting the upregulation of apoptotic factors such as Snail, slug, TCF-/ZEB1, and Bax [27, 36]. If Nrf2 can control so many factors critical in apoptosis and necrosis, it stands to reason that upregulation of Nrf2 by CDDO compounds may provide protection and/or ablation of cytotoxic ROS-induced death in normal cells while causing cancerous or abnormal cells to die.

In prostate cancer cells, CDDO-Me was reported to activate caspases 3, 8, and 9 while disrupting NF-κB signaling through direct inhibition of iκB kinase, killing the cancer cells [37, 38]. It was also documented that CDDO-Me induced prostate cancer cell death via suppression of Akt [39]. Similar results were found in ovarian cancer cells and rat kidney reperfusion injury [40–42]. In acute myeloid leukemia (AML) cells, CDDO-Me has been reported to suppress phosphorylation of ERK1/2 through the activation of p38/MAPK (43). Intriguingly, another report showed that, in AML, CDDO-Me could sensitize cells to pro-apoptotic TRAIL while downregulating anti-apoptotic FLIP levels and that CDDO strongly upregulates caspase 8 [44, 45]. In iMycEμ mice that are prone to B and plasma cell neoplasms (viz. lymphoma), CDDO-Im treatment caused upregulation of Fmo4 and P450 oxygenases with downregulation of c-Myc and apoptosis [46]. Yates et al. demonstrated that CDDO-Im mitigates the aflatoxin-induced oxidative stress in the liver with an increase in GSTA2, GSTA5, AFAR, and EPHX1 antioxidant genes [47, 48]. Bey et al. [49] reported that NQO1, which is a primary transcriptional target of Nrf2 and is upregulated upon CDDO treatment, is required for PARP1-programmed necrosis in breast cancers, which can be apoptosis resistant. On the flip side of ROS-induced injury and cellular protection, Li et al. [50] have reported that doxorubicin-induced cardiac necrosis can be ameliorated by Nrf2 increases. Treatment with CDDO could provide the increased Nrf2 necessary to ablate doxorubicin-induced cardiac injury. In the normal liver, caspases intimately associated with apoptosis and necrosis have been shown to be downregulated by lipoic acid which activates Nrf2, especially caspase-3 [31]. In normal hearts and in early-stage heart disease, Nrf2 is also very protective [16, 27, 51]. It is therefore important to note that CDDO compounds in published studies show protective effects to normal or injured cells but kill cancerous cells. Interestingly, a report that compared Keap1 knockout mice to CDDO-Im-treated mice show that both genetic and pharmacological activation of Nrf2 regulates many metabolism genes, including lipid and carbohydrate metabolism (particularly the pentose phosphate pathway to sustain Nrf2 activity) [52, 53]. This indicates that cancerous cells, which often show defects in metabolic pathways, may be adversely affected by Nrf2 upregulation forcing upregulation of apoptotic factors in these and not normal cells or cells with minor injury. In fact, a recent report by Qin et al. [54] has found a solid link between the action of Nrf2 and the functional status of autophagy: Nrf2 activation is cardioprotective when myocardial autophagy is intact whereas Nrf2 acts as a mediator of cardiac maladaptive remodeling and dysfunction when myocardial autophagy is impaired. Bernstein et al. showed a similar effect in B-cell lymphoma cells via CDDO treatment/Nrf2 activation and inhibition of the Lon protease system, which clears mitochondrial proteins [55–57].

This proves that a critical link exists between metabolism (specifically autophagy) and the effect of Nrf2 on a cell. Upon Nrf2 activation, normal cells (and even the retina) with normal autophagic function receive protection in the form of upregulated antioxidant defense while abnormal cells with autophagy impairment may see deleterious effects [58, 59]. Other oleanolic acid derivatives have also been shown to cause this induction of autophagy in normal cells that, in cells with dysfunctional autophagic machinery, can cause early death [60, 61].

5 Other Targets of CDDO: Heat Shock Protein, Telomerase, and MTOR

Although the strongest transcriptional effects from CDDO treatment come from Nrf2 activation, there have been several other direct targets reported in the literature. Suh et al. [62] reported that CDDO-Im and CDDO-ethyl amide were able to induce chondrogenesis in newborn mice by upregulating SOX9 and collagen. However, as there was no in-depth exploration as to the effect of Nrf2 on these genes, it is yet unclear as to whether or not CDDO had direct effects on upstream elements in the chondrogenic pathway. Telomerase (hTERT) activity is a critical part of cancer cell proliferation and there is a report that CDDO-Me targets hTERT in prostate cancer cells, with knockdown of hTERT increasing apoptosis upon CDDO treatment [63]. Heat shock protein 90 (hsp90) was found by Qin et al. [64] to directly target hsp90 in an ovarian cancer cell model, inhibiting it and reducing cell proliferation. This was shown by thermal shift assay and can be blocked by dithiothreitol [64]. Although several putative targets have been reported, only the hsp90 interaction has been shown to be a direct effect of CDDO and not as a Nrf2-mediated effect. Although these several reports have shown some potential of CDDO to target alternate pathways directly, the majority of evidence points to a primarily Nrf2-mediated mechanism of action. However, the specificity of CDDO for Nrf2 makes it useful in isolating Nrf2-related pathways and mechanisms with little interference from other upstream regulators.

6 Diseases

The goal of CDDO as a therapy is to exploit its ability to upregulate Nrf2 and Nrf2's ability to protect healthy cells from necrosis while destroying abnormal ones by apoptosis. Because CDDO and its derivatives are fairly nontoxic, they lend themselves well to testing as therapies for various diseases.

6.1 Cardiac Disease/Vascular Dysfunction

Much work has been done in animal models with CDDO in the prevention of cardiopulmonary disease and injury. Sussan et al. [16] reported that, in mice, cigarette smoke-induced cardiac dysfunction and emphysema modeling chronic obstructive pulmonary disease (COPD) could be reduced by CDDO-Im treatment. CDDO-Im has also been shown to ameliorate obesity in mice fed a high-fat diet, showing potential for reducing a major cause of cardiovascular disease [65]. CDDO could also play a key role in attenuating lesion formation and loss of tone in vascular disease, especially as FLIP/TRAIL and Myc, lesion forming factors regulated by Nrf2, play a role in VSMC-mediated neointimal formation [46, 66–68]. Wang reviews several preclinical trials that indicate that CDDO-Me can reduce blood vessel inflammatory responses by regulating the endothelin pathway and that this may be due to involvement of NF-κB in the endothelin pathway which Nrf2 can counter [69]. It is well established in the literature that iNOS and cytokines like IFNγ produced by macrophages activated by periodontal diseases or LPS can cause inflammatory damage in blood vessels, recruiting more macrophages in an M1 response and amplifying vascular damage [3, 70, 71]. CDDO-dhTFEA (dh404) and CDDO-Me have been shown to suppress the inflammatory responses in macrophages, thereby providing protection to the vascular system [71, 72]. Regarding future cardiac studies, vital cardiac adaptation has been shown to rely on a Nrf2/autophagy axis, while clearance of toxic proteins relies on Nrf2, making CDDO treatment a distinct possibility to upregulate those protective features [51, 73].

Studies in humans with CDDO compounds have been completed up to Phase II. A review by Wang lists several Phase I studies that evaluated several pharmacokinetic parameters of CDDO-Me administration in healthy volunteers [69]. Subsequent Phase II trials have either been terminated or withdrawn. A CDDO-Me evaluation in patients with pulmonary hypertension is currently recruiting patients (clinicaltrials.gov NCT02036970). Clearly, CDDO usage in humans carries some kind of cardiovascular risk and the knowledge of autophagic sufficiency for CDDO efficacy in the cardiovascular system may provide a critical insight on targeting upstream regulators of both Nrf2 and autophagy.

6.2 Kidney Disease

Another realm of intense research into CDDO and related compounds is in chronic kidney disease (CKD). Impacting almost 13 % of the US population, CKD is a reduction in estimated glomerular filtration rate (eGFR) along with albuminuria (protein in the urine) that eventually results in a need for renal replacement and sequelae such as anemia and metabolic bone disease [74]. In fact, cardiovascular complications from CKD anemia such as left ventricular hypertrophy due to maladaptation can affect the kidneys further, creating a vicious loop of escalating damage termed "cardiorenal anemia syndrome" that drastically reduces patient long-term survivability by 30 % [74]. To ameliorate the multiple effects of CKD, CDDO in its multiple forms has been extensively tested in animals and clinical trials have been held in humans. In rats, CKD studies have shown improvement in the areas of ROS, inflammation, and fibrosis, with CDDO-TFEA and CDDO-Me [41, 75]. Liu et al. [76] have found CDDO-Im to protect kidneys from ischemic reperfusion injury, which models the damage of CKD, and this protection is entirely dependent on Nrf2 as Nrf2-knockout mice treated with CDDO-Im showed no improvement. Wu et al. [77] showed that CDDO was able to ameliorate lupus-induced nephritis by reduction in ERK, STAT3, and Nf-κB, resulting in decreased CD4 T cell activation. Shelton et al. [78] conducted an extensive proteomic and transcriptomic analysis of wild type and Nrf2 knockout mice treated with CDDO-Me and found that CDDO-Me via Nrf2 upregulation positively regulated proteins related to redox homeostasis and NADPH regulation. The authors also concluded that CDDO would be useful in countering xenobiotics (such as cisplatin or cyclosporin) that generate large amounts of nephrotoxic molecules as well as chronic kidney insults from heavy metals [78, 79]. This clearly points to CDDO's potential to protect the kidneys during chemotherapy which Aleksunes et al. [80] explored in mice, finding that CDDO-Im could protect from cisplatin-induced nephrotoxicity. On the structural level, Aminzadeh et al. [81] found that CDDO-TFEA could ameliorate damage due to the cardiorenal axis with restoration of endothelial function in CKD rat aortic rings as measured by acetylcholine-mediated relaxation response. Additionally, CKD-induced aortic upregulation of MCP-1 angiotensin II and NADPH oxidases was all ameliorated by CDDO-TFEA [81].

These animal studies serve to illustrate that CDDO compounds are of great value in renal protection against chronic diseases. Indeed, in a Phase I trial conducted by Hong et al. in 2012, 47 patients diagnosed with solid tumors and lymphomas were given CDDO-Me in microcrystalline form for 21 consecutive days out of a 28-day cycle, with multiple cycles and saw an increase in eGFR estimated at 26 % in all patients with a 33.9 % increase in the highest dosage [7]. Clearly, CDDO-Me improved kidney health that may have been ravaged by antineoplastics and other chemotherapeutics. A Reata Pharmaceuticals-funded Phase II trial from 2008 to 2009 (clincaltrials.gov NCT00811889) found significant improvement in eGFR in patients treated with CDDO-Me at 24 weeks, with up to 10.5 additional ml (per minute per 1.73 m^2 body surface area) in the 75 mg dosage range [82]. Another Phase II study in 2010 by Reata (clinicaltrials.gov NCT01053936) evaluating CDDO-Me in eGFR in type 2 diabetes as well as another study (clinicaltrials.gov NCT00664027) was completed with no published data. Unfortunately, after initial Phase II success, a Phase III trial in 2014 (clinicaltrials.gov NCT013516750) was terminated due to an increase in cardiovascular adverse events, even though eGFR, renal function, and body weight improved significantly [83] (Table 2).

Table 2 Human studies involving CDDO-Me

Disease	References
Type 2 diabetes/CKD	[12, 82, 83]
Solid tumors	[7]

Table 3 Oncogenic targets of CDDO compounds

Target	References
Akt	[39, 100]
P38/MAPK	[43]
FLIP/TRAIL	[44, 45]
p42	[85]
hTERT	[63, 94]
mTOR	[95, 100]
ICAM	[96]
PDP Polymerase	[96]
Nf-κB	[38, 42]
BRCA1	[102]
Bcl	[103]
Hsp90	[64]

6.3 AML

Leukemia, especially acute myeloid leukemia, is defined as an increase in myeloid cells within the bone marrow and a subsequent insufficiency of the hematopoietic cells due to their failure to mature [84]. Ito et al. [45] reported that human AML cells underwent caspase 8-mediated apoptosis when treated with CDDO. Subsequent reports found that CDDO-Me could induce apoptosis in acute myelogenous leukemia, suppress MAPK in these cells, increase TRAIL sensitization, downregulate FLIP, promote hematopoietic progenitor expansion, and upregulate p42 CCAAT enhancer-binding protein alpha in granulocytes [43, 44, 85–87]. Although not yet used in human clinical trials, CDDO compounds show a clear effect in promoting aberrant leukocytes to undergo apoptosis while pushing differentiation/maturation of immature cells forward (Table 3).

6.4 Retinal Blindness

Damage to the eyes of diabetic patients is a well-known diabetic complication. Age-related macular degeneration due to oxidative damage may also be a concern in a rapidly aging population. A cytoprotective effect of CDDO-TFEA, CDDO-Im, and CDDO-Me was seen in retinal cell lines to protect against oxidation-induced retinal degeneration and the lipid phosphatase PTEN was inhibited in mice treated with CDDO-TFEA [59]. Wei et al. [88] found that Nrf2 protects both neurons and capillaries from retinal ischemia-reperfusion injury so the action of CDDO is protective to the retina via upregulation of Nrf2. Xu et al. [89] verified this in a separate report, showing that Nrf2 knockout mice experienced a greater loss of retinal neuron function. Other reports verified that Nrf2 can modulate cigarette smoke-induced complement activation in the retina and that Nrf2 is a critical modulator of oxidation-induced death in the retinal ganglion [90, 91]. Experiments in astrocytes, microglia, and neurons showed that all CDDO compounds are protective against oxidative damage and upregulate antioxidant genes via Nrf2 [92]. Taken together, these results show that CDDO may hold promise for protecting the brain from age-related oxidative stress as well as treating such chronic eye diseases as macular degeneration and tobacco smoke-induced injury.

6.5 Cancer

CDDO compounds have been rigorously tested in multiple rodent cancer models, as its ability to force abnormal cells into apoptosis could form the basis of a chemotherapeutic approach that, unlike current xenobiotics and chemotherapeutics, also simultaneously protects the liver and kidneys. CDDO-Me has been used in colitis-associated colon cancer models in mice to interrupt inflammation-driven downregulation of prostaglandin dehydrogenase as well as the entire suite of inflammatory cytokines such as IL-6, iNOS, IL-1β, and TNFα [93]. A study by Alabran et al. that used CDDO compounds against multiple human neuroblastoma cell lines found that these cells underwent rapid arrest in S-phase, Bax was activated (apoptosis induction), and that CDDO compounds were effective against these cells in low concentrations (IC_{50} 5–170 nM) [9]. CDDO-Me has also been found to downregulate telomerase activity (hTERT) and induce cell death in pancreatic cancer cell lines [94]. However, it is unclear as to whether this hTERT inhibition is a direct interaction or an Nrf2-associated effect. A review by Shanmugam et al. details oleanolic acid derivatives and the genes they primarily affect, such as mTOR, AKT, STAT3, ICAM1, and PADP polymerase—all of which are critical for regulating cellular homeostasis and which may be compromised in transformed cells [95, 96]. As cancer cells use vascular endothelial growth factor (VEGF)-driven angiogenesis to form new capillary feeder networks, it is interesting to note that CDDO-Me has been reported in mice to suppress Matrigel plug angiogenesis in picomolar concentrations [18]. Coupled with induced arrest and apoptosis, a one-two punch of cutting off the blood supply and then inducing tumor cell death is an attractive prospect for a chemotherapeutic drug. It is important to note that CDDO compounds may harm cancerous cells but it must be remembered that normal cells are protected against insult [97]. Again, this may be due to a need for autophagic competency to accompany increased Nrf2 levels in order to be protected or in the mitochondrial Lon protease system, which is inhibited by CDDO [57]. In a rat liver cancer model involving aflatoxin, CDDO-Im proved a powerful and complete protection, with damage almost completely ablated by treatment [98]. Liby et al. [99] found that CDDO-Me and CDDO-ethyl amide could protect A/J mice against vinyl carbamate-induced lung cancer. This proves that CDDO compounds may be a powerful prophylactic against specific types of environmental carcinogens that transform cells by ROS damage.

Table 4 Anticancer mechanisms in cell lines treated with CDDO

Cell types	Cell lines	Mechanism	References
Human neuroblastoma	NB1691, 15 N, LAN-1, SK-N-AS	Apoptosis	[9]
Pancreatic cancer	MiaPaCa2, Panc-1	hTERT	[94]
Kaposi's sarcoma	KS-IMM	Angiogenesis	[18]
Ovarian cancer	CNCaP, PC-3, OVCAR-3, OVCAR-5, SK-OV3, MDAH-2774	Akt, Nf-κB, PPARγ	[39, 100]
Ovarian cancer	H08910	Hsp90	[64]
Esophageal squamous	Ec109, KYSE70, Het1A	Apoptosis and autophagy	[36]
Human breast cancer	SUM159, MDA-MB-231	Stem cell signaling	[104]
Breast cancer and macrophage-like	MCF-7, MDA-MB-231, RAW264.7	Apoptosis and autophagy	[60, 61, 104]

Not only can CDDO protect against somatic cancers but increasing evidence shows that it is effective against gender-specific cancers, as well. Interestingly, a report by Gao et al. revealed that CDDO-Me controls apoptosis in ovarian cancer by inhibiting AKT, NF-κB, and mTOR signaling without affecting PDK1 kinase or PP2A activity [39, 100]. Mammary carcinogenesis in polyoma middle T mice was slowed by CDDO-Me, extending lifespan by roughly 5 weeks, and BRCA1-mediated cancers in mice are delayed by CDDO-Me, as well [101, 102]. In prostate cancer, CDDO-Me regulates Bcl and other survival signals in TRAMP mice and hTERT can also be targeted by CDDO-Me in prostate cancer [63, 103]. There is also evidence that Hsp90 might be targeted by CDDO-Me in cancer cells [64].

There is a recent theory of cancer stem cells, which are cells from a tumor that possess stem cell abilities to differentiate into different cancer types. Current reports show that CDDO-Me can suppress stemness in esophageal cancer lines and triple negative breast cancer cells [36, 104].

Other oleanolic acid derivatives, such as SZC017, CDDO-2P-Im, CDDO-3P-Im, and HIMOXOL, are being evaluated for anticancer effects such as apoptotic induction ability and cancer cell arrest [60, 61, 105]. Also, vehicles for efficient delivery of CDDO by nanoparticles have been explored [106] (Table 4).

There have been several clinical trials for cancer treatment using CDDO-Me. Hong et al. accomplished a Phase I trial which showed promise in hepatoprotection but did not show significant improvement in tumor size as seen in animal models [7]. However, two Phase II studies in patients with advanced solid tumors (clinicaltrials.gov NCT00508807, NCT00529438) were completed but results were not disclosed. Although in vitro and animal models show great promise in using CDDO compounds as cancer treatments, a lack of published data in the two completed clinical trials makes it difficult to evaluate CDDO as a promising chemotherapeutic.

6.6 Liver

The liver is the most critical organ in the body for metabolic processes and detoxification by the cytochrome enzymatic pathways. This makes it susceptible to not just ROS damage but other hepatotoxic molecules that may be generated by medicines, chemical compounds, or alcohols. Shah et al. [107] found that CDDO-Im could protect HepG2 cells against acrolein-induced toxicity by GSH upregulation as well as reducing levels of death markers such as protein carbonyls. A report by Liu as far back as 1993 established that oleanolic acid could rescue large-dosage acetaminophen liver damage in mice and upregulate GSH levels [1]. This led to the logical conclusion that oleanolic acid derivates with even higher Nrf2 stimulating activity could protect the liver even better. As such, CDDO-dhTFEA was reported to induce hepatoprotective genes including thioredoxin reductase (Txnrd), glutamate cysteine ligase catalytic and modifier subunits (Gclc and Gclm), gamma-glutamyl transpeptidase 1 (Ggt1), heme oxygenase-1 (Ho-1), and NAD(P)H quinone oxidoreductase 1 (Nqo1), while also increasing bile flow in rats, as bile is related to GSH levels [108]. A review by Klaassen collates over 15 separate studies in rats and mice where hepatotoxic compounds such as acetaminophen, concavalin A, and high-fat diets saw their damage ameliorated by CDDO-Im or oleanolic acid [26]. This clearly indicates that Nrf2 is strongly hepatoprotective, especially against hepatic damage induced by medications for chronic diseases (e.g., large doses of acetaminophen for arthritis) or metabolic syndrome. Also of note in the Klaassen review is a summary of 6 Nrf2 knockout rodent models for use in studying liver disease and CDDO treatment, such as carbon tetrachloride and arsenic [26]. A comprehensive proteomic report by Walsh et al. [109] has found that CDDO-Me in mice induces cytochrome P4502A5, glutathione-S-transferase, UDP-glucose-6-dehydrogenase, and epoxide hydrolase, prompting the liver to begin detoxification with P450 enzymes while simultaneously protecting from subsequent free radical activity by inducing antioxidant response enzymes. Most importantly, they found that 97 % of the proteins induced by CDDO-Me were specific for Nrf2 signaling, reassuring researchers that non-Nrf2-targeting effects during treatment would be kept to a minimum [78]. As seen in other organs, CDDO compounds provide strong hepatoprotective abilities that may be useful in combatting damage from medications, environmental chronic exposure, and metabolic syndrome.

6.7 Sepsis/Sickle Cell/Lupus

The presence of lipopolysaccharides (LPS) in the bloodstream may produce an aggressive immune response including inflammation. LPS, along with active bacteria, may also induce a massive cytokine release, dilating the capillary network, and causing a severe and often fatal drop in blood pressure. This septic shock is often fatal. Noel et al. [110] explored ex vivo Nrf2 activation by CDDO-Me administration to monocytes obtained from human patients with septic shock. Their results showed a differential activation between purified and peripheral monocytes, with purified monocytes decreasing in IL-6 production and peripheral monocytes increasing IL-6 production [110]. Another study using neutrophils and peripheral monocytes showed strong activation of antioxidant response and attenuation of inflammatory cytokine response (TNFα,MLP, etc.) upon treatment with CDDO-Im and CDDO-Me, revealing that Nrf2 activation may be protective against challenge with LPS [111]. An interesting report by Keleku-Lukwete et al. [112] showed that Nrf2 could modulate the clearance of plasma heme in a mouse sickle cell model with administration of CDDO-Im relieving organ inflammation and failure in the model mice. These studies indicate that CDDO can be useful in sepsis as well as in chronic inflammatory diseases such as sickle cell anemia.

7 Conclusion

Oleanolic acid has been used in China as traditional medicine for liver problems and can be found in many plants and foods [113]. Having shown promise in multiple organ systems, CDDO compounds (by virtue of the ability to strongly upregulate Nrf2) seemed set to serve as a panacea for chronic diseases. In the liver, kidneys, retina, blood, and bone marrow, CDDO works to upregulate Nrf2, which is highly protective against oxidative damage and also to modulate a host of signaling pathways, including Akt/PI3 K, mTOR, FLIP/TRAIL, and Myc. CDDO-mediated upregulation of Nrf2 in these organs and in cancer cell lines and animal models induces apoptosis of aberrant cells and protects normal cells against insult from both oxidative stress and environmental insult.

Unfortunately, CDDO has not shown promise in the amelioration of cardiovascular disease or human cancers. Although in vitro and in vivo animal studies have shown excellent results, systemic effects of CDDO have not been fully elucidated and, in human clinical trials, CDDO has actually shown deleterious effects in the heart. Although multiple studies have shown that, at least early on in heart disease, Nrf2 upregulation is cardioprotective, a seminal finding in mice has shown very strong evidence that a lack of Nrf2 response in later stage heart disease is actually protective [51, 114, 115]. Recent literature has dubbed this effect as "reductive stress" (RS) as opposed to "oxidative stress" (OS) and that too many antioxidants can actually cause damage to the tissue as they reduce (donate electrons to reduce charge as opposed to steal them and add charge) [116]. DNA, with a negatively charged backbone, could be easily damaged by reductive attack, damaging it repair. Clinical reports are filtering in that finding reductive stress can occur in post-surgical complications such as restenosis of balloon angioplasty and stenting (BAS) and post-exercise [117, 118]. Additionally, in cancer, high antioxidant responses may be protective to the cancer cells against ROS-inducing chemotherapy as well as ROS generated by their much higher basal metabolic rate. Nrf2 can also cause upregulation of genes that metabolize chemotherapeutics as well as upregulate the pentose phosphate pathway, increasing tumor cell proliferation and survival [28, 52, 53, 78].

Intriguingly, recent reports have found that the functional integrity of autophagy is needed to reap positive benefits from Nrf2 regulation, with upregulation of Nrf2 and autophagic dysfunction associated with negative outcomes [119]. It may be that Nrf2 upregulation can increase scavenging of free radicals but can also damage cells by reductive stress from which they cannot recover without autophagy to recycle reduced membrane or other cell components. In fact, since some antioxidants can be more damaging than free radicals (e.g., ECGC as reported by Lu et al.), it is entirely possible that a lack of autophagy is a necrotic death sentence for a reductively damaged cell [120]. In this case, it would be critical to regulate both Nrf2 and autophagy simultaneously by regulating a common upstream element. The deubiquitinase CYLD is a master key in the NF-κB pathway regulating inflammation and immune development, but has been shown to affect many other pathways such as TLR-mediated signaling, Wnt/Catenin, and Snail [121]. CYLD has been recently shown in a seminal report to regulate Nrf2 transcriptionally, repressing it via downregulation of the p38 MAPK/ERK pathway [122]. If CYLD could also be shown to negatively regulate autophagy, then it would be possible to downregulate CYLD locally in the heart and preserve autophagic function along with Nrf2 activation which would be the best of both worlds. Since there are critical autophagic components, such as p62 and HDAC6, that are K63 polyubiquitinated, it may be possible that CYLD can control autophagy by enzymatic action on p62 or some other component of the pathway [123, 124]. In conclusion, CDDO holds some promise for certain types of chronic diseases, but cardiovascular and cancer therapies might benefit if master upstream elements like CYLD could be exploited to control both Nrf2 and autophagic mechanisms to prevent damage from reductive stress.

References

1. Liu J, Liu Y, Madhu C, Klaassen CD (1993) Protective effects of oleanolic acid on acetaminophen-induced hepatotoxicity in mice. J Pharmacol Exp Ther 266(3):1607–1613
2. Honda T, Finlay HJ, Gribble GW, Suh N (1997) MBS. New enone derivatives of oleanolic acid and ursolic acid as inhibitors of nitric oxide production in mouse macrophages. Bioorg Med Chem Lett 7(13):1623–1628
3. Honda T, Suh N (1998) Bioorganic Med Chem Lett 8:2711–2714
4. Suh N, Wang Y, Honda T, Gribble GW, Dmitrovsky E, Hickey WF et al (1999) A novel synthetic oleanane triterpenoid, 2-cyano-3,12-dioxoolean-1,9-dien-28-oic acid, with potent differentiating, antiproliferative, and anti-inflammatory activity. Cancer Res 59(2):336–341
5. Couch RD, Browning RG, Honda T, Gribble GW, Wright DL, Sporn MB et al (2005) Studies on the reactivity of CDDO, a promising new chemopreventive and chemotherapeutic agent: implications for a molecular mechanism of action. Bioorganic Med Chem Lett. 15 (9):2215–2219
6. Fu L, Gribble GW (2013) Efficient and scalable synthesis of bardoxolone methyl (cddo-methyl ester). Org Lett 15(7):1622–1625
7. Hong DS, Kurzrock R, Supko JG, He X, Naing A, Wheler J et al (2012) A phase I first-in-human trial of bardoxolone methyl in patients with advanced solid tumors and lymphomas. Clin Cancer Res 18(12):3396–3406

8. Yates MS, Tauchi M, Katsuoka F, Flanders KC, Liby KT, Honda T et al (2007) Pharmacodynamic characterization of chemopreventive triterpenoids as exceptionally potent inducers of Nrf2-regulated genes. Mol Cancer Ther 6(1):154–162
9. Alabran JL, Cheuk A, Liby K, Sporn M, Khan J, Letterio J et al (2008) Human neuroblastoma cells rapidly enter cell cycle arrest and apoptosis following exposure to C-28 derivatives of the synthetic triterpenoid CDDO. Cancer Biol Ther 7(5):709–717
10. Noker Patricia E, Gorman Gregory S, Schweikart Karen M, Tomaszewski Joseph E, Sporn MB, Page JG (2004) Pharmacokinetics and toxicity of CDDO, a synthetic triterpenoid, in rats and dogs. Cancer Res 45:471
11. Perez HL, Junnotula V, Knecht D, Nie H, Sanchez Y, Boehm JC et al (2014) Analytical approaches for quantification of a Nrf2 pathway activator: overcoming bioanalytical challenges to support a toxicity study. Analyst. 139(8):1902–1912
12. Thomas M (2012) A preliminary evaluation of bardoxolone methyl for the treatment of diabetic nephropathy. Expert Opin Drug Metab Toxicol. 8(8):1015–1022
13. Jaramillo MC, Zhang DD (2013) The emerging role of the Nrf2-Keap1 signaling pathway in cancer. Genes Dev 27(20):2179–2191
14. Ma Q (2013) Role of nrf2 in oxidative stress and toxicity. Annu Rev Pharmacol Toxicol 53:401–426
15. Cleasby A, Yon J, Day PJ, Richardson C, Tickle IJ, Williams PA et al (2014) Structure of the BTB domain of Keap1 and its interaction with the triterpenoid antagonist CDDO. PLoS ONE 9(6):e98896
16. Sussan TE, Rangasamy T, Blake DJ, Malhotra D, El-Haddad H, Bedja D et al (2009) Targeting Nrf2 with the triterpenoid CDDO-imidazolide attenuates cigarette smoke-induced emphysema and cardiac dysfunction in mice. Proc Natl Acad Sci USA 106(1):250–255
17. Ogura T, Tong KI, Mio K, Maruyama Y, Kurokawa H, Sato C et al (2010) Keap1 is a forked-stem dimer structure with two large spheres enclosing the intervening, double glycine repeat, and C-terminal domains. Proc Natl Acad Sci USA 107(7):2842–2847
18. Vannini N, Lorusso G, Cammarota R, Barberis M, Noonan DM, Sporn MB et al (2007) The synthetic oleanane triterpenoid, CDDO-methyl ester, is a potent antiangiogenic agent. Mol Cancer Ther 6(12 Pt 1):3139–3146
19. Winkel AF, Engel CK, Margerie D, Kannt A, Szillat H, Glombik H et al (2015) Characterization of RA839, a non-covalent small-molecule binder to Keap1 and selective activator of Nrf2 signalling. J Biol Chem 17:jbc.M115.678136
20. Kobayashi A, Kang M-I, Okawa H, Ohtsuji M, Zenke Y, Chiba T et al (2004) Oxidative stress sensor Keap1 functions as an adaptor for Cul3-based E3 ligase to regulate proteasomal degradation of Nrf2. Mol Cell Biol 24(16):7130–7139
21. Chen W, Sun Z, Wang X-J, Jiang T, Huang Z, Fang D et al (2009) Direct Interaction between Nrf2 and p 21Cip1/WAF1 upregulates the Nrf2-mediated antioxidant response. Mol Cell 34 (6):663–673
22. Lau A, Wang X-J, Zhao F, Villeneuve NF, Wu T, Jiang T et al (2010) A noncanonical mechanism of Nrf2 activation by autophagy deficiency: direct interaction between Keap1 and p62. Mol Cell Biol 30(13):3275–3285
23. Itoh K, Wakabayashi N, Katoh Y, Ishii T, O'Connor T, Yamamoto M (2003) Keap1 regulates both cytoplasmic-nuclear shuttling and degradation of Nrf2 in response to electrophiles. Genes Cells 8(4):379–391
24. Sporn MB, Liby KT (2012) NRF2 and cancer: the good, the bad and the importance of context. Nat Rev Cancer 12(8):564–571
25. Kansanen E, Kuosmanen SM, Leinonen H, Levonen A-L (2013) The Keap1-Nrf2 pathway: mechanisms of activation and dysregulation in cancer. Redox Biol 1(1):45–49
26. Klaassen CD, Reisman S (2010) Nrf2 the rescue: effects of the antioxidative/electrophilic response on the liver. Toxicol Appl Pharmacol 244(1):57–65
27. Xing Y, Niu T, Wang W, Li J, Li S, Janicki JS et al (2012) Triterpenoid dihydro-CDDO-trifluoroethyl amide protects against maladaptive cardiac remodeling and dysfunction in mice: a critical role of Nrf2. PLoS ONE 7(9):e44899

28. Leinonen HM, Kansanen E, Pölönen P, Heinäniemi M, Levonen A-L (2014) Role of the Keap1-Nrf2 pathway in cancer. Adv Cancer Res 122:281–320
29. Tanigawa S, Fujii M, Hou D-X (2007) Action of Nrf2 and Keap1 in ARE-mediated NQO1 expression by quercetin. Free Radic Biol Med 42(11):1690–1703
30. Ahmed MAE, El-Awdan SA (2015) Lipoic acid and pentoxifylline mitigate nandrolone decanoate-induced neurobehavioral perturbations in rats via re-balance of brain neurotransmitters, up-regulation of Nrf2/HO-1 pathway, and down-regulation of TNFR1 expression. Horm Behav 73:186–199
31. Valdecantos MP, Prieto-Hontoria PL, Pardo V, Módol T, Santamaría B, Weber M et al (2015) Essential role of Nrf2 in the protective effect of lipoic acid against lipoapoptosis in hepatocytes. Free Radic Biol Med 84:263–278
32. Deng C, Sun Z, Tong G, Yi W, Ma L, Zhao B et al (2013) α-Lipoic acid reduces infarct size and preserves cardiac function in rat myocardial ischemia/reperfusion injury through activation of PI3 K/Akt/Nrf2 pathway. PLoS ONE 8(3):e58371
33. Na H-K, Surh Y-J (2008) Modulation of Nrf2-mediated antioxidant and detoxifying enzyme induction by the green tea polyphenol EGCG. Food Chem Toxicol 46(4):1271–1278
34. Moallem SA, Hales BF (1998) The role of p53 and cell death by apoptosis and necrosis in 4-hydroperoxycyclophosphamide-induced limb malformations. Development 125(16):3225–3234
35. Ouyang L, Shi Z, Zhao S, Wang FT, Zhou TT, Liu B et al (2012) Programmed cell death pathways in cancer: a review of apoptosis, autophagy and programmed necrosis. Cell Prolif 45(15):487–498
36. Wang Y-Y, Yang Y-X, Zhao R, Pan S-T, Zhe H, He Z-X et al (2015) Bardoxolone methyl induces apoptosis and autophagy and inhibits epithelial-to-mesenchymal transition and stemness in esophageal squamous cancer cells. Drug Des Devel Ther 9:993–1026
37. Wang Y-Y, Zhe H, Zhao R (2014) Preclinical evidences toward the use of triterpenoid CDDO-Me for solid cancer prevention and treatment. Mol Cancer 13:30
38. Yore MM, Liby KT, Honda T, Gribble GW, Sporn MB (2006) The synthetic triterpenoid 1-[2-cyano-3,12-dioxooleana-1,9(11)-dien-28-oyl]imidazole blocks nuclear factor- B activation through direct inhibition of I B kinase. Mol Cancer Ther 5(12):3232–3239
39. Liu Y, Gao X, Deeb D, Gautam SC (2012) Oleanane triterpenoid CDDO-Me inhibits Akt activity without affecting PDK1 kinase or PP2A phosphatase activity in cancer cells. Biochem Biophys Res Commun. 417(1):570–575
40. Gao X, Liu Y, Deeb D, Arbab AS, Guo AM, Dulchavsky SA et al (2011) Synthetic oleanane triterpenoid, CDDO-Me, induces apoptosis in ovarian cancer cells by inhibiting prosurvival AKT/NF-κB/mTOR signaling. Anticancer Res 31(11):3673–3681
41. Kocak C, Kocak EF, Akcilar R, Bayat Z, Aras B, Metineren MH et al (2015) Effects of captopril, telmisartan, and bardoxolone methyl (CDDO-Me) in ischemia reperfusion-induced acute kidney injury in rats: an experimental comparative study. Clin Exp Pharmacol Physiol
42. Deeb D, Gao X, Dulchavsky SA, Gautam SC (2007) CDDO-me induces apoptosis and inhibits Akt, mTOR and NF-kappaB signaling proteins in prostate cancer cells. Anticancer Res 27(5A):3035–3044
43. Konopleva M, Contractor R, Kurinna SM, Chen W, Andreeff M, Ruvolo PP (2005) The novel triterpenoid CDDO-Me suppresses MAPK pathways and promotes p 38 activation in acute myeloid leukemia cells. Leukemia 19(8):1350–1354
44. Suh W-S, Kim YS, Schimmer AD, Kitada S, Minden M, Andreeff M et al (2003) Synthetic triterpenoids activate a pathway for apoptosis in AML cells involving downregulation of FLIP and sensitization to TRAIL. Leuk Off J Leuk Soc Am Leuk Res Fund UK 17 (11):2122–2129
45. Ito Y, Pandey P, Place A, Sporn MB, Gribble GW, Honda T et al (2000) The novel triterpenoid 2-cyano-3,12-dioxoolean-1,9-dien-28-oic acid induces apoptosis of human myeloid leukemia cells by a caspase-8-dependent mechanism. Cell Growth Differ 11(5):261–267

46. Han S-S, Peng L, Chung S-T, DuBois W, Maeng S-H, Shaffer AL et al (2006) CDDO-Imidazolide inhibits growth and survival of c-Myc-induced mouse B cell and plasma cell neoplasms. Mol Cancer. 5:22
47. Shen H, Liu J, Wang Y, Lian H, Wang J, Xing L et al (2013) Aflatoxin G1-induced oxidative stress causes DNA damage and triggers apoptosis through MAPK signaling pathway in A549 cells. Food Chem Toxicol 62:661–669
48. Yates MS (2006) Potent protection against aflatoxin-induced tumorigenesis through induction of Nrf2-regulated pathways by the triterpenoid 1-[2-cyano-3-,12-dioxooleana-1,9 (11)-dien-28-oyl]imidazole. Cancer Res 66(4):2488–2494
49. Bey EA, Reinicke KE, Srougi MC, Varnes M, Anderson VE, Pink JJ et al (2013) Catalase abrogates β-lapachone-induced PARP1 hyperactivation-directed programmed necrosis in NQO1-positive breast cancers. Mol Cancer Ther 12(10):2110–2120
50. Li S, Wang W, Niu T, Wang H, Li B, Shao L et al (2014) Nrf2 deficiency exaggerates doxorubicin-induced cardiotoxicity and cardiac dysfunction. Oxid Med Cell Longev
51. Wang W, Li S, Wang H, Li B, Shao L, Lai Y et al (2014) Nrf2 enhances myocardial clearance of toxic ubiquitinated proteins. J Mol Cell Cardiol 72:305–315
52. Yates MS, Tran QT, Dolan PM, Osburn WO, Shin S, McCulloch CC et al (2009) Genetic versus chemoprotective activation of Nrf2 signaling: Overlapping yet distinct gene expression profiles between Keap1 knockout and triterpenoid-treated mice. Carcinogenesis 30(6):1024–1031
53. Heiss EH, Schachner D, Zimmermann K, Dirsch VM (2013) Glucose availability is a decisive factor for Nrf2-mediated gene expression. Redox Biol 1(1):359–365
54. Qin Q, Qu C, Niu T, Zang H, Qi L, Lyu L et al (2016) Nrf2-mediated cardiac maladaptive remodeling and dysfunction in a setting of autophagy insufficiency. Hypertension 67(1):107–117
55. Bernstein SH, Venkatesh S, Li M, Lee J, Lu B, Hilchey SP et al (2012) The mitochondrial ATP-dependent Lon protease: a novel target in lymphoma death mediated by the synthetic triterpenoid CDDO and its derivatives. Blood 119(14):3321–3329
56. Ngo JK, Pomatto LCD, Davies KJA (2013) Upregulation of the mitochondrial Lon Protease allows adaptation to acute oxidative stress but dysregulation is associated with chronic stress, disease, and aging. Redox Biol. 1:258–264
57. Gibellini L, Pinti M, Bartolomeo R, De Biasi S, Cormio A, Musicco C et al (2015) Inhibition of Lon protease by triterpenoids alters mitochondria and is associated to cell death in human cancer cells. Oncotarget. 6(28):25466–25483
58. Hsieh M-J, Yang S-F, Hsieh Y-S, Chen T-Y, Chiou H-L (2012) Autophagy inhibition enhances apoptosis induced by dioscin in huh7 cells. Evid Based Complement Alternat Med 2012:134512
59. Pitha-Rowe I, Liby K, Royce D, Sporn M (2009) Synthetic triterpenoids attenuate cytotoxic retinal injury: cross-talk between Nrf2 and PI3K/AKT signaling through inhibition of the lipid phosphatase PTEN. Invest Ophthalmol Vis Sci 50(11):5339–5347
60. Gao L, Wang Y, Xu Z, Li X, Wu J, Liu S et al (2015) SZC017, a novel oleanolic acid derivative, induces apoptosis and autophagy in human breast cancer cells. Apoptosis 20 (12):1636–1650
61. Lisiak N, Paszel-Jaworska A, Bednarczyk-Cwynar B, Zaprutko L, Kaczmarek M, Rybczyńska M (2014) Methyl 3-hydroxyimino-11-oxoolean-12-en-28-oate (HIMOXOL), a synthetic oleanolic acid derivative, induces both apoptosis and autophagy in MDA-MB-231 breast cancer cells. Chem Biol Interact 5(208):47–57
62. Suh N, Paul S, Lee HJ, Yoon T, Shah N, Son AI et al (2012) Synthetic triterpenoids, CDDO-Imidazolide and CDDO-Ethyl amide, induce chondrogenesis. Osteoarthritis Cartilage 20(5):446–450
63. Liu Y, Gao X, Deeb D, Arbab AS, Gautam SC (2012) Telomerase reverse transcriptase (TERT) is a therapeutic target of oleanane triterpenoid CDDO-Me in prostate cancer. Molecules 17(12):14795–14809

64. Qin D-J, Tang C-X, Yang L, Lei H, Wei W, Wang Y-Y et al (2015) Hsp90 is a novel target molecule of CDDO-Me in inhibiting proliferation of ovarian cancer cells. PLoS ONE 10(7): e0132337
65. Shin S, Wakabayashi J, Yates MS, Wakabayashi N, Dolan PM, Aja S et al (2009) Role of Nrf2 in prevention of high-fat diet-induced obesity by synthetic triterpenoid CDDO-Imidazolide. Eur J Pharmacol 620(1–3):138–144
66. Clempus RE, Griendling KK (2006) Reactive oxygen species signaling in vascular smooth muscle cells. Cardiovasc Res 71:216–225
67. Chan J, Prado-Lourenco L, Khachigian LM, Bennett MR, Di Bartolo BA, Kavurma MM (2010) TRAIL promotes VSMC proliferation and neointima formation in a FGF-2-, Sp1 phosphorylation-, and NFkappaB-dependent manner. Circ Res 106(6):1061–1071
68. Mannion JD, Ormont ML, Magno MG, O'Brien JE, Shi Y, Zalewski A (1998) Sustained reduction of neointima with c-myc antisense oligonucleotides in saphenous vein grafts. Ann Thorac Surg 66(6):1948–1952
69. Wang Y-Y, Yang Y-X, Zhe H, He Z-X, Zhou S-F (2014) Bardoxolone methyl (CDDO-Me) as a therapeutic agent: an update on its pharmacokinetic and pharmacodynamic properties. Drug Des Devel Ther 8:2075–2088
70. Miyajima S, Naruse K, Kobayashi Y, Nakamura N, Nishikawa T, Adachi K et al (2014) Periodontitis-activated monocytes/macrophages cause aortic inflammation. Sci Rep. 4:5171
71. Li B, Abdalrahman A, Lai Y, Janicki JS, Ward KW, Meyer CJ et al (2014) Dihydro-CDDO-trifluoroethyl amide suppresses inflammatory responses in macrophages via activation of Nrf2. Biochem Biophys Res Commun 444(4):555–561
72. Onyango EO, Fu L, Cao M, Liby KT, Sporn MB, Gribble GW (2014) Synthesis and biological evaluation of amino acid methyl ester conjugates of 2-cyano-3,12-dioxooleana-1,9 (11)-dien-28-oic acid against the production of nitric oxide (NO). Bioorg Med Chem Lett 24 (2):532–534
73. Li S, Wang W, Niu T, Wang H, Li B, Shao L et al (2014) Nrf2 deficiency exaggerates doxorubicin-induced cardiotoxicity and cardiac dysfunction. Oxid Med Cell Longev 2014:748524
74. Thomas R, Kanso A, Sedor JR (2008) Chronic kidney disease and its complications. Prim Care Clin Off Pract 35(2):329–344
75. Aminzadeh MA, Reisman SA, Vaziri ND, Khazaeli M, Yuan J, Meyer CJ (2014) The synthetic triterpenoid RTA dh404 (CDDO-dhTFEA) restores Nrf2 activity and attenuates oxidative stress, inflammation, and fibrosis in rats with chronic kidney disease. Xenobiotica 44(6):570–578
76. Liu M, Reddy NM, Higbee EM, Potteti HR, Noel S, Racusen L et al (2014) The Nrf2 triterpenoid activator, CDDO-imidazolide, protects kidneys from ischemia-reperfusion injury in mice. Kidney Int 85(1):134–141
77. Wu T, Ye Y, Min S-Y, Zhu J, Khobahy E, Zhou J et al (2014) Prevention of murine lupus nephritis by targeting multiple signaling axes and oxidative stress using a synthetic triterpenoid. Arthritis Rheumatol (Hoboken, NJ) 66(11):3129–3139
78. Shelton LM, Lister A, Walsh J, Jenkins RE, Wong MHL, Rowe C et al (2015) Integrated transcriptomic and proteomic analyses uncover regulatory roles of Nrf2 in the kidney. Kidney Int 1261–1273
79. Shelton LM, Park BK, Copple IM (2013) Role of Nrf2 in protection against acute kidney injury. Kidney Int 84(6):1090–1095
80. Aleksunes LM, Goedken MJ, Rockwell CE, Thomale J, Manautou JE, Klaassen CD (2010) Transcriptional regulation of renal cytoprotective genes by Nrf2 and its potential use as a therapeutic target to mitigate cisplatin-induced nephrotoxicity. J Pharmacol Exp Ther 335 (1):2–12
81. Aminzadeh MA, Reisman SA, Vaziri ND, Shelkovnikov S, Farzaneh SH, Khazaeli M et al (2013) The synthetic triterpenoid RTA dh404 (CDDO-dhTFEA) restores endothelial function impaired by reduced Nrf2 activity in chronic kidney disease. Redox Biol 1:527–531

82. Pergola PE, Raskin P, Toto RD, Meyer CJ, Huff JW, Grossman EB et al (2011) Bardoxolone methyl and kidney function in CKD with type 2 diabetes. N Engl J Med 365(4):327–336
83. de Zeeuw D, Akizawa T, Audhya P, Bakris GL, Chin M, Christ-Schmidt H et al (2013) Bardoxolone methyl in type 2 diabetes and stage 4 chronic kidney disease. N Engl J Med 369 (26):2492–2503
84. Lowenberg B, Downing JR, Burnett A (1999) Acute myeloid leukemia. N Engl J Med 341 (14):1051–1062
85. Konopleva M (2002) Novel triterpenoid CDDO-Me is a potent inducer of apoptosis and differentiation in acute myelogenous leukemia. Blood 99(1):326–335
86. Koschmieder S, D'Alò F, Radomska H, Schöneich C, Ji SC, Konopleva M et al (2007) CDDO induces granulocytic differentiation of myeloid leukemic blasts through translational up-regulation of p42 CCAAT enhancer-binding protein alpha. Blood 110(10):3695–3705
87. Ames E, Harouna S, Meyer C, Welniak LA, Murphy WJ (2012) The triterpenoid CDDO-Me promotes hematopoietic progenitor expansion and myelopoiesis in mice. Biol Blood Marrow Transplant 18(3):396–405
88. Wei Y, Gong J, Yoshida T, Eberhart CG, Xu Z, Kombairaju P et al (2011) Nrf2 has a protective role against neuronal and capillary degeneration in retinal ischemia-reperfusion injury. Free Radic Biol Med 51(1):216–224
89. Xu Z, Cho H, Hartsock MJ, Mitchell KL, Gong J, Wu L et al (2015) Neuroprotective role of Nrf2 for retinal ganglion cells in ischemia-reperfusion. J Neurochem 133(2):233–241
90. Wang L, Kondo N, Cano M, Ebrahimi K, Yoshida T, Barnett BP et al (2014) Nrf2 signaling modulates cigarette smoke-induced complement activation in retinal pigmented epithelial cells. Free Radic Biol Med 70:155–166
91. Himori N, Yamamoto K, Maruyama K, Ryu M, Taguchi K, Yamamoto M et al (2013) Critical role of Nrf2 in oxidative stress-induced retinal ganglion cell death. J Neurochem 127 (5):669–680
92. Graber DJ, Park PJ, Hickey WF, Harris BT (2011) Synthetic triterpenoid CDDO derivatives modulate cytoprotective or immunological properties in astrocytes, neurons, and microglia. J Neuroimmune Pharmacol. 6(1):107–120
93. Choi SH, Kim B-G, Robinson J, Fink S, Yan M, Sporn MB et al (2014) Synthetic triterpenoid induces 15-PGDH expression and suppresses inflammation-driven colon carcinogenesis. J Clin Invest 124(6):2472–2482
94. Deeb D, Gao X, Liu Y, Kim S-H, Pindolia KR, Arbab AS et al (2012) Inhibition of cell proliferation and induction of apoptosis by oleanane triterpenoid (CDDO-Me) in pancreatic cancer cells is associated with the suppression of hTERT gene expression and its telomerase activity. Biochem Biophys Res Commun 422(4):561–567
95. Shanmugam MK, Dai X, Kumar AP, Tan BKH, Sethi G, Bishayee A (2014) Oleanolic acid and its synthetic derivatives for the prevention and therapy of cancer: preclinical and clinical evidence. Cancer Lett 346(2):206–216
96. Taguchi K, Motohashi H, Yamamoto M (2011) Molecular mechanisms of the Keap1–Nrf2 pathway in stress response and cancer evolution. Genes Cells 16(2):123–140
97. El-Ashmawy M, Delgado O, Cardentey A, Wright WE, Shay JW (2014) CDDO-Me protects normal lung and breast epithelial cells but not cancer cells from radiation. PLoS ONE 9(12): e115600
98. Johnson NM, Egner PA, Baxter VK, Sporn MB, Wible RS, Sutter TR et al (2014) Complete protection against aflatoxin B(1)-induced liver cancer with a triterpenoid: DNA adduct dosimetry, molecular signature, and genotoxicity threshold. Cancer Prev Res (Phila) 7 (7):658–665
99. Liby K, Royce DB, Williams CR, Risingsong R, Yore MM, Honda T et al (2007) The synthetic triterpenoids CDDO-methyl ester and CDDO-ethyl amide prevent lung cancer induced by vinyl carbamate in A/J mice. Cancer Res 67(6):2414–2419
100. Gao X, Liu Y, Deeb D, Arbab AS, Guo AM, Dulchavsky SA et al (2011) Synthetic oleanane triterpenoid, CDDO-Me, induces apoptosis in ovarian cancer cells by inhibiting prosurvival AKT/NF-kappaB/mTOR signaling. Anticancer Res 31(11):3673–3681

101. Tran K, Risingsong R, Royce D, Williams CR, Sporn MB, Liby K (2012) The synthetic triterpenoid CDDO-methyl ester delays estrogen receptor-negative mammary carcinogenesis in polyoma middle T mice. Cancer Prev Res (Phila) 5(5):726–734
102. Kim E-H, Deng C, Sporn MB, Royce DB, Risingsong R, Williams CR et al (2012) CDDO-methyl ester delays breast cancer development in BRCA1-mutated mice. Cancer Prev Res (Phila) 5(1):89–97
103. Deeb D, Gao X, Liu Y, Jiang D, Divine GW, Arbab AS et al (2011) Synthetic triterpenoid CDDO prevents the progression and metastasis of prostate cancer in TRAMP mice by inhibiting survival signaling. Carcinogenesis 32(5):757–764
104. So JY, Lin JJ, Wahler J, Liby KT, Sporn MB, Suh N (2014) A synthetic triterpenoid CDDO-Im inhibits tumorsphere formation by regulating stem cell signaling pathways in triple-negative breast cancer. PLoS ONE 9(9):e107616
105. Cao M, Onyango EO, Williams CR, Royce DB, Gribble GW, Sporn MB, et al. Novel synthetic pyridyl analogues of CDDO-Imidazolide are useful new tools in cancer prevention. Pharmacol Res. Elsevier Ltd; 2015;100:135–47
106. Zhao Y, Huo M, Xu Z, Wang Y, Huang L (2015) Nanoparticle delivery of CDDO-Me remodels the tumor microenvironment and enhances vaccine therapy for melanoma. Biomaterials 68:54–66
107. Shah H, Speen AM, Saunders C, Brooke EA, Nallasamy P, Zhu H et al (2015) Protection of HepG2 cells against acrolein toxicity by 2-cyano-3,12-dioxooleana-1,9-dien-28-imidazolide via glutathione-mediated mechanism. Exp Biol Med (Maywood) 240(10):1340–1351
108. Reisman SA, Ward KW, Klaassen CD, Meyer CJ (2013) CDDO-9,11-dihydro-trifluoroethyl amide (CDDO-dhTFEA) induces hepatic cytoprotective genes and increases bile flow in rats. Xenobiotica 43(7):571–578
109. Walsh J, Jenkins RE, Wong M, Olayanju A, Powell H, Copple I et al (2014) Identification and quantification of the basal and inducible Nrf2-dependent proteomes in mouse liver: biochemical, pharmacological and toxicological implications. J Proteomics. 28(108):171–187
110. Noel S, Zheng L, Navas-Acien A, Fuchs RJ (2014) The effect of ex vivo CDDO-Me activation on nuclear factor erythroid 2-related factor 2 pathway in white blood cells from patients with septic shock. Shock. 42(5):392–399
111. Thimmulappa RK, Fuchs RJ, Malhotra D, Scollick C, Traore K, Bream JH et al (2007) Preclinical evaluation of targeting the Nrf2 pathway by triterpenoids (CDDO-Im and CDDO-Me) for protection from LPS-induced inflammatory response and reactive oxygen species in human peripheral blood mononuclear cells and neutrophils. Antioxid Redox Signal 9(11):1963–1970
112. Keleku-Lukwete N, Suzuki M, Otsuki A, Tsuchida K, Katayama S, Hayashi M et al (2015) Amelioration of inflammation and tissue damage in sickle cell model mice by Nrf2 activation. Proc Natl Acad Sci 112(39):12169–12174
113. Hastings J, de Matos P, Dekker A, Ennis M, Harsha B, Kale N et al (2013) The ChEBI reference database and ontology for biologically relevant chemistry: enhancements for 2013. Nucleic Acids Res 41(Database issue):D456–D463
114. Zhou S, Sun W, Zhang Z, Zheng Y (2014) The role of Nrf2-mediated pathway in cardiac remodeling and heart failure. Oxid Med Cell Longev 2014:260429
115. Kannan S, Muthusamy VR, Whitehead KJ, Wang L, Gomes AV, Litwin SE et al (2013) Nrf2 deficiency prevents reductive stress-induced hypertrophic cardiomyopathy. Cardiovasc Res 100(1):63–73
116. Seifirad S, Ghaffari A, Amoli MM (2014) The antioxidants dilemma: are they potentially immunosuppressants and carcinogens? Front Physiol 5:245
117. de Haan JB (2014) Limiting reductive stress for treating in-stent stenosis: the heart of the matter? J Clin Invest 124(12):5092–5094
118. Margaritelis NV, Kyparos A, Paschalis V, Theodorou AA, Panayiotou G, Zafeiridis A et al (2014) Reductive stress after exercise: the issue of redox individuality. Redox Biol 2:520–528

119. Qin Q, Qu C, Niu T, Zang H, Qi L, Lyu L et al (2016) Nrf2-mediated cardiac maladaptive remodeling and dysfunction in a setting of autophagy insufficiency. Hypertension 67(1):107–117
120. Lu LY, Ou N, Lu Q-B (2013) Antioxidant induces DNA damage, cell death and mutagenicity in human lung and skin normal cells. Sci Rep. 3:3169
121. Mathis BJ, Lai Y, Qu C, Janicki JS, Cui T (2015) CYLD-mediated signaling and diseases. Curr Drug Targets 16(4):284–294
122. Wang H, Lai Y, Mathis BJ, Wang W, Li S, Qu C et al (2015) Deubiquitinating enzyme CYLD mediates pressure overload-induced cardiac maladaptive remodeling and dysfunction via downregulating Nrf2. J Mol Cell Cardiol 84:143–153
123. Linares JF, Duran A, Yajima T, Pasparakis M, Moscat J, Diaz-Meco MT (2013) K63 polyubiquitination and activation of mTOR by the p62-TRAF6 complex in nutrient-activated cells. Mol Cell 51(3):283–296
124. Yao T-P (2010) The role of ubiquitin in autophagy-dependent protein aggregate processing. Genes Cancer. 1(7):779–786
125. Wang Y-Y, Zhang C-Y, Ma Y-Q, He Z-X, Zhe H, Zhou S-F (2015) Therapeutic effects of C-28 methyl ester of 2-cyano-3,12-dioxoolean-1,9-dien-28-oic acid (CDDO-Me; bardoxolone methyl) on radiation-induced lung inflammation and fibrosis in mice. Drug Des Devel Ther 9:3163–3178
126. Ai Y, Kang F, Huang Z, Xue X, Lai Y, Peng S et al (2015) Synthesis of CDDO–amino acid-nitric oxide donor trihybrids as potential antitumor agents against both drug-sensitive and drug-resistant colon cancer. J Med Chem 58(5):2452–2464
127. To C, Ringelberg CS, Royce DB, Williams CR, Risingsong R, Sporn MB et al (2015) Dimethyl fumarate and the oleanane triterpenoids, CDDO-imidazolide and CDDO-methyl ester, both activate the Nrf2 pathway but have opposite effects in the A/J model of lung carcinogenesis. Carcinogenesis 36(7):769–781
128. Liby KT (2014) Synthetic triterpenoids can protect against toxicity without reducing the efficacy of treatment with carboplatin and paclitaxel in experimental lung cancer. Dose Response 12(1):136–151
129. Gao X, Deeb D, Liu Y, Liu P, Zhang Y, Shaw J et al (2015) CDDO-Me inhibits tumor growth and prevents recurrence of pancreatic ductal adenocarcinoma. Int J Oncol 47(6):2100–2106
130. Kitsukawa M, Tsuchiyama H, Maeda A, Oshida K, Miyamoto Y (2014) Immunosuppressive potential of bardoxolone methyl using a modified murine local lymph node assay (LLNA). J Toxicol Sci 39(4):545–550
131. Perez HL, Junnotula V, Knecht D, Nie H, Sanchez Y, Boehm JC et al (2014) Analytical approaches for quantification of a Nrf2 pathway activator: overcoming bioanalytical challenges to support a toxicity study. Analyst. 139:1902–1912
132. Fitzpatrick LR, Stonesifer E, Small JS, Liby KT (2014) The synthetic triterpenoid (CDDO-Im) inhibits STAT3, as well as IL-17, and improves DSS-induced colitis in mice. Inflammopharmacology 22(6):341–349
133. Reisman SA, Buckley DB, Tanaka Y, Klaassen CD (2009) CDDO-Im protects from acetaminophen hepatotoxicity through induction of Nrf2-dependent genes. Toxicol Appl Pharmacol 236(1):109–114
134. Osburn WO, Yates MS, Dolan PD, Chen S, Liby KT, Sporn MB et al (2008) Genetic or pharmacologic amplification of nrf2 signaling inhibits acute inflammatory liver injury in mice. Toxicol Sci 104(1):218–227
135. Kensler KH, Slocum SL, Chartoumpekis DV, Dolan PM, Johnson NM, Ilic Z et al (2014) Genetic or pharmacologic activation of Nrf2 signaling fails to protect against aflatoxin genotoxicity in hypersensitive GSTA3 knockout mice. Toxicol Sci 139(2):293–300
136. Zhang F, Wang S, Zhang M, Weng Z, Li P, Gan Y et al (2012) Pharmacological induction of heme oxygenase-1 by a triterpenoid protects neurons against ischemic injury. Stroke 43(5):1390–1397

137. Furusawa Y, Uruno A, Yagishita Y, Higashi C, Yamamoto M (2014) Nrf2 induces fibroblast growth factor 21 in diabetic mice. Genes Cells 19(12):864–878
138. Neymotin A, Calingasan NY, Wille E, Naseri N, Petri S, Damiano M et al (2011) Neuroprotective effect of Nrf2/ARE activators, CDDO ethylamide and CDDO trifluoroethylamide, in a mouse model of amyotrophic lateral sclerosis. Free Radic Biol Med 51(1):88–96
139. Getachew Y, Cusimano FA, Gopal P, Reisman SA, Shay JW (2015) The synthetic triterpenoid RTA 405 (CDDO-EA) halts progression of liver fibrosis and reduces hepatocellular carcinoma size resulting in increased survival in an experimental model of chronic liver injury. Toxicol Sci 405:kfv213

Evodiamine and Its Role in Chronic Diseases

Qunyou Tan and Jingqing Zhang

Abstract Evodiamine (EVO) is a major alkaloid compound extracted from the dry unripened fruit Evodiae fructus (*Evodia rutaecarpa* Benth., Rutaceae). EVO has a variety of pharmacological activities, such as anti-obesity, anti-allergenic, analgesic, anti-tumor, anti-ulcerogenic, and neuroprotective activities. EVO has varying efficacies in animal models and humans. Here, the physicochemical properties of EVO are presented, and the EVO's functions and mechanisms of action in various chronic diseases are reviewed. EVO is worth exploring in more depth in the future for its potential use in various chronic diseases.

Keywords Evodiamine · Physico-chemical properties · Cell signaling pathways · Pharmacologicalactivities · Mechanisms of action · Chronic diseases

1 Introduction

Evodiamine (EVO) is the main bioactive component extracted from the dry unripened fruit of Evodiae fructus (Chinese name is Wu-Chu-Yu) or other Tetradium genus of plants. EVO has a variety of pharmacological activities, such as anti-obesity, anti-inflammatory, and anti-tumor. The role of EVO in various chronic diseases and its possible mechanisms of action are outlined here.

Q. Tan (✉)
Department of Thoracic Surgery, Institute of Surgery Research, Daping Hospital, Third Military Medical University, Chongqing 400042, China
e-mail: tanqy001@163.com

J. Zhang (✉)
Chongqing Research Center for Pharmaceutical Engineering, Chongqing Medical University, Chongqing 400016, China
e-mail: zjqrae01@163.com

S.C. Gupta et al. (eds.), *Drug Discovery from Mother Nature*,
Advances in Experimental Medicine and Biology 929,
DOI 10.1007/978-3-319-41342-6_14

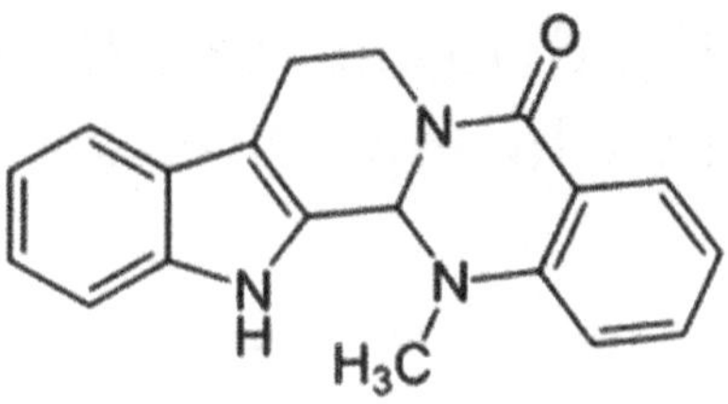

Fig. 1 Structure of evodiamine

2 Physicochemical Properties of Evodiamine

EVO (CAS: 518-17-2) is a plant alkaloid and its systematic name is 21-methyl-3,13,21-triazapentacyclo[11.8.0.02,10.04,9.015,20] henicosa-2(10),4,6, 8,15,17,19-heptaen-14-one (Fig. 1). EVO is a pale yellow crystal with no perceptible odor or taste. The main physicochemical parameters of EVO are listed in Table 1. EVO can be assayed using an ultraviolet spectrophotometer at 225 nm or by a high-performance liquid chromatography system using an internal standard method [1].

3 Modulation of Cell Signaling Pathways by Evodiamine

3.1 Anti-obese Action

EVO induces the phosphorylation of EGFR, PKCα, and ERK, and it inhibits adipogenesis via the EGFR–PKCα–ERK signaling pathway [2]. EVO inhibits adipocyte differentiation in 3T3-L1 and C3H10T1/2 cells [3]. The anti-obese mechanism of action of EVO is reported to be similar to that of capsaicin [4].

3.2 Anti-inflammatory and Anti-allergenic Action

EVO exerts an anti-inflammation activity on human umbilical vein endothelial cells (HUVEC) with high glucose by suppressing the P2X4 receptor (P2X4R) signaling pathway, accompanied by the downregulation of NF-κB, TNFR-α, P2X4R, and intracellular reactive oxygen species (ROS), and upregulation of the nitric oxide

Table 1 The main physicochemical parameters of evodiamine

Molecular formula	Molecular weight	Appearance	Solubility	Melting point	Boiling point	Density	Refractive index	Storage temperature
C19H17N3O	303.36	Fine powder	Insoluble	263–265 °C	575.1 °C	1.39 g/cm^3	1.764	2–8 °C

(NO) level [5]. EVO inhibits the secretion of interleukin (IL)-10 and decreases production of IL-2 from the LPS-stimulated endothelial cells [6]. EVO inhibits LIGHT-induced migration via the suppression of ROS production and NADPH oxidase activation in human monocytes [7]. EVO represses hypoxia-induced COX-2 expression by inhibiting hypoxia-inducible factor 1-alpha which is mediated by the dephosphorylation of Akt and p70S6K in RAW264.7 cells [8]. EVO exerts an anti-allergenic effect by inhibiting the protein levels of TNF-α and IL-4 induced by the IgE–antigen complex in RBL-2H3 cells [9].

3.3 Analgesic Effect

EVO induces significant increases in intracellular calcium and inward currents in dorsal root ganglion neurons and the transient receptor potential (TRP) V1-transfected HEK293 cells, which suggests that EVO suppresses thermal hyperalgesia by activating TRPV1 channels [10].

3.4 Mechanistic Aspects of Evodiamine in Cancer Cells

EVO has a high binding affinity and selectivity to potential vanilloid-1 (TRPV1). It may be used for the treatment of cancer cells by acting as a TRPV1 agonist [11] or aryl hydrocarbon receptor (AhR) antagonist [12].

3.4.1 Respiratory System Tumor Cells

Lung Cancer Cells

EVO inhibits the A549 cell proliferation via metadherin suppression and apoptosis activation [13]. EVO induces arrest at G2/M phase and apoptosis via the mitochondrial and endoplasmic reticulum pathways in H446 and H1688 cells [14].

Nasopharyngeal Carcinoma Cells

EVO inhibits the invasion and metastasis of NPC cells via repressing the expression and activity of MMP2 and attenuating the phosphorylation level of ERK1/2 [15].

3.4.2 Circulating Tumor Cells

Leukemia Cells and Resistant Leukemia Cells

EVO inhibits the K562 cell proliferation by regulating the peroxisome proliferator-activated receptor-gamma (PPARγ) pathway via downregulating cell cycle control protein cyclin D1 and upregulating cyclin-dependent kinase inhibitor p21 [16].

Resistant Leukemia Cells

EVO exhibits increased inhibition against camptothecin-resistant K562, THP-1, CCRF-CEM, and CCRF-CEM/C1 cells by acting as a dual catalytic inhibitor of topoisomerases I and II [17].

3.4.3 Digestive System Tumor Cells

Gastric Cancer Cells and Cancer Stem Cells

EVO inhibited proliferation and induced apoptosis in SGC7901 cells via suppressing survivin and increasing caspase-3 mRNA [18]. EVO inhibits proliferation and sphere formation ability of gastric cancer stem cells (GCSCs) via repressing the Wingless and INT-1 (Wnt)/β-catenin signaling pathway and represses the induced pluripotent stem cell factors and epithelial-to-mesenchymal transition (EMT) factors [19].

Oral Cancer Cells

EVO inhibits MC3 and HSC4 cell proliferation and induces apoptosis by reducing phosphorylated AKT expression [20].

Colorectal Cancer Cells

EVO exerts anti-proliferative effects by downregulating IGF-1/HIF-1α expression in LoVo cells [21]. In HCT-116 cells, EVO inhibits proliferation, induces S and G2/M arrest, induces apoptosis via the p53 signaling pathway, and inhibits migration by downregulating the expression of matrix metalloproteinase 3 (MMP3) by inactivating the JAK2/STAT3 pathway [22]. In HCT-116/L-OHP cells, EVO inhibited growth and induced apoptosis in a dose- and time-dependent manner, reduced the accumulation of rhodamine 123 and the activity of ATPase, and inhibited phosphorylation of the NF-κB pathway, such as p50/p65. Thus, EVO may suppress ABCG2-mediated drug resistance (MDR) by inhibiting the p50/NF-κB pathway [23].

Pancreatic Cancer Cells

EVO increases the anti-pancreatic cancer effect of gemcitabine in SW1990 cells via downregulating PI3K/Akt pathway [24].

Hepatocellular Carcinoma Cells

EVO inhibits STAT3 tyrosine 705 signaling by inducing phosphatase shatterproof 1 in HepG2 cells [25].

3.4.4 Urologic Cancer Cells

Renal Proximal Tubular Epithelial Cells

EVO inhibited transforming growth factor (TGF)-β1-induced epithelial–mesenchymal transition (EMT) in rat NRK52E cells. Smad-2 and the PPARγ signal pathway participated in promoting the effects of evodiamine [26].

Bladder Cancer Cells

EVO enhances tumor necrosis factor-related apoptosis-inducing ligand (TRAIL)-induced apoptosis in 253J and T24 cells through an mTOR/S6K1-mediated reduction of Mcl-1 levels [27].

3.4.5 Genital Carcinoma Cells

Breast Cancer Cells and Resistant Breast Cancer Cells

As a topoisomerase-1 inhibitor, EVO facilitates the formation of topoisomerase I-DNA cleavable complex in MCF-7 breast cancer cells [28]. EVO induces apoptosis of doxorubicin (DOX)-sensitive MCF-7 and DOX-resistant MCF-7/ADR cells by increasing cleaved poly(ADP-ribose) polymerase (PARP), caspase-7/9, and caspase activities, as well as inhibiting the Ras/MEK/ERK cascade and inhibitors of apoptosis (IAPs) [29].

Ovarian Cancer Cells

EVO has anti-proliferative effects on ovarian epithelial cancer cells, A2780 and A2780/PTX(R), induces G2/M arrest mediated by cyclin B1 and Cdc2, and, via the

MAPK signaling pathway, improves chemo-resistance by downregulating MDR-1 expression [30].

3.4.6 Brain Tumor Cells

Glioblastoma Cells

EVO stimulates U87 cells to tumor necrosis factor-α-related apoptosis-inducing ligand (TRAIL) via the death receptor pathway by increasing the death receptor (DR) 4, DR5, caspase-8, and cleaved caspase-3 [31].

Neuronal Cells

When tested against the S, XS [11], L(G), L(A), XL [17], and XL [18] alleles, 2 μM EVO increased 5-HTT promoter (the serotonin transporter) activities by 220, 80, 310, 180, 175, and 102 %, respectively. EVO increased promoter activity depending on the genetic variation of the 5-HTTLPR polymorphism [32].

3.4.7 Osteosarcoma Cells

EVO inhibits OS 143B cell proliferation by upregulating phosphatase and tensin homolog (PTEN) levels through blocking PI3K/Akt signaling [33].

3.5 Antibacterial Effect

Through inhibiting topoisomerase I and supercoiled plasmid DNA relaxation, EVO has a significantly lower minimal inhibitory concentration (MIC) compared with five antibiotics including cefotaxime and aztreonam (128 vs. >512 μg/mL) against the clinical isolate of *Klebsiella pneumoniae* [34].

3.6 Anti-virus Effect

EVO acts against influenza A virus (IAV) by markedly inhibiting IAV replication and IAV-induced autophagy via the AMPK/TSC2/mTOR signal pathway, blocking LC3-II, p62 and EGFP-LC3 aggregation; retarding Atg5–Atg12/Atg16 heterotrimer formation; decreasing Atg5, Atg7, and Atg12 expressions; and blocking TNF-α, IL-1β, IL-6, and IL-8 cytokine release [35].

3.7 *Effects on Cerebral or Cardiac Ischemia*

EVO induces transient receptor potential vanilloid-1 (TRPV1) and calcium-mediated protective autophagy through a calcium/c-Jun N-terminal kinase (JNK) pathway in U87-MG astrocytes [36]. EVO inhibits β1-AR activity by downregulating cAMP and PKA in Chinese hamster ovary cells with high expression levels of β1-AR (β1-AR/CHO-S cells) [37]. EVO may prevent cardiac ischemia–reperfusion injury via energy modulation [37].

3.8 *Insulin-Sensitizing Effect or Insulin Resistance*

EVO activates AMP-activated protein kinase (AMPK) via the Ca(2+)-dependent PI3K/Akt/CaMKII signaling pathway and promotes the high molecular weight adiponectin multimerization in 3T3-L1 adipocytes [38].

4 Role of Evodiamine in Chronic Diseases

EVO is an indole alkaloid extracted from the traditional Chinese medicinal herb *Evodia rutaecarpa* (Rutaceae family). EVO and *E. rutaecarpa* are currently used for the treatment of headaches, abdominal pain, vomiting, colds, and reduced blood circulation in the clinic practices of doctors of traditional Chinese medicine in some southeast countries such as China, Japan, and Korea.

Chronic disease is defined by the World Health Organization as a generally slow-progressing disease of long duration. EVO plays positive roles in curing some chronic diseases, such as cancer, diabetes, and cardiovascular diseases [39], by intervening on the risk factors and underlying determinants linked with chronic diseases. EVO may be a potential therapeutic drug against other chronic diseases such as renal tubulointerstitial fibrosis [26], atherogenesis [7], hypoxia [8], glioma [31], hypomotility disorders [40], and IgE-induced allergenic diseases, including atopic dermatitis and rhinitis [9]. EVO may prevent cardiac ischemia–reperfusion injury via energy modulation [37].

5 Biological Activities of Evodiamine in Animal Models

EVO possesses a variety of biological activities, such as anti-obesity, anti-inflammatory, anti-nociceptive, anti-cancer, antibacterial, and antidepressant-like effects. The biological effects of EVO are tested in various animal models.

5.1 Anti-obese Effect

EVO suppresses neuropeptide Y (NPY) and agouti gene-related protein (AgRP) mRNA level in the hypothalamus and decreases the food intake in male rats [41]. EVO acts as a nonpungent vanilloid receptor agonist. When the mice were fed evodiamine as 0.03 % of their diet for 12 days or the rats were given with evodiamine-containing ethanol extract of Evodia fruits at 0.02 % for 21 days, the body weights, perirenal and epididymal fat weights, the levels of free fatty acid in sera, and total lipids, triglyceride and cholesterol in the liver decreased markedly compared with the control group [4]. EVO influences lipid metabolism by decreasing the expression of lipogenesis genes, such as the expression of peroxisome proliferator-activated receptor-g (PPARg), sterol-regulatory element binding protein (SREBP-1c), and fatty acid synthase, as well as increasing the expression of lipolysis genes, such as the expression of hormone-sensitive lipase. In addition, EVO reduces body weight and heat [42]. EVO reduces body weight gain and the blood glucose levels in db/db mice [3].

5.2 Anti-allergic Effect

EVO has anti-allergic effects and inhibits passive cutaneous anaphylaxis (PCA) reaction and scratching behaviors in ICR mice [9].

5.3 Analgesic Effect

EVO pretreatment decreased thermal hyperalgesia induced by intraplantar injection of capsaicin in adult rats [10]. The analgesic effect of EVO may be due to the desensitization of TRPV1 in sensory neurons [10].

5.4 Anti-tumor Effects

EVO (20 mg/kg/day) significantly inhibited xenograft HepG2 tumor growth in nude mice by blocking STAT3 signaling after 13 days being orally administered [25].

5.5 Anti-ulcerogenic Activity

Pretreatment of EVO markedly suppressed the Rho, Rho-kinase 1 and 2, and cytosolic and nucleic necrosis factor (NF)-κBp65 expression against ethanol-induced gastric ulcer in mice [43]. Evodiamine pretreatment obviously increased the glutathione, superoxide dismutase, and catalase levels in sera and lowered the malonaldehyde level and myeloperoxidase activity in the stomachs of mice [43].

5.6 Neuroprotective Effect

EVO protects the brain from cerebral ischemic damage in mice through upregulating pAkt, pGSK3β, and claudin-5, downregulating NF-κB expression, and ameliorating blood–brain barrier permeability [44].

5.7 Antidepressant-Like Effect

EVO can reverse the chronic unpredictable mild stress-induced behavioral deficits and biochemical changes in chronic unpredictable mildly stressed rats. The mechanisms are related to the modulation of the monoamine transmitters and brain-derived neurotropic factor tropomyosin-related kinase B [45].

5.8 Alzheimer's Disease

EVO improves the learning ability and memory in transgenic mice with Alzheimer's disease by reversing the glucose uptake inhibition and decreasing IL-1β, IL-6, TNF-α, and COX-2 expression [46].

5.9 Prevention of Insulin Resistance

EVO reduces the insulin-stimulated mammalian target of rapamycin and ribosomal S6 protein kinase (mTOR-S6K) signaling and insulin receptor substrate 1 (IRS1) serine phosphorylation in white adipose tissues and improves glucose tolerance in obese/diabetic KK-Ay mice [47].

5.10 Cardiotonic Effect or Remedy for Cardiac Diseases

EVO evokes transient positive inotropic and chronotropic effects on the atria of the guinea pig, which is due to its interaction with the vanilloid receptors and the release of the calcitonin gene-related peptide antagonist (CGRP) [4]. EVO attenuates myocardial infarct size, improves metabolism disorders between fatty acids and glucose, increases ATP and Ca(2+)-ATPase activity, and reduces the peroxisome proliferator-activated receptor-α (PPARα) protein level in the myocardial ischemia–reperfusion (I/R) rats [37].

5.11 Other Effects

EVO exerts stimulatory effects on rat jejunal contractility, exhibiting its potential role in relieving hypomotility disorders [40]. EVO improves the undesirable effects of some drugs while preserving their pharmacological activities. For example, the side effects (adipogenesis, body weight gain, and hepatotoxicity) of rosiglitazone can be attenuated by being co-administered with EVO, but the blood glucose-lowering effect of rosiglitazone is still well preserved [3].

6 Biological Activities of Evodiamine in Humans

There are few reports of the biological activities of EVO in humans. Evodiae fructus is reported to be used as an analgesic in traditional Chinese medicine [10]. The typical commercial preparation of traditional Chinese medicines containing EVO is the Zuojin pill. The Zuojin pill is composed of Evodiae fructus and Rhizoma (the mass ratio is 1:6). The Zuojin pill inhibits gastric emptying and the secretion of gastric acid. The Zuojin pill also has an obvious anti-ulcer effect [48]. The Zuojin pill is officially listed in the Chinese Pharmacopoeia.

7 Conclusions

EVO is a major bioactive alkaloid isolated and purified from the Chinese herbal drug "Wu-Chu-Yu" (Evodiae fructus). It possesses a multitude of positive effects, such as anti-cancer and anti-nociceptive effects on different cells, including stem cells, animals, and humans through modulating diverse targeting regions or through various signaling pathways. Evodiae fructus or the extraction of Evodiae fructus, such as ethanol, methanol, and chloroform extracts, exhibits some effects similar to those of EVO [49]. EVO can be used alone or in combination with other drugs. The combination therapy of EVO with gemcitabine augments its therapeutic effects [24]. Furthermore, EVO shows little toxicity against normal cells [50] in contrast to its positive effects.

In the future, three measures are recommended to be pursued in order to promote the clinical application of EVO in the treatment of chronic diseases: First is to develop a new EVO delivery system, such as a supermolecular nanoemulsion [51] or a phospholipid complex [1], in order to modify the pharmacokinetic behavior and increase the bioavailability of EVO; second is to chirally separate two EVO stereoisomers because sometimes the S-(+) EVO is more effective than the R-(−) evodiamine [52]; third is to synthesize new derivatives with much better potency and less toxicity [53], such as carbamates [54], compared with the parent drug EVO.

References

1. Tan Q, Liu S, Chen X, Wu M, Wang H, Yin H, He D, Xiong H, Zhang J (2012) Design and evaluation of a novel evodiamine-phospholipid complex for improved oral bioavailability. AAPS Pharm Sci Tech 13(2):534–547
2. Wang T, Wang Y, Yamashita H (2012) Evodiamine inhibits adipogenesis via the EGFR-PKCalpha-ERK signaling pathway. FEBS Lett 583(22):3655–3659
3. Bak EJ, Park HG, Kim JM, Kim JM, Yoo YJ, Cha JH (2010) Inhibitory effect of evodiamine alone and in combination with rosiglitazone on in vitro adipocyte differentiation and in vivo obesity related to diabetes. Int J Obes (Lond). 34(2):250–260
4. Kobayashi Y, Nakano Y, Kizaki M, Hoshikuma K, Yokoo Y, Kamiya T (2001) Capsaicin-like anti-obese activities of evodiamine from fruits of *Evodia rutaecarpa*, a vanilloid receptor agonist. Planta Med 67(7):628–633
5. Lv Q, Xue Y, Li G, Zou L, Zhang X, Ying M, Wang S, Guo L, Gao Y, Li G, Xu H, Liu S, Xie J, Liang S (2015) Beneficial effects of evodiamine on P2X4-mediated inflammatory injury of human umbilical vein endothelial cells due to high glucose. Int Immunopharmacol 28 (2):1044–1049
6. Hu Y, He K, Zhu H (2015) Chinese herbal medicinal ingredients affect secretion of NO, IL-10, ICAM-1 and IL-2 by endothelial cells. Immunopharmacol Immunotoxicol 37(3):324–328
7. Heo SK, Yun HJ, Yi HS, Noh EK, Park SD (2009) Evodiamine and rutaecarpine inhibit migration by LIGHT via suppression of NADPH oxidase activation. J Cell Biochem 107 (1):123–133
8. Liu YN, Pan SL, Liao CH, Huang DY, Guh JH, Peng CY, Chang YL, Teng CM (2009) Evodiamine represses hypoxia-induced inflammatory proteins expression and hypoxia-inducible factor 1alpha accumulation in RAW264.7. Shock. 32(3):263–269
9. Shin YW, Bae EA, Cai XF, Lee JJ, Kim DH (2007) In vitro and in vivo antiallergic effect of the fructus of *Evodia rutaecarpa* and its constituents. Biol Pharm Bull 30(1):197–199
10. Iwaoka E, Wang S, Matsuyoshi N, Kogure Y, Aoki S, Yamamoto S, Noguchi K, Dai Y (2016) Evodiamine suppresses capsaicin-induced thermal hyperalgesia through activation and subsequent desensitization of the transient receptor potential V1 channels. J Nat Med 70(1):1–7
11. Ivanova B, Spiteller M (2014) Evodiamine and rutaecarpine alkaloids as highly selective transient receptor potential vanilloid 1 agonists. Int J Biol Macromol 65:314–324
12. Yu H, Tu Y, Zhang C, Fan X, Wang X, Wang Z, Liang H (2010) Evodiamine as a novel antagonist of aryl hydrocarbon receptor. Biochem Biophys Res Commun 402(1):94–98
13. Zou Y, Qin X, Xiong H, Zhu F, Chen T, Wu H (2015) Apoptosis of human non-small-cell lung cancer A549 cells triggered by evodiamine through MTDH-dependent signaling pathway. Tumour Biol 36(7):5187–5193
14. Fang C, Zhang J, Qi D, Fan X, Luo J, Liu L, Tan Q (2014) Evodiamine induces G2/M arrest and apoptosis via mitochondrial and endoplasmic reticulum pathways in H446 and H1688 human small-cell lung cancer cells. PLoS ONE 9(12):e115204

15. Peng X, Zhang Q, Zeng Y, Li J, Wang L, Ai P (2015) Evodiamine inhibits the migration and invasion of nasopharyngeal carcinoma cells in vitro via repressing MMP-2 expression. Cancer Chemother Pharmacol 76(6):1173–1184
16. Sun C, Zhang G, Luan S, Luan C, Shao H, Dong F, Liu X (2015) Evodiamine inhibits the proliferation of leukemia cell line K562 by regulating peroxisome proliferators-activated receptor gamma (PPARγ) pathway. J Recept Signal Transduct Res. doi:10.3109/10799893.2015.1122040
17. Pan X, Hartley JM, Hartley JA, White KN, Wang Z, Bligh SW (2012) Evodiamine, a dual catalytic inhibitor of type I and II topoisomerases, exhibits enhanced inhibition against camptothecin resistant cells. Phytomedicine 19(7):618–624
18. Shen H, Zhao S, Xu Z, Zhu L, Han Y, Ye J (2015) Evodiamine inhibits proliferation and induces apoptosis in gastric cancer cells. Oncol Lett. 10(1):367–371
19. Wen Z, Feng S, Wei L, Wang Z, Hong D, Wang Q (2015) Evodiamine, a novel inhibitor of the Wnt pathway, inhibits the self-renewal of gastric cancer stem cells. Int J Mol Med 36(6):1657–1663
20. Sachita K, Kim Y, Yu HJ, Cho SD, Lee JS (2015) In vitro assessment of the anticancer potential of evodiamine in human oral cancer cell lines. Phytother Res 29(8):1145–1151
21. Huang J, Chen ZH, Ren CM, Wang DX, Yuan SX, Wu QX, Chen QZ, Zeng YH, Shao Y, Li Y, Wu K, Yu Y, Sun WJ, He BC (2015) Antiproliferation effect of evodiamine in human colon cancer cells is associated with IGF-1/HIF-1α downregulation. Oncol Rep. doi:10.3892/or.2015.4309
22. Zhao LC, Li J, Liao K, Luo N, Shi QQ, Feng ZQ, Chen DL (2015) Evodiamine induces apoptosis and inhibits migration of HCT-116 human colorectal cancer cells. Int J Mol Sci 16(11):27411–27421
23. Sui H, Zhou LH, Zhang YL, Huang JP, Liu X, Ji Q, Fu XL, Wen HT, Chen ZS, Deng WL, Zhu HR, Li Q (2015) Evodiamine suppresses ABCG2 mediated drug resistance by inhibiting p50/NF-κB pathway in colorectal cancer. J Cell Biochem. doi:10.1002/jcb.25451
24. Wei WT, Chen H, Wang ZH, Ni ZL, Liu HB, Tong HF, Guo HC, Liu DL, Lin SZ (2012) Enhanced antitumor efficacy of gemcitabine by evodiamine on pancreatic cancer via regulating PI3K/Akt pathway. Int J Biol Sci. 8(1):1–14
25. Yang J, Cai X, Lu W, Hu C, Xu X, Yu Q, Cao P (2013) Evodiamine inhibits STAT3 signaling by inducing phosphatase shatterproof 1 in hepatocellular carcinoma cells. Cancer Lett 328(2):243–251
26. Wei J, Li Z, Yuan F (2014) Evodiamine might inhibit TGF-beta1-induced epithelial-mesenchymal transition in NRK52E cells via Smad and PPAR-gamma pathway. Cell Biol Int 38(7):875–880
27. Zhang T, Qu S, Shi Q, He D, Jin X (2014) Evodiamine induces apoptosis and enhances TRAIL-induced apoptosis in human bladder cancer cells through mTOR/S6K1-mediated downregulation of Mcl-1. Int J Mol Sci 15(2):3154–3171
28. Chan AL, Chang WS, Chen LM, Lee CM, Chen CE, Lin CM, Hwang JL (2009) Evodiamine stabilizes topoisomerase I-DNA cleavable complex to inhibit Chan topoisomerase I activity. Molecules 14(4):1342–1352
29. Wang S, Wang L, Shi Z, Zhong Z, Chen M, Wang Y (2014) Evodiamine synergizes with doxorubicin in the treatment of chemoresistant human breast cancer without inhibiting P-glycoprotein. PLoS ONE 9(5):e97512
30. Zhong ZF, Tan W, Wang SP, Qiang WA, Wang YT (2015) Anti-proliferative activity and cell cycle arrest induced by evodiamine on paclitaxel-sensitive and -resistant human ovarian cancer cells. Sci Rep. 5:16415
31. Khan M, Bi Y, Qazi JI, Fan L, Gao H (2015) Evodiamine sensitizes U87 glioblastoma cells to TRAIL via the death receptor pathway. Mol Med Rep. 11(1):257–262
32. Hu Y, Ehli EA, Hudziak JJ, Davies GE (2012) Berberine and evodiamine influence serotonin transporter (5-HTT) expression via the 5-HTT-linked polymorphic region. Pharmacogenomics J. 12(5):372–378

33. Meng ZJ, Wu N, Liu Y, Shu KJ, Zou X, Zhang RX, Pi CJ, He BC, Ke ZY, Chen L, Deng ZL, Yin LJ (2015) Evodiamine inhibits the proliferation of human osteosarcoma cells by blocking PI3K/Akt signaling. Oncol Rep 34(3):1388–1396
34. Wu JY, Chang MC, Chen CS, Lin HC, Tsai HP, Yang CC, Yang CH, Lin CM (2013) Topoisomerase I inhibitor evodiamine acts as an antibacterial agent against drug-resistant *Klebsiella pneumoniae*. Planta Med 79(1):27–29
35. Dai JP, Li WZ, Zhao XF, Wang GF, Yang JC, Zhang L, Chen XX, Xu YX, Li KS (2012) A drug screening method based on the autophagy pathway and studies of the mechanism of evodiamine against influenza A virus. PLoS ONE 7(8):e42706
36. Liu AJ, Wang SH, Hou SY, Lin CJ, Chiu WT, Hsiao SH, Chen TH, Shih CM (2013) Evodiamine induces transient receptor potential vanilloid-1-mediated protective autophagy in U87-MG astrocytes. Evid Based Complement Alternat Med 2013:354840
37. Xue H, Cheng Y, Wang X, Yue Y, Zhang W, Li X (2015) Rutaecarpine and evodiamine selected as β1-AR inhibitor candidates using β1-AR/CMC-offline-UPLC/MS prevent cardiac ischemia-reperfusion injury via energy modulation. J Pharm Biomed Anal 115:307–314
38. Liu LH, Xie JY, Guo WW, Wu GY, Chen ZF, Yi JY, Zhang L, Zhang ZJ, Li Z (2014) Evodiamine activates AMPK and promotes adiponectin multimerization in 3T3-L1 adipocytes. J Asian Nat Prod Res 16(11):1074–1083
39. Wei J, Ching LC, Zhao JF, Shyue SK, Lee HF, Kou YR, Lee TS (2013) Essential role of transient receptor potential vanilloid type 1 in evodiamine-mediated protection against atherosclerosis. Acta Physiol (Oxf) 207(2):299–307
40. Xiong YJ, Chen DP, Peng JY, Wang JY, Lv BC, Liu FF, Lin Y (2015) Characteristics of evodiamine-exerted stimulatory effects on rat jejunal contractility. Nat Prod Res 29(4):388–391
41. Shi J, Yan J, Lei Q, Zhao J, Chen K, Yang D, Zhao X, Zhang Y (2009) Intragastric administration of evodiamine suppresses NPY and AgRP gene expression in the hypothalamus and decreases food intake in rats. Brain Res 1247:71–78
42. Jiang DF, Li WT, Yang HL, Zhang ZZ, Chen D, Sun C (2014) Long-term effects of evodiamine on expressions of lipogenesis and lipolysis genes in mouse adipose and liver tissues. Genet Mol Res 13(1):1038–1046
43. Zhao Z, Gong S, Wang S, Ma C (2015) Effect and mechanism of evodiamine against ethanol-induced gastric ulcer in mice by suppressing Rho/NF-κB pathway. Int Immunopharmacol 28(1):588–595
44. Zhao T, Zhang X, Zhao Y, Zhang L, Bai X, Zhang J, Zhao X, Chen L, Wang L, Cui L (2014) Pretreatment by evodiamine is neuroprotective in cerebral ischemia: up-regulated pAkt, pGSK3β, down-regulated NFκB expression, and ameliorated BBB permeability. Neurochem Res 39(8):1612–1620
45. Jiang ML, Zhang ZX, Li YZ, Wang XH, Yan W, Gong GQ (2015) Antidepressant-like effect of evodiamine on chronic unpredictable mild stress rats. Neurosci Lett 588:154–158
46. Yuan SM, Gao K, Wang DM, Quan XZ, Liu JN, Ma CM, Qin C, Zhang LF (2011) Evodiamine improves congnitive abilities in SAMP8 and APP(swe)/PS1(ΔE9) transgenic mouse models of Alzheimer's disease. Acta Pharmacol Sin 32(3):295–302
47. Wang T, Kusudo T, Takeuchi T, Yamashita Y, Kontani Y, Okamatsu Y, Saito M, Mori N, Yamashita H (2013) Evodiamine inhibits insulin-stimulated mTOR-S6K activation and IRS1 serine phosphorylation in adipocytes and improves glucose tolerance in obese/diabetic mice. PLoS ONE 8(12):e83264
48. Doe J (2015) http://www.wiki8.com/zuojinwan_23586. Accessed 23 Dec 2015
49. Matsuda H, Wu JX, Tanaka T, Iinuma M, Kubo M (1997) Antinociceptive activities of 70 % methanol extract of evodiae fructus (fruit of *Evodia rutaecarpa* var. bodinieri) and its alkaloidal components. Biol Pharm Bull 20(3):243–248
50. Liao CH, Pan SL, Guh JH, Chang YL, Pai HC, Lin CH, Teng CM (2005) Antitumor mechanism of evodiamine, a constituent from Chinese herb Evodiae fructus, in human multiple-drug resistant breast cancer NCI/ADR-RES cells in vitro and in vivo. Carcinogenesis 26(5):968–975

51. Hu J, Sun L, Zhao D, Zhang L, Ye M, Tan Q, Fang C, Wang H, Zhang J (2014) Supermolecular evodiamine loaded water-in-oil nanoemulsions: enhanced physicochemical and biological characteristics. Eur J Pharm Biopharm 88(2):556–564
52. De Petrocellis L, Schiano Moriello A, Fontana G, Sacchetti A, Passarella D, Appendino G, Di Marzo V (2014) Effect of chirality and lipophilicity in the functional activity of evodiamine and its analogues at TRPV1 channels. Br J Pharmacol 171(10):2608–2620
53. Wang S, Fang K, Dong G, Chen S, Liu N, Miao Z, Yao J, Li J, Zhang W, Sheng C (2015) Scaffold diversity inspired by the natural product evodiamine: discovery of highly potent and multitargeting antitumor agents. J Med Chem 58(16):6678–6696
54. Huang G, Kling B, Darras FH, Heilmann J, Decker M (2014) Identification of a neuroprotective and selective butyrylcholinesterase inhibitor derived from the natural alkaloid evodiamine. Eur J Med Chem 81:15–21

Guggulsterone and Its Role in Chronic Diseases

Takanori Yamada and Ken Sugimoto

Abstract Guggulsterone is a plant sterol derived from gum resin of *Commiphora wightii*. The gum resin from guggul plants has been used for thousand years in Ayurveda to treat various disorders, including internal tumors, obesity, liver disorders, malignant sores and ulcers, urinary complaints, intestinal worms, leucoderma, sinuses, edema, and sudden paralytic seizures. Guggulsterone has been identified a bioactive components of this gum resin. This plant steroid has been reported to work as an antagonist of certain nuclear receptors, especially farnesoid X receptor, which regulates bile acids and cholesterol metabolism. Guggulsterone also mediates gene expression through the regulation of transcription factors, including nuclear factor-kappa B and signal transducer and activator of transcription 3, which plays important roles in the development of inflammation and tumorigenesis. Guggulsterone has been shown to downregulate the expression of proteins involved in anti-apoptotic, cell survival, cell proliferation, angiogenic, metastatic, and chemoresistant activities in tumor cells. This review aimed to clarify the cell signal pathways targeted by guggulsterone and the bioactivities of guggulsterone in animal models and humans.

Keywords Guggul · Guggulsterone · Cancer · Inflammation · Hyperlipidemia · Chemoprevention

---

T. Yamada (✉)
Department of Gastroenterology, Iwata City Hospital, 512-3, Okubo, Iwata 438-8550, Japan
e-mail: tky@hospital.iwata.shizuoka.jp

K. Sugimoto
First Department of Medicine, Hamamatsu University School of Medicine, Hamamatsu 431-3192, Japan

S.C. Gupta et al. (eds.), *Drug Discovery from Mother Nature*, Advances in Experimental Medicine and Biology 929,
DOI 10.1007/978-3-319-41342-6_15

1 Introduction

Cancers or vascular events are major causes of death all over the world. Both of these critical conditions are considered to be associated with chronic inflammation and obesity. In spite of huge efforts to control them, these disorders are still highly prevalent. Generally, modern medicines tend to be mono-targeted, focusing on a single gene product or pathway. However, most chronic diseases develop and progress in a multistep process. The discrepancy between the design concept of modern medicine and disease progression processes may be one of the reasons why modern medicine has not yet overcome these disorders.

Guggul is one of the very ancient Ayurvedic drugs and has been used for several thousand years. Guggulsterone is the major bioactive compound of guggul. According to the Sushruta Samhita, a well-known Ayurvedic medical text, guggul when taken orally, is a curative for obesity, liver disorder, internal tumors, malignant sores and ulcers, urinary complaints, fistula-in-ano, intestinal worms, leucoderma, sinus, edema, and sudden paralytic seizures [77, 84]. It has been revealed that guggulsterone acts as an antagonist of the farnesoid X receptor (FXR) and has hypolipidemic effects [97]. Guggulsterone has also been reported to inhibit pro-inflammatory signals, including transcription factor nuclear factor-kappa B (NF-κB) [82]. Furthermore, guggulsterone suppressed tumor progression in multistep cell growth, proliferation, invasion, metastasis, and angiogenesis. This review describes the cell signaling pathways targeted by guggulsterone and its bioactivities in animal models and humans [85].

2 Physicochemical Properties of Guggulsterone

The guggul tree (*Commiphora mukul*) is native to India and its neighboring countries. The oleogum resin of this species is a yellowish substance that is tapped during winter, and each tree yields about 700–900 g of resin [76]. Guggul is a complex mixture of gum, minerals, essential oils, terpenes, sterols, ferrulates, flavanones, and sterones. When extracted with ethyl acetate, the extraction yields two fractions: 45 % soluble and 55 % insoluble fractions. The bioactive components found in the ethyl acetate soluble fraction, known as gugulipid, consist of diterpenoids, triterpenoids, steroids, lignans, and fatty tetrol esters. Further fractionation of the soluble fraction with pH gradients yielded a 4 % acidic fraction, 1 % basic fraction, and 95 % neutral fraction. Additional fractionation of the neutral fraction led to the isolation of a major nonketonic (88 %) and a small ketonic fraction (12 %). The ketonic fraction contained a number of steroids including the two isomers E-(*cis*-) and Z-(*trans*-)guggulsterone (4, 17(20)-pregnadiene-3, 16-dione)

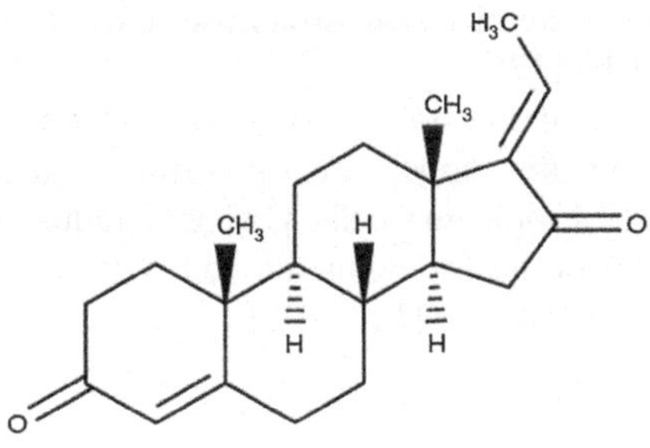

E- (cis-) guggulsterone

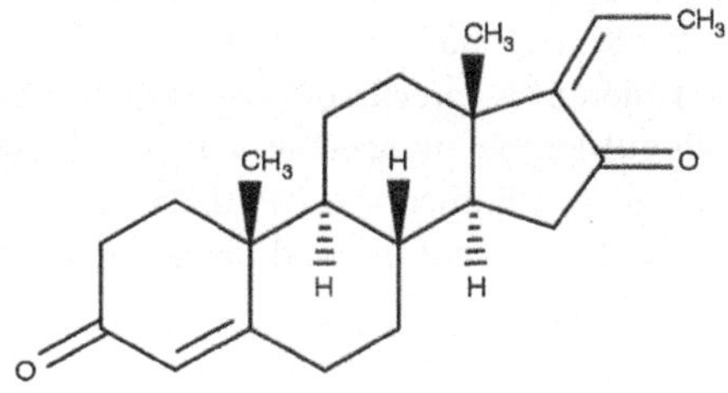

Z- (trans-) guggulsterone

Fig. 1 Chemical structure of guggulsterone isomers. **a** [4,17[20]-(*cis*)-pregnadiene-3,16-dione] is E-guggulsterone. **b** [4,17[20]-(*trans*)-pregnadiene-3,16-dione] is Z-guggulsterone

(Fig. 1). The guggulsterones constitute approximately 2 % of gum guggul and 5 % of gugulipid by weight [19, 83].

Molecular docking simulation studies reported that guggulsterone bound to FXR and NF-κB. Guggulsterone cloud docks into two noncanonical binding sites of FXR, helix 1-loop-helix 2 loop and parts of helix–helix 8 including helix 8-loop-helix 9 [62, 111]. Guggulsterone also binds to the NF-κB precursor protein p105 on its RH domain, which contains sequences important for DNA binding and dimerization, which might be the reason for its NF-κB inhibitory activities [38].

3 Modulation of the Cell Signaling Pathway by Guggulsterone

3.1 Farnesoid X Receptor

FXR is a member of the nuclear hormone receptor superfamily and is expressed in the liver, intestine, kidney, adrenals, stomach, fat, and heart [113]. The physiological ligands of FXR are bile acids [58, 71, 99], and it is involved in the regulation of bile acids, cholesterol [69], triglyceride [87], and glucose [114] metabolism. Guggulsterone is a highly efficacious antagonist of FXR, and guggulsterone treatment decreased hepatic cholesterol in wild-type mice fed a high-cholesterol diet but was not effective in FXR-null mice. The inhibition of FXR activation may be the basis for the cholesterol-lowering activity of guggulsterone [97].

In HepG2 cells, in the presence of an FXR agonist such as chenodeoxycholate or GW4064, guggulsterone enhanced endogenous bile salt export pump (BSEP) expression with maximal induction of 400–500 % by the FXR agonist alone. Gugulipid treatment in rats increased expression of BSEP and small heterodimer partner (SHP) but not cholesterol 7α1 (*Cyp 7α1*), sterol 12α-hydroxylase (*Cyp 8b1*), or intestinal bile acid-binding protein (I-BABP) [17].

FXR may have a role in the development of intestinal metaplasia, which is considered a precursor lesion of cancer in the upper gastrointestinal tract. Guggulsterone induced apoptosis in Barrett's esophagus cells [18] and reduced caudal type homeobox 2 (Cdx2) expression in rat gastric epithelial cells (RGM-1) and in human gut-derived adenocarcinoma cells (Bic-1) [107, 108].

3.2 Other Nuclear Receptors

Nuclear receptors are ligand-modulated transcription factors that bind to DNA and regulate the expression of adjacent genes.

Both E- and Z-guggulsterone displayed high affinity for FXR as well as other steroid receptors, including the androgen, glucocorticoid, and progesterone receptors [8]. Guggulsterone functions as an efficacious constitutive androstane receptor inverse agonist. The ratio of constitutive androstane receptor to PXR determined the activity of guggulsterone against the Cyp2b10 promoter [21].

3.3 Nuclear Factor-κB

NF-κB, a proinflammatory transcription factor, can promote the development of tumors. Various inflammatory agents, carcinogens, tumor promoters, and the tumor microenvironment activate NF-κB. NF-κB proteins themselves and proteins regulated by it have been linked to cellular transformation, proliferation, apoptosis suppression, invasion, angiogenesis, and metastasis. Constitutively activated NF-κB is common in a wide variety of tumors. Furthermore, there exists genetic evidence that NF-κB mediates tumorigenesis. Thus, suppression of NF-κB activation should be effective in the prevention and treatment of cancer [1].

Guggulsterone suppressed DNA binding of NF-κB induced by multistimulation in lung carcinoma cells through inhibition of IκB kinase activation, and it also suppressed induced and constitutive NF-κB activation in most tumor cells. Guggulsterone decreased the expression gene products involved in anti-apoptosis (IAP1, xIAP, Bfl-1/A1, Bcl-2, cFLIP, and survivin), proliferation (cyclin D1 and c-Myc), and metastasis (matrix metalloproteinase [MMP]-9, cyclooxygenase-2 [COX-2], and vascular endothelial growth factor [VEGF]) [82]. These results suggested that guggulsterone suppresses NF-κB and NF-κB-regulated gene products, which many explain its anti-inflammatory and anti-tumor activities.

4 Signal Transducer and Activator of Transcription

Signal transducer and activator of transcription (STAT) 3 is a member of a family of transcription factors. This factor is associated with inflammation, cellular transformation, survival, proliferation, invasion, angiogenesis, and cancer metastasis. Various types of carcinogens, radiation, viruses, growth factors, oncogenes, and inflammatory cytokines have been found to activate STAT3. STAT3 is constitutively active in most tumor cells but not in normal cells [2].

Guggulsterone inhibited angiogenesis by blocking STAT3 and VEGF expression in colon cancer cells (HT-29). It also reduced MMP-2 and MMP-9 enzyme activity in colon cancer cells. The recruitment of STAT3 and anyl hydrocarbon receptor nuclear translocator, but not hypoxia-inducible factor (HIF)-1α, to the VEGF promoter was inhibited by guggulsterone treatment. Human umbilical vein endothelial cells (HUVECs) produced much foreshortened and severely broken tubes and showed decreased migration activity as a result of guggulsterone treatment [43].

Guggulsterone also inhibits interleukin (IL)-6-induced STAT3 activation through the induction of SHP-1 in human multiple myeloma cells (U226). Downregulation of the expression of STAT3-regulated anti-apoptotic (Bcl-2, Bcl-xL, Mcl-1), proliferative (cyclin D1), and angiogenetic (VEGF) gene products occurred in response to guggulsterone treatment; and this correlated with the suppression of proliferation, accumulation of cells in subG1 phase of the cell cycle, and induction of apoptosis [4].

5 Mitogen-Activated Protein Kinase

Mitogen-activated protein kinase (MAPK) pathways are evolutionarily conserved kinase modules that link extracellular signals to the machinery that controls fundamental cellular processes such as growth, proliferation, differentiation, migration, and apoptosis. To date, six distinct groups of MAPKs have been characterized in mammals: extracellular signal-regulated kinase (ERK)1/2, ERK3/4, ERK5, ERK7/8, c-Jun N-terminal kinase (JNK)1/2/3, and the p38 isoforms. Generally, the effect of MAPKs is anti-proliferative and proapoptotic, but dependent on the cellular context they may also contribute to tumorigenesis [20].

Guggulsterone-induced cell death in human prostate cancer cells (PC-3 and LNCaP) was regulated by reactive oxygen intermediate (ROI)-dependent activation of JNK, but independent of ERK1/2 or p38. Guggulsterone did not generate ROIs in normal prostate cancer cells (PrEC) [89], but it inhibited 12-*O*-tetradecanoylphorbol-13-acetate-mediated skin edema and hyperplasia in mice. Treatment with guggulsterone also inhibited 12-*O*-tetradecanoylphorbol-13-acetate-induced phosphorylation of ERK1/2, JNK, and p38 [75], and it suppressed the activation of ERK1/2 and JNK in the pancreas of cerulein-induced murine pancreatitis [41]. MAPKs likely show different responses according to conditions, e.g., stimuli or cell types.

6 PI3K/Akt Signaling

The PI3K-Akt signaling pathway has been firmly established as a critical contributor toward tumorigenesis. This pathway is involved in cell growth, survival, and proliferation within tumors [53].

Guggulsterone-induced apoptosis was related to inactivation of Akt followed by activation of JNK in human monocytic leukemia cells (U937) [85]. Additionally, it inhibited angiogenesis by suppressing the VEGF-VEGF-R2-Akt signaling in HUVECs [101].

7 Inducible Nitric Oxygen Synthase

Nitric oxide (NO) is involved in various physiological functions, and its role in tumorigenesis has been well studied. A large majority of human and experimental tumors appear to progress owing to NO resulting from inducible NO synthase (iNOS), further stimulated by proinflammatory cytokines [33].

Z- and E-guggulsterone were more potent inhibitors of NO production (IC50 = 1.1 and 3.3 μM, respectively) compared with curcumin (IC50 = 12.3 μM) in lipopolysaccharide (LPS)-activated murine macrophages (J774.1) [61]. Guggulsterone prevented cytokines-induced NO correlated with reduced level of iNOS expression in rat insulinoma cells (RINm5F) [54]. It also reduced LPS-induced iNOS mRNA expression in mouse inner medullary collecting duct cells (mIMCD-3) [42].

8 Cyclooxygenase-2

COX-2 converts arachidonic acid to prostaglandins and prostanoids through stimulation. COX-2 has been shown to be one of the key players in the induction of inflammation and tumorigenesis.

Guggulsterone prevented IL-1β-induced and interferon (IFN)-γ-induced COX-2 expression and prostaglandin E2 (PGE2) production in rat insulinoma cells (RINm5F) [54]. It suppressed deoxycholic acid (DCA)-induced and constitutive COX-2 expression and PGE2 production in esophageal adenocarcinoma cells (OE19, OE33) [109].

9 Wnt/Beta (β)-Catenin Signaling

Wnt signaling is involved in virtually every aspect of embryonic development and also controls homeostatic self-renewal in a number of adult tissues. Germline mutations in the Wnt/β-catenin pathway cause several hereditary diseases, and somatic mutations are associated with cancer of the intestine and a variety of other tissues [15].

Guggulsterone reduced β-catenin/T-cell factor 4 complex and Wnt/β-catenin targeting genes, such as cyclin D1, C-myc, and T-cell factor 4 in breast cancer cells (MCF-7, MDA-MB-231), indicating that the β-catenin signaling pathway is the target for gugulipid-induced growth inhibition and apoptosis in human breast cancer [34] (Tables 1 and 2).

10 P-glycoprotein

P-glycoprotein (P-gp) is expressed in many normal human tissues and cancers. P-gp plays a major role in the distribution and excretion of drugs and is involved in the intrinsic and acquired drug resistance of cancers [12]. Targeting the regulation of P-gp and related resistance mechanisms is a potential therapeutic approach against cancer.

Guggulsterone showed a dual inhibitory effect on the function of P-gp and in multidrug-resistant human cells (KB-C2) [65]. When guggulsterone was combined with doxorubicin, it significantly promoted the sensitivity of doxorubicin-resistant human myelogenous leukemia cells (K562/DOX) toward doxorubicin. The inhibitory effect of guggulsterone on P-gp activity was the major cause of increased stagnation of doxorubicin inside K562/DOX cells, indicating that guggulsterone may effectively reverse multidrug resistance in K562/DOX cells via inhibiting the expression and drug transport function of P-gp [105].

11 Role of Guggulsterone in Chronic Diseases

11.1 Hypolipidemic and Anti-adipogenesis Effects

The hypolipidemic effects of guggulsterone have been well established in clinical trials compared with the other bioactivities of guggulsterone. Several animal model studies revealed that guggulsterone attenuates hyperlipidemia in the animals fed a high-fat diet.

Treatment with guggulsterone decreased hepatic cholesterol in wild-type mice fed a high-cholesterol diet but was not effective in FXR-null mice. The inhibition of FXR activation is the basis for the cholesterol-lowering activity of guggulsterone

Table 1 Effects of guggulsterone on diseases other than tumors

Disease	Mechanism/effect	Cells	Animal models
Hypolipidemia	FXR↓, BSEP↑, cholesterol↓ (total, LDL, VLDL), triglyceride↓, HDL↑		FXR-null mice, rats, rabbits, chickens, pigs, monkeys
Diabetes	NO↓, iNOS↓, LI-1β↓, IFNγ↓, COX-2↓, PGE2↓, prevention of β-cell size reduction in high-fat-fed rats, improvement of glucose tolerance in ob/ob mice	RINm5F	Rats, ob/ob mice
Kidney injury	NF-κB↓, iNOS↓, COX-2↓, IL-6↓, TNF-α↓	mIMCD-3	
Drug resistance	P-gp↓, MRP1↓, reversal of doxorubicin resistance	K567/DOX, KB-C2	Xenograft
Obesity	C/EBPs↓, PPATγ↓, FABP↓, SREEBP-1c↓, adipoQ↓, SOCS-3↓ induction caspase-dependent apoptosis in adipocytes	3T3−L1	
Thyroid dysfunction	Increase in iodine uptake by the thyroid		Rats
Cardiovascular disorders	FXR↓, TF↑, PAI-1↓, VCAM-1↓, reversal of metabolic changes, reduction of caspase-dependent apoptosis	H9C2, neonatal rat cardiac myocytes, HAECs	Murine MI/R model
Hepatitis	ICAM-1↓, NF-κB↓, HIF-1α↓, decrease in collagen deposition, hepatic stellate cell apoptosis, blocking upregulated by bile acids, and basal level of hepatic C virus replication	HepG2, LX-2, Huh-7, Hul	Mice
Inflammatory bowel disease	ICAM-1↓, NF-κB↓, IKK↓, IL-2↓, IL-4↓, IFN-γ↓, IL-12↓, TNFα↓	Caco-2, COLO205, BMDC	DSS-, TNBS- or oxazolone-IBD mice, IL-10K/O mice
Pancreatitis	Reduction in pancreas weight/body weight ratio, serum lipase, infiltrations of macrophages and neutrophils		Mice
Arthritis	NF-κB↓, RANTES↓, ENA-78↓, MMP-1↓, MMP-3↓, reversal of thickness and swelling in joints	Fibroblast-like synoviocytes	Rabbits
Neurological disorder	AChe↓, protection of memory deficit, induction of neural stem cells into dopaminergic neurons		Mice
Melanogenesis in skin	Tyrosinase↓, TRP-1↓	B16/10	
Uveitis	NF-κB, ↓NO↓, iNOS↓, COX-2↓, PGE2↓, MMP-2↓	HNPECs	Rats
Respiratory disorder	Reversal of effect by FXR agonist on respiratory rhythm		Rats

↑ indicates upregulation of expression or activation by guggulsterone
↓ indicates downregulation of expression or activation by guggulsterone

[97]. Guggulsterone also showed the ability to enhance the action of agonists of BSEP expression, because gugulipid treatment in rats lowered serum triglyceride and raised high-density lipoprotein (HDL) levels in vivo [17].

Guggulsterone reversed adipogenesis-related gene, CAAT/enhancer-binding protein (C/EBPs), and peroxisome proliferator-activated receptor (PPAR) γ, fatty acid-binding protein, sterol regulatory element binding protein-1c (SREBP-1c), and adipoQ, mRNA expression induced by a FXR ligand in preadipocytes (3T3-L1) [74]. It also induced caspase-dependent apoptosis, reduced the lipid content in adipocytes (3T3-L1), and downregulated the adipocyte-specific transcription factors PPARγ2, C/EBPα, and C/EBPβ [70, 110].

11.2 Diabetes Mellitus

Several studies have implicated guggulsterone is a potential remedy for diabetes. Treatment with guggulsterone prevented IL-1β- and IFN-γ-induced β-cell damage, as well as NO and PGE2 production, and these effects were related to reduced levels of iNOS and COX-2 expression. Guggulsterone prevented cytokines-induced NO and PGE2 production, iNOS and COX-2 expression, Janus kinase/STAT activation, downregulated suppressor of cytokine signaling-3, and impaired glucose-stimulated insulin secretion [54]. It also attenuated the reduction in pancreatic β-cell size, increase in adipocytes, and steatosis of the liver in high-fat-diet-fed rats. Guggulsterone inhibited 3T3-L1 preadipocytes differentiation, and it had both hypoglycemic and hypolipidemic effects that can help to cure type 2 diabetes [80].

Bile acids acutely stimulate insulin secretion by mouse β-cells via FXR activation and K_{ATP} channel inhibition, but guggulsterone suppressed this effect. FXR in pancreatic β-cell may contribute to a pharmaceutical strategy for the treatment of type 2 diabetes mellitus [24]. Furthermore, gugulipid (20 g/kg diet) improved glucose tolerance in female Lep(ob)/Lep(ob) mice [16].

11.3 Thyroid Stimulatory Effects

Guggulsterone showed a strong thyroid stimulatory action, but not through pituitary activation, in rats [94, 95].

11.4 Cardiovascular Protection

Several studies have reported cardioprotective effects of guggulsterone both in vitro and in vivo.

Table 2 Effects of guggulsterone on tumors

Disease/condition	Mechanism/effect	Cells	Animal models
Leukemia	NF-κB↓, COX-2↓, MMP-9↓, cyclinD1↓, Akt↑, JNK↓, cyclinD1↓, cdc2↓, Bfl-1↓, cFLIP↓, Bcl-XL↓, Bcl-2↓, xIAP↓, cMcl1↓, survivin↓, c-Myc↓, caspase-dependent apoptosis	U937	
Head and neck cancer	STAT3↓, HIF-1α↓, NF-κB↓, COX-2↓, VEGF↓, PP2A↑, 14-3-3ζ↓, Bad↓, Bcl-2↓, xIAP↓, cMcl1↓, survivin↓, cyclin D1↓, c-Myc↓, caspase-dependent apoptosis, reduction of tumor xenograft size, enhancing chemotherapy effect	1482, UM-22A, UM-22B, SCC4, HSC2,	Xenograft
Breast cancer	NF-κB↓, AP-1↓, β-catenin↓, cyclinD1↓, c-Myc↓ TCF-4↓, HO-1↑, Nrf2↑, VEGFR2↑	MCF-7, MDA-MB-231, MCF10A	
Lung cancer	NF-κB↓, COX-2↓, MMP-9↓, VEGF↓, cyclinD1↓, IAP1↓, XIAP↓, Bfl-1/A1↓, Bcl-2↓, TRAF1↓, cFLIP↓, survivin↓, induction of apoptosis	H1299	
Intestinal metaplasia	Cdx2↓, MUC-2↓	CP-18821, RGM-1, Bic-1, OE19, OE33,	
Esophageal adenocarcinoma	COX-2↓, PGE2↓, IBABP↓, SHP↓, IL-8↓, MIP3α↓, caspase-dependent apoptosis, reduction of tumor xenograft size	OE19, OE33, TE-7	Xenograft
Colorectal cancer	STAT3↓, VEGF↓, ARNT↓, MMP-2↓, MMP-9↓, caspase-dependent apoptosis, reduction of tumor xenograft size	HT-29	Xenograft
Pancreatobiliary cancer	FXR↓, SrC↓, Jak/STAT↓, MUC4↓, JNK↓, NF-κBp65↓VEGF-c↓, MMP-2↓, enhancement of chemotherapy effect	MIA-PaCa2, PANC-1, CD18/HPAF, Capan1, TGBC1, TGBC2	Xenograft
Hepatoma	Sensitization to TRAIL	Hep3B, HepG2	
Prostate cancer	ROI↑, JNK↓, ACLY/Akt↓, reduction of tumor xenograft size	PC-3, LNCaP, PrEC	Xenograft
Brain tumor	Ras↓, NF-κB↓, sensitization to SANT-1	A172, U87MG, T98G	
Bone metastasis	NF-κB↓, RANKL↓, RUNX2↓, interference with osteoblastic differentiation, prevention of migration	MDA-MB-468, U226, BMSC, MG63	
Radiosensitivity	NF-κB↓, IGF-Rα↓, ERα↓, inhibition of DNA double-strand break repair	PC-Sw, MFC-7, HT-29	
Drug resistance	P-gp↓, MRP1↓, reversal of doxorubicin resistance	MCF-7/DOX, KB-C2	Xenograft

↑ indicates upregulation of expression or activation by guggulsterone
↓ indicates downregulation of expression or activation by guggulsterone

A marked protective effect was shown by guggulsterone on cardiac enzymes and the P450 system against myocardial necrosis induced by isoproterenol in rats [37]. Guggulsterone showed marked reversal of the metabolic change in the heart, with increased phospholipase, decreased cardiac glycogen, and increased cytosolic lipid peroxide, related to ischemia of the heart induced by isoproterenol in rats [10].

Guggulsterone reduced DOX-induced apoptosis and cell death in cardiomyocytes (H9C2). Pretreatment using guggulsterone reversed DOX-induced decreases in PARP, caspase-3, and bcl-2 and increases in Bax, cytochrome C release, cleaved-PERP, and cleaved caspase-3 [100].

siRNA-mediated silencing of endogenous FXR or guggulsterone reduced post-ischemic myocardial apoptosis in murine myocardial ischemia. FXR acted as a novel functional receptor in cardiac tissue, regulated apoptosis in cardiomyocytes, and contributed to myocardial ischemia/reperfusion injury [72].

Guggulsterone inhibited TNF-α-induced endothelial tissue factor protein and mRNA expression and surface activity in human aortic endothelial cells. It enhanced endothelial tissue factor pathway inhibitor and impaired plasminogen activator inhibitor-1 as well as vascular cell adhesion molecule-1 (VCAM-1) protein. Guggulsterone offers a novel therapeutic option, in particular in inflammatory disease associated with an increased risk of thrombosis [26].

11.5 Hepatoprotective Effects

Treatment with guggulsterone inhibited intracellular adhesion molecule-1 expression by GW4064, a FXR selective agonist, in human hepatocytes (HepG2) [73]. Guggulsterone attenuated activation and survival of hepatic stellate cells (LX-2) by inhibiting NF-κB activation and inducing apoptosis. High-dose guggulsterone decreased the extent of collagen deposition and the percentage of activated hepatic stellate cells undergoing apoptosis in mice [40]. HIF-1α expression was also reduced by guggulsterone in hypoxic conditions in hepatocytes (HepG2) [64].

The bile acid-mediated increase in HCV RNA in hepatocytes (Huh-7, GS4.1) was reduced by guggulsterone [11], and it blocked upregulation by bile acids and basal levels of hepatic C virus replication in an HCV replication model (Hul cells) [79].

11.6 Kidney Protection Effects

LPS treatment of mouse inner medullary collecting cells produced pro-inflammatory molecules such as iNOS, COX-2, IL-6, and TNF-α; however, guggulsterone treatment inhibited this process. Guggulsterone inhibited the degradation of Iκ-Bα and translocation of NF-κB and could inhibit inflammatory responses in collecting duct cells, which may contribute to kidney injury due to systemic infection [42].

11.7 Inflammatory Bowel Disease

Several in vitro and in vivo studies implicated guggulsterone as an attractive therapeutic option in the treatment of inflammatory bowel disease.

Guggulsterone significantly inhibited LPS- or IL-1β-induced intracellular adhesion molecule-1 gene expression, NF-κB transcriptional activity, IκB phosphorylation/degradation, and NF-κB DNA binding activity in colon cancer cells (Caco-2) or rat intra-epithelial cells (IEC-18). Moreover, guggulsterone strongly blocked IKK activity [13] and attenuated the generation of IL-2 and IL-4 and IFN-γ as well as T-cell proliferation (Mencarel[52].

GG-52, a guggulsterone derivative, blocked NF-κB activation in colon cancer cells (COLO 205) [44], and LPS-induced IL-12p40 and TNF-α gene expression, IκBα degradation, and NF-κB DNA binding activity in bone marrow-derived dendritic cells [44].

Both guggulsterone and GG-52 have also been reported to attenuate different murine inflammatory bowel disease models in vivo [13, 36, 44, 60].

11.8 Pancreatitis

Pre-treatment with guggulsterone attenuated histological damage, reduced pancreas weight/body weight ratio, decreased serum lipase levels, inhibited infiltration of macrophages and neutrophils, and suppressed cytokine production in murine cerulei-induced acute pancreatitis [41].

11.9 Arthritis

Guggulsterone blocked IL-1β-mediated inflammatory proteins, such as regulated in activation normal T-cell expressed and secreted, epithelial neutrophil activating peptide-78, MMP-1 and MMP-3 by suppressing NF-κB activation in fibroblast-like synoviocytes [50].

Guggul decreased the thickness of joint swelling in an experimental rabbit arthritis model resembling rheumatoid arthritis in humans [81].

In a human study, 30 male and female participants with arthritis received gum guggul. Participants showed significantly improved Western Ontario and MacMaster Osteoarthritis Index total scores after taking the supplement for

1 month and continued to improve at the 2-month time point and during follow-up [88].

11.10 Neuroprotective Effects

Gugulipid (p.o.) treatment showed improvements in scopolamine-induced deficits in a passive avoidance test in mice. Gugulipid (i.c.) treatment had protective effects in a streptozotocin-induced memory deficit model of dementia that can be attributed to antioxidant and anti-acetylcholinesterase (AChE) activities of gugulipid. These observations suggested gugulipid as a potential anti-dementia drug [78].

In addition, guggulsterone was found to be highly effective. These neurons have been extensively characterized and shown to be functional. This new approach may offer a practical route to creating neurons of sufficient quality to be used to treat Parkinson's disease [28].

11.11 Nodulocystic Acne

Treatment with gugulipid (50 mg guggulsterone) for 3 months resulted in a 68 % decrease inflammatory lesions in patients with nodulocystic acne. Patients with oily faces responded remarkably to gugulipid [93].

11.12 Melanogenesis in Skin

Treatment with guggulsterone dose dependently inhibited isobutylmethylxanthine-induced melanogenesis and cellular tyrosinase activity with no cytotoxicity in melanoma cells (B16/F10). Decreased melanin biosynthesis was accompanied by the reduced expression of melanogenesis-related genes, such as tyrosinase, microphthalmia-associated transcription factor, tyrosinase-related protein (TRP) 1, and TRP-2 [45].

11.13 Uveitis

Guggulsterone prevented the expression of endotoxin-induced uveitis (EIU)-induced inflammatory markers, such as MMP-2, NO, and PGE2 in rats. It also prevented the expression of MMP-2, iNOS, and COX-2 proteins and of IκB and NF-κB in various eye tissues of rats. Treatment with guggulsterone inhibited LPS-induced expression of inflammatory proteins in human primary nonpigment ciliary epithelial cells. Guggulsterone could be a novel option for the treatment of ocular inflammation [35].

11.14 *Respiratory Diseases*

FXR agonists are able to regulate respiratory rhythm, and guggulsterone completely reversed the effect of FXR agonists in neonatal rat brainstem medulla oblongata slices. FXR is a potential therapeutic target in treating respiratory diseases [115].

11.15 *Anti-tumor*

Treatment with guggulsterone suppressed DNA binding of NF-κB induced by multistimulation in lung carcinoma cells (H1299) through inhibition of IκB kinase activation. Guggulsterone suppressed induced and constitutive NF-κB activation in most tumor cells (A549, KBM-5, Jurkat, U266, MDA1986). Guggulsterone decreased the expression of gene products involved in anti-apoptosis (IAP1, xIAP, Bfl-1/A1, Bcl-2, cFLIP, and survivin), proliferation (cyclin D1 and c-Myc), and metastasis (MMP-9, COX-2, and VEGF) [82, 85].

Guggulsterone inhibited angiogenesis by blocking STAT3 and VEGF expression, which play important roles in angiogenesis, in colon cancer cells (HT-29) and neck squamous cell carcinoma cells (SCC4, HSC2) [43, 56].

Therefore, guggulsterone is considered as a promising option for chemoprevention as well as therapy against tumors.

11.16 *Leukemia*

Guggulsterone inhibited the proliferation of human leukemia cells (U937, jurkat, KBM-5, and K562). It induced S-phase arrest correlated with a decrease in cyclin D1 and cdc2, and induced caspase-dependent apoptosis through activation of JNK and suppression of the Akt pathway in leukemia cells (U937). [82].

11.17 *Head and Neck Cancer*

The effect of bortezomib to induce cell death through STAT3 inhibition was enhanced by guggulsterone in neck squamous cell carcinoma cells (PCI-37a, UM-22b, and 1483) [51].

Guggulsterone induced apoptosis and cell cycle arrest, inhibited invasion, and enhanced the efficacy of erlotinib, cetuximab, and cisplatin in human head and neck squamous cell carcinoma cells (HNSCCs) (1483, UM-22A, and UM-22B). It decreased total and phosphotyrosine STAT3 as well as HIF-1α in HNSCCs. In a xenograft model of HNSCCs, guggulsterone treatment increased apoptosis and decreased expression of STAT3. Guggulsterone-mediated inhibition of STAT3 and HIF-1α provided a biologic rationale for further clinical investigation in the treatment of HNSCCs [52]. Treatment with guggulsterone in HNSCCs (SCC4, HSC2) abrogated both smokeless tobacco- and nicotine-induced nuclear activation of NF-κB and pSTAT3 proteins and their downstream targets COX-2 and VEGF. Guggulsterone treatment decreased the level of ST- and nicotine-induced secreted interleukin-6 in culture media of HNSCCs [56].

Treatment with guggulsterone released Bad from the inhibitory action of 14-3-3 ζ(zeta) in proliferating SCC4 cells by activating protein phosphatase 2A (PP2A). These events initiated the intrinsic mitochondrial pathway of apoptosis. Guggulsterone treatment reduced the expression of anti-apoptotic proteins, Bcl-2, xIAP, Mcl1, survivin, cyclin D1, and c-Myc, thus committing cells to apoptosis. These events were followed by activation of caspase-9, caspase-8, and caspase-3. 14-3-zeta, a multifunctional phospho-serine/phospho-threonine binding protein, was a molecular target in guggulsterone-induced apoptosis in head and neck cancer cells (SCC4) [55].

11.18 Breast Cancer

E- and Z-guggulsterone downregulated MMP-9 expression and tumor invasion through the IKK/NF-κB pathway and MAPK/activator protein-1, respectively, in breast cancer cells (MCF-7). A combination of these isomers exerted an additive effect in the inhibition of cell invasion [66].

E-guggulsterone induced heme oxygenase-1 expression through inhibition of AKT phosphorylation and NF-E2-related factor 2 activation in human mammary cells (MCF10A) [5].

Deoxycholate promoted the expression of vascular endothelial growth factor receptor 2 (VEGFR2) and decreased ceramide-mediated apoptosis of breast cancer progenitor cells (4T1). Guggulsterone reduced VEGFR2 expression and angiogenesis in endothelial cell culture [46].

Z-guggulsterone reduced β-catenin/TCF-4 complex and Wnt/β-catenin targeting genes, such as cyclin D1, c-Myc, and TCF-4, in breast cancer cells, indicating that β-catenin signaling pathway is the target for gugulipid-induced growth inhibition and apoptosis in human breast cancer (MCF-7, MDA-MB-231) [34].

11.19 Lung Cancer

Guggulsterone has been also reported to suppress NF-κB activation induced by tumor necrosis factor (TNF), phorbol ester, okadaic acid, cigarette smoke condensate, hydrogen peroxide or IL-1 through inhibition of IκB degradation in non-small lung cancer cells (H1299). Guggulsterone also suppressed COX-2, MMP-9, VEGF, and cyclin D1 expression, as well as inhibiting proliferation and inducing apoptosis [82].

11.20 Intestinal Metaplasia

The effects of chenodeoxycholic acid and GW4064, an FXR antagonist, on mRNA expression of Cdc2 and goblet-specific gene mucin 2 were abolished by guggulsterone in normal rat gastric epithelial cells (RGM-1) [107].

11.21 Esophageal Cancer

FXR was significantly overexpressed in Barrett's esophagus compared with normal mucosa, esophagitis, and esophageal adenocarcinoma. Guggulsterone induced apoptosis and caspase-3 activity in Barrett's esophagus-derived cells (CP-18821) [18]. Expression of FXR, the bile acid metabolism genes I-BABP and SHP, and the chemokines IL-8 and macrophage inflammatory protein 3α were increased in Barrett's epithelium. DCA induced FXR, I-BABP, macrophage inflammatory protein 3α, and IL-8 mRNA expression in an esophageal cell line (TE7), and guggulsterone abolished DCA-induced mRNA expression [9]. Inhibition of FXR by FXR shRNA or guggulsterone suppressed esophageal cancer cell viability and induced apoptosis in vitro and reduced tumor formation and growth in nude mouse xenografts in vivo [30].

Guggulsterone suppressed DCA-induced and NF-κB-dependent activation of Cdx2 and COX-2 expression. Furthermore, guggulsterone also reduced the viability of esophageal adenocarcinoma cells. Guggulsterone may serve as candidate for preventing and treating esophageal adenocarcinoma as well as Barrett's esophagus [109].

11.22 Colorectal Cancer

Treatment with guggulsterone significantly increased apoptosis in colon cancer cells (HT-29) by activating caspase-3 and caspase-8. The size of tumors in guggulsterone-treated mice was significantly smaller than the size of tumors in control mice [6]. Guggulsterone also inhibited angiogenesis by blocking STAT3 and VEGF expression, and reducing MMP-2 and MMP-9 enzyme activity in HT-29 cells [43].

Thus, there is a potential therapeutic use for guggulsterone in the treatment of colorectal cancer.

11.23 Pancreatobiliary Cancer

FXR overexpression in pancreatic cancer tissue with lymph node metastasis is associated with poor patient survival. siRNA-mediated downregulation of FXR and guggulsterone-mediated FXR inhibition resulted in marked reduction in cell migration and invasion human pancreatic cells (MIA-PaCa2, PANC-1) [49]. Guggulsterone inhibited proliferation, decreased motility and invasion, and induced apoptosis in pancreatic cancer cells (CD18/HPAF, Capan1). These anti-tumor effects of guggulsterone possibly involve multiple networks including inhibition of Src and Jak/STAT signaling, alteration in Bad phosphorylation, recognition of actin cytoskeleton, and down-regulation of MUC4, which is involved in chemoresistance [57].

In vitro, the combination treatment of guggulsterone with gemcitabine resulted in more growth inhibition and apoptosis through the downregulation of NFκ-B activity with Akt and Bcl-2 and through the activation of JNK and Bax in pancreatic cancer cells. In vivo, combination therapy amended tumor growth inhibition through the same mechanism as in tumor tissue. The combination therapy with guggulsterone and gemcitabine has the potential to become a valuable strategy for the treatment of pancreatic cancer [3].

Guggulsterone inhibited the proliferation and suppressed migration and invasion of gallbladder cancer cells (TGBC1, TGBC2), and it decreased NF-κB p65, VEGF-C, and MMP-2 activities. Gallbladder cancer cells treated with a combination of guggulsterone and gemcitabine demonstrated inhibition of cell proliferation and invasion compared with treatment with gemcitabine alone. Guggulsterone could be a potential therapeutic option for patients with gallbladder cancer [112].

11.24 Hepatoma

Death receptor DR5 induction via eukaryotic initiation factor-2α and C/EBF homologous transcription factor was crucial for the marked synergetic effects induced by TNF-related apoptosis including ligand and guggulsterone in human hepatocellular carcinoma cells (Hep3B, HepG). Guggulsterone- /TNF-related apoptosis, including ligand combination, could represent a novel tool for cancer therapy [63].

11.25 Prostate Cancer

Guggulsterone induced caspase-dependent apoptosis in part mediated by Bax and Bak in prostate cancer cells (PC-3) [90]. Guggulsterone-induced cell death in human prostate cancer cells (PC-3 and LNCaP) was regulated by ROI-dependent activation of JNK but not in normal prostate cancer cells (PrEC) [89]. Gugulipid-induced apoptosis was associated with ROS production and was regulated by JNK signaling axis in human prostate cancer cells. Representative normal prostate epithelial cells (PrEC) were relatively more resistant to gugulipid-mediated cellular responses compared with prostate cancer cells [102]. Guggulsterone inhibited prostate cancer growth also via inactivation of Akt regulation by ATP citrate lyase signaling in human prostate cancer cells (PC-3 and LNCaP) [25].

11.26 Brain Tumors

Although the sonic hedgehog pathway effector Gli1 is overexpressed in gliomas, a sonic hedgehog inhibitor, SANT-1, failed to induce apoptosis in glioblastoma cells (A172, U87MG, T98G). However, guggulsterone inhibited Ras and NF-κB activity and sensitized glioblastoma cells to SANT-1-induced apoptosis [22].

11.27 Bone Metastasis

Receptor activator of NF-κB ligand (RANKL), a member of the TNF superfamily, was implicated as a major mediator of bone resorption, suggesting that agents that can suppress RANKL signaling have the potential to inhibit bone resorption or osteoclastogenesis. Guggulsterone suppressed RANKL-activated NFκ-B activation and differentiation of monocytes into osteoclasts. Guggulsterone completely suppressed differentiation of monocytes into osteoclasts induced by co-incubation of human breast tumor cells (MDA-MB-468) or human multiple myeloma cells (U266). Guggulsterone suppressed RANKL and tumor cell-induced osteoclastogenesis by suppressing the activation of NF-κB [31]. Chenodeoxycholic acid stimulated the expression osteoblast marker genes (bone sialoprotein, osteocalcin, osteopontin, and alkaline phosphatase), as well as DNA binding activity of the bone transcription factor RUNX2 in human bone marrow stromal cells (BMSCs). Guggulsterone inhibited alkaline phosphatase activity, calcium deposition, DNA binding RUNX2, and bone marker expression, indicating that guggulsterone interfered with osteoblastic differentiation [32].

Deoxycholate released from human osteoblast-like MG63 cells or bone tissue promoted cell survival and induced the migration of metastatic human breast cancer cells (MDA-MA-231). Guggulsterone prevented the migration of these cells and induced apoptosis [86].

11.28 Radiosensitivity

Radiation-induced NF-κB activation was inhibited by guggulsterone and this enhanced radiosensitivity in pancreatic cells (PC-Sw), and it reduced both cell cycle movement and growth. Guggulsterone reduced ERα protein levels in breast cancer cells (MFC-7) and insulin-like growth factor receptor β-protein in colon cancer cells (HT-29) and pancreatic cancer cells (PC-Sw) and inhibited DNA double-strand break repair following radiation. The ability of guggulsterone to modulate radiosensitivity in human cancer cell lines needs further study [14].

11.29 Drug Resistance

Co-administration of guggulsterone (10 μM) resulted increases the chemosensitivity of MCF-7/DOX cells to doxorubicin, compared with doxorubicin treatment alone [103]. When doxorubicin and guggulsterone were co-administered, their anti-tumor activities were augmented in MCF-7/DOX xenografts. Examining body weight, hematological parameters, hepatic cardiac, and gastrointestinal tract histopathology revealed that no significant signs of toxicity were related to guggulsterone. Guggulsterone might reverse doxorubicin resistance in vivo, without severe side effect [104].

Co-administration of guggulsterone increased chemosensitivity of imatinib-resistant K562 cells (K562/IMA) to imatinib compared with imatinib treatment alone. Guggulsterone induced apoptosis by inhibiting COX-2 and PGE2 and downregulating P-gp expression [106].

12 Biological Activities of Guggulsterone in Animal Models

12.1 Hypolipidemic Effects

A primary study reported that administration of gum guggul lowered serum cholesterol levels in hypercholesterolemic rabbits. Hypercholesterolemia was induced in male albino rabbits by the administration of cholesterol (500 mg/kg body weight). The experimental group was fed gum guggul 2 g/kg body weight daily for 6 weeks. In both the control and experimental cholesterol treated groups, an increase in serum and tissue cholesterol level was observed; however, the gum guggul-treated group exhibited significantly lower serum and liver cholesterol levels. In this study, a significant decrease in the body weight of the rabbits fed gum guggul was observed [77]. However, an effect of guggul on triglyceride was not shown in this study.

Another experiment showed that treatment with guggulsterone (25 mg/kg body weight for 10 days) resulted in a 27 % decrease of serum cholesterol and a 31 % decrease in serum triglyceride levels in rats. In the same study, membranes prepared from the livers of guggulsterone-treated rats exhibited up to an 87 % increase in binding sites [91]. Guggulsterone treatment improved fasting blood glucose, glucose tolerance, plasma insulin level, level of harmful lipid (total, low-density lipoprotein [LDL], very low-density lipoprotein [VLDL] cholesterol, and triglyceride), expression profiles of various genes involved in lipid metabolism in high-fat-diet-fed mice [80]. The hypolipidemic effect of guggul has been reported in several other animal models, including chicken [7], Indian domestic pig [39], Presbytis monkey [23], and albino rat [48].

Guggulsterone treatment decreased hepatic cholesterol in wild-type mice fed a high-cholesterol diet but was not effective in FXR-null mice. The inhibition of FXR activation is the basis for the cholesterol-lowering activity of guggulsterone [97].

Gugulipid treatment in rats lowered serum triglyceride and increased HDL levels. Guggulsterone is considered as a novel class of FXR ligand characterized by antagonist activities in coactivator association assays but with the ability to enhance the action of agonists on BSEP expression in vivo (Fisher rats) [17].

12.2 Diabetes Mellitus

Treatment with guggulsterone improved fasting blood glucose, glucose tolerance, plasma insulin level, level of harmful lipids, expression profiles of various genes involved in carbohydrate, and lipid metabolism (phosphoenol pyruvate carboxykinase, glucose-6-phosphatase, glucose transporter-4, PPARγ, and TNF-α) in high-fat-diet-fed mice. Guggulsterone also attenuated reductions in pancreatic β-cell size, increases in adipocytes, steatosis of the liver in high-fat-diet-fed mice. Guggulsterone had both hypoglycemic and hypolipidemic effects that can help to treat type 2 diabetes [80]. In addition, gugulipid (20 g/kg diet) improved glucose tolerance in female Lep(ob)/Lep(ob) mice [16].

12.3 Thyroid Stimulatory Effects

Guggulsterone showed a strong thyroid stimulatory action when administered to albino rats. Its administration (1 mg/100 g body weight) brought about an increase in iodine uptake by the thyroid and enhanced activities by thyroid peroxidase and protease as well as oxygen consumption by isolated slices of liver and biceps muscle [94]. The thyroid was not stimulated by guggulsterone through pituitary activation in rats pretreated with carbimazole (10 mg/kg body weight) [95].

12.4 Cardiovascular Protection

Treatment with guggulsterone (50 mg/kg body weight orally [p.o.] for 5 days) showed a marked protective effect on cardiac enzymes and the P450 system against myocardial necrosis induced by isoproterenol in rats [37]. Treatment with both isomers of guggulsterone (50 mg/kg body weight p.o.) protected against cardiac damage induced by isoproterenol as assessed by the reversal of blood and heart biochemical parameters in rats [10].

Commiphora mukul (100, 200 and 400 mg/kg body weight p.o. for 30 days) was administered. On the 29th and 30th days, animals in the isoprenaline control and *Commiphora mukul* pretreatment groups were administered isoprenaline (85 mg/kg subcutaneously [s.c.]), consecutively at an interval of 24 h. *Commiphora mukul* pretreatment reversed the isoprenaline-induced oxidative changes in the rat myocardium. Furthermore, histopathological examination showed a reduction in necrosis, edema, and inflammation after *Commiphora mukul* pretreatment [68].

Guggulsterone or siRNA-mediated silencing of endogenous FXR reduced post-ischemic myocardial apoptosis in a murine model of myocardial ischemia/reperfusion injury [72].

In addition, guggulsterone inhibited tissue factor activity and photochemical injury induced by thrombotic occlusion of the carotid artery in mice. These findings indicated that guggulsterone may be a novel therapeutic option for the prevention of thrombosis [26].

13 Hepatoprotective Effects

High-dose guggulsterone (50 mg/kg in 5 % dextrose [0.1 ml] by gavage 5 days per week for 5 weeks) decreased the extent of collagen deposition and the percentage of activated hepatic stellate cells undergoing apoptosis in liver fibrosis model mice (thioacetamine 200 mg/kg body weight 3 times per week for 6 weeks). This suggests that guggulsterone may be useful as an antifibrotic agent in chronic liver diseases [40].

13.1 Inflammatory Bowel Disease

Several animal studies have been reported to show the potential of guggulsterone as a therapeutic option for inflammatory bowel disease.

Administration of guggulsterone significantly reduced the severity of dextran sulfate sodium (DSS)-induced murine colitis as assessed by clinical disease activity score, colon length, and histology. Furthermore, tissue upregulation of IκB and IKK phosphorylation induced by DSS was attenuated in guggulsterone-treated mice [13].

E-guggulsterone effectively attenuated the severity of wasting disease, fecal score, and colon inflammation in murine colitis induced by trinitro-benzene sulfonic acid and oxazolone [52].

In addition, GG-52 blocked and attenuated DSS-induced acute murine colitis and in an IL-$10^{-/-}$ mouse model chronic colitis [36, 44]. Both GG-52 and guggulsterone are potential therapeutic agents for inflammatory bowel disease.

13.2 Pancreatitis

In an analysis of pancreatitis, guggulsterone was administered (10, 25, or 50 mg/kg body weight intraperitoneal [i.p.]) 1 h before the first cerulein treatment (50 mg/kg body weight i.p. hourly for 6 h). Mice were sacrificed 6 h after the final cerulein injection. Pretreatment with guggulsterone attenuated cerulein-induced histological damage, reduced pancreas weight/body weight ratio, decreased serum lipase levels, inhibited infiltrations of macrophages and neutrophils, and suppressed cytokine production. In addition, guggulsterone treatment suppressed the activation of ERK and JNK in the pancreas in cerulein-induced pancreatitis. In conclusion, our results suggested that guggulsterone could attenuate pancreatitis via inactivation of ERK and JNK [41].

13.3 Arthritis

Guggul administration (500 mg/kg body weight daily p.o. for 5 months) decreased the thickness of the joint swelling during the course of drug treatment. These results indicated the beneficial role of guggul in experimental rabbit arthritis resembling rheumatoid arthritis in humans [81].

13.4 Neuroprotective Effects

Gugulipid (12.5, 25, and 50 mg/kg, p.o.) showed dose-dependent improvements in scopolamine-induced deficits in a passive avoidance test. Intracerebral (i.c.) injections of streptozotocin (0.5 mg/kg, 1st and 3rd day) caused murine dementia. Pre- and post-treatment against streptozotocin (i.c.) with gugulipid (50 mg/kg, p.o.) significantly attenuated memory deficit and dementia activity, respectively. Gugulipid treatment caused significant decreases in AChE activity compared with vehicle administration in streptozotocin (i.c.)-treated mice. The study demonstrated that gugulipid had a significant protective affect against streptozotocin-induced memory deficits in a model of dementia that can be attributed to the antioxidant and anti-AChE activity of gugulipid. These observations suggested gugulipid as a potential anti-dementia drug [78].

13.5 Uveitis

EIU was induced by subcutaneous injection of LPS (150 mg) into rats treated with guggulsterone (30 mg/kg body weight i.p.) or control. After 24 h, the rats were sacrificed, eyes were enucleated, and aqueous humor was collected. The expression levels of MMP-2, iNOS, COX-2, phospho-IκB, and phospho-NF-κB were determined immunohistochemically. Compared with the control, the EIU rat eye aqueous humor had a significantly higher number of infiltrating cells and inflammatory markers, such as MMP-2, NO, and PGE2, and treatment with guggulsterone prevented EIU-induced increases. Guggulsterone also prevented the expression of MMP-2, iNOS, and COX-2 proteins and of IκB and NF-κB in various eye tissues. These results suggested that the supplementation of guggulsterone could be a novel approach for the treatment of ocular inflammation [35].

13.6 Anticancer Effects

In a xenograft model of HNSCCs, guggulsterone treatment resulted in increased apoptosis and decreased expression of STAT3. In vivo treatment with gugulipid resulted in decreased rates of tumor growth and enhancement of cetuximab activity [51].

Gastroesophageal reflux is a risk factor for esophageal adenocarcinoma, and bile acids and their receptor, FXR, have been implicated in esophageal tumorigenesis. Inhibition of FXR by FXR shRNA or guggulsterone suppressed esophageal cancer cell (SKGT-4) viability and induced apoptosis in vitro and reduced tumor formation and growth in nude mouse xenografts [30].

Guggulsterone reduced the size of colon cancer cell (HT-29) xenograft tumors in guggulsterone-treated mice more than tumors in control mice [6].

The combination of guggulsterone with gemcitabine enhanced antitumor efficacy through apoptosis in a pancreatic cancer cell (MiaPaCa-2) xenograft model using nude mice [3].

Oral gavage of guggulsterone significantly retarded the growth of prostate cancer cell (PC-3) xenografts in athymic mice without causing weight loss or any other side effects. The guggulsterone-induced apoptosis was associated with downregulation of ATP citrate lyase/Akt signaling [25].

When doxorubicin and guggulsterone were co-administrated, their antitumor activities were augmented in MCF-7/DOX xenografts. Examining body weight, hematological parameters, and hepatic, cardiac, and gastrointestinal tract histopathology revealed that no significant signs of toxicity were related to guggulsterone. Guggulsterone might reverse doxorubicin resistance in vivo with no severe side effects [104].

14 Biological Activities of Guggulsterone in Humans

14.1 Hypolipidemic Effects

Several clinical trials have been conducted to evaluate the hypolipidemic effect of gum guggul, gugulipid, ethyl acetate extract, ether soluble fraction of guggul and guggulsterone. Although most of these studies have shown that guggul lowers serum cholesterol and triglycerides, some studies failed to show hypolipidemic effects. These variations in outcomes remain unexplained.

A clinical trial was reported in 1971 that the ether extract (fraction A) of gum guggul (0.5 g daily) was given to 20 patients with elevated lipid levels for 12 weeks. Serum cholesterol, triglyceride, and phospholipid levels were lowered by 27, 29, and 18 %, respectively [59]. In one double-blind randomized controlled study in obese subjects, gum guggul extract (1 g twice daily) was given to obese patients for 3 weeks. The study showed reduced serum lipid levels in hyperlipidemic subjects [47].

Treatment with gum guggul (3 g three times daily) and fraction A (0.5 g daily) for 21 days decreased serum lipid levels in hypercholesterolemic and hyperlipidemic patients but not in obese hyperlipidemic patients. When the study was repeated with obese subjects, guggul extract significantly reduced the serum lipid levels in hyperlipidemic non-obese patients; however, the hypolipidemic effects were not observed in obese subjects [96]. In 13 of 22 patients with hyperlipidemia, administration of gugulipid (0.5 g 3 times daily for 6 weeks) also lowered the serum cholesterol levels by 25 % and serum triglyceride levels by 25 % [29]. Another double-blind randomized controlled study in 10 healthy subjects fed guggulsterone (25 mg daily for 8 weeks) showed a significant decrease in total serum cholesterol levels [27]. It was found that total cholesterol and triglyceride levels were decreased by 22 and 27 %, respectively, and HDL-cholesterol level was increased by 36 % in 40 patients suffering from hyperlipidemia received gum guggul (4.5 g daily 16 weeks) [98].

In the largest multicenter clinical trial and a double-blind crossover study, the efficacy of gugulipid alongside clofibrate was tested. In total, 205 subjects completed a 12-week open trial receiving gugulipid (0.5 g daily) or placebo following an 8-week diet. Gugulipid reduced serum cholesterol and triglyceride levels in 70–80 % of the subjects. Average reductions in the levels of serum cholesterol and triglycerides with gugulipid treatment were 11 and 16.8 %, respectively. Hypercholesterolemic patients responded better to gugulipid than hypertriglyceridemic patients who responded better to clofibrate therapy. In mixed hyperlipidemic patients, the response to both drugs was similar. HDL level increased in 60 % of cases who responded to gugulipid therapy; however, clofibrate had no effect on HDL [96]. The first study was published in Western medical literature. In another randomized, double-blind study, 61 patients with hypercholesterolemia divided into two groups received either gugulipid (50 mg twice daily) or placebo for 24 weeks after a low-fat diet with fruits and vegetables for 12 weeks prior to the treatment. Treatment with gugulipid decreased total cholesterol levels by 11.7 %, LDL by 12.5 %, triglycerides by 12.0 %, and total cholesterol/HDL ratio by 11.1 % from the post-diet levels, whereas the levels were unchanged in the placebo group. HDL-cholesterol levels showed no changes in the two groups. After a 12-week washout period, subjects treated with gugulipid exhibited substantial increases in total cholesterol by 6.5 %, LDL by 6.6 %, and triglyceride by 7.7 %, whereas such increases were not observed in the placebo group [96].

The first clinical trial in the USA, a double-blind, randomized, placebo-controlled trial, was carried out with 103 healthy adults with hypercholesterolemia to evaluate the short-term efficacy of gugulipid in a Western population. The subjects received an oral dose of 1 g or 2 g gugulipid or placebo 3 times daily for 8 weeks. The study reported no significant changes in the levels of total serum cholesterol, HDL, VLDL, or triglyceride following the treatment. In this study, only 18 % of subjects showed a 5 % decrease in LDL. In total, 45 subjects with high baseline LDL levels who received 2 g or 1 g gugulipid showed 14 and 10 % reductions in serum triglyceride, respectively [92]. The double-blind, randomized, placebo-controlled study in Norwegian subjects was carried out to evaluate the efficacy of guggul extract on healthy adults with moderately increased cholesterol. Thirty-four subjects randomized into two groups received 2160 mg guggul or placebo for 12 weeks. After 12 weeks, mean levels of total cholesterol and HDL in the active-treatment group were reduced compared with the placebo group. However, the mean levels of LDL, triglycerides, and total cholesterol/HDL ratio between the two groups did not change significantly [67].

The differences in study outcomes may be attributed to differences in ethnic and genetic backgrounds, dietary habits, lifestyle, and the kinds of guggul extract examined.

14.2 Arthritis

Thirty male and female participants with arthritis were administered gum guggul in capsule form (500 mg concentrated) along with food. On the primary measure, the Western Ontario and MacMaster Osteoarthritis Index total score, participants showed significant improvement ($p < 0.0001$) after taking the supplement for 1 month and continued to improve at the 2-month marker and follow-up. There were no side effects reported during the trial. Gum guggul appeared to be a relatively safe and effective supplement to reduce the symptoms of osteoarthritis [88].

14.3 Nodulocystic Acne

Twenty patients with nodulocystic acne were randomly allocated to one of two treatment schedules tetracycline (500 mg) or gugulipid (equivalent to 25 mg guggulsterone). Both were taken twice daily for 3 months, and gugulipid and tetracycline reduced inflammatory lesions by 65.2 and 68 %, respectively; this difference was not statistically significant ($p > 0.05$). Follow-up at 3 months showed a relapse in 4 cases on tetracycline and 2 cases on gugulipid. An interesting observation was that the patients with oily faces responded remarkably better to gugulipid [93].

15 Conclusion

According to the indications of guggul for various disorders in the ancient Ayurveda and the recent accumulation of data provided by in vitro experiments, guggulsterone seems to have multiple pharmacological activities, especially hypolipidemic, anti-inflammatory, and anti-tumor effects. Although some animal models and clinical trials showed the hypolipidemic effects of guggulsterone, other clinical studies did not confirm these hypolipidemic effects. The variations among results of these clinical trials could be attributed to the differences in study design, sample size, subject population, dose, and the kind of guggul extract. Larger and well-designed clinical studies are necessary to demonstrate the efficacy of guggulsterone in hypolipidemic therapy as well as to find a biomarker for the selection of guggulsterone therapy responders.

In contrast to a certain amount of clinical trials on its hypolipidemic effect, there have been few clinical trials in anti-inflammation or anti-tumor effects of guggulsterone. Further studies, including clinical trials, are required to confirm the clinical usefulness of guggulsterone. However, numerous studies have demonstrated that guggulsterone modulates several transcription factors, enzymes, cytokines, and anti-apoptotic proteins that are involved in inflammation and carcinogenesis. These studies strongly suggest that guggulsterone has substantial potential as a chemopreventive and therapeutic agent against inflammation and tumors.

References

1. Aggarwal BB (2004) Nuclear factor-kappaB: the enemy within. Cancer Cell 6(3):203–208
2. Aggarwal BB, Kunnumakkara AB, Harikumar KB, Gupta SR, Tharakan ST, Koca C, Dey S, Sung B (2009) Signal transducer and activator of transcription-3, inflammation, and cancer: how intimate is the relationship? Ann N Y Acad Sci 1171:59–76
3. Ahn DW, Seo JK, Lee SH, Hwang JH, Lee JK, Ryu JK, Kim YT, Yoon YB (2012) Enhanced antitumor effect of combination therapy with gemcitabine and guggulsterone in pancreatic cancer. Pancreas 41(7):1048–1057
4. Ahn KS, Sethi G, Sung B, Goel A, Ralhan R, Aggarwal BB (2008) Guggulsterone, a farnesoid X receptor antagonist, inhibits constitutive and inducible STAT3 activation through induction of a protein tyrosine phosphatase SHP-1. Cancer Res 68(11):4406–4415
5. Almazari I, Park JM, Park SA, Suh JY, Na HK, Cha YN, Surh YJ (2012) Guggulsterone induces heme oxygenase-1 expression through activation of Nrf2 in human mammary epithelial cells: PTEN as a putative target. Carcinogenesis 33(2):368–376
6. An MJ, Cheon JH, Kim SW, Kim ES, Kim TI, Kim WH (2009) Guggulsterone induces apoptosis in colon cancer cells and inhibits tumor growth in murine colorectal cancer xenografts. Cancer Lett 279(1):93–100
7. Baldwa VS, Bhasin V, Ranka PC, Mathur KM (1981) Effects of *Commiphora mukul* (Guggul) in experimentally induced hyperlipemia and atherosclerosis. J Assoc Phys India 29 (1):13–17
8. Burris TP, Montrose C, Houck KA, Osborne HE, Bocchinfuso WP, Yaden BC, Cheng CC, Zink RW, Barr RJ, Hepler CD, Krishnan V, Bullock HA, Burris LL, Galvin RJ, Bramlett K, Stayrook KR (2005) The hypolipidemic natural product guggulsterone is a promiscuous steroid receptor ligand. Mol Pharmacol 67(3):948–954
9. Capello A, Moons LM, Van De Winkel A, Siersema PD, Van Dekken H, Kuipers EJ, Kusters JG (2008) Bile acid-stimulated expression of the farnesoid X receptor enhances the immune response in Barrett esophagus. Am J Gastroenterol 103(6):1510–1516
10. Chander R, Rizvi F, Khanna AK, Pratap R (2003) Cardioprotective activity of synthetic guggulsterone (E and Z-isomers) in isoproterenol induced myocardial ischemia in rats: a comparative study. Indian J Clin Biochem 18(2):71–79
11. Chang KO, George DW (2007) Bile acids promote the expression of hepatitis C virus in replicon-harboring cells. J Virol 81(18):9633–9640
12. Chen KG, Sikic BI (2012) Molecular pathways: regulation and therapeutic implications of multidrug resistance. Clin Cancer Res 18(7):1863–1869
13. Cheon JH, Kim JS, Kim JM, Kim N, Jung HC, Song IS (2006) Plant sterol guggulsterone inhibits nuclear factor-kappaB signaling in intestinal epithelial cells by blocking IkappaB kinase and ameliorates acute murine colitis. Inflamm Bowel Dis 12(12):1152–1161
14. Choudhuri R, Degraff W, Gamson J, Mitchell JB, Cook JA (2011) Guggulsterone-mediated enhancement of radiosensitivity in human tumor cell lines. Front Oncol 1:19
15. Clevers H (2006) Wnt/beta-catenin signaling in development and disease. Cell 127(3): 469–480
16. Cornick CL, Strongitharm BH, Sassano G, Rawlins C, Mayes AE, Joseph AN, O'dowd J, Stocker C, Wargent E, Cawthorne MA, Brown AL, Arch JR (2009) Identification of a novel agonist of peroxisome proliferator-activated receptors alpha and gamma that may contribute to the anti-diabetic activity of guggulipid in Lep(ob)/Lep(ob) mice. J Nutr Biochem 20 (10):806–815

17. Cui J, Huang L, Zhao A, Lew JL, Yu J, Sahoo S, Meinke PT, Royo I, Pelaez F, Wright SD (2003) Guggulsterone is a farnesoid X receptor antagonist in coactivator association assays but acts to enhance transcription of bile salt export pump. J Biol Chem 278(12):10214–10220
18. De Gottardi A, Dumonceau JM, Bruttin F, Vonlaufen A, Morard I, Spahr L, Rubbia-Brandt L, Frossard JL, Dinjens WN, Rabinovitch PS, Hadengue A (2006) Expression of the bile acid receptor FXR in Barrett's esophagus and enhancement of apoptosis by guggulsterone in vitro. Mol Cancer 5:48
19. Deng R (2007) Therapeutic effects of guggul and its constituent guggulsterone: cardiovascular benefits. Cardiovasc Drug Rev 25(4):375–390
20. Dhillon AS, Hagan S, Rath O, Kolch W (2007) MAP kinase signalling pathways in cancer. Oncogene 26(22):3279–3290
21. Ding X, Staudinger JL (2005) The ratio of constitutive androstane receptor to pregnane X receptor determines the activity of guggulsterone against the Cyp2b10 promoter. J Pharmacol Exp Ther 314(1):120–127
22. Dixit D, Ghildiyal R, Anto NP, Ghosh S, Sharma V, Sen E (2013) Guggulsterone sensitizes glioblastoma cells to Sonic hedgehog inhibitor SANT-1 induced apoptosis in a Ras/NFkappaB dependent manner. Cancer Lett 336(2):347–358
23. Dixit VP, Joshi S, Sinha R, Bharvava SK, Varma M (1980) Hypolipidemic activity of guggal resin (*Commiphora mukul*) and garlic (*Alium sativum* linn.) in dogs (*Canis familiaris*) and monkeys (Presbytis entellus entellus Dufresne). Biochem Exp Biol 16(4):421–424
24. Dufer M, Horth K, Wagner R, Schittenhelm B, Prowald S, Wagner TF, Oberwinkler J, Lukowski R, Gonzalez FJ, Krippeit-Drews P, Drews G (2012) Bile acids acutely stimulate insulin secretion of mouse beta-cells via farnesoid X receptor activation and K(ATP) channel inhibition. Diabetes 61(6):1479–1489
25. Gao Y, Zeng Y, Tian J, Islam MS, Jiang G, Xiao D (2014) Guggulsterone inhibits prostate cancer growth via inactivation of Akt regulated by ATP citrate lyase signaling. Oncotarget
26. Gebhard C, Stampfli SF, Gebhard CE, Akhmedov A, Breitenstein A, Camici GG, Holy EW, Luscher TF, Tanner FC (2009) Guggulsterone, an anti-inflammatory phytosterol, inhibits tissue factor and arterial thrombosis. Basic Res Cardiol 104(3):285–294
27. Ghorai M, Mandal SC, Pal M, Pal SP, Saha BP (2000) A comparative study on hypocholesterolaemic effect of allicin, whole germinated seeds of bengal gram and guggulipid of gum gugglu. Phytother Res 14(3):200–202
28. Gonzalez R, Garitaonandia I, Abramihina T, Wambua GK, Ostrowska A, Brock M, Noskov A, Boscolo FS, Craw JS, Laurent LC, Snyder EY, Semechkin RA (2013) Deriving dopaminergic neurons for clinical use. A practical approach. Sci Rep 3:1463
29. Gopal K, Saran RK, Nityanand S, Gupta PP, Hasan M, Das SK, Sinha N, Agarwal SS (1986) Clinical trial of ethyl acetate extract of gum gugulu (gugulipid) in primary hyperlipidemia. J Assoc Physicians India 34(4):249–251
30. Guan B, Li H, Yang Z, Hoque A, Xu X (2013) Inhibition of farnesoid X receptor controls esophageal cancer cell growth in vitro and in nude mouse xenografts. Cancer 119(7): 1321–1329
31. Ichikawa H, Aggarwal BB (2006) Guggulsterone inhibits osteoclastogenesis induced by receptor activator of nuclear factor-kappaB ligand and by tumor cells by suppressing nuclear factor-kappaB activation. Clin Cancer Res 12(2):662–668
32. Id Boufker H, Lagneaux L, Fayyad-Kazan H, Badran B, Najar M, Wiedig M, Ghanem G, Laurent G, Body JJ, Journe F (2011) Role of farnesoid X receptor (FXR) in the process of differentiation of bone marrow stromal cells into osteoblasts. Bone 49(6):1219–1231
33. Janakiram NB, Rao CV (2012) iNOS-selective inhibitors for cancer prevention: promise and progress. Future Med Chem 4(17):2193–2204
34. Jiang G, Xiao X, Zeng Y, Nagabhushanam K, Majeed M, Xiao D (2013) Targeting beta-catenin signaling to induce apoptosis in human breast cancer cells by z-guggulsterone and Gugulipid extract of Ayurvedic medicine plant *Commiphora mukul*. BMC Complement Altern Med 13:203

35. Kalariya NM, Shoeb M, Reddy AB, Zhang M, Van Kuijk FJ, Ramana KV (2010) Prevention of endotoxin-induced uveitis in rats by plant sterol guggulsterone. Invest Ophthalmol Vis Sci 51(10):5105–5113
36. Kang SJ, Kim JM, Koh SJ, Kim SH, Im JP, Jung HC, Kim JS (2013) The guggulsterone derivative GG-52 inhibits NF-kappaB signaling in bone marrow-derived dendritic cells and attenuates colitis in IL-10 knockout mice. Life Sci 92(22):1064–1071
37. Kaul S, Kapoor NK (1989) Cardiac sarcolemma enzymes and liver microsomal cytochrome P450 in isoproterenol treated rats. Indian J Med Res 90:62–68
38. Khan MK, Ansari IA, Khan MS (2013) Dietary phytochemicals as potent chemotherapeutic agents against breast cancer: inhibition of NF-kappaB pathway via molecular interactions in rel homology domain of its precursor protein p105. Pharmacogn Mag 9(33):51–57
39. Khanna DS, Agarwal OP, Gupta SK, Arora RB (1969) A biochemical approach to anti-atherosclerotic action of Commiphora-mukul: an Indian indigenous drug in Indian domestic pigs (*Sus scrofa*). Indian J Med Res 57(5):900–906
40. Kim BH, Yoon JH, Yang JI, Myung SJ, Lee JH, Jung EU, Yu SJ, Kim YJ, Lee HS, Kim CY (2013) Guggulsterone attenuates activation and survival of hepatic stellate cell by inhibiting nuclear factor kappa B activation and inducing apoptosis. J Gastroenterol Hepatol 28 (12):1859–1868
41. Kim DG, Bae GS, Choi SB, Jo IJ, Shin JY, Lee SK, Kim MJ, Kim MJ, Jeong HW, Choi CM, Seo SH, Choo GC, Seo SW, Song HJ, Park SJ (2015) Guggulsterone attenuates cerulein-induced acute pancreatitis via inhibition of ERK and JNK activation. Int Immunopharmacol 26(1):194–202
42. Kim DG, Bae GS, Jo IJ, Choi SB, Kim MJ, Jeong JH, Kang DG, Lee HS, Song HJ, Park SJ (2015) Guggulsterone attenuated lipopolysaccharide-induced inflammatory responses in mouse inner medullary collecting duct-3 cells. Inflammation 39:87–95
43. Kim ES, Hong SY, Lee HK, Kim SW, An MJ, Kim TI, Lee KR, Kim WH, Cheon JH (2008) Guggulsterone inhibits angiogenesis by blocking STAT3 and VEGF expression in colon cancer cells. Oncol Rep 20(6):1321–1327
44. Kim JM, Kang HW, Cha MY, Yoo D, Kim N, Kim IK, Ku J, Kim S, Ma SH, Jung HC, Song IS, Kim JS (2010) Novel guggulsterone derivative GG-52 inhibits NF-kappaB signaling in intestinal epithelial cells and attenuates acute murine colitis. Lab Invest 90 (7):1004–1015
45. Koo JH, Rhee KS, Koh HW, Jang HY, Park BH, Park JW (2012) Guggulsterone inhibits melanogenesis in B16 murine melanoma cells by downregulating tyrosinase expression. Int J Mol Med 30(4):974–978
46. Krishnamurthy K, Wang G, Rokhfeld D, Bieberich E (2008) Deoxycholate promotes survival of breast cancer cells by reducing the level of pro-apoptotic ceramide. Breast Cancer Res 10(6):R106
47. Kuppurajan K, Rajagopalan SS et al (1973) Effect of guggul (*Commiphora mukul*) on serum lipids in obese subjects. J Res India Med 8:8
48. Lata S, Saxena KK, Bhasin V, Saxena RS, Kumar A, Srivastava VK (1991) Beneficial effects of *Allium sativum*, *Allium cepa* and *Commiphora mukul* on experimental hyperlipidemia and atherosclerosis—a comparative evaluation. J Postgrad Med 37(3):132–135
49. Lee JY, Lee KT, Lee JK, Lee KH, Jang KT, Heo JS, Choi SH, Kim Y, Rhee JC (2011) Farnesoid X receptor, overexpressed in pancreatic cancer with lymph node metastasis promotes cell migration and invasion. Br J Cancer 104(6):1027–1037
50. Lee YR, Lee JH, Noh EM, Kim EK, Song MY, Jung WS, Park SJ, Kim JS, Park JW, Kwon KB, Park BH (2008) Guggulsterone blocks IL-1beta-mediated inflammatory responses by suppressing NF-kappaB activation in fibroblast-like synoviocytes. Life Sci 82(23–24):1203–1209
51. Leeman-Neill RJ, Wheeler SE, Singh SV, Thomas SM, Seethala RR, Neill DB, Panahandeh MC, Hahm ER, Joyce SC, Sen M, Cai Q, Freilino ML, Li C, Johnson DE, Grandis JR (2009) Guggulsterone enhances head and neck cancer therapies via inhibition of signal transducer and activator of transcription-3. Carcinogenesis 30(11):1848–1856

52. Li C, Zang Y, Sen M, Leeman-Neill RJ, Man DS, Grandis JR, Johnson DE (2009) Bortezomib up-regulates activated signal transducer and activator of transcription-3 and synergizes with inhibitors of signal transducer and activator of transcription-3 to promote head and neck squamous cell carcinoma cell death. Mol Cancer Ther 8(8):2211–2220
53. Luo J, Manning BD, Cantley LC (2003) Targeting the PI3K-Akt pathway in human cancer: rationale and promise. Cancer Cell 4(4):257–262
54. Lv N, Song MY, Kim EK, Park JW, Kwon KB, Park BH (2008) Guggulsterone, a plant sterol, inhibits NF-kappaB activation and protects pancreatic beta cells from cytokine toxicity. Mol Cell Endocrinol 289(1–2):49–59
55. Macha MA, Matta A, Chauhan S, Siu KM, Ralhan R (2010) 14-3-3 zeta is a molecular target in guggulsterone induced apoptosis in head and neck cancer cells. BMC Cancer 10:655
56. Macha MA, Matta A, Chauhan SS, Siu KW, Ralhan R (2011) Guggulsterone (GS) inhibits smokeless tobacco and nicotine-induced NF-kappaB and STAT3 pathways in head and neck cancer cells. Carcinogenesis 32(3):368–380
57. Macha MA, Rachagani S, Gupta S, Pai P, Ponnusamy MP, Batra SK, Jain M (2013) Guggulsterone decreases proliferation and metastatic behavior of pancreatic cancer cells by modulating JAK/STAT and Src/FAK signaling. Cancer Lett 341(2):166–177
58. Makishima M, Okamoto AY, Repa JJ, Tu H, Learned RM, Luk A, Hull MV, Lustig KD, Mangelsdorf DJ, Shan B (1999) Identification of a nuclear receptor for bile acids. Science 284(5418):1362–1365
59. Malhotra SC, Ahuja MM (1971) Comparative hypolipidaemic effectiveness of gum guggulu (*Commiphora mukul*) fraction 'A', ethyl-P-chlorophenoxyisobutyrate and Ciba-13437-Su. Indian J Med Res 59(10):1621–1632
60. Mencarelli A, Renga B, Palladino G, Distrutti E, Fiorucci S (2009) The plant sterol guggulsterone attenuates inflammation and immune dysfunction in murine models of inflammatory bowel disease. Biochem Pharmacol 78(9):1214–1223
61. Meselhy MR (2003) Inhibition of LPS-induced NO production by the oleogum resin of *Commiphora wightii* and its constituents. Phytochemistry 62(2):213–218
62. Meyer U, Costantino G, Macchiarulo A, Pellicciari R (2005) Is antagonism of E/Z-guggulsterone at the farnesoid X receptor mediated by a noncanonical binding site? A molecular modeling study. J Med Chem 48(22):6948–6955
63. Moon DO, Park SY, Choi YH, Ahn JS, Kim GY (2011) Guggulsterone sensitizes hepatoma cells to TRAIL-induced apoptosis through the induction of CHOP-dependent DR5: involvement of ROS-dependent ER-stress. Biochem Pharmacol 82(11):1641–1650
64. Moon Y, Choi SM, Chang S, Park B, Lee S, Lee MO, Choi HS, Park H (2015) Chenodeoxycholic acid reduces hypoxia inducible factor-1alpha protein and its target genes. PLoS ONE 10(6):e0130911
65. Nabekura T, Yamaki T, Ueno K, Kitagawa S (2008) Effects of plant sterols on human multidrug transporters ABCB1 and ABCC1. Biochem Biophys Res Commun 369(2): 363–368
66. Noh EM, Chung EY, Youn HJ, Jung SH, Hur H, Lee YR, Kim JS (2013) *Cis*-guggulsterone inhibits the IKK/NF-kappaB pathway, whereas trans-guggulsterone inhibits MAPK/AP-1 in MCF7 breast cancer cells: guggulsterone regulates MMP9 expression in an isomer-specific manner. Int J Mol Med 31(2):393–399
67. Nohr LA, Rasmussen LB, Straand J (2009) Resin from the mukul myrrh tree, guggul, can it be used for treating hypercholesterolemia? A randomized, controlled study. Complement Ther Med 17(1):16–22
68. Ojha S, Bhatia J, Arora S, Golechha M, Kumari S, Arya DS (2011) Cardioprotective effects of *Commiphora mukul* against isoprenaline-induced cardiotoxicity: a biochemical and histopathological evaluation. J Environ Biol 32(6):731–738
69. Owsley E, Chiang JY (2003) Guggulsterone antagonizes farnesoid X receptor induction of bile salt export pump but activates pregnane X receptor to inhibit cholesterol 7alpha-hydroxylase gene. Biochem Biophys Res Commun 304(1):191–195

70. Pal P, Kanaujiya JK, Lochab S, Tripathi SB, Sanyal S, Behre G, Trivedi AK (2013) Proteomic analysis of rosiglitazone and guggulsterone treated 3T3-L1 preadipocytes. Mol Cell Biochem 376(1–2):81–93
71. Parks DJ, Blanchard SG, Bledsoe RK, Chandra G, Consler TG, Kliewer SA, Stimmel JB, Willson TM, Zavacki AM, Moore DD, Lehmann JM (1999) Bile acids: natural ligands for an orphan nuclear receptor. Science 284(5418):1365–1368
72. Pu J, Yuan A, Shan P, Gao E, Wang X, Wang Y, Lau WB, Koch W, Ma XL, He B (2013) Cardiomyocyte-expressed farnesoid-X-receptor is a novel apoptosis mediator and contributes to myocardial ischaemia/reperfusion injury. Eur Heart J 34(24):1834–1845
73. Qin P, Borges-Marcucci LA, Evans MJ, Harnish DC (2005) Bile acid signaling through FXR induces intracellular adhesion molecule-1 expression in mouse liver and human hepatocytes. Am J Physiol Gastrointest Liver Physiol 289(2):G267–G273
74. Rizzo G, Disante M, Mencarelli A, Renga B, Gioiello A, Pellicciari R, Fiorucci S (2006) The farnesoid X receptor promotes adipocyte differentiation and regulates adipose cell function in vivo. Mol Pharmacol 70(4):1164–1173
75. Sarfaraz S, Siddiqui IA, Syed DN, Afaq F, Mukhtar H (2008) Guggulsterone modulates MAPK and NF-kappaB pathways and inhibits skin tumorigenesis in SENCAR mice. Carcinogenesis 29(10):2011–2018
76. Satyavati GV (1988) Gum guggul (*Commiphora mukul*)–the success story of an ancient insight leading to a modern discovery. Indian J Med Res 87:327–335
77. Satyavati GV, Dwarakanath C, Tripathi SN (1969) Experimental studies on the hypocholesterolemic effect of *Commiphora mukul* Engl. (Guggul). Indian J Med Res 57 (10):1950–1962
78. Saxena G, Singh SP, Pal R, Singh S, Pratap R, Nath C (2007) Gugulipid, an extract of Commiphora whighitii with lipid-lowering properties, has protective effects against streptozotocin-induced memory deficits in mice. Pharmacol Biochem Behav 86(4):797–805
79. Scholtes C, Diaz O, Icard V, Kaul A, Bartenschlager R, Lotteau V, Andre P (2008) Enhancement of genotype 1 hepatitis C virus replication by bile acids through FXR. J Hepatol 48(2):192–199
80. Sharma B, Salunke R, Srivastava S, Majumder C, Roy P (2009) Effects of guggulsterone isolated from *Commiphora mukul* in high fat diet induced diabetic rats. Food Chem Toxicol 47(10):2631–2639
81. Sharma JN, Sharma JN (1977) Comparison of the anti-inflammatory activity of *Commiphora mukul* (an indigenous drug) with those of phenylbutazone and ibuprofen in experimental arthritis induced by mycobacterial adjuvant. Arzneimittelforschung 27(7):1455–1457
82. Shishodia S, Aggarwal BB (2004) Guggulsterone inhibits NF-kappaB and IkappaBalpha kinase activation, suppresses expression of anti-apoptotic gene products, and enhances apoptosis. J Biol Chem 279(45):47148–47158
83. Shishodia S, Azu N, Rosenzweig JA, Jackson DA (2015) Guggulsterone for chemoprevention of cancer. Curr Pharm Des 22:294–306
84 Shishodia S, Harikumar KB, Dass S, Ramawat KG, Aggarwal BB (2008) The guggul for chronic diseases: ancient medicine, modern targets. Anticancer Res 28(6a):3647–3664
85. Shishodia S, Sethi G, Ahn KS, Aggarwal BB (2007) Guggulsterone inhibits tumor cell proliferation, induces S-phase arrest, and promotes apoptosis through activation of c-Jun N-terminal kinase, suppression of Akt pathway, and downregulation of antiapoptotic gene products. Biochem Pharmacol 74(1):118–130
86. Silva J, Dasgupta S, Wang G, Krishnamurthy K, Ritter E, Bieberich E (2006) Lipids isolated from bone induce the migration of human breast cancer cells. J Lipid Res 47(4):724–733
87. Sinal CJ, Tohkin M, Miyata M, Ward JM, Lambert G, Gonzalez FJ (2000) Targeted disruption of the nuclear receptor FXR/BAR impairs bile acid and lipid homeostasis. Cell 102(6):731–744
88. Singh BB, Mishra LC, Vinjamury SP, Aquilina N, Singh VJ, Shepard N (2003) The effectiveness of *Commiphora mukul* for osteoarthritis of the knee: an outcomes study. Altern Ther Health Med 9(3):74–79

89. Singh SV, Choi S, Zeng Y, Hahm ER, Xiao D (2007) Guggulsterone-induced apoptosis in human prostate cancer cells is caused by reactive oxygen intermediate dependent activation of c-Jun NH_2-terminal kinase. Cancer Res 67(15):7439–7449
90. Singh SV, Zeng Y, Xiao D, Vogel VG, Nelson JB, Dhir R, Tripathi YB (2005) Caspase-dependent apoptosis induction by guggulsterone, a constituent of Ayurvedic medicinal plant *Commiphora mukul*, in PC-3 human prostate cancer cells is mediated by Bax and Bak. Mol Cancer Ther 4(11):1747–1754
91. Singh V, Kaul S, Chander R, Kapoor NK (1990) Stimulation of low density lipoprotein receptor activity in liver membrane of guggulsterone treated rats. Pharmacol Res 22(1):37–44
92. Szapary PO, Wolfe ML, Bloedon LT, Cucchiara AJ, Dermarderosian AH, Cirigliano MD, Rader DJ (2003) Guggulipid for the treatment of hypercholesterolemia: a randomized controlled trial. JAMA 290(6):765–772
93. Thappa DM, Dogra J (1994) Nodulocystic acne: oral gugulipid versus tetracycline. J Dermatol 21(10):729–731
94. Tripathi YB, Malhotra OP, Tripathi SN (1984) Thyroid stimulating action of Z-guggulsterone obtained from *Commiphora mukul*. Planta Med 50(1):78–80
95. Tripathi YB, Tripathi P, Malhotra OP, Tripathi SN (1988) Thyroid stimulatory action of (Z)-guggulsterone: mechanism of action. Planta Med 54(4):271–277
96. Ulbricht C, Basch E, Szapary P, Hammerness P, Axentsev S, Boon H, Kroll D, Garraway L, Vora M, Woods J, Natural Standard Research C (2005) Guggul for hyperlipidemia: a review by the Natural Standard Research Collaboration. Complement Ther Med 13(4):279–290
97. Urizar NL, Liverman AB, Dodds DT, Silva FV, Ordentlich P, Yan Y, Gonzalez FJ, Heyman RA, Mangelsdorf DJ, Moore DD (2002) A natural product that lowers cholesterol as an antagonist ligand for FXR. Science 296(5573):1703–1706
98. Verma SK, Bordia A (1988) Effect of *Commiphora mukul* (gum guggulu) in patients of hyperlipidemia with special reference to HDL-cholesterol. Indian J Med Res 87:356–360
99. Wang H, Chen J, Hollister K, Sowers LC, Forman BM (1999) Endogenous bile acids are ligands for the nuclear receptor FXR/BAR. Mol Cell 3(5):543–553
100. Wang WC, Uen YH, Chang ML, Cheah KP, Li JS, Yu WY, Lee KC, Choy CS, Hu CM (2012) Protective effect of guggulsterone against cardiomyocyte injury induced by doxorubicin in vitro. BMC Complement Altern Med 12:138
101. Xiao D, Singh SV (2008) Z-guggulsterone, a constituent of Ayurvedic medicinal plant *Commiphora mukul*, inhibits angiogenesis in vitro and in vivo. Mol Cancer Ther 7(1): 171–180
102. Xiao D, Zeng Y, Prakash L, Badmaev V, Majeed M, Singh SV (2011) Reactive oxygen species-dependent apoptosis by gugulipid extract of ayurvedic medicine plant *Commiphora mukul* in human prostate cancer cells is regulated by c-Jun N-terminal kinase. Mol Pharmacol 79(3):499–507
103. Xu HB, Li L, Liu GQ (2011) Reversal of multidrug resistance by guggulsterone in drug-resistant MCF-7 cell lines. Chemotherapy 57(1):62–70
104. Xu HB, Shen ZL, Fu J, Xu LZ (2014) Reversal of doxorubicin resistance by guggulsterone of *Commiphora mukul* in vivo. Phytomedicine 21(11):1221–1229
105. Xu HB, Xu LZ, Li L, Fu J, Mao XP (2012) Reversion of P-glycoprotein-mediated multidrug resistance by guggulsterone in multidrug-resistant human cancer cell lines. Eur J Pharmacol 694(1–3):39–44
106. Xu HB, Xu LZ, Mao XP, Fu J (2014) Guggulsterone of *Commiphora mukul* resin reverses drug resistance in imatinib-resistant leukemic cells by inhibiting cyclooxygenase-2 and P-glycoprotein. Phytomedicine 21(7):1004–1009
107. Xu Y, Watanabe T, Tanigawa T, Machida H, Okazaki H, Yamagami H, Watanabe K, Tominaga K, Fujiwara Y, Oshitani N, Arakawa T (2010) Bile acids induce cdx2 expression through the farnesoid x receptor in gastric epithelial cells. J Clin Biochem Nutr 46(1):81–86
108. Yamada T, Osawa S, Hamaya Y, Furuta T, Hishida A, Kajimura M, Ikuma M (2010) Guggulsterone suppresses bile acid-induced and constitutive caudal-related homeobox 2 expression in gut-derived adenocarcinoma cells. Anticancer Res 30(6):1953–1960

109. Yamada T, Osawa S, Ikuma M, Kajimura M, Sugimoto M, Furuta T, Iwaizumi M, Sugimoto K (2014) Guggulsterone, a plant-derived inhibitor of NF-TB, suppresses CDX2 and COX-2 expression and reduces the viability of esophageal adenocarcinoma cells. Digestion 90(3):208–217
110. Yang JY, Della-Fera MA, Baile CA (2008) Guggulsterone inhibits adipocyte differentiation and induces apoptosis in 3T3-L1 cells. Obesity (Silver Spring) 16(1):16–22
111. Yang L, Broderick D, Jiang Y, Hsu V, Maier CS (2014) Conformational dynamics of human FXR-LBD ligand interactions studied by hydrogen/deuterium exchange mass spectrometry: insights into the antagonism of the hypolipidemic agent Z-guggulsterone. Biochim Biophys Acta 1844(9):1684–1693
112. Yang MH, Lee KT, Yang S, Lee JK, Lee KH, Moon IH, Rhee JC (2012) Guggulsterone enhances antitumor activity of gemcitabine in gallbladder cancer cells through suppression of NF-kappaB. J Cancer Res Clin Oncol 138(10):1743–1751
113. Zhang Y, Kast-Woelbern HR, Edwards PA (2003) Natural structural variants of the nuclear receptor farnesoid X receptor affect transcriptional activation. J Biol Chem 278(1):104–110
114. Zhang Y, Lee FY, Barrera G, Lee H, Vales C, Gonzalez FJ, Willson TM, Edwards PA (2006) Activation of the nuclear receptor FXR improves hyperglycemia and hyperlipidemia in diabetic mice. Proc Natl Acad Sci U S A 103(4):1006–1011
115. Zhao C, Wang X, Cong Y, Deng Y, Xu Y, Chen A, Yin Y (2014) Effects of bile acids and the bile acid receptor FXR agonist on the respiratory rhythm in the in vitro brainstem medulla slice of neonatal Sprague-Dawley rats. PLoS ONE 9(11):e112212

Deguelin and Its Role in Chronic Diseases

Jonathan Boyd and Alice Han

Abstract Deguelin is one of four major naturally occurring rotenoids isolated from root extracts and is best recognized as a NADH: ubiquinone oxidoreductase (complex I) inhibitor, resulting in significant alterations in mitochondrial function. Deguelin has also been implicated as a regulator of apoptosis through signaling pathways, such as the (PI3K)/Akt pathway, as well as an initiator of cell cycle arrest. Consequently, this compound has accrued great interest as a potential chemopreventive and chemotherapeutic. Additionally, deguelin exposure has been linked to Parkinson's disease (PD). PD is a neurodegenerative disorder, characterized by a substantial loss of dopaminergic neurons in the substantia nigra, as well the manifestation of symptoms such as bradykinesia, rigidity, and rest tremor. While exploring the genetic impact of PD is imperative, environmental factors, such as exposure to pesticides, herbicides, and insecticides, have also been connected to the development of PD. The etiology and pathogenesis of PD are yet to be fully understood and elucidated, but mitochondrial dysfunction is gaining recognition as a molecular hallmark of PD. In fact, deguelin has been reported to elicit PD-like symptoms (degeneration of the dopaminergic pathway) in rats administered with deguelin (6 mg/kg/day for 6 days), possibly through the inhibition of mitochondrial complex I. Further research investigating the mechanisms by which deguelin inhibits central cellular processes is essential in order to advance any prospective research addressing potential applications and risks of deguelin.

Keywords Deguelin · Mitochondrial complex I inhibitor · Apoptosis · Cell cycle arrest · Chemopreventive · Chemotherapeutic · Parkinson's disease

J. Boyd (✉) · A. Han
C. Eugene Bennett Department of Chemistry, West Virginia University, Morgantown, WV, USA
e-mail: Jonathan.boyd@mail.wvu.edu

S.C. Gupta et al. (eds.), *Drug Discovery from Mother Nature*, Advances in Experimental Medicine and Biology 929,
DOI 10.1007/978-3-319-41342-6_16

1 Introduction

Deguelin (Fig. 1) is one of four major naturally produced rotenoids isolated from Cubé resin, a root extract from plant species such as *Lonchocarpus utilis* and *Lonchocarpus urucu* [16]. Cubé resin has been applied as an insecticide, acaricide, and piscicide [40, 47] and additionally has been investigated for potential use as a chemotherapeutic [37] and chemopreventive [26], but has also been investigated for its potential toxicological threat [19]. Deguelin research was first published in 1930, investigating the insecticidal potencies of components derived from root extracts [13]. Since then, a tremendous increase in information describing how it affects central cellular processes has been reported. For instance, deguelin has most recently been implicated in the disruption of cell growth [3] and the suppression of select proteins [39]. In this chapter, we will present known physicochemical properties of deguelin, discuss pertinent cell signaling pathways, identify certain diseases associated with deguelin, and highlight central responses in both animal models and humans.

2 Physicochemical Properties of Deguelin

Several pertinent physicochemical properties of deguelin have been determined, providing the necessary information to appropriately conduct experiments and interpret data. Known information retrieved from the PubChem Compound database is presented in Table 1. There is, however, a serious lack of accessible data detailing the physical and chemical properties of deguelin. For instance, boiling point, flammability, relative density, water solubility, viscosity, and oxidizing properties are all fundamental data that cannot be found in any Material Safety Data Sheet. There are also cases of inconsistent data: For instance, the melting point of deguelin, directly extracted from a root, was reported as 171 °C in a publication

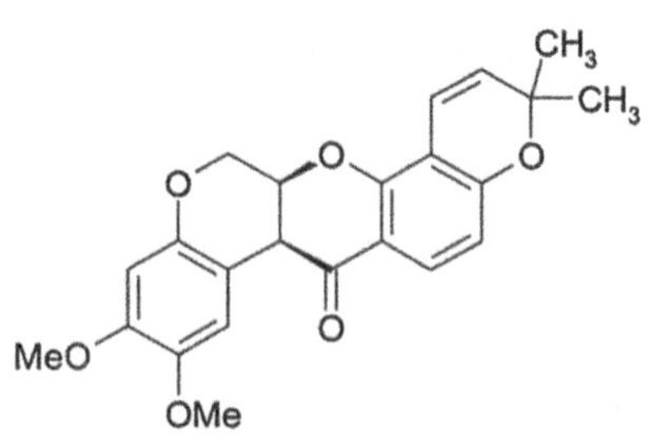

Fig. 1 Deguelin, also known as (7aS,13aS)-13,13a-dihydro-9,10-dimethoxy-3,3-dimethyl-3H-bis [1]benzopyrano [3,4-b:6′,5′-3]pyran-7(7aH)-one, can be found in derris roots and possesses potential chemotherapeutic properties for its ability to inhibit cellular processes involved in cell proliferation

Table 1 Physical and chemical properties of deguelin from the PubChem Compound database

Molecular weight	394.41718 g/mol
Molecular formula	$C_{23}H_{22}O_6$
Log *P* value	3.7
Hydrogen bond donor count	0
Hydrogen bond acceptor count	6
Rotatable bond count	2
Topological polar surface area	63.2 A^2
Heavy atom count	29
Formal charge	0
Isotope atom count	0
Defined atom stereocenter count	2
Undefined atom stereocenter count	0
Defined bond stereocenter count	0
Undefined bond stereocenter count	0
Covalently bonded unit count	1

National Center for Biotechnology Information. PubChem Compound database; CID = 107,935, https://pubchem.ncbi.nlm.nih.gov/compound/107935 (accessed Nov. 16, 2015)

from 1931 [10] and has been listed as so in many documents. In other sources, however, the melting point has been reported to range between 85 and 87 °C (Sigma Aldrich, MSDS [15]). The observed discrepancy may be due to differences between a synthesized product and a natural extracted product, but there is currently no provided clarification. Regardless of the reasons behind inconsistent and lacking data, it is clear that not only is there limited information on the physicochemical properties of deguelin, but great caution must be taken in acquiring appropriate values.

3 Modulation of Cell Signaling Pathways by Deguelin

3.1 Apoptosis and Cell Cycle Arrest

Apoptosis initiated by deguelin exposure is a mechanism that has been investigated at length for its potential application as a chemotherapeutic and chemopreventive. Significant signaling pathways have been identified and implicated as key features in the induction of cell death. First, the phosphatidylinositol 3-kinase (PI3K)/Akt pathway has been identified in multiple cells lines and tissue types to possess a key role in apoptosis triggered by deguelin. The (PI3K)/Akt pathway is involved in a wide array of cellular processes regulating cell proliferation, apoptosis, metabolism, survival, angiogenesis, transcription, and protein synthesis [20]. Activation of Akt, prompted by phosphorylation at Thr308 and Ser473, can promote cell survival through direct inhibition of pro-apoptotic proteins or by stimulating pro-survival pathways through activation of NF-κB [33]. (PI3K)/Akt pathway-dependent apoptosis, following deguelin exposures ranging from 0.001 to 20 μM, has been confirmed in many different cell lines, such as malignant human bronchial epithelial [9], metastatic mammary gland [8], and gastric carcinoma cell lines [29]. A conserved decrease in Akt expression or activation (through phosphorylation), coupled with the presence of apoptosis indicators (caspases, pro-apoptotic factors, DNA fragmentation, apoptotic morphology, phosphatidylserine translocation) was observed in those studies, further offering evidence that deguelin causes Akt pathway-mediated apoptosis. While Akt appears to be a central hub in regulating cell death, upstream and downstream events that ultimately lead to apoptosis are slowly being elucidated. For instance, a recent study discovered 1.0–10 μM deguelin results in apoptosis via insulin-like growth factor (IGF-1)- and epidermal growth factor (EGF)-induced Akt activation [1]. Heat-shock protein (Hsp90), which is known to assist with proper function and stabilization of many proteins (including Akt), was also suppressed in H1299 lung cancer cells when dosed with 100 nM deguelin [42]. Proteins downstream of Akt, such as NF-κB in colon cancer cell lines [25] and phosphorylation of Glycogen synthase kinase-3 β/β-catenin (GSK-3β/β-catenin) in prostate cancer cells [46], were additionally downregulated, following 50–300 and 50–100 nM deguelin exposure, respectively.

In addition to inducing apoptosis, deguelin may also initiate a concurrent process of cell cycle arrest. In fact, cell arrest at all cell cycle phases and checkpoints have been observed, but have varied depending on the cell type. Cell arrest in the G_1/S phase was detected in colon cancer cells through analysis of regulatory protein expression: Levels of cyclin E, which is characteristically expressed in the G_1/S phase transition, were significantly reduced upon exposure to 1 μM deguelin [37]. Cells were also found to be arrested in both G_1/S and G_2/M phases, evidenced by a downregulation in cyclin D1, P21, and pRb in lymphoma cells after 20–160 nM exposure to deguelin [52]. Other studies have found cell proliferation inhibition of breast cancer cells after 1 μM treatments of deguelin via cell arrest at the S phase [36]. It is evident that cell cycle arrest is a significant response to deguelin exposure, but the mechanism has yet to be fully understood.

3.2 Mitochondrial Complex I Inhibition

Deguelin is actually classically categorized as a NADH: ubiquinone oxidoreductase (complex I) inhibitor and therefore is anticipated to affect mitochondrial activity or induce dysfunction. Mitochondrial complex I is an essential component of the electron transport chain (ETC) that functions to pass electrons from NADH to ubiquinone, while concurrently transferring protons across the inner mitochondrial membrane [43]. Inhibition of complex I and the consequent disruption of processes regulating electron and proton movement can be detrimental to the cell: The most apparent outcome is the discontinued production of adenosine triphosphate (ATP), one of the most fundamental biomolecules and energy sources involved in regulating cellular processes. The mechanism by which deguelin inhibits complex I is uncertain, but rotenone, a similarly structured complex I inhibitor, is believed to bind to the piericidin A and the capsaicin site of the complex [43]. NADH: ubiquinone oxidoreductase inhibition is also associated with the obstruction of ornithine decarboxylase (ODC) activity, which is closely involved in cell proliferation and tumor promotion processes [16]. As expected, in the presence of deguelin and similar rotenoid analogs, both NADH: ubiquinone oxidoreductase and ODC activity have been observed to significantly decrease [5]. The reduction in ODC activity may also be attributed to the loss of mitochondrial energetics, as a result of arrested ATP production due to an inhibited complex I [18].

In altering mitochondrial function through inhibition of complex I, a number of adverse outcomes are expected to occur. For instance, studies have shown dose-dependent (1.0–100 μM) decreases in oxygen consumption [50] and time-dependent decreases in ATP levels, as well increases in the ADP/ATP ratio, after dosing with 100 nM deguelin [24]. As the availability of ATP is reduced, some cells (especially cancerous cells) can survive by utilizing aerobic glycolysis, instead of oxidative phosphorylation to replenish ATP stores [51]. Under hypoxic conditions, or in the absence of oxygen, many cells may be prompted to undergo apoptosis if aerobic glycolysis is not a viable option. Changes in post-translational phosphorylation are additional potential outcomes from deguelin exposure resulting from the cell's decision to initiate pro-apoptotic or cell survival signaling cascades. In one study, Vrana et al. [50] examined phosphorylation responses of proteins closely associated with cell death or survival signaling pathways, such as Akt, ERK1/2, JNK, p38MAPK, HSP27, IκBα, p53, and p90RSK. They found that relative p38MAPK phosphorylation was significantly increased over a wide dosing range of deguelin (0.1–10 μM), while oxygen consumption was decreased for similar dosing ranges in hepatocellular carcinoma cells. When p38MAPK phosphorylation was inhibited by co-exposing cells with deguelin and SB202190 (a p38 MAPK inhibitor), oxygen consumption levels were relatively increased compared to levels found when only deguelin was present. These results indicated p38MAPK possesses a significant role in mediating one of the adverse effects of deguelin exposure.

3.3 Reactive Oxygen Species and Oxidative Stress

The mitochondria is one of the major sites of reactive oxygen species (ROS) production. ROS were initially believed to be harmful byproducts of aerobic processes, but are now recognized as central features in cellular signaling [35]. Complex I inhibitors have been associated with an increase in ROS concentrations [31]. In some cases, electrons that leak from this complex can ultimately reduce oxygen and form superoxide anions [17]. In addition, ROS can be produced from complex I by NADH dehydrogenase found in the matrix side of the inner membrane [7]. It has also been postulated that the levels and relative ratios of NADH and NAD+ regulate the formation of ROS: Lower concentrations of NAD+ have been linked to increased superoxide production [27]. When complex I is inhibited, the transfer of electron from NADH to ubiquinone is prohibited and NAD + concentration decreases, raising the likelihood of ROS production and subsequently causing cellular oxidative stress. In accordance with what is known about complex I inhibition, studies have shown increased ROS production upon exposure to deguelin. For instance, ROS concentrations, such as intracellular hydrogen peroxide, have been observed to increase in H1299 cells, a human lung carcinoma cell line after exposure to 100 nM deguelin [42].

3.4 Cytokines

Functioning as key contributors of cellular signaling, cytokines are known to be indispensably involved in vital mechanisms, such as cell proliferation. Their role in the cellular response to deguelin has been briefly addressed, highlighting growth factor cytokines as key contributors of inhibited cell growth. Kang et al. [25] determined that interleukin-8 (IL-8) expression was significantly decreased in colon cancer cells, following 50 and 300 nM deguelin exposures, and discussed that this decrease may be a resulting effect of the inhibition of NF-κB by deguelin. Inhibition of NF-κB is clearly known to be associated with deguelin-induced apoptosis [3] and the subsequent inhibition of IL-8 may be another step in the signaling cascade which ultimately leads to cell death. In fact, IL-8 is well known to be a crucial mediator of cell survival and proliferation [30].

4 Role of Deguelin in Chronic Diseases

4.1 Parkinson's Disease Overview

To date, the only disease that has been associated with deguelin exposure is Parkinson's disease (PD). PD is a neurodegenerative disorder, which is characterized by a substantial loss of dopaminergic neurons in the substantia nigra, along with the manifestation of symptoms such as bradykinesia, rigidity, and rest tremor [14]. While a genetic role of the onset of PD has been explored (identifying certain associated genetic mutations) [2], environmental factors, such as exposure to pesticides, herbicides, and insecticides, have also been linked to the development of PD [44, 49]. In some cases, traces of insecticides or pesticides have been found in postmortem brains [11] and in the serum of individuals afflicted with PD [45]. In actuality, most instances of PD are classified as sporadic, while familial, or hereditary cases are very rare [38].

4.2 Molecular Features of Parkinson's Disease

PD is associated with the death of different types of neurons, but the greatest loss is observed with dopaminergic neurons. The reduction of neurons results in a significant decrease in dopamine levels, which is thought to be responsible for the development of symptoms related to motor control, such as bradykinesia or tremors. The formation of Lewy bodies (LB), or abnormal aggregates of protein that develop inside nerve cells, is also a standard indication of a deteriorating brain. Cellular mutations that directly initiate abnormal protein folding or inhibit the ability of the cell to detect and degrade misfolded proteins may be involved in the loss of dopaminergic neurons. It is, however, unknown whether the formation of LBs is a protective mechanism or further promotes neurodegeneration [12].

4.3 Mitochondrial Dysfunction

The etiology and pathogenesis of PD are still unclear, but mitochondrial dysfunction is gaining recognition as molecular hallmark of PD. One of the first reported cases of PD caused by mitochondrial dysfunction was described in the 1980s: Young drug abusers injected themselves with an opiate MPPP (1-methyl-4-phenyl-4-propionoxypiperidine) and started to exhibit signs of PD. It was revealed that a byproduct of the synthesized drug, MPTP (1-methyl-4-phenyl-1,2,3,6-tetrahydropyridine), was responsible for the development of PD-like symptoms [28] and subsequent studies discovered that MPTP inhibits mitochondrial respiration at complex I of the ETC [41]. Presently, MPTP is one of the neurotoxins used to model PD in animal studies. These findings suggest that any substance which behaves like MPTP can potentially contribute to the onset of PD [38]. For instance, deguelin is a well-known complex I inhibitor and has been reported to elicit PD-like symptoms in rats administered with deguelin (6 mg/kg/day for 6 days) [6]. Caboni et al., observed degeneration of the dopaminergic pathway in the substantia nigra, in the form of reduced tyrosine hydroxylase immunoreactivity.

4.4 Deguelin and Cancer

While deguelin does not promote the development of cancer, there is a prominent association between deguelin exposure and cancerous diseases. Deguelin is known to possess anticancer properties through the inhibition of central cellular metabolic processes [50], coupled with the activation of pro-apoptotic mechanisms [8]. The exact science behind how deguelin acts to inhibit cancer growth and destroy cancerous cells is yet to be clearly defined, but many animal and human model studies have observed the promising effects of deguelin as an anticancer agent.

These findings are presented in the subsequent sections of this chapter, *Biological activities of Deguelin in animal models* and *Biological activities of Deguelin in humans.*

5 Biological Activities of Deguelin in Animal Models

5.1 Pharmacokinetic Properties in Animals

Pharmacokinetic properties describe how a compound is absorbed, distributed, metabolized, and excreted. These values are important in assessing the potential toxicity of a compound and it metabolites, evaluating the efficacy and risks of a drug, or even determining the appropriate dosage of a drug. Presently, the following pharmacokinetic properties of deguelin have been determined in female Sprague Dawley rats [48]. It is important to note that all of the listed values are reported from one study that used a very specific set of conditions to investigate initial pharmacokinetics of deguelin. Briefly, Udeani et al. administered single doses of 0.25 mg/kg (intravenous) or 4 mg/kg (intragastric) of deguelin to female Sprague Dawley rats and monitored them for a maximum of 5 days. There are currently no other publications that have examined pharmacokinetic properties of deguelin at any other conditions or exposure concentrations in a live model. There are many in vivo and in vitro studies that identify cell type- and concentration-dependent responses, but complete analyses from exposure to excretion are limited.

The following pharmacokinetic parameters were identified by Udeani et al.: Mean residence time (MRT)—6.98 h; terminal half-life—9.26 h; area under the curve (AUC)—57.3 ng h/mL; total clearance (Cl)—4.37 l/h/kg; volume of distribution—3.421 l/kg; volume of distribution (at steady state)—30.46 l/kg. Brief descriptions of each pharmacokinetic parameter are listed in Table 2. It was also discovered that following an intragastric administration of deguelin, approximately 58.1 and 14.4 % were eliminated through feces and urine, respectively. The remaining percentage of deguelin is assumed to be distributed in tissues, such as the heart, liver, lung, kidney, brain, and colon [48].

5.2 Toxicological Properties in Animal Models

Toxicological properties, also referred to as health hazard information, describe all issues related to the potential toxicity of a chemical or substance. This dataset can address acute and chronic toxicity, skin corrosion/irritation, eye damage/irritation, respiratory or skin sensitization, germ cell mutagenicity, carcinogenicity, reproductive toxicity, specific target organ toxicity—single/repeated exposure, aspiration hazards, and symptoms of various routes of exposure. Unfortunately, the general consensus is that the current available data concerning deguelin toxicity are

Table 2 Definitions of pharmacokinetic parameters

Parameter	Definition
Mean residence time (MRT)	Amount of time compound stays in the body
Terminal half-life	Time required for the plasma concentration to decrease by 50 % during the elimination phase
Area under the curve	An estimated exposure of the drug over time, after one administration of the compound
Total clearance	The removal of drug from a volume of plasma per time
Volume of distribution	Theoretical plasma volume needed to contain the total amount of an administered dose in the body
Volume of distribution (at steady state)	Accounts for the actual blood and tissue volume into which a drug is administered and the relative binding of drug to proteins

insufficient to define *all* issues listed above. There are, however, a few pieces of useful toxicity data: The lethal dose, which eliminates 50 % of the population (LD_{50}), is reported as 300, 3200, and 980 mg/kg for the mouse, rabbit, and rat, respectively. These distinctly different LD_{50} values among three different species convey the importance of understanding intraspecies variability. Caution must be taken in comparing results, especially when different animal models are involved.

5.3 Deguelin as a Chemotherapeutic and Chemopreventive in Animal Models

Many studies on deguelin have focused on the potential chemotherapeutic and chemopreventive applications. Both animal in vitro and in vivo investigations have revealed deguelin to be a promising candidate for reducing tumor sizes and inhibiting growth. For instance, 2 mg/kg deguelin treatment drastically inhibited the growth of murine mammary cancer cells in mice and no additional indications of cytotoxicity were observed, demonstrating the effectiveness, yet nontoxic nature of deguelin, at the dose used in the study [34]. In vitro studies assess the effectiveness of deguelin by measuring the extent of apoptosis or cell proliferation inhibition. Li et al. [32] found deguelin induced a time (24–72 h)- and dose (0–2000 ng/mL)-dependent decrease in cell proliferation in murine myeloma cells, coupled with decreased levels of Akt phosphorylation and upregulation of pro-apoptotic factors. A myriad of other studies in animal models demonstrating the effectiveness of deguelin as a chemotherapeutic in different cell types and of distinct growth abnormalities warrants further investigation of deguelin as a potential anticancer agent [22, 23, 53].

6 Biological Activities of Deguelin in Humans

6.1 *Toxicity in Humans*

A thorough toxicity assessment of deguelin in humans, from the point of administration to excretion, has yet to be completed. There have, however, been reported cases of vomiting, acute congestive cardiac failure, weak pulse, dilated pupils, and even fatality after consumption of derris roots, which is high in concentration of deguelin and rotenone [21]. How much of the toxicity was induced by solely deguelin is unclear. Presently, researchers have concluded that deguelin has a relatively nontoxic effect on human cell lines through results that demonstrate no decreases in survival rates or increases in apoptosis in healthy, noncancerous cells, after dosing with deguelin [4]. These findings are, of course, specific for the type of cell line, the dose of deguelin administered, and the total time of exposure. There is therefore no definitive threshold of toxicity in humans at this time.

6.2 *Deguelin as a Chemotherapeutic and Chemopreventive in Human Models*

The majority of deguelin studies address its potential anticancer applications due to its ability to inhibit several cellular processes that are involved in cell proliferation. While deguelin has not been approved yet for clinical testing on human subjects, a variety of different cancerous human cell lines have been assessed after treatment with deguelin and have demonstrated promising chemotherapeutic results. Ranging from human colon cancer cell lines [25] to malignant human bronchial epithelial and non-small-cell lung cancer cell lines [26], a decrease in cell growth or an increase in apoptosis is observed after dosing with deguelin concentrations ranging from 50 to 300 nM. These studies offer justification to further investigate the potential anticancer applications of deguelin.

7 Conclusions

Deguelin, while a naturally produced compound, has been reported to elicit adverse effects in humans. In-depth investigations of this root extracted substance have generated interest in using it for its anticancer properties: Deguelin has demonstrated in a variety of both human and animal cancerous cell lines, as well as in vivo animal models, the ability to inhibit cell proliferation and induce apoptosis. Unfortunately, high doses of deguelin have also been associated with the development of PD through the inhibition of mitochondrial complex I. Additional research elucidating the mechanisms by which deguelin inhibits central cellular processes, as well as a detailed profiling of its toxicological effects, is required in order to move forward with future research addressing potential applications and risks of deguelin.

References

1. Baba Y, Fujii M, Maeda T, Suzuki A, Yuzawa S, Kato Y (2015) Deguelin induces apoptosis by targeting both EGFR-Akt and IGF1R-Akt pathways in head and neck squamous cell cancer cell lines. Biomed Res Int 2015:657179
2. Bekris LM, Mata IF, Zabetian CP (2010) The genetics of Parkinson disease. J Geriatr Psychiatry Neurol 23:228–242
3. Boreddy SR, Srivastava SK (2013) Deguelin suppresses pancreatic tumor growth and metastasis by inhibiting epithelial-to-mesenchymal transition in an orthotopic model. Oncogene 32:3980–3991
4. Bortul R, Tazzari PL, Billi AM, Tabellini G, Mantovani I, Cappellini A, Grafone T, Martinelli G, Conte R, Martelli AM (2005) Deguelin, A PI3K/AKT inhibitor, enhances chemosensitivity of leukaemia cells with an active PI3K/AKT pathway. Br J Haematol 129:677–686
5. Boyd J, Saksena A, Patrone JB, Williams HN, Boggs N, Le H, Theodore M (2011) Exploring the boundaries of additivity: mixtures of NADH: quinone oxidoreductase inhibitors. Chem Res Toxicol 24:1242–1250
6. Caboni P, Sherer TB, Zhang N, Taylor G, Na HM, Greenamyre JT, Casida JE (2004) Rotenone, deguelin, their metabolites, and the rat model of Parkinson's disease. Chem Res Toxicol 17:1540–1548
7. Chen Q, Vazquez EJ, Moghaddas S, Hoppel CL, Lesnefsky EJ (2003) Production of reactive oxygen species by mitochondria: central role of complex III. J Biol Chem 278:36027–36031
8. Chu ZH, Liang XH, Zhou XL, Huang RF, Zhan Q, Jiang JW (2011) Effects of deguelin on proliferation and apoptosis of MCF-7 breast cancer cells by phosphatidylinositol 3-kinase/Akt signaling pathway. Zhong Xi Yi Jie He Xue Bao 9:533–538
9. Chun KH, Kosmeder JW, Sun S, Pezzuto JM, Lotan R, Hong WK, Lee HY (2003) Effects of deguelin on the phosphatidylinositol 3-kinase/Akt pathway and apoptosis in premalignant human bronchial epithelial cells. J Natl Cancer Inst 95:291–302
10. Clark EP (1931) Deguelin. I. The preparation, purification and properties of deguelin, a constituent of certain tropical fish-poisoning plants. J Am Chem Soc 53:313–317
11. Corrigan FM, Wienburg CL, Shore RF, Daniel SE, Mann D (2000) Organochlorine insecticides in substantia nigra in Parkinson's disease. J Toxicol Environ Health A 59:229–234
12. Dauer W, Przedborski S (2003) Parkinson's disease: mechanisms and models. Neuron 39:889–909
13. Davidson WM (1930) The relative value as contact insecticides of some constituents of Derris. J Econ Entomol 23:877–879
14. Davie CA (2008) A review of Parkinson's disease. Br Med Bull 86:109–127
15. Deguelin; MSDS [Online]; Sigma-Aldrich 06/27/2014. Accessed 16 Nov 2015
16. Fang N, Casida JE (1999) Cubé resin insecticide: identification and biological activity of 29 rotenoid constituents. J Agric Food Chem 47:2130–2136
17. Fato R, Bergamini C, Bortolus M, Maniero AL, Leoni S, Ohnishi T, Lenaz G (2009) Differential effects of mitochondrial complex I inhibitors on production of reactive oxygen species. Biochim Biophys Acta 1787:384–392
18. Gerhäuser C, Lee SK, Kosmeder JW, Moriarty RM, Hamel E, Mehta RG, Moon RC, Pezzuto JM (1997) Regulation of ornithine decarboxylase induction by deguelin, a natural product cancer chemopreventive agent. Cancer Res 57:3429–3435

19. Gersdorff WA (1931) A study of the toxicity of toxicarol, deguelin and tephrosin using the goldfish as the test animal. J Am Chem Soc 53:1897–1901
20. Hers I, Vincent EE, Tavare JM (2011) Akt signalling in health and disease. Cell Signal 23:1515–1527
21. Holland EA (1938) Suicide by ingestion of derris root sp. in New Ireland. Trans Roy Soc Trop Med Hyg 32:293–294
22. Hsu YC, Chiang JH, Yu CS, Hsia TC, Wu RS, Lien JC, Lai KC, Yu FS, Chung JG (2015) Antitumor effects of deguelin on H460 human lung cancer cells in vitro and in vivo: roles of apoptotic cell death and H460 tumor xenografts model. Environ Toxicol
23. Hu J, Ye H, Fu A, Chen X, Wang Y, Ye X, Xiao W, Duan X, Wei Y, Chen L (2010) Deguelin–an inhibitor to tumor lymphangiogenesis and lymphatic metastasis by downregulation of vascular endothelial cell growth factor-D in lung tumor model. Int J Cancer 127:2455–2466
24. Jin Q, Feng L, Behrens C, Bekele BN, Wistuba II, Hong WK, Lee HY (2007) Implication of AMP-activated protein kinase and Akt-regulated survivin in lung cancer chemopreventive activities of deguelin. Cancer Res 67:11630–11639
25. Kang HW, Kim JM, Cha MY, Jung HC, Song IS, Kim JS (2012) Deguelin, an Akt inhibitor, down-regulates NF-kappaB signaling and induces apoptosis in colon cancer cells and inhibits tumor growth in mice. Dig Dis Sci 57:2873–2882
26. Kim WY, Chang DJ, Hennessy B, Kang HJ, Yoo J, Han SH, Kim YS, Park HJ, Seo SY, Mills G, Kim KW, Hong WK, Suh YG, Lee HY (2008) A novel derivative of the natural agent deguelin for cancer chemoprevention and therapy. Cancer Prev Res (Phila) 1:577–587
27. Kussmaul L, Hirst J (2006) The mechanism of superoxide production by NADH: ubiquinone oxidoreductase (complex I) from bovine heart mitochondria. Proc Natl Acad Sci U S A 103:7607–7612
28. Langston JW, Ballard P, Tetrud JW, Irwin I (1983) Chronic parkinsonism in humans due to a product of meperidine-analog synthesis. Science 219:979–980
29. Lee H, Lee JH, Jung KH, Hong SS (2010) Deguelin promotes apoptosis and inhibits angiogenesis of gastric cancer. Oncol Rep 24:957–963
30. Li A, Dubey S, Varney ML, Dave BJ, Singh RK (2003) IL-8 directly enhanced endothelial cell survival, proliferation, and matrix metalloproteinases production and regulated angiogenesis. J Immunol 170:3369–3376
31. Li N, Ragheb K, Lawler G, Sturgis J, Rajwa B, Melendez JA, Robinson JP (2003) Mitochondrial complex I inhibitor rotenone induces apoptosis through enhancing mitochondrial reactive oxygen species production. J Biol Chem 278:8516–8525
32. Li Z, Wu J, Wu C, Jiang J, Zheng X, Xu B, Li M (2012) Deguelin, a natural rotenoid, inhibits mouse myeloma cell growth in vitro via induction of apoptosis. Oncol Lett 4:677–681
33. Lopiccolo J, Blumenthal GM, Bernstein WB, Dennis PA (2008) Targeting the PI3K/Akt/mTOR pathway: effective combinations and clinical considerations. Drug Resist Updat 11:32–50
34. Mehta RR, Katta H, Kalra A, Patel R, Gupta A, Alimirah F, Murillo G, Peng X, Unni A, Muzzio M, Mehta RG (2013) Efficacy and mechanism of action of deguelin in suppressing metastasis of 4T1 cells. Clin Exp Metastasis 30:855–866
35. Mittler R, Vanderauwera S, Suzuki N, Miller G, Tognetti VB, Vandepoele K, Gollery M, Shulaev V, van Breusegem F (2011) ROS signaling: the new wave? Trends Plant Sci 16:300–309
36. Murillo G, Peng X, Torres KE, Mehta RG (2009) Deguelin inhibits growth of breast cancer cells by modulating the expression of key members of the Wnt signaling pathway. Cancer Prev Res (Phila) 2:942–950
37. Murillo G, Salti GI, Kosmeder JW, Pezzuto JM, Mehta RG (2002) Deguelin inhibits the growth of colon cancer cells through the induction of apoptosis and cell cycle arrest. Eur J Cancer 38:2446–2454
38. Nagatsu T, Sawada M (2006) Cellular and molecular mechanisms of Parkinson's disease: neurotoxins, causative genes, and inflammatory cytokines. Cell Mol Neurobiol 26:781–802

39. Nair AS, Shishodia S, Ahn KS, Kunnumakkara AB, Sethi G, Aggarwal BB (2006) Deguelin, an Akt inhibitor, suppresses IkappaBalpha kinase activation leading to suppression of NF-kappaB-regulated gene expression, potentiation of apoptosis, and inhibition of cellular invasion. J Immunol 177:5612–5622
40. Negherbon WO (1959) Handbook of toxicology, vol III. Insecticides
41. Nicklas WJ, Vyas I, Heikkila RE (1985) Inhibition of NADH-linked oxidation in brain mitochondria by 1-methyl-4-phenyl-pyridine, a metabolite of the neurotoxin, 1-methyl-4-phenyl-1,2,5,6-tetrahydropyridine. Life Sci 36:2503–2508
42. Oh SH, Woo JK, Yazici YD, Myers JN, Kim WY, Jin Q, Hong SS, Park HJ, Suh YG, Kim KW, Hong WK, Lee HY (2007) Structural basis for depletion of heat shock protein 90 client proteins by deguelin. J Natl Cancer Inst 99:949–961
43. Okun JG, Lummen P, Brandt U (1999) Three classes of inhibitors share a common binding domain in mitochondrial complex I (NADH: ubiquinone oxidoreductase). J Biol Chem 274:2625–2630
44. Priyadarshi A, Khuder SA, Schaub EA, Priyadarshi SS (2001) Environmental risk factors and Parkinson's disease: a metaanalysis. Environ Res 86:122–127
45. Richardson JR, Shalat SL, Buckley B, Winnik B, O'Suilleabhain P, Diaz-Arrastia R, Reisch J, German DC (2009) Elevated serum pesticide levels and risk of Parkinson disease. Arch Neurol 66:870–875
46. Thamilselvan V, Menon M, Thamilselvan S (2011) Anticancer efficacy of deguelin in human prostate cancer cells targeting glycogen synthase kinase-3 beta/beta-catenin pathway. Int J Cancer 129:2916–2927
47. Tomlin CDS (1997) The pesticide manual, 11 edn. xliii+1606p–xliii+1606p
48. Udeani GO, Zhao GM, Shin YG, Kosmeder JW, Beecher CW, Kinghorn AD, Moriarty RM, Moon RC, Pezzuto JM (2001) Pharmacokinetics of deguelin, a cancer chemopreventive agent in rats. Cancer Chemother Pharmacol 47:263–268
49. van der Mark M, Brouwer M, Kromhout H, Nijssen P, Huss A, Vermeulen R (2012) Is pesticide use related to Parkinson disease? Some clues to heterogeneity in study results. Environ Health Perspect 120:340–347
50. Vrana JA, Boggs N, Currie HN, Boyd J (2013) Amelioration of an undesired action of deguelin. Toxicon 74:83–91
51. Warburg O (1956) On the origin of cancer cells. Science 123:309–314
52. Xiong JR, Liu HL (2013) Regulatory effects of deguelin on proliferation and cell cycle of Raji cells. J Huazhong Univ Sci Technol Med Sci 33:491–495
53. Yan Y, Wang Y, Tan Q, Lubet RA, You M (2005) Efficacy of Deguelin and Silibinin on Benzo(a)pyrene-Induced Lung Tumorigenesis in A/J Mice1. Neoplasia 7:1053–1057

Quercetin and Its Role in Chronic Diseases

Ganiyu Oboh, Ayokunle O. Ademosun and Opeyemi B. Ogunsuyi

Abstract Quercetin, a member of the flavonoid class of polyphenol, is one of the most abundantly distributed flavonoids found in various food sources such as fruits, vegetables, nuts, wine and seeds. Quercetin and quercetin-rich foods have been reported to have wide range of health promoting effects, especially in the prevention and management of several diseases; however, the subject of its solubility and bioavailability has limited its use. This section will therefore, consider quercetin as a food-rich flavonoid, the various food sources, the limitations in its use and new approaches at improving its solubility and bioavailability. The therapeutic potentials of quercetin at the prevention/management of some degenerative diseases such as diabetes, hypertension and neurodegenerative diseases, as well as the underlying biochemical mechanisms such as free radical scavenging and enzyme inhibition will also be discussed.

Keywords Quercetin · Flavonoids · Bioavailability · Degenerative diseases · Antioxidant

1 Quercetin; Abundance, Metabolism and Bioavailability

Our everyday diet often contain a wide variety of health promoting constituents which has been linked to the prevention and management of many diseases. Furthermore, data from epidemiological studies have provided useful information on the relationship between increased intake of flavonoid rich diets and decreased risk of chronic diseases including certain cancers [56]. Quercetin (3,3′,4′,5,7-pentahydroxyflavone) (Fig. 1) is a flavonoid found ubiquitously in the form of a glycoside in various vegetables, fruits, seeds, nuts, tea and red wine; it has gained significant attention over the years for its potential antiproliferative,

G. Oboh (✉) · A.O. Ademosun · O.B. Ogunsuyi
Functional Foods and Nutraceuticals Unit, Department of Biochemistry, Federal University of Technology, P.M.B. 704, Akure 340001, Ondo State, Nigeria
e-mail: Goboh2001@yahoo.com

S.C. Gupta et al. (eds.), *Drug Discovery from Mother Nature*,
Advances in Experimental Medicine and Biology 929,
DOI 10.1007/978-3-319-41342-6_17

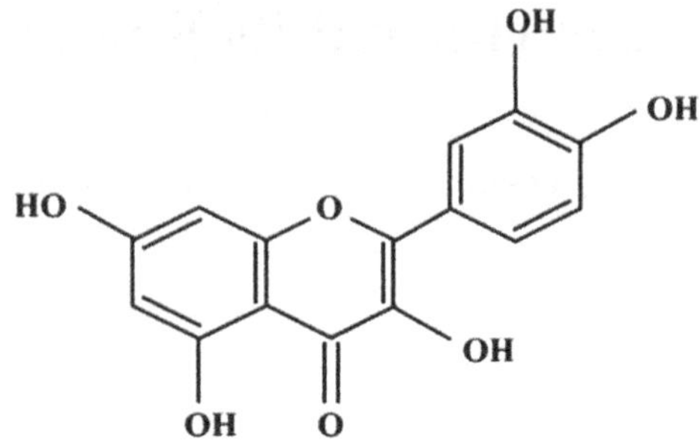

Fig. 1 Structure of quercetin

chemopreventive, anti-inflammatory, and anticarcinogenic activities and gene expression-modulating potential [43]. Most often, research on flavonoids is inclined towards quercetin (QUR). Nevertheless, studies have also shown that QUR has potentially toxic effects such as its mutagenicity, pro-oxidant activity, mitochondrial toxicity, and inhibition of key enzymes involved in hormone metabolism [37].

The medicinal use of QUR has been greatly limited by its poor water solubility, short biological half-life, and low oral bioavailability [28, 39]. The bioavailability of QUR is greatly dependent on its metabolism in the gut and liver, and thereafter distributed across the different animal tissues [9]. Therefore, efforts at increasing the bioavailability of QUR has been largely on improving its solubility; nevertheless, it relatively high molecular weight and melting point seams a major obstacle. Consequently, since QUR glycosides are metabolized in the intestinal tracts [15], it is believed that a novel delivery system could help improve the solubility and hence, bioavailability of this flavonoid.

2 Quercetin and Oxidative Stress

Oxidative stress occurs as a consequent of an imbalance in the body antioxidant defense mechanisms and free radical generation, often shifting to an excess of the latter. Free radicals has been implicated in the pathogenesis and progression of many diseases such as diabetes, atherosclerosis, hypertension, neurodegenerative diseases, inflammation, erectile dysfunction, and cancer [67]. Therefore, dietary antioxidant sources such as polyphenols which could augment the endogenous antioxidant machineries have been well studied and reported as possible therapeutic target for many of these diseases. Generally, flavonoid family of antioxidants reduce the deleterious effects of free radicals by hydrogen atom transfer to stabilize the radicals; a feature which has structure-function relationship [9]. QUR has been well characterized for its antioxidant and free radical scavenging abilities. QUR is one of the flavonoids with the most potent antioxidant properties by scavenging reactive oxygen species produced during normal cellular oxidative metabolism or obtained from exogenous sources [43, 51]; as well as bind transition metal ions, while being simultaneously oxidized to the unstable semiquinone radical [9]. Semiquinone radical is equally oxidized to quercetin quinone which reacts readily with protein thiols and eliminated by conjugation with glutathione [49]. Nevertheless, the glycosylation of QUR reduces its antioxidant activities [9]. In addition, depending on concentration, QUR can act as both antioxidant and pro-oxidant. At low concentration (10–10 μM), QUR have shown protective effect against DNA oxidative damage (in vitro) in human lymphocytes [68]. According to a study by Spencer et al. [61], QUR at a concentration of up to 10 μM showed protective effect against oxidative stress induced fibroblast damage while on the contrary, cytotoxicity was observed at a concentration of 30 μM.

The structural aspect of free radical scavenging ability of QUR majorly hinges on its 3-OH substituent [11] which has been associated with increased stability of the flavonoid radical [9]. In addition, the catechol group is also responsible largely for the ability of QUR to chelate transition metals and thus prevent their induction of free radical induced cellular damage [43]. The mechanism by which QUR prevents free radical induced cellular damage is multifaceted; one of such ways is by direct free radicals scavenging [43]. By such radical scavenging ability, QUR is able to inhibit the oxidation of LDL cholesterol and thus prevent the formation of atherosclerotic plaques [38]. Furthermore, the ability of QUR to scavenge free radicals can also be linked to reduction in ischemia-reperfusion injury via modification of the endothelial nitric oxide system [58]. The endothelial cells produce NO at physiological concentration for maintaining the dilation of the blood vessels via the nitric oxide synthase system [30]. However, at higher concentration, NO can react with superoxide free radicals to produce the highly reactive peroxynitrite [43]. Peroxynitrite is highly damaging and can react directly with many macromolecules including LDL to produce an irreversible damage to cell membranes [43]. Therefore, QUR can act to protect such cellular damage by either scavenging the superoxide radicals and thus prevent them from reacting with NO to produce peroxynitrite and/or scavenge NO itself.

Free radicals also contribute to the pathogenesis of chronic inflammatory diseases by activation of transcription factors which in turn induce the production of pro-inflammatory cytokins [14]. However, it has been shown that QUR has the potential to reduce inflammation by scavenge free radicals [9]. Furthermore, apart from excessive free radicals generated endogenously, oxidative stress can also be induced when exposed to exogenous sources of free radicals such as environmental pollutants. For example, free radicals generated from cigarette smoke tar has been reported to cause membrane damage in erythrocytes [9]. However, studies have shown that quercetin aglycone and its conjugate metabolites (Quercetin -3-O-β-glucuronide and Quercetin -3-O- β-glucoside) were able to prevent smoking induced erythrocyte cell membrane damage [13].

3 Quercetin and Neurodegenerative Diseases

Neurodegenerative diseases are group of chronic diseases characterized by progressive, selective and strategic decline in neuronal and cognitive functions, found in about 5 % of reported cases of brain diseases [48]. The unique pattern by which each neurodegenerative disease cause progressive neuronal decline and their ability to produce disease-specific cellular biomarkers have been of importance in the classification of these diseases [53]. Alzheimer's disease is a neurodegenerative disease characterized by marked decline in acetylcholine neurotransmitter, deposition of senile plaques, neurofibrillary tangles and progressive loss of cognitive function [48, 53]. Another typical neurodegenerative disease is Parkinson's disease characterized by generation of Lewy bodies and depletion of dopamine neurotransmitter while cellular inclusions and swollen motor axons are found in amyotrophic lateral sclerosis [16]. Huntington's disease features loss of neurons containing gamma- aminobutyric acid [18].

QUR has been reported to offer protection against neurodegenerative diseases such as Alzheimer's disease where it shows inhibitory effect against acetylcholinesterase [20]. Furthermore, it has also been reported that QUR attenuates oxidative stress induced in rat's striatum neuronal cells by 6-hydroxydopamine [27]. QUR also show antidepressant effect in vivo in animal models and also improve social interaction time and behavioral indices in experimental animal models. In vitro and in vivo studies have however, shown that QUR's mood improvement properties could be by mechanisms such as monoamine oxidase A inhibition [22, 59]. This may also qualify it as an effective adjunct in the use of L-dopa for the treatment of Parkinson-like symptoms [59]. In addition, QUR could induce the activation of GABA receptors; this is believed to enhance the ability of QUR to significantly induce non-rapid eye movement (non-REM) sleep in rats during dark periods while it also significantly attenuates REM sleep [35]. Alzheimer's disease (AD) is characterized by the formation of amyloid-beta plagues and neurofibrillary tangles. QUR offers neuroprotective properties against AD by inhibiting the formation of these amyloid-beta plaques [65]. In an experiment conducted to assess the effect of chronic administration of QUR on the cognitive function of ethanol intoxicated mice, it was observed that QUR significantly attenuate the impairments in cognitive functions induced by the exposure to ethanol [60]. QUR also show positive effect in the treatment of neuroleptic-induced extrapyramidal side effects, such as seen in the use of haloperidol [52].

4 Quercetin and Diabetes

Diabetes Mellitus (DM) is a chronic metabolic disease resulting in an impaired metabolism of carbohydrates, protein and lipid as a result of either insufficient secretion of insulin as seen in type 1 or increased insulin resistance by cells as characteristic of type 2 diabetes. Type 2 diabetes mellitus (T2DM) accounts for over 90 % of all DM cases [19]. Reducing rise in blood glucose after meal, via inhibition of carbohydrate hydrolyzing enzymes (alpha-amylase and alpha-glucosidase) present in the gastro-intestinal tract is one of the major management therapy [1]. However, management therapies which are mostly inhibitors of these enzymes, often come with several side effects [2], as well as associated financial constraint. Hence, the search for potent but cheap alternative/ complementary therapies, with little or no side effect has been endless. Furthermore, pancreatic cellular damage induced by free radicals is one of the causes of T2DM [17]. Reports of elevated malondialdehyde (MDA) content in pancreatic tissue in vitro [2, 3, 55] and in vivo in diabetic animal models [4, 32] caused by lipid peroxidation also substantiate the role of free radicals in pathogenesis and progression of T2DM. Nevertheless, the use of phytochemicals such as flavonoids to augment endogenous antioxidants which help to effectively protect biological cells against deleterious effect caused by oxidative stress, has been reported in both in vitro and in vivo studies [54].

Several in vitro studies have sought to elucidate the mechanisms behind the antidiabetic properties of QUR. One of such study reported that QUR significantly inhibited the activities of both alpha amylase and alpha glucosidase concentration dependently, as well as also prevent the lipid peroxidation of pancreatic tissue homogenates [55]. The inhibition of these two carbohydrate metabolizing enzymes could slow down the rise in blood glucose level while prevention of pancreatic lipid peroxidation could prevent further cellular damage to the pancreas which could further impair insulin production and secretion. Another of such study showed that QUR is able to slow down the absorption of glucose in Caco-2E intestinal cell culture by inhibition of the glucose transporter (GLUT2) dose dependently up to a concentration of 200 μM [42]. Another mechanism behind QUR antidiabetic properties could be as a result of its influence on insulin secretion. Youl et al. [69], reported that QUR potentiate both glucose and glibenclamide-induced insulin secretion in insulin-secreting cell line INS-1 β; these observations were also recorded when isolated islets of Langerhans from rat were used. Furthermore, diabetes is associated with a number of complications such as neuropathy, retinopathy, diabetic cataracts, and nephropathy. These complications often arise as a result of build of sorbitol, a sugar alcohol which is produced from glucose catalyzed by the enzyme aldose reductase [37]. QUR has been reported to inhibit the activity of aldose reductase and thus slow does the build-up of sorbitol. For example the quercetin glycoside (quercitrin) significantly reduced sorbitol accumulation in lens of rodents to a level less significant to induce cataracts [37]; hence, QUR may offer therapeutic benefits in the management of diabetes [36].

Likewise, studies on diabetic animal models have shown that QUR can cause a decrease in plasma glucose level, protect the cellular and functional integrity of pancreatic beta cells as well as prevent some diabetic complications such as neuropathy and nephropathy [6]. Supplementation of diet with 0.08 % QUR in C57BL/KsJdb-db mice fed for 49 days resulted in reduced serum glucose level and blood glycated haemoglobin but not serum insulin level [41] and the reduced blood glucose was attributed to the inhibition of maltase activity in the small intestine. Nevertheless, the long term use of QUR especially as a supplement in the management of diabetes has been a subject of major concern. In a study by Hsieh et al. [29], carried out by administering QUR to streptozotocin-induced diabetic rats for 29 days, the authors reported elevated cases of cataract and impaired renal function especially in groups administered QUR; the authors suggested that long term use of QUR could act as pro-oxidant during progression of diabetes. While such report remains at best speculative, it has called for more research into finding out the effect of chronic use of QUR in diabetic human subjects [37]. Also, Jung et al. [34], compared the possible benefits of QUR supplementation and food rich in QUR in diabetic rat models. Animals were fed on HFD supplemented with either 1 % onion peel extract (OPE) (containing 0.1 % of QUR) or 0.1 % of QUR alone for 8 weeks. While OPE administration led to significantly improved oral glucose tolerance, QUR alone did not have this effect.

5 Quercetin and Cardiovascular Disorders

The cardiovascular system exist in a delicate state of homeostasis tightly regulated by the vascular endothelium A distortion in such equilibrium could induce endothelial dysfunction, a risk factor for cardiovascular diseases leading to hypertension, atherosclerosis, ischemia and platelet aggregation [44]. Endothelial dysfunction is the main risk factor for cardiovascular diseases and is characterized by impaired endothelium-dependent vasodilatation, reduced NO activity and a prothrombotic and proinflammatory state of endothelial cells [44].

Hypertension is one of the most prevalent risk factors of several cardiovascular diseases and a major health problem globally [21]. The renin-angiotensin system plays an important role in blood pressure regulation [66]; hence, the regulation of this pathway is of great pharmacological significance blood pressure control [5]. Unique to the Renin-angiotensin pathway id the Angiotensin I converting enzyme (ACE) which cleaves angiotensin I to angiotensin II, a powerful vasoconstrictor, and also inhibits bradykinin, a vasodilator [12, 50]. Hence, ACE inhibitors are widely used as standard blood pressure lowering drug owing to its vasodilatory effect [63]. Nevertheless, the complications such as dry cough and angioneuroticedema, arising from the use of these inhibitors cannot be entirely ignored [70].

Oxidative stress which is induced by excessive free radical generation is another known etiology of endothelial dysfunction-induced hypertension and other cardiovascular diseases [57]. These free radicals can cause cellular damage by oxidation of biomolecules such as lipids, proteins and DNA [8], and have been associated with the development and progression of several diseases, including hypertension [47]. Hence, attempts at attenuating oxidative stress could be one practical way to ensure holistic management of hypertension and other cardiovascular diseases [5].

Endothelial dysfunction is a common feature in the pathogenesis of cardiovascular diseases. The endothelium releases several vasoactive substances including vasodilators such as nitric oxide (NO) and vasoconstrictors such as endothelin-1 (ET-1), with which it regulates blood flow and vascular tone (). Depletion of NO to counteract the vasoconstricting effect of ET-1 is often the hallmark of endothelial dysfunction [44]. Hence, a positive approach at management of CVDs is often to prevent/manage endothelial dysfunction.

Early understandings based experimental data from animal models on the blood pressure lowering ability of QUR has been on attenuation of oxidative stress [44]. While several animal models have shown reduced blood pressure and improvement in antioxidant status following administration of QUR, data emanating from studies on human subjects have not be too convincing. The major challenge however seams to hinge on the bioavailability of QUR at tissue and cellular levels. In a study [33], it was reported that rats supplemented with 150 mg QUR/kg (plasma QUR metabolite level = 3.96 μg/mL) resulted in reduced liver malondialdehyde content, there was neither change in plasma antioxidant power nor urinary isoprostanes in QUR humans subjects supplemented with about 8.1 mg QUR/kg (plasma QUR metabolite level = 0.48 μg/mL) [24]. These observations may bring to bear the challenge of bioavailability of QUR in tissues and cells which could have negatively impaired its antioxidant functions. While higher doses of QUR produces significant antioxidant properties in animal models, such is not for humans based on available data. For example. Egert et al. [25] in their study in which they administered QUR supplementation to healthy and normotensive human subjects for 14 days did not affect plasma antioxidant indices. Another study in which 730 mg/day QUR supplements was administered to pro-hypertensive and stage 1 hypertensive human subjects also produced no significant influence on plasma antioxidant indices [44]. All these hence may incline that the observed antihypertensive properties of QUR especially reported in human studies may depend more largely on other mechanisms other than the antioxidant properties of QUR.

Endothelium- and NO-dependent relaxation has been reported for several isolated flavonoids [10, 56]. QUR have been shown to have vasodilatory effect which is partially endothelium-dependent and associated with the release of endothelium-derived relaxing factors [7, 40]. QUR seems to have a varying and complex effects on NO depending on the prevailing conditions. In a cell-free system, QUR undergoes oxidation to generate superoxide radical which reacts rapidly to inactivate NO [45]. However, in the presence of endothelial cells and absence of oxidative stress, QUR was reported to potentiate the production of NO as measured by an amperometric electrode [64]; whereas, no increment was observed when NO production was monitored with electron paramagnetic resonance spectroscopy [62]. In addition, QUR has been reported to inhibit the activity of endothelial nitric oxide synthase (eNOS) [31].

In vivo studies have also substantiated the modulatory effects of QUR on the endothelial system. It was reported in one study that QUR reduced blood pressure in spontaneously hypertensive rats (SHR) with a concomitant improvement in endothelium-dependent vasodilation of isolated aorta [23]. In another study, hypertensive animal models created by feeding with high fat and high sucrose diet for 28 days were supplemented with QUR which led to reduction in systemic hypertension, improved aortic NOS activity and increased urinary NO metabolites (Yamamoto et al.). These studies have shown that QUR is able to ameliorate endothelial dysfunction and its associated cardiovascular diseases by increasing the bioavailability of NO.

Investigation into the modulatory effect of QUR on ACE activity as a possible mechanism behind its protective effect against cardiovascular diseases and especially, hypertension has gained significant prominence. In a study by Mackraj et al. [46], they compared the antihypertensive effects of QUR to that of captopril (a standard ACE inhibitor) in Dahl salt sensitive rats for 28 days. They observed that groups treated with QUR and captopril showed a significant reduction in blood pressure compared to the control group. However, while it could be concluded that the antihypertensive effect of captopril observed in this study was due to ACE inhibition, the inability of authors to monitor ACE activity could not make it substantive to opine that QUR also reduce blood pressure via ACE inhibition. Hackl et al. [26], however reported a 31 % reduction in ACE activity in QUR administered normotensive Wister rats placed on infusion of bradykinin and angiotensin-1. The infusions of bradykinin and angiotensin-1 significantly induced a hypertensive state marked by elevated blood pressure which was ameliorated by QUR. This study therefore reveals that QUR has an actual ACE inhibitory effect which could contribute significantly to its antihypertensive properties. However, there is still lack of data on the efficacy or possibility of this mechanism, applying to the blood pressure lowering effect of QUR in human hypertensive subjects.

References

1. Abirami A, Nagarani G, Siddhuraju P (2014) In vitro antioxidant, anti-diabetic, cholinesterase and tyrosinase inhibitory potential of fresh juice from *Citrus hystrix* and *C. maxima* fruits. Food Sci Hum Wellness 3:16–25
2. Adefegha SA, Oboh G (2012) Inhibition of key enzymes linked to type 2 diabetes and sodium nitroprusside-induced lipid peroxidation in rat pancreas by water extractable phytochemicals from some tropical spices. Pharm Biol 50:857–865
3. Ademiluyi AO, Oboh G, Aragbaiye FP, Oyeleye SI, Ogunsuyi OB (2015) Antioxidant properties and in vitro α-amylase and α-glucosidase inhibitory properties of phenolics constituents from different varieties of *Corchorus* spp. J Taibah Univ Med Sci 10:278–287
4. Ademiluyi AO, Oboh G, Boligon AA, Athayde ML (2014) Effect of fermented soybean condiment supplemented diet on α-amylase and α-glucosidase activities in Streptozotocin-induced diabetic rats. J Funct Foods 9:1–9
5. Ademiluyi AO, Oboh G, Ogunsuyi OB, Oloruntoba FM (2015) A comparative study on antihypertensive and antioxidant properties of phenolic extracts from fruit and leaf of some guava (*Psidium guajava* L.) varieties. Comp Clin Pathol. doi:10.1007/s00580-015-2192-y
6. Aguirre L, Arias N, Macarulla MT, Gracia A, Portillo MP (2011) Beneficial effects of quercetin on obesity and diabetes. Open Nutraceuticals J 4:189–198
7. Ajay M, Gilani AU, Mustafa MR (2003) Effects of flavonoids on vascular smooth muscle of the isolated rat thoracic aorta. Life Sci 74:603–612

8. Ajila CM, Prasada UJS (2008) Protection against hydrogen peroxide induced oxidative damage in rat erythrocytes by Mangifera indica L. peel extract. Food Chem Toxicol 46: 303–309
9. Alrawaiq NS, Abdullah A (2014) A review of flavonoid quercetin: metabolism, bioactivity and antioxidant properties. Int J Pharm Tech Res 6:933–941
10. Andriambeloson E, Magnier C, Haan-Archipoff G, Lobstein A, Anton R, Beretz A, Stoclet JC, Andriantsitohaina R (1998) Natural dietary polyphenolic compounds cause endothelium-dependent vasorelaxation in rat thoracic aorta. J Nutr 128:2324–2333
11. Arora A, Nair MG, Strasburg GM (1998) Structure–activity relationships for antioxidant activities of a series of flavonoids in a liposomal system. Free Radic Biol Med 24(9): 1355–1363
12. Balasuriya BWN, Rupasinghe HPV (2011) Plant flavonoids as angiotensin converting enzyme inhibitors in regulation of hypertension. Funct Foods Health Dis 1:172–188
13. Begum AN, Terao J (2002) Protective effect of quercetin against cigarette tar extract-induced impairment of erythrocyte deformability. J Nutr Biochem 13(5):265–272
14. Boots AW, Haenen GR, Bast A (2008) Health effects of quercetin: from antioxidant to nutraceutical. Eur J Pharmacol 585(2):325–337
15. Bose S, Michniak-Kohn B (2013) Preparation and characterization of lipid based nanosystems for topical delivery of quercetin. Eur J Pharm Sci 48(3):442–452
16. Brown RH (1998) Amyotrophic lateral sclerosis and the inherited motor neuron diseases. In: Martin JB (ed) Molecular neurology. Scientific American, New York, pp 223–238
17. Brownlee M (2005) The pathobiology of diabetic complications: a unifying mechanism. Diabetes 54:1615–1625
18. Centonze D, Rossi S, Prosperetti C, Tscherter A, Bernardi G, Maccarrone M, Calabresi P (2005) Abnormal sensitivity to cannabinoid receptor stimulation might contribute to altered gamma-aminobutyric acid transmission in the striatum of R6/2 Huntington's disease mice. Biol Psychiatry 57(12):1583–1589
19. Centre for Disease Control (2014) [Cited 2014 March]. Available from http://www.cdc.gov/diabetes/consumer/learn.htm
20. Choi GN, Kim JH, Kwak JH, Jeong C-H, Jeong HR, Lee U, Heo HJ (2012) Effect of quercetin on learning and memory performance in ICR mice under neurotoxic trimethyltin exposure. Food Chem 132:1019–1024
21. Crews DE (2007) Senescence, aging and disease. J Physiol Anthropol 26:365–372
22. Dimpfel W (2009) Rat electropharmacograms of the flavonoids rutin and quercetin in comparison to those of moclobemide and clinically used reference drugs suggest antidepressive and/or neuroprotective action. Phytomedicine 16:287–294
23. Duarte J, Perez-Palencia R, Vargas F, Ocete MA, Perez-Vizcaino F, Zarzuelo A, Tamargo J (2001) Antihypertensive effects of the flavonoid quercetin in spontaneously hypertensive rats. Br J Pharmacol 133:117–124
24. Edwards RL, Lyon T, Litwin SE, Rabovsky A, Symons JD, Jalili T (2007) Quercetin reduces blood pressure in hypertensive subjects. J Nutr 137(11):2405–2411
25. Egert S, Bosy-Westphal A, Seiberl J, Kurbitz C, Settler U, Plachta-Danielzik S, Wagner AE, Frank J, Schrezenmeir J, Rimbach G, Wolffram S, Muller MJ (2009) Quercetin reduces systolic blood pressure and plasma oxidised low-density lipoprotein concentrations in overweight subjects with a high-cardiovascular disease risk phenotype: a double-blinded, placebo-controlled cross-over study. Br J Nutr 2009(102):1–10
26. Hackl LP, Cuttle G, Dovichi SS, Lima-Landman MT, Nicolau M (2002) Inhibition of angiotensin-converting enzyme by quercetin alters the vascular response to Bradykinin and angiotensin I. Pharmacology 65:182–186
27. Haleagrahara N, Siew CJ, Ponnusamy K (2013) Effect of quercetin and desferrioxamine on 6-hydroxydopamine (6-OHDA) induced neurotoxicity in striatum of rats. J Toxicol Sci 38:25–33

28. Hollman PC, Gaag MV, Mengelers MJ, Van Trijp JM, De Vries JH, Katan MB (1996) Absorption and disposition kinetics of the dietary antioxidant quercetin in man. Free Radic Biol Med 21(5):703–707
29. Hsieh CL, Peng CC, Cheng YM, Lin LY, Ker YB, Chang CH, Peng RY (2010) Quercetin and ferulic acid aggravate renal carcinoma in long-term diabetic victims. J Agric Food Chem 58(16):9273–9280
30. Huk I, Brovkovych V, Nanobash Vili J, Weigel G, Neumayer C, Partyka L, Malinski T (1998) Bioflavonoid quercetin scavenges superoxide and increases nitric oxide concentration in ischaemia–reperfusion injury: an experimental study. Br J Surg 85(8):1080–1085
31. Jackson SJ, Venema RC (2006) Quercetin inhibits eNOS, microtubule polymerization, and mitotic progression in bovine aortic endothelial cells. J Nutr 136:1178–1184
32. Jaganjac M, Tirosh O, Cohen G, Sasson S, Zarkovic N (2013) Reactive aldehydes-second messengers of free radicals in diabetes mellitus. Free Radic Res 47:39–48
33. Jalili T, Carlstrom J, Kim S, Freeman D, Jin H, Wu TC, Symons JD (2006) Quercetin-supplemented diets lower blood pressure and attenuate cardiac hypertrophy in rats with aortic constriction. J Cardiovasc Pharmacol 47(4):531–541
34. Jung JY, Lim Y, Moon MS, Kim JY, Kwon O (2011) Onion peel extracts ameliorate hyperglycemia and insulin resistance in high fat diet/streptozotocin-induced diabetic rats. Nutr Metab (Lond) 8(1):18
35. Kambe D, Kotani M, Yoshimoto M, Kaku S, Chaki S, Honda K (2010) Effects of quercetin on the sleep–wake cycle in rats: involvement of gamma-aminobutyric acid receptor type A in regulation of rapid eye movement sleep. Brain Res 1330:83–88
36. Kawahara T, Kawaguchi-Ihara N, Okuhashi Y, Itoh M, Nara N, Tohda S (2009) Cyclopamine and quercetin suppress the growth of leukemia and lymphoma cells. Anticancer Res 29(11):4629–4632
37. Kelly GS (2011) Quercetin. Altern Med Rev 16(2):172–194
38. Kerry NL, Abbey M (1997) Red wine and fractionated phenolic compounds prepared from red wine inhibit low density lipoprotein oxidation in vitro. Atherosclerosis 135(1):93–102
39. Khaled KA, El-Sayed YM, Al-Hadiya BM (2003) Disposition of the flavonoid quercetin in rats after single intravenous and oral doses. Drug Dev Ind Pharm 29(4):397–403
40. Khoo NK, White CR, Pozzo-Miller L, Zhou F, Constance C, Inoue T, Patel RP, Parks DA (2010) Dietary flavonoid quercetin stimulates vasorelaxation in aortic vessels. Free Radic Biol Med 49:339–347
41. Kim JH, Kang MJ, Choi HN, Jeong SM, Lee YM, Kim JI (2011) Quercetin attenuates fasting and postprandial hyperglycemia in animal models of diabetes mellitus. Nutr Res Prac 5(2):107–111
42. Kwon O, Eck P, Chen S, Corpe CP, Lee JH, Kruhlak M, Levine M (2007) Inhibition of the intestinal glucose transporter GLUT2 by flavonoids. FASEB J 21(2):366–377
43. Lakhanpal P, Rai DK (2007) Quercetin: a versatile flavonoid. Internet J Med Update 2(2):22–37
44. Larson AJ, Symons JD, Jalili T (2010) Quercetin: a treatment for hypertension?—A review of efficacy and mechanisms. Pharmaceuticals 3(1):237–250
45. Lopez-Lopez G, Moreno L, Cogolludo A, Galisteo M, Ibarra M, Duarte J, Lodi F, Tamargo J, Perez-Vizcaino F (2004) Nitric oxide (NO) scavenging and NO protecting effects of quercetin and their biological significance in vascular smooth muscle. Mol Pharmacol 65:851–859
46. Mackraj I, Govender T, Ramesar S (2008) The antihypertensive effects of quercetin in a salt-sensitive model of hypertension. J Cardiovasc Pharmacol 51:239–245
47. Manso MA, Marta M, Jeanne E, Rosario H, Amaya A, Rosina L (2008) Effect of the long-term intake of an egg white hydrolysate on the oxidative status and blood lipid profile of spontaneously hypertensive rats. Food Chem 109:361–367
48. Martin JB (1999) Molecular basis of the neurodegenerative disorders. N Engl J Med 340(25):1970–1980
49. Metodiewa D, Jaiswal AK, Cenas N, Dickancaité E, Segura-Aguilar J (1999) Quercetin may act as a cytotoxic prooxidant after its metabolic activation to semiquinone and quinoidal product. Free Radic Biol Med 26(1):107–116

50. Miguel M, Aleixandre MA, Ramos M, López- Fandiño R (2006) Effect of simulated gastrointestinal digestion on the antihypertensive properties of ACE-inhibitory peptides derived from ovalbumin. J Agric Food Chem 54:726–731
51. Moskaug JØ, Carlsen H, Myhrstad M, Blomhoff R (2004) Molecular imaging of the biological effects of quercetin and quercetin-rich foods. Mech Ageing Dev 125(4):315–324
52. Naidu PS, Kulkarni SK (2004) Quercetin, a bioflavonoid, reverses haloperidol induced catalepsy. Methods Find Exp Clin Pharmacol 26(5):323–326
53. Nieoullon A (2011) Neurodegenerative diseases and neuroprotection: current views and prospects. J Appl Biomed 9(4):173–183
54. Oboh G, Ademiluyi AO, Akinyemi AJ, Henle T, Saliu J, Schwarzenbolz U (2012) Inhibitory effect of polyphenol-rich extracts of jute leaf (*Corchorus olitorius*) on key enzyme linked to type 2 diabetes (a-amylase and a-glucosidase) and hypertension (angiotensin I converting) in vitro. J Funct Foods 4:450–458
55. Oboh G, Ademosun AO, Ayeni PO, Omojokun OS, Bello F (2014) Comparative effect of quercetin and rutin on α-amylase, α-glucosidase, and some pro-oxidant-induced lipid peroxidation in rat pancreas. Comp Clin Pathol 24:1–8
56. Perez-Vizcaino F, Duarte J (2010) Flavonols and cardiovascular disease. Mol Aspects Med 31(6):478–494
57. Schiffrin EL (2010) Antioxidants in hypertension and cardiovascular diseases. Mol Inter 10:354–362
58. Shoskes DA (1998) Effect of bioflavonoids quercetin and curcumin on ischemic renal injury: a new class of renoprotective agents1. Transplantation 66(2):147–152
59. Singh A, Naidu PS, Kulkarni SK (2003) Quercetin potentiates L-Dopa reversal of drug-induced catalepsy in rats: possible COMT/MAO inhibition. Pharmacology 68:81–88
60. Singh A, Naidu PS, Kulkarni SK (2003) Reversal of aging and chronic ethanol—induced cognitive dysfunction by quercetin a bioflavonoid. Free Radic Res 37(11):1245–1252
61. Spencer J, Kuhnle G, Williams R, Rice-Evans C (2003) Intracellular metabolism and bioactivity of quercetin and its in vivo metabolites. Biochem J 372:173–181
62. Stoclet JC, Kleschyov A, Andriambeloson E, Diebolt M, Andriantsitohaina R (1999) Endothelial no release caused by red wine polyphenols. J Physiol Pharmacol 50:535–540
63. Taler SJ, Agarwal R, Bakris GL, Flynn JT, Nilsson PM, Rahman M, Sanders PW, Textor SC, Weir MR, Townsend RR (2013) KDOQI US commentary on the 2012 KDIGO clinical practice guideline for management of blood pressure in CKD. Am J Kidney Dis 62(2):201–213
64. Taubert D, Berkels R, Klaus W, Roesen R (2002) Nitric oxide formation and corresponding relaxation of porcine coronary arteries induced by plant phenols: essential structural features. J Cardiovasc Pharmacol 40:701–713
65. Tzeng SH, Ko WC, Ko FN, Teng CM (1991) Inhibition of platelet aggregation by some flavonoids. Thromb Res 64:91–100
66. Umamaheswari M, Ajith MP, Asokkumar K, Sivashanmugam T, Subhadradevi V, Jagannath P, Madeswaran A (2012) In vitro angiotensin converting enzyme inhibitory and antioxidant activities of seed extract of *Apium graveolens* Linn. Ann Biol Res 3:1274–1282
67. Valko M, Leibfritz D, Moncol J, Cronin MT, Mazur M, Telser J (2007) Free radicals and antioxidants in normal physiological functions and human disease. Int J Biochem Cell Biol 39(1):44–84
68. Wilms LC, Hollman PC, Boots AW, Kleinjans JC (2005) Protection by quercetin and quercetin-rich fruit juice against induction of oxidative DNA damage and formation of BPDE-DNA adducts in human lymphocytes. Mutat Res/Genetic Toxicol Environ Mutagen 582(1):155–162
69. Youl E, Bardy G, Magous R, Cros G, Sejalon F, Virsolvy A, Bataille D (2010) Quercetin potentiates insulin secretion and protects INS-1 pancreatic β-cells against oxidative damage via the ERK1/2 pathway. Br J Pharmacol 161(4):799–814
70. Zhang Z-L, Lia Q-L, Lia B-G, Zhangb Y, Gaob X-P, Lia C-Q (2008) Three angiotensin-converting enzyme inhibitors from *Rabdosia coetsa*. Phytomedicine 15:386–388

Eucalyptol and Its Role in Chronic Diseases

Geun Hee Seol and Ka Young Kim

Abstract Patients with chronic diseases such as cardiovascular diseases, chronic respiratory diseases, and neurological diseases have been shown to benefit from treatments such as aromatherapy in addition to medication. Most chronic diseases are caused by chronic inflammation and oxidative stress as well as harmful factors. Eucalyptol (1,8-cineole), a terpenoid oxide isolated from *Eucalyptus* species, is a promising compound for treating such conditions as it has been shown to have anti-inflammatory and antioxidant effects in various diseases, including respiratory disease, pancreatitis, colon damage, and cardiovascular and neurodegenerative diseases. Eucalyptol suppresses lipopolysaccharide (LPS)-induced proinflammatory cytokine production through the action of NF-κB, TNF-α, IL-1β, and IL-6 and the extracellular signal-regulated kinase (ERK) pathway, and reduces oxidative stress through the regulation of signaling pathways and radical scavenging. The effects of eucalyptol have been studied in several cell and animal models as well as in patients with chronic diseases. Furthermore, eucalyptol can pass the blood–brain barrier and hence can be used as a carrier to deliver drugs to the brain via a microemulsion system. In summary, the various biological activities of eucalyptol such as its anti-inflammatory and antioxidant properties, as well as its physicochemical characteristics, make this compound a potentially important drug for the treatment of chronic diseases.

Keywords Eucalyptol · Chronic disease · Anti-inflammatory · Antioxidant

G.H. Seol (✉)
Department of Basic Nursing Science, School of Nursing, Korea University, Seoul 02841, Republic of Korea
e-mail: ghseol@korea.ac.kr

K.Y. Kim
Department of Nursing Science, School of Nursing, Gachon University, Incheon 21936, Republic of Korea

S.C. Gupta et al. (eds.), *Drug Discovery from Mother Nature*, Advances in Experimental Medicine and Biology 929,
DOI 10.1007/978-3-319-41342-6_18

1 Introduction

Patient with chronic disease such as cardiovascular diseases, cancers, chronic respiratory diseases, diabetes, and mental illness needs to be constantly managed because the patient may be impacted by various factors including smoking, lack of physical activity, and poor eating habits [5]. Furthermore, the prevalence of chronic diseases tends to increase with age. Chronic diseases may result from various causes including chronic inflammation and oxidative stress [4, 16]. Chronic inflammation is regarded as one of the main causes of cancers, diabetes, cardiovascular diseases, autoimmune diseases, and other age-related diseases [16]. Moreover, it facilitates neoplastic transformation through inflammatory processes, including injury, repair, resolution, and oxidative stress [6]. Age-related diseases and cardiovascular diseases are characterized by inflammatory pathogenesis and oxidative stress [3, 7, 25].

Alternative medicines such as aromatherapy with aromatic plant oils including essential oils and plant materials may be helpful in the continuous care and management of patients with chronic disease. Natural plant-derived components have been widely used in a wide variety of diseases including chronic disease [8]. Eucalyptol, which has anti-inflammatory and antioxidant activities, has been used to treat lung inflammation and respiratory diseases including bronchitis, sinusitis, bronchial asthma, and chronic obstructive pulmonary disease (COPD) [11, 12, 17, 33, 34]. Furthermore, eucalyptol showed neuroprotective effects in an ischemic stroke model [20] and anti-inflammatory effects in neurodegenerative diseases such as Alzheimer's disease as well as significantly reducing preoperative anxiety in patients undergoing surgery [18].

This review describes the role of eucalyptol in chronic diseases through its regulation of cell signaling pathways and biological activities in animal models and humans.

2 Physicochemical Properties of Eucalyptol

Eucalyptol, also known as 1,8-cineole, is a terpenoid oxide isolated from Eucalyptus species such as *Eucalyptus globules* Labill. and *Eucalyptus tereticornis* Sm. Eucalyptol is derived from the leaf oil of these plants, which contains various volatile organic components [1]. Terpenes such as eucalyptol are lipophilic molecules that disturb intracellular lipids and increase drug penetration [21]. A lipid-based microemulsion system of eucalyptol has been utilized for transdermal drug delivery. Eucalyptol is metabolized to 2-exo-hydroxy-1,8-cineole by rat and human liver microsomal P450 enzymes and eliminated in the urine [22]. Moreover, eucalyptol can easily pass through the blood–brain barrier and may have direct action on receptors and enzymes in the brain [24].

Eucalyptol has been reported to have antimicrobial, anti-inflammatory, antioxidant, analgesic, and spasmolytic effects in various diseases including colds, influenza, other respiratory infections, rhinitis, and sinusitis [28]. Eucalyptol acted as a strong inhibitor of proinflammatory cytokines such as tumor necrosis factor (TNF)-α and interleukin (IL)-1β and showed an analgesic effect in an inflammatory model [28]. Eucalyptol significantly increased the beat frequency of nasal cilia in mucus membranes and had bronchodilation effects [33]. In addition, it decreased exacerbation in asthma, sinusitis, and COPD symptoms by inhibiting cytokine-induced airway mucus hypersecretion [28]. It exhibits antioxidant activity by radical scavenging [30] and reduces Ca^{2+} influx via calcium channels in cardiac muscle [31].

3 Eucalyptol Modulation of Cell Signaling Pathways

Chronic diseases are closely associated with chronic inflammation and oxidative stress [4, 16]. The pathological features of chronic inflammation include the production of inflammatory cytokines and tissue damage [16]. Oxidative stress disturbs the normal functions of lipids, proteins, and DNA and is therefore toxic to cells and tissues. Free radicals cause mutations and damage DNA in cancer and age-related diseases. Oxidative stress regulates signaling pathways that induce the production of proinflammatory cytokines and chemokines [16, 26].

Lipopolysaccharide (LPS) plays an important role in inflammatory processes by activating the NF-κB and MAPK signaling pathways [10]. Eucalyptol was shown to inhibit LPS-induced cytokine production by human lymphocytes and monocytes [28] and to reduce LPS-induced NF-κB activity and to increase IκBα protein levels in the human astrocyte U373 and HeLa cell lines [8]. In a BALB/C mouse model, eucalyptol reduced the number of inflammatory cells, expression of matrix metalloproteinase-9 (MMP-9), and production of cytokines including TNF-α and IL-6 as well as nitric oxide and NF-κB [17]. Moreover, early growth response factor-1 (Egr-1) mediates LPS-induced tissue factor and TNF-α gene expression in human monocytic cells [9]. Eucalyptol inhibited LPS-stimulated expression of Egr-1 through the extracellular signal-regulated kinase (ERK) pathway in human monocyte THP-1 cells, without affecting NF-κB expression [35]. Eucalyptol injection improved cerulein-induced acute pancreatitis and significantly reduced the histological damage induced by cerulein, including pancreatic edema, as well as the expression of NF-κB, myeloperoxidase (MPOs), malondialdehyde (MDA), and proinflammatory cytokines, including TNF-α, IL-1β, and IL-6 [20]. Moreover, eucalyptol exerted an anti-inflammatory effect by regulating NF-κB and MAPK in LPS-induced inflammatory models.

In addition to the above effects, studies in rat neurons and glia found that eucalyptol reduced oxygen glucose deprivation/reoxygenation (OGD/R)-induced ischemic injury by decreasing oxidative stress [27]. In a cell model of Alzheimer's disease, pretreatment of PC12 cells with eucalyptol reduced mitochondrial membrane potential and the levels of ROS, NO, COX-2, NF-κB, and the proinflammatory cytokines TNF-α, IL-β, and IL-6 induced by $A\beta_{25\text{-}35}$ [15].

4 Role of Eucalyptol in Chronic Diseases

Eucalyptol was shown to have effects in various inflammatory diseases including respiratory diseases, pancreatitis, and cardiovascular and neurodegenerative disease as well as reducing colon damage [11, 15, 20, 23, 29, 34]. In particular, it is reported that eucalyptol has been studied in animal and human model-related chronic disease (Table 1). Eucalyptol is used in inflammatory airway diseases as a mucolytic agent. Eucalyptol treatment significantly reduced dyspnea and enhanced lung function and quality of life relative to placebo in patients with stable COPD [33]. Eucalyptol treatment also resulted in improvements in patients with asthma, a disease characterized by a chronic inflammatory process, by enhancing lung function and general health [32]. Moreover, eucalyptol has been used to treat chronic bronchitis, sinusitis, and rhinitis.

The protective effects of eucalyptol in neurodegenerative diseases may be due to its anti-inflammatory activities [15]. Eucalyptol also showed antihypertensive effects by increasing nitrite levels and reducing MDA activity [23]. Eucalyptol was also reported to reduce heart rate through a parasympathetic mechanism and to induce hypotension by vasorelaxation in cardiovascular diseases [19].

5 Biological Activities of Eucalyptol in Animal Models

The anti-inflammatory and antihypertensive effects of eucalyptol have been studied in several animal models. Eucalyptol inhalation suppressed the inflammatory process in airways of ovalbumin-challenged guinea pigs [2]. Eucalyptol also showed anti-inflammatory effects in bronchoalveolar fluid of mice with LPS-induced lung inflammation [17] and suppressed acute pulmonary inflammation by reducing the levels of TNF-α, IL-1β, NF-κB p65, and toll-like receptor 4 (TLR4) in mice [34]. Eucalyptol improved cerulein-induced acute pancreatitis through an anti-inflammatory mechanism and antioxidative activity in mice [20] and reduced colonic damage in rats with acute trinitrobenzene sulfonic acid (TNBS)-induced colitis [29].

Moreover, eucalyptol was found to lower blood pressure through the regulation of NO and lipid peroxidation in a rat model of hypertension induced by chronic exposure to nicotine [23]. Eucalyptol was also reported to relax bronchial and vascular smooth muscle by reducing isometric contractions in rat ventricular papillary muscle [31].

Table 1 Summary of the effects of eucalyptol in chronic diseases

Related chronic disease	Model/methods	Measurement parameter	Results	Reference
Asthma	32 patients with steroid-dependent bronchial asthma in a double-blind, placebo-controlled trial	Lung function using ATS guideline	Eucalyptol treatment maintained lung function four times longer despite administering lower dosages of prednisolone	[12]
	Administered as eucalyptol 200 mg t.i.d. or placebo capsules at 3, 6, 9, 12 weeks as outpatients	Mini-Wright peak-flow meter to measure PEFR (peak expiratory flow rate)	Reductions in daily prednisolone dosage of 36 % with active treatment versus a decrease of only 7 % in the placebo group were tolerated	
	Glucocorticosteroid dose reduced by 2.5 mg every 3 weeks	Scores for frequency of dyspnea	Eucalyptol treatment did not tolerate any reduction in glucocorticosteroid dosage showed steroid-saving effects in asthma	
COPD	242 patients with stable COPD in double-blind trial Eucalyptol 200 mg 3 times as concomitant therapy for 6 months	Frequency, duration, severity, and symptoms of exacerbations	The number ($p = 0.0016$), degree ($p = 0.0031$), and severity ($p = 0.0025$) of exacerbations by Wei-Lachin test procedure were statistically significant in eucalyptol. Eucalyptol decreased the frequency, severity, and duration of exacerbations in lung function	[33]
		Lung function, respiratory symptoms, and quality of life	Eucalyptol increased the forced vital capacity (FVC) by 62 ml (2.7 %) compared with placebo of a reduction of 25 ml (1.1 %)	
		Spirometric measurements: before the beginning of the study to determine the reversibility of the airflow limitation, determination of forced expiratory volume in 1 s (FEV1), forced vital capacity (FVC), and vital capacity (VC) at commencement and after 3 and 6 months	The improvement of SGRQ total symptoms score was statistically significant in the eucalyptol group ($p = 0.0224$)	
		Symptom score for dyspnea, weekly frequency of dyspnea, general condition, and cough	The increase in FEV1, improvement of dyspnea, and total SGRQ score were statistically significant by the Wei-Lachin test procedure for multiple criteria ($p = 0.0024$)	

(continued)

Table 1 (continued)

Related chronic disease	Model/methods	Measurement parameter	Results	Reference
Airway inflammatory disease	Male guinea pigs that were sensitized by means of three intraperitoneal injections of ovalbumin (OVA, 10 mg/kg) every other day	Inflammatory parameters such as mucociliary clearance, tracheal responsiveness to carbachol, cytokine levels (TNF-α, IL-1β, IL-10), and myeloperoxidase activity on bronchoalveolar lavage fluid (BALF)	Eucalyptol inhalation before OVA administration reduced tracheal contractions than inhaled eucalyptol before administration of saline	[2]
			Proinflammatory cytokine levels including TNF-α and IL-1β were decreased in BALF of eucalyptol group	
			Eucalyptol treatment reduced the increase in myeloperoxidase (MPO) activity	
			In OVA-challenged guinea pigs, the number of inflammatory cells was smaller in BALF of eucalyptol-treated guinea pigs than in BALF that did not treat eucalyptol	
			Pretreatment with eucalyptol completely abrogated the OVA-induced increase in TNF- α and IL-1 levels after antigen challenge	
	OVA-sensitized conscious guinea pigs inhaled a single dose of eucalyptol for 15 min		Eucalyptol inhibited the decrease of the mucociliary clearance in antigen-induced changes	
Asthma	247 asthmatic patients that receive the concomitant therapy with eucalyptol	Lung function, asthma symptoms, and quality of life: nocturnal asthma scores, diagnosis-related quality of life by Asthma Quality of Life Questionnaire (AQLQ), forced vital capacity (FVC) and vital capacity (VC), symptom scores for dyspnea frequency and intensity during rest and after exercise, coughing and propensity to cough, scores for quantity of secretion	Lung function, symptoms of asthma, cough, hypersecretion, and Asthma Quality of Life Questionnaire (AQLQ) were improved by concomitant therapy with eucalyptol	[32]
			After 6 months of eucalyptol treatment, Wei-Lachin test procedures including forced expiratory volume in 1 s (FEV1), asthma symptoms, and AQLQ were significant as $p = 0.0398$, $p = 0.0325$, and 0.0475, respectively	

(continued)

Table 1 (continued)

Related chronic disease	Model/methods	Measurement parameter	Results	Reference
			In lung function, the difference between the mean increase of FVC and the increase of peak-flow rate was significant in the eucalyptol compared to the placebo group ($p = 0.0226$, $p = 0.0197$)	
			The perceived difference was significant for dyspnea at rest ($p = 0.0198$) and dyspnea during exercise ($p = 0.0446$)	
			At 6 months, the mean improvement of quality of life according to AQLQ was significant ($p = 0.0475$)	
	Administered as eucalyptol 200 mg 3 times for 6 months in a double-blind, placebo-controlled trial		The differences of hypersecretion ($p = 0.0015$) and coughing ($p = 0.0007$) at multiple endpoints were significantly in the eucalyptol group	
Cardiovascular disease	The hypertension model using male Sprague–Dawley rats induced chronically by 0.8 mg/kg nicotine for 21 days, followed by 3 mg/kg nicotine the next day	Systolic blood pressure, plasma nitrite concentration, and plasma corticosterone concentration were measured by a tail-cuff transducer, nitrite assay, and enzyme immunoassay, respectively	Eucalyptol decreased the nicotine-induced increase in systolic blood pressure ($p = 0.011$)	[23]
			Eucalyptol (0.1 mg/kg) effectively inhibited the increase in SBP induced by nicotine	
	Eucalyptol was injected intraperitoneally at 0.01, 0.1, and 1 mg/kg		Eucalyptol reduced the concentration of plasma nitrite ($p = 0.03$) and plasma corticosterone ($p = 0.05$) that was increased in nicotinic rat model	

6 Biological Activities of Eucalyptol in Humans

Eucalyptol has been reported to have anti-inflammatory and analgesic effects in clinical studies. Eucalyptol treatment of patients with asthma significantly increased lung function and overall health condition and reduced dyspnea [32]. Systemic therapy with eucalyptol for 12 weeks had anti-inflammatory effects in patients with steroid-dependent bronchial asthma [12]. Moreover, eucalyptol decreased the discomforts of non-purulent rhinosinusitis in acute rhinosinusitis patients [14], and showed anti-inflammatory effects in various chronic respiratory diseases in a clinical study.

Eucalyptol has been found to have analgesic and antianxiety effects in humans. Inhalation of eucalyptus oil, which is mainly composed of eucalyptol, effectively reduced pain and blood pressure in patients who underwent total knee replacement [13]. A randomized clinical trial found that inhalation of eucalyptol significantly reduced anxiety in patients before selective nerve root block (SNRB) [18].

7 Conclusions

Eucalyptol exerts anti-inflammatory and antioxidative effects by regulating the NF-κB and MAPK signaling pathways in several diseases, including chronic diseases. These beneficial effects of eucalyptol have been observed in clinical studies and in several animal models. Eucalyptol, which has lipophilic properties and exerts various actions on receptors and enzymes, may be a potentially important drug in the treatment of chronic diseases.

References

1. Aparicio S, Alcalde R, Davila MJ, Garcia B, Leal JM (2007) Properties of 1,8-cineole: a thermophysical and theoretical study. J Phys Chem B 111(12):3167–3177. doi:10.1021/jp067405b
2. Bastos VP, Gomes AS, Lima FJ, Brito TS, Soares PM, Pinho JP, Magalhaes PJ (2011) Inhaled 1,8-cineole reduces inflammatory parameters in airways of ovalbumin-challenged Guinea pigs. Basic Clin Pharmacol Toxicol 108(1):34–39. doi:10.1111/j.1742-7843.2010.00622.x
3. Dhalla NS, Temsah RM, Netticadan T (2000) Role of oxidative stress in cardiovascular diseases. J Hypertens 18(6):655–673
4. Edwards T (2005) Inflammation, pain, and chronic disease: an integrative approach to treatment and prevention. Altern Ther Health Med 11(6), 20–27; quiz 28, 75
5. Elwood P, Galante J, Pickering J, Palmer S, Bayer A, Ben-Shlomo Y, Gallacher J (2013) Healthy lifestyles reduce the incidence of chronic diseases and dementia: evidence from the Caerphilly cohort study. PLoS ONE 8(12):e81877. doi:10.1371/journal.pone.0081877
6. Federico A, Morgillo F, Tuccillo C, Ciardiello F, Loguercio C (2007) Chronic inflammation and oxidative stress in human carcinogenesis. Int J Cancer 121(11):2381–2386. doi:10.1002/ijc.23192

7. Franceschi C, Campisi J (2014) Chronic inflammation (inflammaging) and its potential contribution to age-associated diseases. J Gerontol A Biol Sci Med Sci 69(Suppl 1):S4–S9. doi:10.1093/gerona/glu057
8. Greiner JF, Muller J, Zeuner MT, Hauser S, Seidel T, Klenke C, Kaltschmidt C (2013) 1,8-Cineol inhibits nuclear translocation of NF-kappaB p65 and NF-kappaB-dependent transcriptional activity. Biochim Biophys Acta 1833(12):2866–2878. doi:10.1016/j.bbamcr.2013.07.001
9. Guha M, O'Connell MA, Pawlinski R, Hollis A, McGovern P, Yan SF, Mackman N (2001) Lipopolysaccharide activation of the MEK-ERK1/2 pathway in human monocytic cells mediates tissue factor and tumor necrosis factor alpha expression by inducing Elk-1 phosphorylation and Egr-1 expression. Blood 98(5):1429–1439
10. He X, Wei Z, Zhou E, Chen L, Kou J, Wang J, Yang Z (2015) Baicalein attenuates inflammatory responses by suppressing TLR4 mediated NF-kappaB and MAPK signaling pathways in LPS-induced mastitis in mice. Int Immunopharmacol 28(1):470–476. doi:10.1016/j.intimp.2015.07.012
11. Juergens UR (2014) Anti-inflammatory properties of the monoterpene 1.8-cineole: current evidence for co-medication in inflammatory airway diseases. Drug Res (Stuttg), 64(12), 638–646. doi:10.1055/s-0034-1372609
12. Juergens UR, Dethlefsen U, Steinkamp G, Gillissen A, Repges R, Vetter H (2003) Anti-inflammatory activity of 1.8-cineol (eucalyptol) in bronchial asthma: a double-blind placebo-controlled trial. Respir Med 97(3):250–256
13. Jun YS, Kang P, Min SS, Lee JM, Kim HK, Seol GH (2013) Effect of eucalyptus oil inhalation on pain and inflammatory responses after total knee replacement: a randomized clinical trial. Evid Based Complement Alternat Med 2013:502727. doi:10.1155/2013/502727
14. Kehrl W, Sonnemann U, Dethlefsen U (2004) Therapy for acute nonpurulent rhinosinusitis with cineole: results of a double-blind, randomized, placebo-controlled trial. Laryngoscope 114(4):738–742. doi:10.1097/00005537-200404000-00027
15. Khan A, Vaibhav K, Javed H, Tabassum R, Ahmed ME, Khan MM, Islam F (2014) 1,8-cineole (eucalyptol) mitigates inflammation in amyloid Beta toxicated PC12 cells: relevance to Alzheimer's disease. Neurochem Res 39(2):344–352. doi:10.1007/s11064-013-1231-9
16. Khansari N, Shakiba Y, Mahmoudi M (2009) Chronic inflammation and oxidative stress as a major cause of age-related diseases and cancer. Recent Pat Inflamm Allergy Drug Discov 3(1):73–80
17. Kim KY, Lee HS, Seol GH (2015) Eucalyptol suppresses matrix metalloproteinase-9 expression through an extracellular signal-regulated kinase-dependent nuclear factor-kappa B pathway to exert anti-inflammatory effects in an acute lung inflammation model. J Pharm Pharmacol 67(8):1066–1074. doi:10.1111/jphp.12407
18. Kim KY, Seo HJ, Min SS, Park M, Seol GH (2014) The effect of 1,8-cineole inhalation on preoperative anxiety: a randomized clinical trial. Evid Based Complement Alternat Med 2014:820126. doi:10.1155/2014/820126
19. Lahlou S, Figueiredo AF, Magalhaes PJ, Leal-Cardoso JH (2002) Cardiovascular effects of 1,8-cineole, a terpenoid oxide present in many plant essential oils, in normotensive rats. Can J Physiol Pharmacol 80(12):1125–1131
20. Lima PR, de Melo TS, Carvalho KM, de Oliveira IB, Arruda BR, de Castro Brito GA, Santos FA (2013) 1,8-cineole (eucalyptol) ameliorates cerulein-induced acute pancreatitis via modulation of cytokines, oxidative stress and NF-kappaB activity in mice. Life Sci 92(24–26):1195–1201. doi:10.1016/j.lfs.2013.05.009
21. Liu CH, Chang FY (2011) Development and characterization of eucalyptol microemulsions for topic delivery of curcumin. Chem Pharm Bull (Tokyo) 59(2):172–178
22. Miyazawa M, Shindo M, Shimada T (2001) Oxidation of 1,8-cineole, the monoterpene cyclic ether originated from eucalyptus polybractea, by cytochrome P450 3A enzymes in rat and human liver microsomes. Drug Metab Dispos 29(2):200–205

23. Moon HK, Kang P, Lee HS, Min SS, Seol GH (2014) Effects of 1,8-cineole on hypertension induced by chronic exposure to nicotine in rats. J Pharm Pharmacol 66(5):688–693. doi:10.1111/jphp.12195
24. Moss M, Oliver L (2012) Plasma 1,8-cineole correlates with cognitive performance following exposure to rosemary essential oil aroma. Ther Adv Psychopharmacol 2(3):103–113. doi:10.1177/2045125312436573
25. Osiecki H (2004) The role of chronic inflammation in cardiovascular disease and its regulation by nutrients. Altern Med Rev 9(1):32–53
26. Ryan KA, Smith MF Jr, Sanders MK, Ernst PB (2004) Reactive oxygen and nitrogen species differentially regulate Toll-like receptor 4-mediated activation of NF-kappa B and interleukin-8 expression. Infect Immun 72(4):2123–2130
27. Ryu S, Park H, Seol GH, Choi IY (2014) 1,8-Cineole ameliorates oxygen-glucose deprivation/reoxygenation-induced ischaemic injury by reducing oxidative stress in rat cortical neuron/glia. J Pharm Pharmacol 66(12):1818–1826. doi:10.1111/jphp.12295
28. Sadlon AE, Lamson DW (2010) Immune-modifying and antimicrobial effects of Eucalyptus oil and simple inhalation devices. Altern Med Rev 15(1):33–47
29. Santos FA, Silva RM, Campos AR, De Araujo RP, Lima Junior RC, Rao VS (2004) 1,8-cineole (eucalyptol), a monoterpene oxide attenuates the colonic damage in rats on acute TNBS-colitis. Food Chem Toxicol 42(4):579–584. doi:10.1016/j.fct.2003.11.001
30. Singh HP, Mittal S, Kaur S, Batish DR, Kohli RK (2009) Characterization and antioxidant activity of essential oils from fresh and decaying leaves of *Eucalyptus tereticornis*. J Agric Food Chem 57(15):6962–6966. doi:10.1021/jf9012407
31. Soares MC, Damiani CE, Moreira CM, Stefanon I, Vassallo DV (2005) Eucalyptol, an essential oil, reduces contractile activity in rat cardiac muscle. Braz J Med Biol Res 38(3): 453–461. doi:10.1590//S0100-879X2005000300017
32. Worth H, Dethlefsen U (2012) Patients with asthma benefit from concomitant therapy with cineole: a placebo-controlled, double-blind trial. J Asthma 49(8):849–853. doi:10.3109/02770903.2012.717657
33. Worth H, Schacher C, Dethlefsen U (2009) Concomitant therapy with Cineole (Eucalyptole) reduces exacerbations in COPD: a placebo-controlled double-blind trial. Respir Res 10:69. doi:10.1186/1465-9921-10-69
34. Zhao C, Sun J, Fang C, Tang F (2014) 1,8-cineol attenuates LPS-induced acute pulmonary inflammation in mice. Inflammation 37(2):566–572. doi:10.1007/s10753-013-9770-4
35. Zhou JY, Wang XF, Tang FD, Zhou JY, Lu GH, Wang Y, Bian RL (2007) Inhibitory effect of 1,8-cineol (eucalyptol) on Egr-1 expression in lipopolysaccharide-stimulated THP-1 cells. Acta Pharmacol Sin 28(6):908–912. doi:10.1111/j.1745-7254.2007.00555.x

Auraptene and Its Role in Chronic Diseases

Giuseppe Derosa, Pamela Maffioli and Amirhossein Sahebkar

Abstract Auraptene (7-geranyloxycoumarin) is the best known and most abundant prenyloxycoumarin present in nature. It is synthesized by various plant species, mainly those of the Rutaceae and Umbeliferae (Apiaceae) families, comprising many edible fruits and vegetables such as lemons, grapefruit and orange. Auraptene has shown a remarkable effect in the prevention of degenerative diseases, in particular it has been reported to be one the most promising known natural chemopreventive

G. Derosa (✉) · P. Maffioli
Department of Internal Medicine and Therapeutics, University of Pavia, Fondazione IRCCS Policlinico San Matteo, P.le C. Golgi, 2-27100 Pavia, Italy
e-mail: giuseppe.derosa@unipv.it

P. Maffioli
e-mail: pamelamaffioli@hotmail.it

G. Derosa · P. Maffioli
Center for Prevention, Surveillance, Diagnosis and Treatment of Rare Diseases, Fondazione IRCCS Policlinico San Matteo, Pavia, Italy

G. Derosa
Center for the Study of Endocrine-Metabolic Pathophysiology and Clinical Research, University of Pavia, Pavia, Italy

G. Derosa
Laboratory of Molecular Medicine, University of Pavia, Pavia, Italy

P. Maffioli
PhD School in Experimental Medicine, University of Pavia, Pavia, Italy

A. Sahebkar
Biotechnology Research Center, Mashhad University of Medical Sciences, Mashhad, Iran

A. Sahebkar
School of Medicine and Pharmacology, Metabolic Research Centre, Royal Perth Hospital, University of Western Australia, Perth, Australia

A. Sahebkar (✉)
Department of Medical Biotechnology, School of Medicine, Mashhad University of Medical Sciences, P.O. Box: 91779-48564, Mashhad, Iran
e-mail: sahebkara@mums.ac.ir; amir_saheb2000@yahoo.com

S.C. Gupta et al. (eds.), *Drug Discovery from Mother Nature*,
Advances in Experimental Medicine and Biology 929,
DOI 10.1007/978-3-319-41342-6_19

agents against several types of cancer. The aim of this chapter is to review the effects of auraptene in the prevention and treatment of different chronic diseases.

Keywords Auraptene · Chemoprevention · Degenerative diseases · Hypertension · Lipid profile

1 Introduction

Several lines of evidence suggest that increasing the consumption of fruits and vegetables in diet reduces the risk of cancer [1]. It has been suggested that certain phytochemicals present in fruits and vegetables inhibit or reverse the process of cancer development. In this regard, citrus peels contain a number of coumarins that possess mevalonate-derived side chains with various oxidation levels. Auraptene (7-geranyloxycoumarin (Fig. 1)) is the best known and most abundant prenyloxycoumarin identified. Auraptene is synthesized by various plant species, mainly those of the Rutaceae and Umbeliferae (Apiaceae) families, comprising many edible fruits and vegetables such as lemons, grapefruit and orange. It was first isolated from members of the genus *Citrus*, including the peels of *Citrus kawachiensis* (Kawachi Bankan), which is one of the citrus products of Ehime, Japan [2]. Auraptene is well known for its antioxidant properties, for its contribution to the protection of deoxyribonucleic acid (DNA) and macromolecules and for its protective effect against cancers of liver, skin, tongue, oesophagus and colon in rodent models. Auraptene has also protective effects in cardiovascular diseases, disorders associated with oxidative stress [3, 4] and a remarkable effect in the prevention of degenerative diseases. For all these different and interesting pharmacological and medicinal properties, auraptene has been proposed as one of the most promising known natural chemopreventive agents against several types of cancer. Despite all these positive effects in animals, however, auraptene actions in humans are not yet known. The aim of this chapter is to review the effects of auraptene in the prevention and treatment of different chronic diseases.

2 Auraptene Effects on Neurodegenerative Diseases

Extracellular signal-regulated kinases 1/2 (ERK1/2) are components of the mitogen-activated protein kinase (MAPK) signalling cascade. Recent studies have shown that ERK1/2 is involved in synaptic plasticity and in the development of

Fig. 1 Auraptene structure

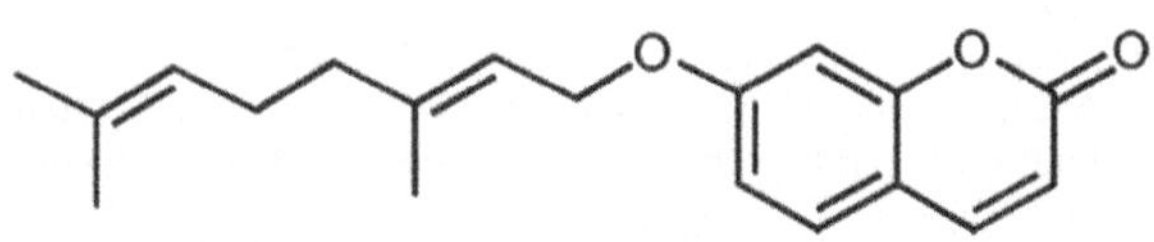

long-term memory in the central nervous system (CNS) [5]. Auraptene was studied to evaluate its beneficial for the treatment of neurodegenerative neurological disorders, and it proved to activate ERK1/2 in cultured cortical neurons [6]. Auraptene has the ability to induce the activation of ERK1/2 not only in cortical neurons, but also in the rat pheochromocytoma cell line (PC12 cells), which is a model system for studies on neuronal proliferation and differentiation. Moreover, auraptene had the ability to promote neurite outgrowth from PC12 cells [7].

Previously published studies reported the effects of auraptene on inflammation, especially in the brain. Okuyama et al. [8] reported that subcutaneously administered auraptene effectively inhibits microglia activation, cyclooxygenase-2 (COX-2) expression by astrocytes and neuronal cell death in the hippocampus. The same authors reported that auraptene could ameliorate lipopolysaccharide (LPS)-induced inflammation in the mouse brain [9]. Regarding the mechanism throughout auraptene acts, there are two hypothesis: some authors think that auraptene passes through the blood–brain barrier and acts directly in the brain as an anti-inflammatory agent, others think that auraptene suppresses the peripheral inflammation, which was followed by the suppression of central inflammation. The most reliable hypothesis is the first: auraptene can penetrate the blood–brain barrier, because it is a hydrophobic small molecule. Considering that inflammatory process in the brain is associated with various neurodegenerative diseases, including Parkinson's disease and Alzheimer's disease [10, 11], as well as with ischaemia and trauma, auraptene might be useful for the reduction of neuroinflammation-related brain diseases.

3 Effects of Auraptene on Periodontal Disease

Periodontal diseases are chronic inflammatory disorders of bacterial origin that affect tooth-supporting tissues. Some agents, including auraptene, have been reported to possess anti-microbial and anti-inflammatory properties, and they may be of interest as therapeutic agents for controlling periodontal diseases, which involve both pathogenic bacteria and host immune responses. Auraptene proved to prevent the adherence of *Porphyromonas gingivalis* to oral epithelial cells, dose dependently reduced the secretion of cytokines (interleukin-8 and tumour necrosis factor-α) and metalloproteinase-8 and metalloproteinase-9 by LPS-stimulated macrophages and inhibited metalloproteinase-9 activity [12]. The exact mechanism by which auraptene inhibits bacterial growth is unknown. However, other natural coumarins inhibit deoxyribonuclease gyrase activity, which results in bacteria death [13]. In addition, auraptene inhibits growth more effectively under iron-limiting conditions, requiring much lower concentrations to significantly reduce the growth of *P. gingivalis*.

4 Effects of Auraptene on Oncogenesis

Naturally occurring coumarins possess anti-carcinogenic activities in part by inducing carcinogen-detoxifying enzymes glutathione S-transferase (GST) and/or NAD(P)H quinone oxidoreductase (NQO1). Auraptene induces murine liver cytosolic GST activities via the Nrf2/ARE mechanism as shown by previous studies [14, 15].

Several other mechanisms have been proposed to possibly explain the positive effects of auraptene on oncogenesis. Pro-inflammatory cytokines were expressed in the colonic tumours and the inflammatory mononuclear cells infiltrated the tumours both internally and peripherally. As the expression of these cytokines may be involved in tumour growth [16, 17], some authors decided to evaluate the effects of dietary 40-geranyloxy-ferulic acid (GOFA)/β-CD and auraptene/β-CD using an inflammation-associated mouse colon carcinogenesis initiated with azoxymethane (AOM) and promoted by colitis-inducing agent, such as dextran sodium sulphate (DSS), on their expression in adenocarcinomas. The treatment with GOFA/β-CD and auraptene/β-CD significantly lowered colonic inflammation induced by DSS. Chronic inflammation is involved in oncogenesis in certain tissues, including the large bowel. The dietary administration with GOFA/β-CD and auraptene/β-CD inhibited colonic inflammation and also modulated proliferation, apoptosis and the expression of several pro-inflammatory cytokines, such as nuclear factor-kappaB, tumour necrosis factor-a, Stat3, NF-E2-related factor 2, interleukin-6 and interleukin-1β, which were induced in the adenocarcinomas [18].

Further results demonstrate that auraptene was able to inhibit the growth and formation of colonospheres of FOLFOX-resistant colon cancer HT-29 cells in vitro [19]. The corresponding parental cells were also similarly affected by auraptene at the same concentration level. The reduction in the growth and colonospheres formation in FOLFOX-resistant HT-29 was also associated with a concomitant decrease in phospho-epidermal growth factor receptor (pEGFR). These findings suggest that auraptene could prevent the re-emergence of colon cancer stem cells.

Positive effects of auraptene were reported also in breast cancer by Krishnan and Kleiner-Hancock [20]. Many mechanisms have been attributed to the chemopreventive effects of auraptene. They include inhibition of polyamine synthesis, induction of detoxifying enzymes, induction of apoptosis, inhibition of metalloproteinase and inhibition of cholesterol esterification. Recently, de Medina and colleagues reported that auraptene modulated genes under the transcriptional control of oestrogen [21]. Cyclin D1 is a key regulatory protein in cell cycle; the D-type cyclins control the G1 to S transition during the cell cycle along with E-type cyclins; in up to 50 % of primary breast cancers, the overexpression of cyclin D1 mRNA and protein has been observed [22]. Thus, cyclin D1 is one of the most overexpressed oncogenes in human breast cancer. Cyclin D1 overexpression is predominantly found in oestrogen-receptor-positive breast cancer, which is a major subtype of human breast cancer. Cyclin D1 protein was significantly reduced in auraptene 500 ppm-treated animals [23].

There are also evidences of a role of auraptene in renal cell carcinoma due to its role of inhibitor of mitochondrial complex I as reported by Jang et al. [24]. The enhancement of VEGF-induced angiogenesis is observed in stages of tumour progression, and auraptene proved to have an anti-angiogenic effect. Jang et al. found that auraptene directly decreased VEGF mRNA expression cells under hypoxic condition; moreover, auraptene inhibited VEGF-induced neovascularization by 10-fold in vivo, consequently reducing tumour cell motility and neovascularization, necessary for renal cell carcinoma progression [24].

Also gastric cancer can benefit of auraptene supplementation as reported by Moon et al. [25]. These authors studied the anti-cancer effects of auraptene as a possible therapeutic candidate in the treatment of human gastric cancer. Auraptene reduced the viability of all types of tested gastric cancer cells in a dose-dependent manner. Among them, SNU-1 was the most sensitive with IC_{50} value ≤ 25 μM. In contrast, auraptene did not pose cytotoxic effects against non-cancer cell lines HEK-293T. Therefore, auraptene has high potential to treat gastric cancer cells without harming normal cells. The PI3K/Akt/mTOR pathway is an intracellular signalling pathway important in cell growth and apoptosis. These authors also examined whether auraptene can regulate the PI3K/Akt/mTOR signalling pathway. Results showed that auraptene could induce p53-dependent cell cycle arrest and apoptosis, and furthermore, it could suppress the proliferation of SNU-1 cells by downregulation of mTOR downstream signalling.

5 Effects of Auraptene on Cystic Fibrosis

Cystic fibrosis is the most common fatal autosomal recessive disease among Caucasian populations and affects multiple organs, most notably in the respiratory and digestive systems. Auraptene seems to have some positive effects on this disease, mainly acting as an agonist of both PPAR-α and PPAR-γ [26]. Auraptene has also been shown to exert anti-inflammatory effects through other mechanisms. These mechanisms include suppression of superoxide anion generation by inflammatory leucocytes, attenuation of LPS-induced expression of both inducible nitric oxide synthase (iNOS) and cyclooxygenase, thereby decreasing the production of nitrite anion and prostaglandin-E2 and suppressing the release of tumour necrosis factor a (TNFa) and IkB degradation. The decrease of prostaglandin-E2 is especially an important effect, since elevated prostaglandin-E2 concentrations have been reported in patients with cystic fibrosis. Throughout these mechanisms, auraptene could have beneficial consequences in decreasing lung inflammation, improving lung function, increasing bone mineral density and normalizing mucus production in cystic fibrosis; however, further studies are needed.

6 Effects of Auraptene on Hypertension

Auraptene proved to have anti-hypertensive effects, as suggested by Razavi et al. [27] that administered for five weeks auraptene (2, 4, 8 and 16 mg/kg/day) and nifedipine (0.25, 0.5, 1, 2 and 4 mg/kg/day) in different groups of normotensive and hypertensive rats (at the end of 3 weeks of treatment by DOCA salt, a compound routinely used to induce hypertension in experimental models). They evaluated the effects on mean systolic blood pressure and mean heart rate. The data indicated that chronic administration of auraptene significantly reduced the mean systolic blood pressure in DOCA salt-treated rats in a dose- and time-dependent manner. The per cent of decreases in mean systolic blood pressure levels by the highest dose of auraptene (16 mg/kg) at the end of 4 th to 8 th weeks were 7.00, 10.78, 16.07, 21.28 and 27.54 %, respectively. Smooth muscle relaxant effects of auraptene and its analogues against some spasmogens including barium ion, acetylcholine and histamine have been reported in another study [28]. This was further confirmed by another study conducted on rats [29]. There is evidence indicating that auraptene inhibits the spontaneous heart beating of cultured mouse myocardial cells via calcium channel antagonist activity which is comparable with that of verapamil [30]. Regarding the hypotensive mechanism of auraptene, there is evidence that there is a suppression of NADPH oxidase, with consequent increase in nitric oxide bioavailability and alleviation of endothelial dysfunction. Decrease in calcium influx and induction of nitric oxide together with vasorelaxation effect have been also observed.

7 Auraptene and Lipid Profile

Throughout its activity of PPAR-α agonist, auraptene could have beneficial effects on lipid profile; PPAR-α is mainly expressed in the liver and skeletal muscle, whose activation induces the mRNA expression of several genes involved in fatty acid (FA) oxidation to reduce circulating lipid level. This was reported by Takahashi et al. [31], which showed that in high-fat-diet (HFD)-fed KK-Ay diabetic obese mice, auraptene treatment suppressed hyperlipidemia and triglyceride accumulation in the liver and skeletal muscle and increased the mRNA expression levels of the PPAR-α target genes involved in fatty acid oxidation in the liver and skeletal muscle. Moreover, the adipocyte size in the auraptene-treated mice was significantly smaller than that in the control HFD-fed mice resulting in the improvement of HFD-induced hyperglycaemia and abnormalities in glucose tolerance. The improvement of glycemia can be partly mediated by the suppression of the increase in the number of hypertrophied adipocytes, which show insulin resistance. In the present study, the size of adipocytes in the auraptene-treated mice decreased, enhancing the expression level of adiponectin, an adipocytokine improving insulin resistance in peripheral tissues.

Table 1 Health promoting effects of auraptene

Health promoting effects of auraptene	Mechanism of action
Effects on neurodegenerative diseases	Activation of ERK1/2
Effects on periodontal disease	Reduction of cytokines secretion
Effects on oncogenesis	Inhibition of polyamine synthesis, induction of detoxifying enzymes, induction of apoptosis, inhibition of metalloproteinase and inhibition of cholesterol esterification
Effects on cystic fibrosis	PPAR-α and PPAR-γ agonism
Effects on hypertension	Suppression of NADPH oxidase, with consequent increase in nitric oxide bioavailability
Effects on lipid profile	PPAR-α agonism

These findings indicate that auraptene treatment may improve abnormalities in lipid and glucose metabolism, suggesting that auraptene is a valuable food-derived compound for managing metabolic disorders. This is in line with what suggested by Sahekbar [4], which proposed auraptene as a potential multifunctional therapeutic agent for nonalcoholic fatty liver disease.

8 Conclusions

From the data reported above, it emerged that auraptene has some potential benefits in the treatment of neurodegenerative diseases, tumours and also metabolic diseases (Table 1). However, further studies are necessary to verify whether these effects observed in animals will be confirmed in humans.

References

1. Ogawa K, Kawasaki A, Yoshida T, Nesumi H, Nakano M, Ikoma Y, Yano M (2000) Evaluation of auraptene content in citrus fruits and their products. J Agric Food Chem 48 (5):1763–1769
2. Furukawa Y, Okuyama S, Amakura Y, Watanabe S, Fukata T, Nakajima M, Yoshimura M, Yoshida T (2012) Isolation and characterization of activators of ERK/MAPK from Citrus plants. Int J Mol Sci 13(2):1832–1845
3. Bravo L (1998) Polyphenols: chemistry, dietary sources, metabolism, and nutritional significance. Nutr Rev 56(11):317–333
4. Sahebkar A (2011) Citrus auraptene: a potential multifunctional therapeutic agent for nonalcoholic fatty liver disease. Ann Hepatol 10(4):575–577

5. Samuels IS, Karlo JC, Faruzzi AN, Pickering K, Herrup K, Sweatt JD, Saitta SC, Landreth GE (2008) Deletion of ERK2 mitogen-activated protein kinase identifies its key roles in cortical neurogenesis and cognitive function. J Neurosci 28(27):6983–6995
6. Furukawa Y, Okuyama S, Amakura Y, Watanabe S, Fukata T, Nakajima M, Yoshimura M, Yoshida T (2012) Isolation and characterization of activators of ERK/MAPK from Citrus plants. Int J Mol Sci 13:1832–1845
7. Furukawa Y, Watanabe S, Okuyama S, Nakajima M (2012) Neurotrophic effect of citrus auraptene: neuritogenic activity in PC12 cells. Int J Mol Sci 13(5):5338–5347
8. Okuyama S, Minami S, Shimada N, Makihata N, Nakajima M, Furukawa Y (2013) Anti-inflammatory and neuroprotective effects of auraptene, a citrus coumarin, following cerebral global ischemia in mice. Eur J Pharmacol 699(1–3):118–123
9. Okuyama S, Yamamoto K, Mori H, Toyoda N, Yoshimura M, Amakura Y, Yoshida T, Sugawara K, Sudo M, Nakajima M, Furukawa Y (2014) Auraptene in the peels of *Citrus kawachiensis* (Kawachi Bankan) ameliorates lipopolysaccharide-induced inflammation in the mouse brain. Evid Based Complement Altern Med, 408503
10. McGeer EG, Klegeris A, McGeer PL (2005) Inflammation, the complement system and the diseases of aging. Neurobiol Aging 26(Suppl 1):94–97
11. Qin L, Wu X, Block ML, Liu Y, Breese GR, Hong JS, Knapp DJ, Crews FT (2007) Systemic LPS causes chronic neuroinflammation and progressive neurodegeneration. Glia 55 (5):453–462
12. Marquis A, Genovese S, Epifano F, Grenier D (2012) The plant coumarins auraptene and lacinartin as potential multifunctional therapeutic agents for treating periodontal disease. BMC Complement Altern Med 12:80
13. Borges F, Roleira F, Milhazes N, Santana L, Uriarte E (2005) Simple coumarins and analogues in medicinal chemistry: occurrence, synthesis and biological activity. Curr Med Chem 12(8):887–916
14. Prince M, Li Y, Childers A, Itoh K, Yamamoto M, Kleiner HE (2009) Comparison of citrus coumarins on carcinogen-detoxifying enzymes in Nrf2 knockout mice. Toxicol Lett 185 (3):180–186
15. Min BK, Hyun DG, Jeong SY, Kim YH, Ma ES, Woo MH (2011) A new cytotoxic coumarin, 7-[(E)-3′,7′-dimethyl-6′-oxo-2′,7′-octadienyl] oxy coumarin, from the leaves of Zanthoxylum schinifolium. Arch Pharmacal Res 34(5):723–726
16. Lewis AM, Varghese S, Xu H, Alexander HR (2006) Interleukin-1 and cancer progression: the emerging role of interleukin-1 receptor antagonist as a novel therapeutic agent in cancer treatment. J Transl Med 4:48
17. Lin WW, Karin M (2007) A cytokine-mediated link between innate immunity, inflammation, and cancer. J Clin Invest 117:1175–1183
18. Tanaka T, de Azevedo MB, Durán N, Alderete JB, Epifano F, Genovese S, Tanaka M, Tanaka T, Curini M (2010) Colorectal cancer chemoprevention by 2 b-cyclodextrin inclusion compounds of auraptene and 40-geranyloxyferulic acid. Int J Cancer 126(4):830–840
19. Epifano F, Genovese S, Miller R, Majumdar AP (2013) Auraptene and its effects on the re-emergence of colon cancer stem cells. Phytotherapy Res 27(5):784–786
20. Krishnan P, Kleiner-Hancock H (2012) Effects of auraptene on IGF-1 stimulated cell cycle progression in the human breast cancer cell line, MCF-7. Int J Breast Cancer, 502092
21. de Medina P, Genovese S, Paillasse MR, Mazaheri M, Caze-Subra S, Bystricky K, Curini M, Silvente-Poirot S, Epifano F, Poirot M (2010) Auraptene is an inhibitor of cholesterol esterification and a modulator of estrogen receptors. Mol Pharmacol 78(5):827–836
22. Sutherland RL, Musgrove EA (2004) Cyclins and breast cancer. J Mammary Gland Biol Neoplasia 9(1):95–104
23. Krishnan P, Yan KJ, Windler D, Tubbs J, Grand R, Li BD, Aldaz CM, McLarty J, Kleiner-Hancock HE (2009) Citrus auraptene suppresses cyclin D1 and significantly delays N-methyl nitrosourea induced mammary carcinogenesis in female Sprague-Dawley rats. BMC Cancer 9:259

24. Jang Y, Han J, Kim SJ, Kim J, Lee MJ, Jeong S, Ryu MJ, Seo KS, Choi SY, Shong M, Lim K, Heo JY, Kweon GR (2015) Suppression of mitochondrial respiration with auraptene inhibits the progression of renal cell carcinoma: involvement of HIF-1α degradation. Oncotarget 6 (35):38127–38138
25. Moon JY, Kim H, Cho SK (2015) Auraptene, a major compound of supercritical fluid extract of phalsak (Citrus Hassaku Hort ex Tanaka), induces apoptosis through the suppression of mTOR pathways in human gastric cancer SNU-1 Cells. Evid Based Complement Altern Med 2015:402385
26. Sahebkar A (2011) Potential benefits of supplementation with auraptene in cystic fibrosis. Clin Nutr 30(2):259–260
27. Razavi BM, Arasteh E, Imenshahidi M, Iranshahi M (2015) Antihypertensive effect of auraptene, a monoterpene coumarin from the genus Citrus, upon chronic administration. Iran J Basic Med Sci 18(2):153–158
28. Yamada Y, Okamoto M, Kikuzaki H, Nakatani N (1997) Spasmolytic activity of auraptene analogs. Biosci Biotechnol Biochem 61:740–742
29. Imenshahidi M, Eghbal M, Sahebkar A, Iranshahi M (2013) Hypotensive activity of auraptene, a monoterpene coumarin from *Citrus* spp. Pharm Biol 51(5):545–549
30. Kakiuchi N, Senaratne LR, Huang SL, Yang XW, Hattori M, Pilapitiya U, Namba T (1991) Effects of constituents of Beli (*Aegle marmelos*) on spontaneous beating and calcium-paradox of myocardial cells. Planta Med 57:43–46
31. Takahashi N, Senda M, Lin S, Goto T, Yano M, Sasaki T, Murakami S, Kawada T (2011) Auraptene regulates gene expression involved in lipid metabolism through PPARα activation in diabetic obese mice. Mol Nutr Food Res 55(12):1791–1797

Author Index

S.C. Gupta et al. (eds.), *Drug Discovery from Mother Nature*,
Advances in Experimental Medicine and Biology 929,
DOI 10.1007/978-3-319-41342-6

The manufacturer's authorised representative in the EU is Springer Nature Customer Service Centre GmbH, Europaplatz 3, 69115 Heidelberg, Germany. If you have any concerns regarding our products, please contact ProductSafety@springernature.com

Printed and bound by CPI Group (UK) Ltd, Croydon, CR0 4YY
22/09/2026
02221052-0001